MEDICAL RADIOLOGY
Diagnostic Imaging

Editors:
A. L. Baert, Leuven
K. Sartor, Heidelberg
J. E. Youker, Milwaukee

Springer-Verlag Berlin Heidelberg GmbH

A. Couture · C. Veyrac

Transfontanellar Doppler Imaging in Neonates

Preface by
F. Brunelle

Foreword by
A. L. Baert

With 400 Figures in 887 Separate Illustrations, 320 in Color and 40 Tables

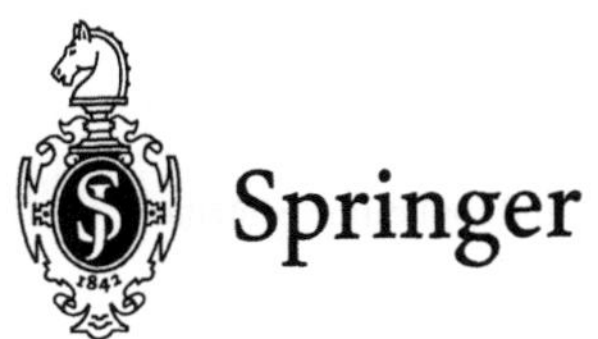

Springer

Alain P. Couture, MD
Corinne Veyrac, MD

Department of Pediatric Radiology
Hôpital Arnaud de Villeneuve
371 Av. Doyen Gaston Giraud
34295 Montpellier Cédex 5
France

Medical Radiology · Diagnostic Imaging and Radiation Oncology

Continuation of
Handbuch der medizinischen Radiologie
Encyclopedia of Medical Radiology

ISBN 978-3-642-62967-9

Library of Congress Cataloging-in-Publication Data
Couture, Alain.
       Transfontanellar Doppler imaging in neonates / A.Couture, C.Veyrac ; preface by
F. Brunelle ; foreword by A. L. Baert.
          p. ; cm – (Medical radiology)
Includes bibliographical references and index.
ISBN 978-3-642-62967-9   ISBN 978-3-642-56724-7 (eBook)
DOI 10.1007/978-3-642-56724-7
1. Doppler ultrasonography. 2. Ultrasonics in obstetrics. 3. Fetus – Ultrasonic imaging.
4. Infants (Newborn)–Diseases–Diagnosis. I. Veyrac, C. (Corinne), 1951 – II. Title. III.
Series.
       [DNLM: 1. Cerebrovascular Disorders–ultrasonography–Infant, Newborn. 2.
Ultrasonography, Doppler, Color–Infant, Newborn. 3. Fetus. 4. Ultrasonography,
Doppler, Pulsed–Infant, Newborn. 5. Ultrasonography, Prenatal. WL 355 C872t 2000]
RG628.3.U58 C68 2000
616.07'543'0832 – dc21   00-038812

http//www.springer.de
© Springer-Verlag Berlin Heidelberg 2001
Originally published by Springer-Verlag Berlin Heidelberg in 2001
Softcover reprint of the hardcover 1st edition 2001
The use of general descriptive names, trademarks, etc.in this publication does not imply, even in the absence of a specific
statement, that such names are exempt from the relevant laws and regulations and therefore free for general use.

Product liability. The publishers cannot guarantee the accuracy of any information about dosage and application contained
in this book. In every case the user must check such information ba consulting the relevant literature.

Cover-Design and Typesetting: Verlagsservice Teichmann, 69256 Mauer
SPIN: 106 747 20   21/3130 – 5 4 3 2 1 0

Foreword

Transfontanellar Doppler imaging was until recently an emerging new diagnostic modality that was not widely used in clinical practice.

Dr. A. Couture and Dr. C. Veyrac have pioneered and incessantly developed the technique of prenatal and neonatal brain scanning until it has now been matured into an indispensable tool for the correct management of infants. Building upon the technical progress in the manufacturing of scanning probes and ultrasonic equipment, the authors have been able to accumulate a unique and exceptional body of knowledge on fetal and neonatal brain scanning.

Their book provides exquisite information not only on the normal neonatal brain, but also on the various pathological conditions and malformations involving the fetal and neonatal brain as provided by ultrasound examination. The book contains numerous illustrative examples, selected from the outstanding personal files of the authors.

Transfontanellar Doppler imaging, because of its great impact on the management of neonates suspected of brain abnormalities, should be available to all pediatric and general radiologists involved in brain scanning in the pediatric age group. They, and also neurologists and neurosurgeons, will find this volume a unique source of information and knowledge.

I congratulate the editors on their outstanding performance and I wish this volume great success within the medical community.

Leuven

ALBERT L. BAERT

Preface

Alain Couture belongs to the breed of pioneers. This requires several unusual traits: orginality, tenacity and vision, and of course hard work.

Alain started to explore the neonatal brain in 1978, a time, it must be remembered, when the brain was a no-man 's land. Very little was known about this undiscovered island.

The only ways to attempt to glimpse the brain were either invasive (pneumoencephalography, angiography) or very rough (transillumination). I was a medical student when Jean Aicardi took me to the black closet with a hydrocephalic patient. He put his special lamp on the head of the macrocephalic newborn and the head of the boy suddenly lit up in the darkness like a Japanese lantern.

Alain discovered the brain anatomy, the diagnosis of hemorrhage, ... This, however, was purely anatomic. Then, when Doppler became available, he discovered the hemodynamics of the neonatal brain. There is probably more to come.

As he was not fully satisfied with his work, he began to apply his skills to the antenatal period. He grew increasingly interested in the transposition of his knowledge to the antenatal brain. He is now regularly invited by the College of Obstetrics, whose members eagerly ask him for clues and new tricks to increase the performance of antenatal US.

Very often, when a specialist has mastered his technique he tends to think that the world can be accounted for (as a whole) through his vision. This mental flaw, ideological totalitarianism, is often seen in science and medicine. Alain Couture, however, is an open-minded, ever young man. He recently became interested in antenatal MRI. His knowledge of the brain anatomy gained through US enabled him rapidly to become an expert in this growing field.

It goes without saying that medicine and pediatric radiology represent only one facet of Alain's life. He recently took it into his head to switch from skiing to snowboarding. He did it – at the price of a wrist fracture to which I was witness. He is a fantastic rock and roll dancer. I am awaiting with trepidation his move to street dancing (I number a good orthopedist among my friends). Egyptology has no secret for him. In short, the appetite of Alain Couture knows no bounds.

Approaching this person gives you more energy than any vitamins. But be warned, you become rapidly addicted. I am proud and fortunate to be one of his friends. The European Society of Pediatric Radiology counts him as one of his diamonds in its crown.

Corinne Veyrac has always worked with Alain. She is his Jiminy Cricket. She would use the pointer and show the slides during meetings, sitting in the front row, while Alain was giving his talk reading his manuscript with his inimitable accent. Corinne has the rigor that keeps the artist alive. She is the coach, he is the actor.

Corinne is a hard worker and an outstanding ultrasonographer. The quality of the images seen in the book, the rigor with which they have been taken, show her hallmark.

The book in your hand represents the unique fruit of this exceptional collaboration. Alain Couture and Corinne Veyrac are two outstanding people who not only love their work, but are delighted to share their passion with others.

You, the reader, will enter this book not only as a scientific compilation of what is known about ultrasound of the head but also, if you can read between the lines, as a doorway to wonderland.

FRANCIS BRUNELLE
Professor of Radiology
Service de Radiologie, Hôpital des Enfants Malades, Paris, France

Contents

Acknowledgements

The following physicians and investigators
contributed to the success of this book:

Dr. C. ADAMSBAUM, Paris
Dr. M. BADR, Montpellier
Dr. C. BAUD, Montpellier
Dr. J-P. BERNARD, Paris
Dr. F. BRUNELLE, Paris
Dr. G. CAMBONIE, Montpellier
Dr. J-F. CHATEIL, Bordeaux
Dr. F. DESCHAMPS, Montpellier
Dr. F. DIDIER, Nancy
Dr. C. FAWER, Lausanne
Dr. J-L. FERRAN, Montpellier
Dr. H. LAURICHESSE-DELMAS, Paris
Dr. F. MONTOYA, Montpellier
Dr. J-E. MORICE, Montpellier
Dr. M-P. QUERE, Nantes
Dr. M. SAGUINTAAH, Montpellier
Dr. I. SIMON, Paris
Dr. C. TALMANT, Nantes
Dr. Y. VILLE, Paris
Dr. U. WILLI, Zurich

1 Doppler Ultrasonography: Technical Considerations

ALAIN P. COUTURE

CONTENTS

Transfontanellar ultrasonography is known as a reliable method to assess brain integrity in the fetus and neonate, and plays a major role in the diagnosis, follow-up, and management of brain damage, whether ischemic-hemorrhagic, infectious, developmental, or tumoral. These morphological data have been established for many years (COUTURE 1994).

Despite its accuracy, ultrasonographic information remains incomplete and insufficient. Because many cerebral lesions are of circulatory origin, it has appeared valuable to study cerebral hemodynamics and to develop different methods, particularly pulsed and color Doppler ultrasonography.

● Of course, some requirements should be respected, that constitute a prerequisite and guide the utilization and interpretation of this imaging.

A. COUTURE, MD
Service de Radiologie Pédiatrique, Hôpital Arnaud de Villeneuve, 371 Av. Doyen Gaston Giraud, 34295 Montpellier Cedex 5, France

1.1 Analysis of Cerebral Hemodynamics is a Necessity

For many years (Lou 1979), we have known that cerebral autoregulation mechanisms are disturbed in the distressed newborn: the capillary bed is directly exposed to hypertensive peaks and may rupture in the germinal matrix, leading to subependymal and intraventricular hemorrhage.

In the same way, cerebral blood flow (CBF) autoregulation is involved during perinatal asphyxia: the blood flow linearly follows changes in systemic arterial blood pressure, and vasodilatation resulting from hypoxemia, hypercapnia, and acidosis is opposed to low blood flow resulting from bradycardia and hypotension. The severity of the ischemic damage depends on the balance between protective vasodilatation and ischemia inducing low blood flow.

These two examples emphasize that most of the neuropathological processes that accompany perinatal brain injury are related to changes in CBF and velocity. Hence, detecting an ischemic-hemorrhagic lesion is important but inadequate, because it comes too late; we should attempt to prevent the damage and understand its mechanisms of occurrence, which are of vascular origin.

1.1.1 Methods

All these data explain why studying fetal and neonatal cerebral hemodynamics is valuable. Many techniques have been proposed in order to quantify blood flow, and many reports have been published during the last 20 years. The ideal method should be noninvasive, nonaggressive, quantitative, continuing, and inexpensive; at present such a method does not exist.

● Several techniques have failed to prove their validity completely:

- Those using inert gas, N_2O or radioactive xenon-133 (Xe133), either by intra-arterial or intravenous injection or by inhalation, are invasive, ionizing, and ethically difficult to propose in normal newborns. They have some methodological limitations including contamination from extracerebral sources and the unknown blood-brain partition of xenon. Nevertheless, the Xe133 clearance method remains useful since it provides normal values for CBF: from 10 ml/100 g min in premature neonates, it reaches 20 ml/100 g min in the term neonate (GREISEN 1992; PRYDS 1996; YOUNKIN 1988).

- **Venous occlusion plethysmography** (COOKE 1977; LEAHY 1979) is used to determine systolic expansion of intracranial volume after brief occlusion of jugular veins. This investigation is noninvasive, may be repeated, but is associated with causes of error that result in underestimation of cerebral blood flow.

- These difficulties explain the paucity of publications concerning the newborn, and those that do exist deal mainly with perinatal asphyxia or distress (GREISEN 1984; Lou 1979). Only plethysmography has been used in the normal newborn. Normal neonatal cerebral blood flow ranges from 20 to 60 ml/100 g/min. During perinatal asphyxia, cerebral blood flow below 10 ml/100 g/min is critical, and is associated with the development of cerebral atrophy and psychomotor retardation (LOU 1979; POWERS 1989).

● Other techniques obviously have a great future, but still belong to the field of research:

- **MR spectroscopy** provides information on cerebral metabolism in animals (CORBETT 1987; PETROFF 1988; YOUNKIN 1984) and human (BOESCH 1989; HOPE 1985; HUPPI 1993). ^{31}P MR spectroscopy, reported after cases of neonatal asphyxia and seizures, confirms earlier animal studies and shows a decrease in phosphocreatine and increase in inorganic phosphate (CADY 1983; YOUNKIN 1985). Demonstration of changes in cerebral metabolites, such as elevation of cerebral lactate, appears to be of great value in the assessment of cerebral disturbances, especially after anoxo-ischemic insult (GRONENDAAL 1994; HANRAHAN 1998; HANRAHAN 1999; SHU 1997).

- **Positron emission tomography** allows in vivo regional physiological and biochemical information about human brain function to be obtained. In the newborn, determination of regional CBF (TAKAHASHI 1999; VOLPE 1985) and glucose metabolism (DOYLE 1983; POWERS 1998) helps our understanding of normal variations of blood flow, brain injury in the term infant with hypoxic-ischemic encephalopathy, and in the premature newborn with major hemorrhage. This method has been used to define the regional distribution of CBF: the highest flows are found in the cortex, thalamus, and brain stem, while the lowest flows are encountered within white matter (VOLPE 1985).

- **Near-infrared spectroscopy** is the most recent of these methods. It obviously has great potential value, since by an optical technique it may provide crucial information concerning cerebral blood volume, CBF, cerebral venous and hemoglobin oxygen saturation, and cerebral oxygen availability. This atraumatic method, assessing blood and brain cells through the skull, allows frequent measurements in the newborn without stopping nursing procedures, and has been reported in several animal and human studies (BENNET 1998; BUCHVALD 1999; CHANG 1999; DIETZ 1999; PRYDS 1990; SAKATANI 1999; WOLF 1998).

● Nevertheless, these high-technology, high-cost techniques remain research techniques. This explains the great interest in the Doppler technique in the last 20 years. First, American groups using continuous-wave Doppler defined the hemodynamic pattern of the normal newborn (VOLPE 1982) (spectral analysis curve, resistive index, area under the curve); they have described the changes in resistive index in patent ductus arteriosus (PERLMAN 1981), pneumothorax (HILL 1982), seizures (PERLMAN 1983), tracheal suctioning (PERLMAN 1983), brain death (MACMENAMIN 1983), hydrocephalus (HILL 1982), bacterial meningitis (MACMENAMIN 1984), and respiratory distress syndrome (PERLMAN 1983). Subsequently, the appearance of pulsed, color, and power Doppler techniques have greatly improved and facilitated the hemodynamic assessment of neonatal brain.

1.1.2
Technical Requirements

● Doppler velocimetry is based on the reflection of sound waves from moving red blood cells that induce a frequency shift, the Doppler effect (DRAYTON 1986).

The frequency shift is proportional to the velocity of the blood cells, but depends also on the angle α of the probe to the axis of blood flow. Mathematically, the principle is expressed as:

$$F = \frac{2foV + cos\,\alpha}{c}$$

where:

F is the frequency shift
fo the transmitted frequency
V the velocity of blood cells
α the angle of the incident sound beam to the vessel axis
c the velocity of sound waves in the tissue.

If c and fo are constant from one study to another, clearly the mean velocity is proportional to the mean frequency shift when the angle of incidence remains unchanged.

A Doppler velocimeter consists of a probe that is obliquely orientated toward the selected vascular territory and contains an emitter and a receptor of ultrasonic waves. The Doppler frequency represents the difference between the emitted (or transmitted) and the received frequencies. This frequency shift is positive or negative, depending on the direction of flow. The choice of Doppler equipment from among the many existing systems has been and remains difficult: continuous-wave Doppler, pulsed-wave Doppler, continuous or pulsed-wave Doppler combined with gray-scale imaging, standard color Doppler, and power Doppler.

1.1.2.1
Continuous-Wave Doppler

Continuous-wave Doppler was the first system to appear (GRAY 1983; PERLMAN 1985; VOLPE 1982) that remains widely used. Representing simple, low-cost technology, its principle is easy to understand. The probe contains two piezoelectric crystals, one of which continuously emits an ultrasonic wave, while the other ensures constant reception of echoes and back-scattered signals.

This system has a major disadvantage for analyzing complex vascular structures such as the vasculature of the brain: if several vessels are simultaneously interrogated by the probe, the resulting Doppler effect is a medley of all vessels; there is no discrimination in depth, and the origin of the Doppler signal is unknown.

1.1.2.2
Pulsed-Wave Doppler

This more sophisticated device overcomes the limitation just mentioned. The probe contains a single piezoelectric crystal that acts alternatively in emission and reception mode. Emission is discontinuous and the delay between the transmitted and the received waves allows calculation of the depth of the reflecting interface. It is possible to select a sample volume as to size and depth along the ultrasonic beam, using an electronic gate; this makes it easy to insonate selected vessels and separate their signals, and a real arterial map may be obtained. This device obviously requires a higher investment.

1.1.2.3
Combition of Doppler with Real-Time B-mode Imaging

The combination of Doppler with real-time imaging represents a decisive advance in the evaluation of cerebral hemodynamics, since the ultrasonic beam and the sample volume may be better adjusted with the real-time B-mode image. With early equipment this image had to be frozen or perhaps refreshed, but recent devices allow the Doppler and B-mode images to be obtained simultaneously.

1.1.2.4
In total

The probe is placed over the anterior fontanel and the following are obtained:
- An audible signal that allows easy location of the vessel
- An immediate curve of blood velocities in the selected vessel
- Determination of the flow direction within the artery or the vein
- With spectral analysis of Doppler signal, distribution of velocities within the vessel, at any time

1.1.2.5.
Color Doppler

Color Doppler represents the most recent and most striking advance in the evaluation of neonatal and fetal brain vasculature. Standard color encoding of blood flow records not only the strength of the received echoes but also the Doppler shift, and provides major information on the direction and speed of circulating red blood cells. This dynamic mapping of blood flows (colored red when flow is moving toward the transducer, and blue when it is moving away from the transducer) gives a two-dimensional image of blood vessels, superimposed on a gray-scale two-dimensional image of the brain (Fig. 1.1).

Although this imaging technique (TAYLOR 1992; WONG 1989) has obvious advantages (easy location of vessels, detection of small vessels, evaluation of the whole venous system, study of the pericerebral vascular environment, improved accuracy of blood velocity measurements), it has also some limitations (the aliasing phenomenon, color noise, dependence on the Doppler angle). This lies behind the recent appearance of power Doppler imaging (RUBIN 1993, 1999) where the *power of the Doppler signal* is encoded in color. This technique, also known as "color Doppler energy" or "amplitude mode color Doppler," provides no information about the speed or direction of flow, but is more sensitive in detecting small vessels with low-velocity flow (BABCOCK 1996; BUDE 1996). As it is relatively independent of the angle of the ultrasonic beam, power Doppler produces vascular mapping of unequaled accuracy (Fig. 1.2), in the neonate (SEIBERT 1998) as in the fetus

1.2
Assessing the Cerebral Hemodynamics

1.2.1
Choice of Ultrasound Equipment

Choosing appropriate apparatus is a major step and should take into account anatomical criteria (the small size of the anterior fontanel), clinical requirements (e.g., the impossibility of moving a ventilated

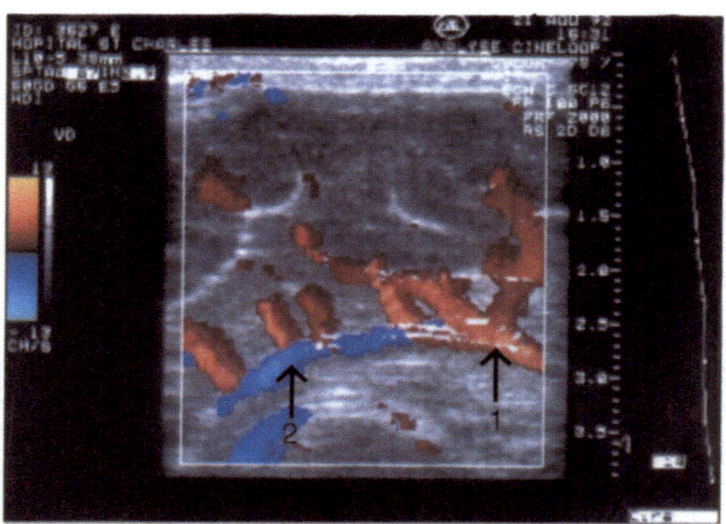

Fig. 1.1. Standard color Doppler. Visualization of the peri-callosal artery. In its proximal portion, coded in red (*1*), flow is toward the transducer, and its distal portion, coded in blue (*2*), flow is away from the transducer

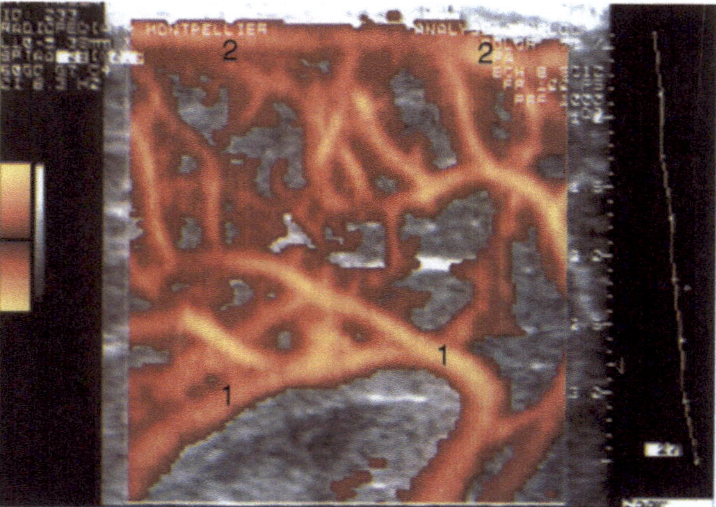

Fig. 1.2. Power Doppler imaging. Vascular mapping is of great quality. The pericallosal artery (*1*) and its branches, and the superior sagittal sinus (*2*) and its cortical venous rami are easily made out

preterm newborn), and technological considerations (continuous-wave Doppler, pulsed-wave Doppler, or color Doppler?).The apparatus must be movable: this must not be overlooked. Distressed newborns are ventilated and cannot be moved. To assess their brain integrity or detect ischemic-hemorrhagic damage using a reliable accurate hemodynamic evaluation is a diagnostic emergency and should be done as early as possible, in the intensive care unit. Modern systems can all be moved, but are complex and likely to break down. This requires unity of place: having the intensive care unit and the Pediatric Radiology Department close together is an obvious advantage.

1.2.2
Choice of probe

In the neonate, the requirements for hemodynamic evaluation are the same as those for morphological assessment of the brain. Small-section probes are necessary because of the small size of the ultrasonic window.

1.2.3
Choice of technology

Everything speaks for the most advanced technology. In the newborn, the cerebral hemodynamic study should be fast, efficient, and complete, since the diagnosis may be urgent and may have consequences for the vital prognosis. Is there low blood flow? Does spectral analysis show intra-cranial hypertension? Is a thrombosis of the superior sagittal sinus or middle cerebral artery confirmed? Is there a fluctuating Doppler. Pulsed and color Doppler are required to answer these questions. This shows why continuous-wave Doppler is too limited: the flows of several arteries may be confused, complete visualization of brain vessels cannot be obtained, and only the anterior cerebral artery is reliably recorded.

To perform a high-quality hemodynamic evaluation and to answer the questions of pediatricians, advanced technology must be used. Pulsed Doppler allows precise location of brain vessels; combining it with real-time imaging improves the reliability and reproducibility of the Doppler angle; while color imaging provides easy visualization of the cerebral vasculature in both neonate and fetus.

Our experience confirms these data. In 1985, we started hemodynamic studies with a Diasonics DRF 400 CV (without color Doppler) which allowed us to learn and become familiar with the difficult technique of pulsed Doppler, which requires a manual dexterity. First, the probe is placed with the Doppler axis and sample volume adjusted according to a real-time two-dimensional image; second, the B-image is frozen and the Doppler mode selected. Complete immobility of the baby's head and of the examinor's hand is obviously important, in order to keep the sample gate on the selected area (Fig. 1.3). Since 1992, these difficulties have decreased, thanks to the possibility of using color Doppler equipment in the intensive care unit (Acuson) and in the Pediatric Radiology Department (ATL UM9 HDI and ATL

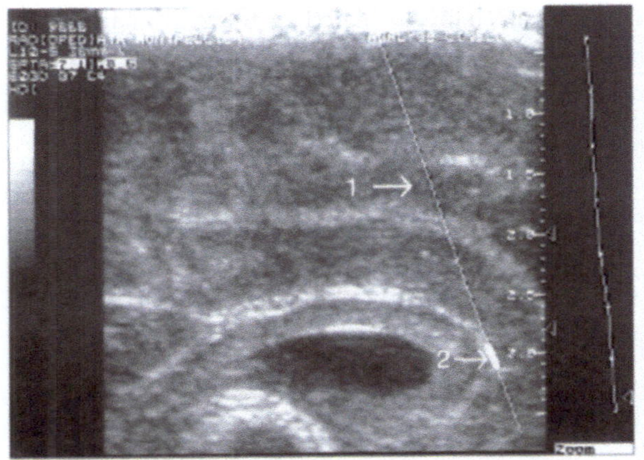
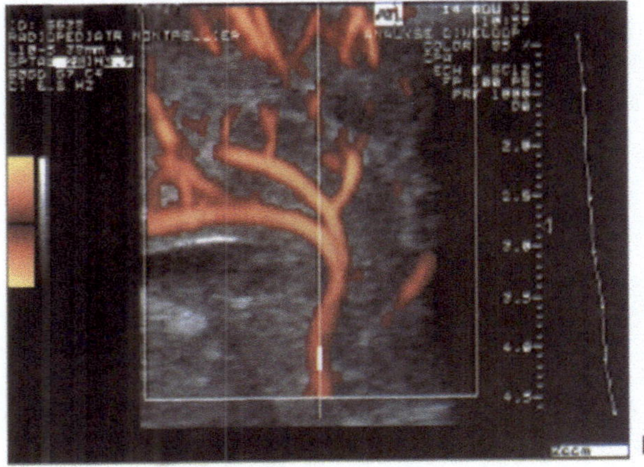

Fig. 1.3a,b. Doppler assessment of cerebral arteries. a Pulsed Doppler: The Doppler beam (1) is positioned, the sample volume is placed on the pulsatile beat of the pericallosal artery along the genu of corpus callosum. The sample volume is very small (2), suited to the size of the artery under study, in order to avoid any interference from adjacent vessels. This technique is time-consuming and difficult, and provides only measurement of the resistive index. b Color Doppler (power Doppler): After color coding of the anterior cerebral artery, the Doppler beam is placed in the vessel axis and the sample volume adjusted. This technique is fast and easy, and allows measurement of flow velocities

3000): the vessel is immediately located, the Doppler beam can be ideally positioned, and arterial and venous velocities reliably measured (Fig. 1.3.).

1.3
Practical Technique

The technique of Doppler investigation is standardized and methodical:
- The newborn or infant is never premedicated. If necessary, the patient is quietened with a bottle or a dummy, while an infrared lamp maintains a good temperature around the baby. For any examination, the baby is seated in a small chair, in an upright position, with the head well centered between two foam cushions (Fig. 1.4.), since Doppler examination requires immobility.
- In cases of neonatal distress, the movable ultrasound apparatus is brought to the intensive care unit. Examination inside the incubator is easy thanks to the flexible connector of the probe (Fig. 1.5). Evidently, the Doppler investigation is always combined with a morphological assessment by ultrasound.

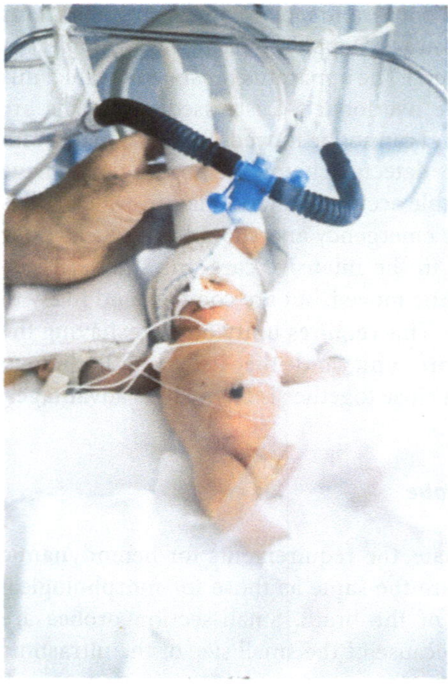

Fig. 1.5. A 28-week premature newborn with perinatal distress. Morphological and Doppler ultrasound evaluation inside the incubator are easy

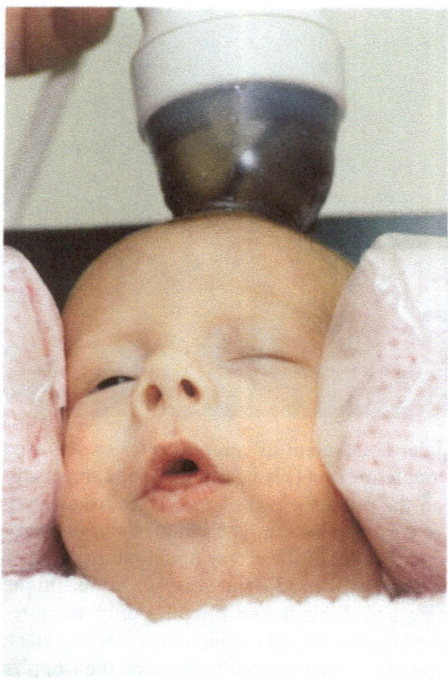

Fig. 1.4. Immobility of the patient is required. Foam cushions provide perfect stability for the infant's head

Since 1992, hemodynamic evaluation has been carried out according to a precise protocol:
- For each neonate and each infant, there is a complete study of the brain vasculature using color Doppler.
- After precise location of the anterior cerebral artery, Doppler recording is carried out in the vessel axis (Fig. 1.3) in order to obtain a reliable spectral analysis curve and to calculate resistive index, peak-systolic (PSV), end-diastolic (EDV), and time average velocities (TAV) (Fig. 1.6). If hemodynamic disturbance is present, spectral analysis of several arteries and veins is performed.
- A main point has been to validate the normal values for resistive index and velocities in dependence on patient age. For this reason, 486 normal newborns and infants have been investigated with depiction of seven vessels: anterior cerebral artery, internal carotid artery, basilar artery, lenticulostriate arteries, internal cerebral vein, straight sinus, and superior sagittal sinus. For each of these vessels, resistive index, pulsatility index, arterial velocities (PSV, EDV, TAV) and venous velocities were determined. The study was performed in the age group ranging from 32 weeks' gestation to 9 months of age.

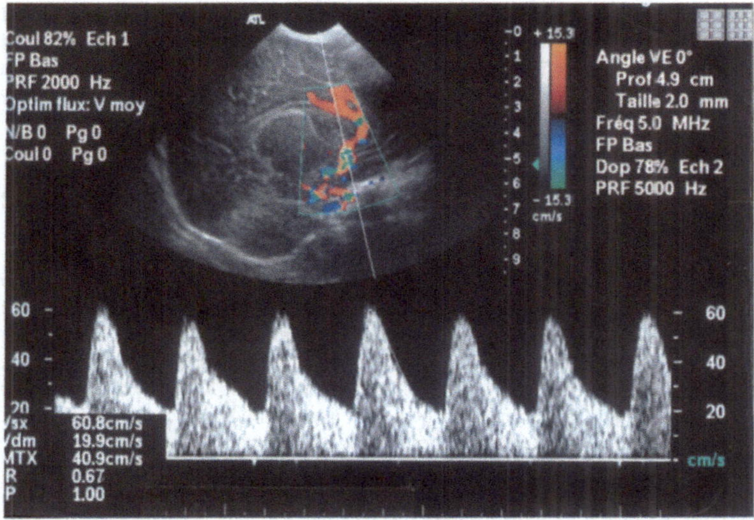

Fig. 1.6. A 2-month-old infant. Spectral analysis curve of the pericallosal artery is accurate. Resistive index (0.67) and arterial velocities are automatically determined: PSV = 60.8 cm/s, EDV = 19.9 cm/s, TAV = 40.0 cm/s

References

Babcock DS, Patriquin H, Lafortune M, Dauzat M (1996) Power Doppler sonography: basic principles and clinical applications in children. Pediatr Radiol 26:109–115

Bennet L, Peebles DM, Edwards AD, Rios A, Hanson MA (1998) The cerebral hemodynamic response to asphyxia and hypoxia in the near-term fetal sheep as measured by near infrared spectroscopy. Pediatr Res 44:951–957

Boesch C, Gritter R, Martin E (1989) Variations in vivo of the 31-phosphorus magnetic resonance spectra of the developing humain brain during postnatal life. Radiology 172:197–199

Buchvald FF, Kesje K, Greisen G (1999) Measurement of cerebral oxyhaemoglobin saturation and jugular blood flow in term healthy newborn infants by near infrared spectroscopy and jugular venous occlusion. Biol Neonate 75:97–103

Bude RO, Rubin JM (1996) Power Doppler sonography. Radiology 200:21–23

Cady EB, Costello AM, Dawson MJ (1983) Noninvasive investigation of cerebral metabolism in newborn infants by phosphorus nuclear magnetic resonance spectroscopy. Lancet 1:1059

Chang YS, Park WS, Lee M, Kim KS, Shin SM, Choi JH (1999) Near infrared spectroscopic monitoring of secondary cerebral energy failure after transient global hypoxia-ischemia in the newborn piglet. Neurol Res 21:216–224

Cooke RW, Rolfe P, Howat P (1977) A technique for the non invasive estimation of cerebral blood flow in the newborn infant. J Med Eng Technol 1:263–266

Corbett RJ, Laptook A, Nunnally RL (1987) The use of the chemical shift of the phosphomonoester P-31 magnetic resonance peak for the determination of intracellular pH in the brains of neonates. Neurology 37:1771–1779

Couture A (1994) Echographie cérébrale par voie transfontanellaire. Impératifs cliniques. In: Couture A, Veyrac C, Baud C (eds) Echographie cérébrale: du foetus au nouveau-né. Imagerie et hémodynamique. Sauramps Médical, Montpellier

Dietz V, Wolf M, Keel M, Siebenthal K, Baezinger O, Bucher H (1999) CO2 reactivity of the cerebral hemoglobin concentration in healthy term newborns measured by near infrared spectrophotometry. Biol Neonate 75:85–90

Doyle LW, Nahmias C, Firnau G (1983) Regional cerebral glucose metabolism of newborn infants measured by positron emission tomography. Dev Med Child Neurol 25:143–151

Drayton MR, Skidmore R (1986) Doppler ultrasound in the neonate. Ultrasound Med Biol 12:761–772

Gray PH, Griffin EA, Drumm JE, Fitzgerald DE, Duignan NM (1983) Continuous wave Doppler ultrasound in evaluation of cerebral blood flow in neonates. Arch Dis Child 58:677–681

Greisen G, Johansen K, Ellison PF, Fredriksen PS, Mali J, Friis-Hansen B (1984) Cerebral blood flow in the newborn infant: comparison of Doppler ultrasound and 133 xenon clearance. J Pediatr 104:411–418

Greisen G (1997) Cerebral blood flow and energy metabolism in the newborn. Clin Perinatol 24:531–545

Greisen G (1992) Effect of cerebral blood flow and cerebrovascular autoregulation on the distribution type and extent of cerebral injury. Brain Pathol 2:223–228

Gronendaal F, Veehoven RH, Van Der Grond J (1994) Cerebral lactate and N-acetyl-aspartate/choline ratios in asphyxiated full-term neonates demonstrated in vitro using proton magnetic resonance spectroscopy. Pediatr Res 35:148–151

Hanrahan JD, Cox IJ, Edwards AD, Cowan FM, Sargentoni J, Bell JD, Bryant DJ, Rutherford MA, Azzopardi D (1998) Persistent increases in cerebral lactate concentration after birth asphyxia. Pediatr Res 44:304–311

Hanrahan JD, Cox IJ, Azzopardi D, Cowan FM, Sargentoni J, Bell JD, Bryant DJ, Edwards AD (1999) Relation between proton magnetic spectroscopy within 18 hours of birth asphyxia and neurodevelopment at 1 year of age. Dev Med Child Neurol 41:76–82

Hill A, Perlman JM, Volpe JJ (1982) Relationship of pneumothorax to the occurrence of intraventricular hemorrhage in the preterm newborn. Pediatrics 69:144–149

Hill A, Volpe JJ (1982) Decrease in pulsatile flow in the anterior cerebral arteries in infantile hydrocephalus. Pediatrics 69:4–7

Hope PL, Reynolds EO (1985) Investigation of cerebral energy metabolism in newborn infants by phosphorus nuclear magnetic resonance spectroscopy. Clin Perinatol 12:261–265

Huppi PS, Posse S, Lazeyras F (1993) ^{1}H-spectroscopy in preterm and term newborns: regional developmental changes in human brain. Pediatr Res 33:205A

Leahy FA, Sankaran K, Cates D (1979) Quantitative noninvasive method to measure cerebral blood flow in newborn infants. Pediatrics 64:277–282

Lou HC, Skow HJ, Pedersen J (1979) Low cerebral blood flow. A risk factor in the neonate. J Pediatr 95:606–609

Lou HC, Lassen NA, Friis-Hansen B (1979) Impaired autoregulation of cerebral blood flow in the distressed newborn infant. J Pediatr 94:118–124

McMenamin JB, Volpe JJ (1983) Doppler ultrasonography in the determination of neonatal brain death. Ann Neurol 14:302–307

McMenamin JB, Volpe JJ (1984) Bacterial meningitis in infants: effects on intracranial pressure and cerebral blood flow velocity. Neurology 34:500–504

Perlman JM (1985) Neonatal cerebral blood flow velocity measurement. Clin Perinatol 12:179–193

Perlman JM, McMenamin JB, Volpe JJ (1983) Fluctuating cerebral blood flow velocity in respiratory distress syndrome. N Engl J Med 308:204–208

Perlman JM, Volpe JJ (1983) Suctioning in the preterm infant: effects on cerebral blood flow velocity, intracranial pressure and arterial blood pressure. Pediatrics 75:329–334

Perlman JM, Volpe JJ (1983) The effect of seizures on cerebral blood flow velocity, intracranial pressure and systolic blood pressure in the preterm infant. J Pediatr 102:288–293

Perlman JM, Hill A, Volpe JJ (1981) The effect of patent ductus arteriosus on flow velocity in the anterior cerebral arteries: ductal steal in the premature newborn infant. J Pediatr 99:767–771

Petroff OAC, Young RSK, Cowan BE (1988) ^{1}H nuclear magnetic resonance spectroscopy study of neonatal hypoglycemia. Pediatr Neurol 4:31–34

Poob RK, Aono T (1996) Transvaginal power Doppler angiography of the fetal brain. Ultrasound Obstet Gynecol 8:417–421

Powers AD, Graeber MC, Smith RR (1989) Transcranial Doppler ultrasonography in the determination of brain death. Neurosurgery 24:884–889

Powers WJ, Rosenbaum JL, Dence CS, Markham J, Videen TO (1998) Cerebral glucose transport and metabolism in preterm human infants. J Cereb Blood Flow Metab 18:632–638

Pryds O, Greisen G, Skov L (1990) Carbon dioxide-related changes in cerebral blood volume and cerebral blood flow in mechanically ventilated preterm neonates: comparison of near infrared spectrophotometry and 133 xenon clearance. Pediatr Res 27:445–449

Pryds O, Edwards D (1996) Cerebral blood flow in the newborn infant. Arch Dis Child 74:F63-F69

Rubin JM, Adler RS (1993) Power Doppler expands standard color capability. Diagn Imaging 12:66–69

Sakatani K, Chen S, Lichty W, Zuo H, Wang YP (1999) Cerebral blood oxygenation changes induced by auditory stimulation in newborn infants measured by near infrared spectroscopy. Early Hum Dev 55:229–236

Seibert JJ, Avva R, Hronas TN, Mocharla R, Vanderzalm T, Cox K, Kinder D, Lidzy B, Knight K (1998) Use of power Doppler in pediatric neurosonography: a pictorial essay. Radiographics 18:879–890

Shu SK, Ashwal S, Holshouser BA, Nystrom G, Hinshaw DB (1997) Prognostic value of ^{1}H-MRS in perinatal CNS insults. Pediatr Neurol 17:309–318

Takahashi T, Shirane R, Sato S, Yoshimoto T (1999) Developmental changes of cerebral blood flow and oxygen metabolism in children. Am J Neuroradiol 20:917–922

Taylor GA (1992) Intracranial venous system in the newborn: evaluation of normal anatomy and flow characteristics with color Doppler US. Radiology 183:449–452

Volpe JJ, Perlman JM, Hill A, McMenamin JB (1982) Cerebral blood flow velocity in the human newborn: the value of its determination. Pediatrics 70:147–152

Volpe JJ, Herscovitch P, Perlman JM (1985) Positron emission tomography in the asphyxiated term newborn: parasagittal impairment of cerebral blood flow. Ann Neurol 17:287–296

Wolf M, Keel M, Schenk D, Dietz V, Von Siebenthal K, Wolf U, Baezinger O, Bucher HU (1998) Comparison of absolute cerebral haemoglobin concentration in neonates measured directly and by the oxygen swing method both based on near infrared spectrophotometry. Adv Exp Med Biol 454:125–129

Wong WS, Tsuruda JS, Liberman RL, Chirino A, Vogt JF, Gangitano E (1989) Color Doppler imaging of intracranial vessels in the neonate. Am J Neuroradiol 10:425–430

Younkin D, Wagerle L, Delivoria-Papadopoulos M (1984) The effects of graded hypoxia on cerebral phosphorus metabolites and intracellular pH in newborn lambs. Ann Neurol 16:383–385

Younkin D, Maris J, Donlon E (1985) The effect of seizures on cerebral metabolites in children. Pediatr Res 19:397

Younkin D, Delivoria-Papadopoulos M, Reivich M, Jaggi J, Obrist W (1988) Regional variations in human newborn cerebral blood flow. J Pediatr 112:104–10

2 Normal Neonatal Brain: Color Doppler and Pulsed Doppler

ALAIN P. COUTURE

CONTENTS

The revolution in the imaging of vascular physiology, the establishing of a diagnosis and the prognostic evaluation of vascular disease lie not in morphological sonographic studies but in the Doppler techniques that can display cerebral vessels in the fetus and neonate. These techniques obviously require

A. COUTURE, MD
Service de Radiologie Pédiatrique, Hôpital Arnaud de Ville-neuve, 371 av. Doyen Gaston Giraud, 34295 Montpellier Cedex, France

long training and an excellent knowledge of the anatomy of the cerebral vasculature. All the same, before being used, they have to be validated. To achieve this, an arterial and venous hemodynamic evaluation should be performed during routine brain ultrasonography in every normal infant.

It is easy to visualize the internal carotid artery on color Doppler imaging; more difficult, though equally important, is to analyze its branches, especially the anterior choroidal artery. It is essential to know the intracerebral vascular map, although literature data are still incomplete.

In the literature, the resistive index (RI) is the most widely used hemodynamic marker, but experience shows that cerebral velocities should be preferred, since they provide more reliable and more accurate criteria in studying the multiple changes of the neonatal period.

2.1
Cerebral Vasculature: Color Doppler

2.1.1
Anatomy of the Cerebral Arteries

The brain arterial supply has two origins: the carotid system with its main branches, the anterior and middle cerebral arteries, and the vertebral system with the basilar artery and its two branches, the posterior cerebral arteries. The multiple imaging tools that are able to visualize this arterial distribution (MORRIS 1996), from the oldest such as intra-arterial angiography, to the most recent, such as MR angiography (Fig. 2.1) have been well described.

The great cerebral arteries are correctly displayed by color Doppler imaging (MITCHELL 1988, 1989; TATSUNO 1990; TAYLOR 1990; WONG 1989), but their branches have been insufficiently analyzed. Today, the technological capabilities of ultrasound equipment enable increasingly complete demonstration of the vascular distribution.

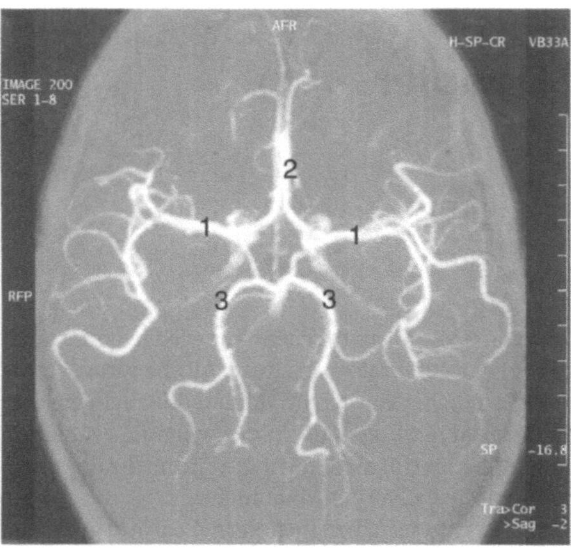

Fig. 2.1. MR angiography in a 8-month old infant: detailed vascular anatomy showing the circle of Willis, middle cerebral arteries (*1*) and their cortical branches, anterior cetebral arteries in the close contact (*2*), and posterior cerebral arteries (*3*), which encircle the brain stem

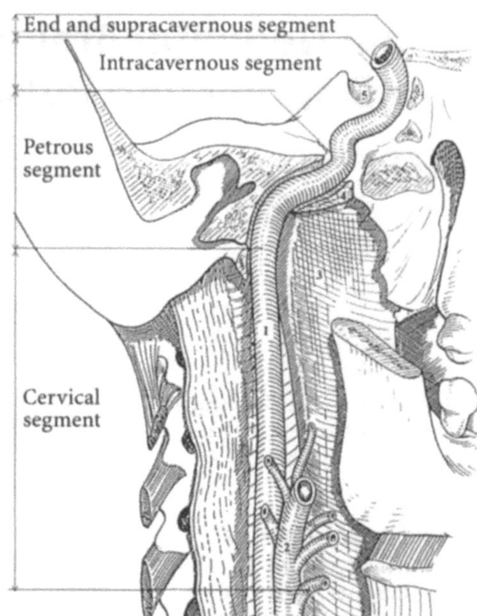

Diagram 2.1. The cervical and intracranial course of the internal carotid artery
> *1* Internal carotid artery
> *2* External carotid artery
> *3* Pharyngeal wall
> *4* Carotid canal
> *5* Sella turcica

2.1.1.1
Internal Carotid Artery

2.1.1.1.1
Course (TAPTAS 1981)

The internal carotid artery begins at the level of the common carotid bifurcation and its course may be divided in four segments: cervical, petrous, cavernous, and supracavernous (Diagram 2.1). It has been well shown by angiography and, more recently, by MR angiography (Fig. 2.2).

The common carotid artery and the cervical portion of its branches (internal and external carotid arteries) are easily visualized with Doppler techniques, but color Doppler can also depict the endocranial course of the internal carotid artery.

● The internal carotid artery enters the base of the brain in the carotid canal (Diagram 2.2) on the posterior exocranial surface of the petrous bone, anterior to the jugular foramen, and courses as a petrous segment.

In the adult, it consists in a short ascending (or tympanic) portion, medial to the basal turn of the cochlea and lateral to the middle ear cavity. Then, a horizontal (or tubal) portion runs anteromedially

along the axis of the petrous bone and ends at the posterior lip of the exocranial foramen lacerum, inferomedially to the edge of the gasserian ganglion within Meckel's cavity, and inferolaterally to the oculomotor nerve (VI). This petrous segment is poorly visualized on color Doppler, probably because the tortuosities of the intracranial internal carotid artery are less pronounced in the neonate (KNOSP 1988). However, on a parasagittal plane, the bony entrance of the petrous segment is well recognized (Fig. 2.3).

● The intracranial portion consists in the carotid siphon and the terminal part of the artery. From its petrous exit to its end, the internal carotid artery exhibits different segments, which are variably designated in the literature (BOUTHILLIER 1996; BRACARD 1997; FISCHER 1938; GIBO 1981). The classification of FISCHER (1938) that distinguishes five segments of the carotid siphon is the best known (Diagram 2.3):
- The precavernous subsellar segment (C5) runs vertically or with a slight superoposterior orientation and shows an anterior curve.
- The intracavernous parasellar segment courses horizontally and anteriorly (C4), followed by a posterior curve (C3). At this level, the artery lies

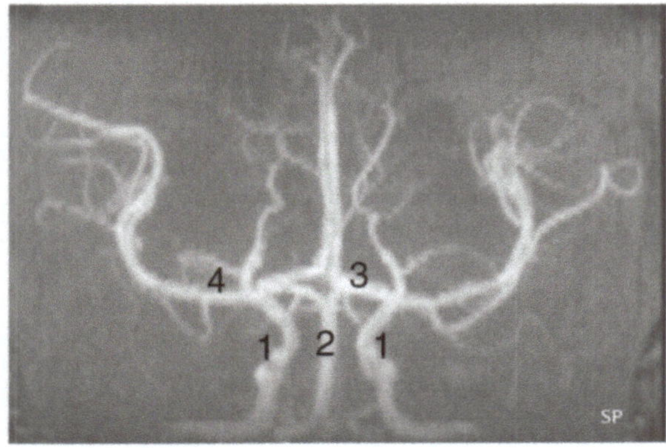

Fig. 2.2. MR angiography. The endocranial course of the internal carotid artery is excellently shown. The two carotid (*1*) arteries encircle the basilar artery (*2*), broadening at their distal part to give rise to the anterior cerebral artery (*3*) and middle cerebral artery (*4*)

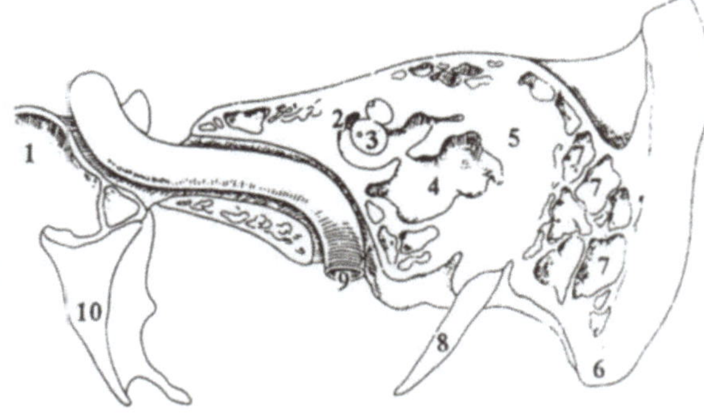

Diagram 2.2. Course of the internal carotid artery (From BOUCHET-CUILLERET 1983)

1 Sphenoidal sinus	*6* Mastoid process
2 Basal turn of cochlea	*7* Mastoid cells
3 Internal auditory canal	*8* Styloid process
4 Tympanic cavity	*9* Internal carotid artery
5 Petrous bone	*10* Pterygoid plate

lateral to the pituitary gland, and inferior and superior to the oculomotor nerves (III, IV and VI), within the cavernous sinus.

– The artery exits from the cavernous sinus into the subarachnoid space, and this supracavernous segment corresponds to C1 and C2 of FISCHER (1938). The second portion of C3 courses superolaterally from the sinus. Near the frontal lobe it lies medial to the optic chiasm and nerve, and divides into terminal branches. C2 is short, posteriorly directed, and runs horizontally or slightly ascending. C1 is vertical and ends the course of the internal carotid artery, which divides into the middle and anterior cerebral arteries (Diagram 2.4) (GRAND 1980).

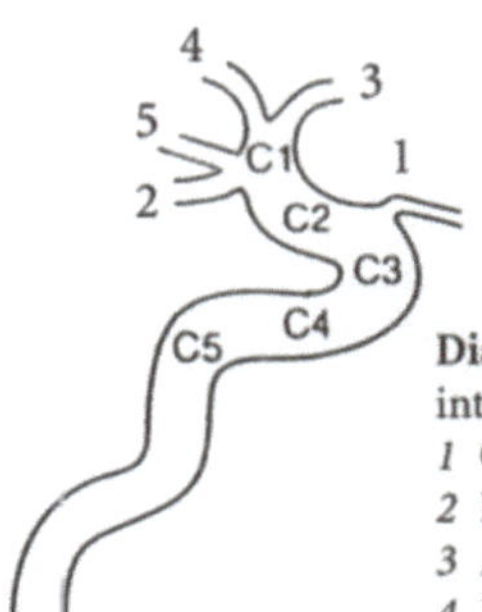

Diagram 2.3. Subdivisions of the internal carotid artery siphon
1 Ophthalmic artery
2 Posterior communicating artery
3 Anterior cerebral artery
4 Middle cerebral artery
5 Anterior choroidal artery

Brain ultrasonography, especially color Doppler, provides complete visualization of the internal carotid artery in its intracranial course.

Since 1989, MITCHELL has used color Doppler to demonstrate the carotid arteries on coronal planes. These data are confirmed by WONG (1989) and TATSUNO (1989), who report good visualization in all of 12 neonates studied.

Although morphological ultrasound (US) easily recognizes the pulsatile beat of the internal carotid artery, it is unable to demonstrate the complete course of the vessel and does not allow reliable hemodynamic assessment by spectral analysis.

The internal carotid artery is visualized on the coronal plane at the level of the sella turcica and sphenoid bone. In the cavernous sinus, the artery

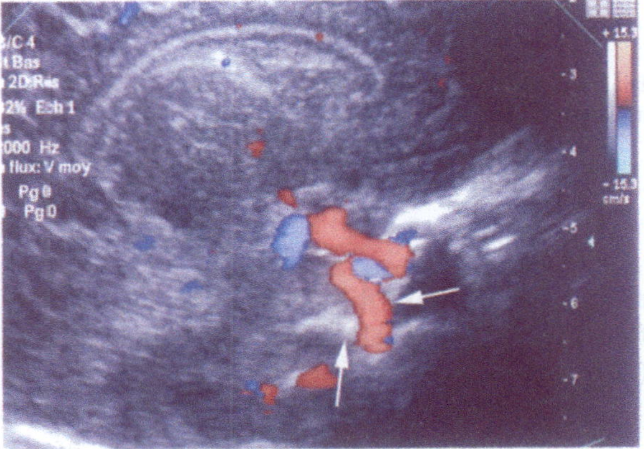

Fig. 2.3. Full-term neonate. Parasagittal scan of right carotid siphon. The intracranial entrance point of the internal carotid artery is well demonstrated (*arrow*)

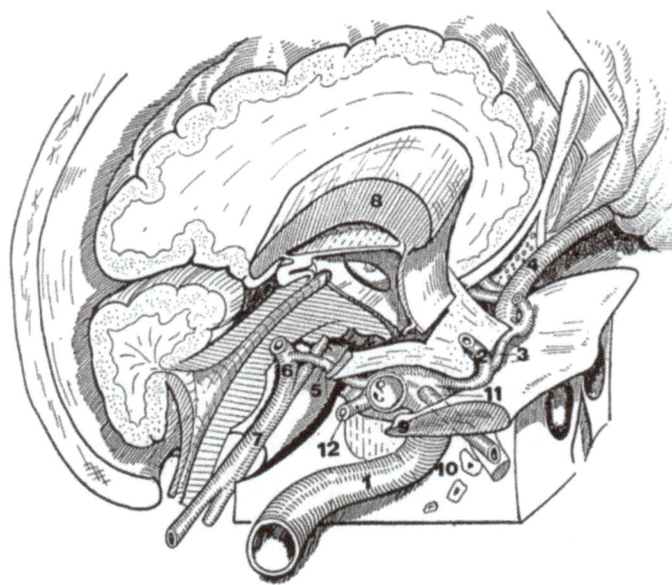

Diagram 2.4. End of the internal carotid artery
  1 Internal carotid artery
  2 Anterior cerebral artery
  3 Anterior communicating artery
  4 Middle cerebral artery
  5 Posterior communicating artery
  6 Posterior cerebral artery
  7 Basilar artery
  8 Corpus callosum
  9 Anterior clinoid process
 10 Sphenoid bone
 11 Ophthalmic artery
 12 Anterior choroidal artery

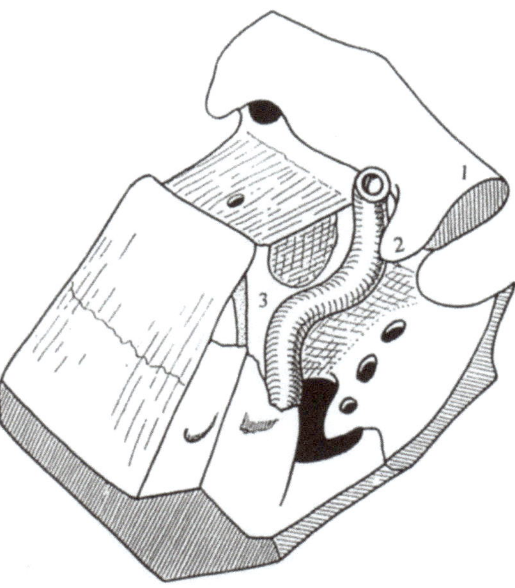

Diagram 2.5. Relations between internal carotid artery
and bony structures
  1 Lesser wing of sphenoid bone
  2 Anterior clinoid process
  3 Sella turcica

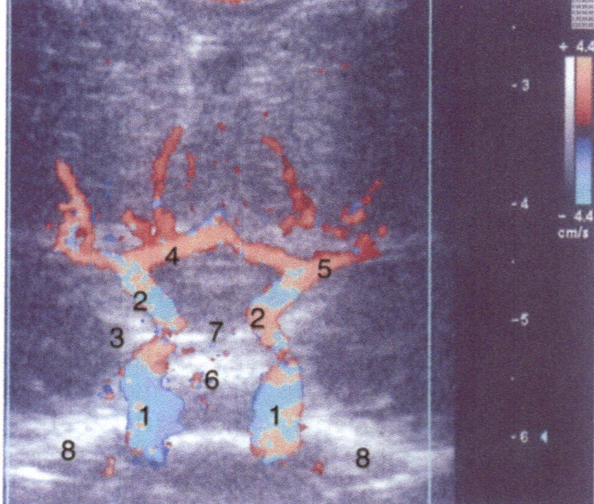

Fig. 2.4. Color imaging of the internal carotid artery. This intracranial segment is completely depicted: the lateral sphenoidal intracavernous segment (*1*) is ideal for hemodynamic investigation; the terminal segment (*2*), close to the anterior clinoid processes (*3*), gives off anterior (*4*) and middle cerebral arteries (*5*). Notice the median protrusion of the sphenoid bone (*6*), inferior to the sella turcica floor (*7*) and medial to the greater wings of the sphenoid bone (*8*)

runs laterally toward the sphenoid body and arises from the sinus, medial to the anterior clinoid process (Diagram 2.5).

In the subarachnoid space, the carotid artery courses superoposteriorly; it is surrounded by the frontal lobe superiorly, the optic chiasm medially, and the clinoid process laterally.

In its last segment, the superolateral orientation of the artery is well seen before its division into middle and anterior cerebral arteries (Fig. 2.4). A parasagittal plane completes the anatomic analysis: the carotid siphon is completely displayed, from C5 to C1 (Fig. 2.5); the posterior and anterior loops appear less tortuous in the newborn than in the adult, with a less pronounced anterior knee (KNOSP 1988) (Fig. 2.6).

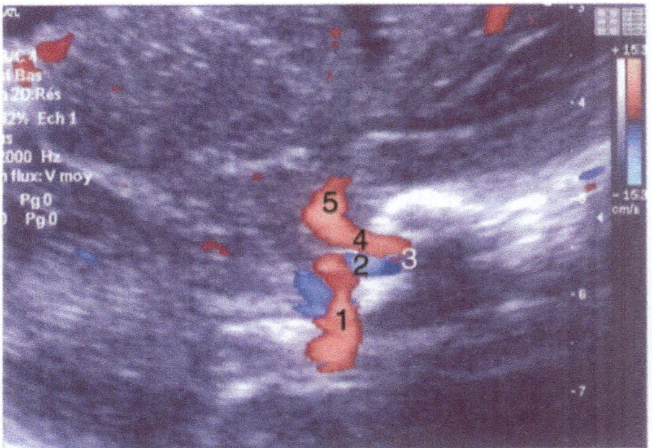

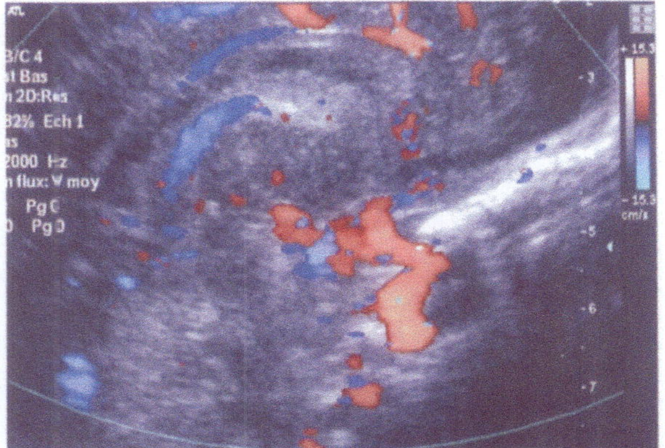

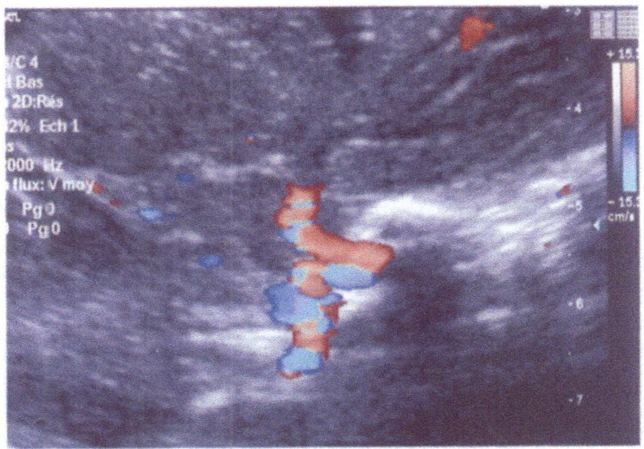

Fig. 2.5. Siphon of internal carotid artery on standard color Doppler imaging. All segments are visualized: the precavernous subsellar vertical segment C5 (*1*) is suitable for pulsed Doppler assessment. Also shown are the intracavernous segments with anteriorly directed C4 (*2*) and posteriorly concave C3 (*3*) and supracavernous segments: posteriorly directed C2 (*4*) and ascending C1 (*5*). When the loops are pronounced, segment C4 is coded *blue*

Fig. 2.6a,b. The course of the carotid siphon differs among children. In this newborn (**a**) the posterior loop of C5 and anterior loop of C3 are poorly marked: the siphon is uniformly coded *red*, contrasting with the swirling flow and the *blue* coding of C4 in this other newborn (**b**), in whom the carotid loops are more pronounced

2.1.1.1.2
Branches

- The intracavernous internal carotid artery gives rise to several branches of great functional importance:
  - The tributaries of the carotid siphon, at the level of C5, usually arise separately, and give off the inferior hypophyseal artery, the clival arteries (which irrigate the dura mater of the dorsal part of the clivus and the cavernous sinus roof), the lateral artery of the gasserian ganglion, and the meningeal artery (which supplies the free margin of the tentorium).
  - The tributaries of segment C4 of the carotid siphon (LASJAUNIAS 1977).
  - The capsular arteries, which feed the dura mater of the pituitary region, the diaphragma sellae, and are very thin arterioles.
  - The inferolateral trunk, which arises at C4 and supplies the oculomotor nerves.
  Despite their important function, these small vessels cannot be identified by color Doppler.

- The supracavernous branches are represented by the superior hypophyseal arteries that feed the pituitary stalk and the anterior lobe of the pituitary gland, and cannot be shown by color US.

  Then, the internal carotid artery gives off the ophthalmic artery, the posterior communicating artery, and the anterior choroidal artery, at the level of C1.

— The ophthalmic artery arises from the anterosuperior surface of C2, in the subarachnoid or, less commonly, intradural space. It courses forward toward the optic canal, inferolateral to the optic nerve. It enters the orbit, crosses the optic nerve, and distributes to the orbital content. On color Doppler, its beginning is commonly visualized for a few millimeters, immediately after the anterior loop of C3. On standard color imaging, it is coded blue (Fig. 2.7).

— The posterior communicating artery (PEDROSA 1987) arises from the dorsal surface of the supracavernous internal carotid artery. It presents a linear posterior course and a variable diameter. It gives off branches toward the thalamus, hypothalamus, optic tract, and posterior limb of the internal capsule. It ends by anastomosing with the posterior cerebral artery.

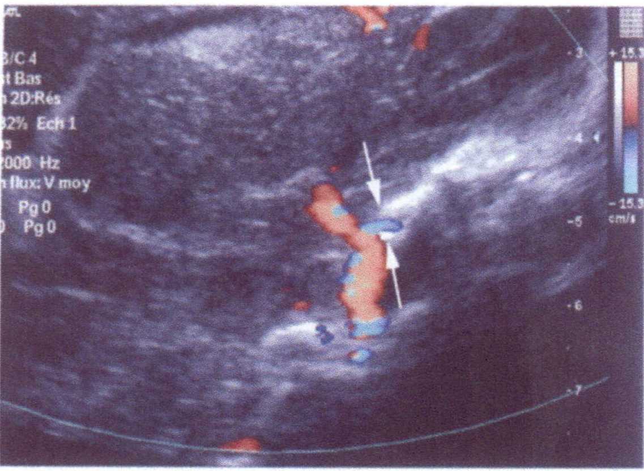

Fig. 2.7. On this scan of the right carotid siphon, the ophthalmic artery, constantly visible, arises from the anterior surface of segment C2 and its subarachnoid course is visible for a few millimeters before it enters the optic canal (*arrow*)

Although the posterior communicating artery is inconstantly visualized on angiography, it is always well displayed by color ultrasonography. The two communicating arteries have been described on transcranial scans (see Fig. 2.14) but the transfontanellar parasagittal planes also provide a good depiction (Fig. 2.8).

— The anterior choroidal artery has an important function since it represents the main arterial feeding of the tela choroidea of the lateral ventricles (Fujii 1980; Rhoton 1979; Théron 1976; Wolfram-Gabel 1987). It arises from the posterior surface of

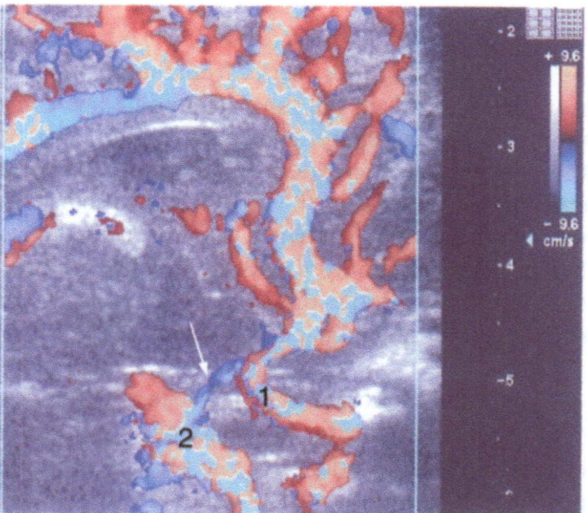

Fig. 2.8. On a slightly parasagittal plane, the posterior communicating artery is easily recognized: it anastomoses with the posterior surface of the supracavernous internal carotid artery (*1*) and the anterior surface of the posterior cerebral artery (*2*)

the carotid siphon (at the level of the C1 segment), a few millimeters above the origin of the posterior communicating artery, and divides into a proximal cisternal segment and a distal plexal segment. Its cisternal segment passes through the optochiasmatic cistern and across the optic tract with a posterolateral course. Then, within the ambient cistern, it ascends slightly and reaches the choroid fissure. It enters the temporal horn of the lateral ventricle with a decreasing diameter.

Its plexal segment ends in branches that run toward the choroid plexus.

It sends important branches; its cisternal segment gives rise to several central arteries toward the globus pallidus, posterior limb of internal capsule, caudate nucleus, ventrolateral thalamus and red nucleus; it also contributes to supply the optic tract.

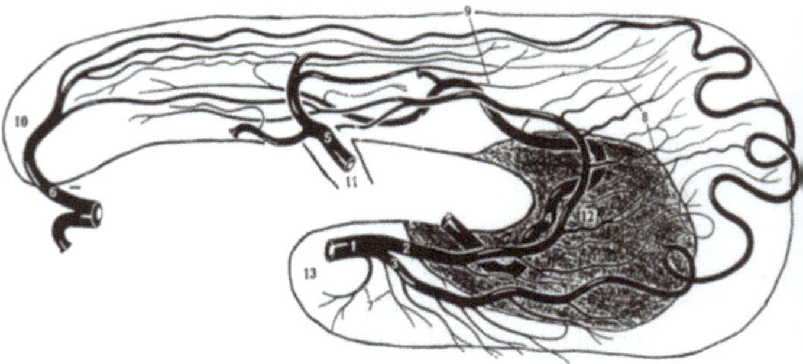

Diagram 2.6. Distribution of arteries within the tela choroidea of the lateral ventricle (From Wolfram-Gabel 1987)
The anterior choroidal artery (*1*) reaches the temporal horn of the lateral ventricle. It divides into two branches, a medial (*2*) and a lateral (*3*). The first branch runs along the attached edge of the tela choroidea, accompanied by the inferior posterolateral choroidal artery (*4*). The second branch, very sinuous, runs along the free edge of the tela. All these arteries reach the interventricular foramen and anastomose with the superior posterolateral choroidal artery (*5*) and with the medial branch of the posteromedial choroidal artery (*6*). The tela choroidea is vascularized by short (*7*), middle (*8*), and long (*9*) choroidal branches. *10* Frontal horn, *11* foramen of Monro, *12* choroid glomus, *13* temporal horn

After entering the anterior part of the temporal horn, it divides into 2 main branches, medial and lateral, that distribute in the lateral ventricle plexus, via short, middle and long choroidal branches (Diagram 2.6).

Color imaging provides accurate information: an oblique parasagittal plane displays the whole course of the anterior choroidal artery (Wolfram-Gabel 1987), from its carotid origin, to its ventricular entrance, where it describes a continuous colored signal that curves around the pulvinar (Fig. 2.9).

2.1.1.2
Basilar Artery
(GRAND 1977; SAEKI 1977)

The basilar artery results from the junction of the vertebral arteries on the anterior surface of the medulla (Diagram 2.7). It runs in the pontomedullary sulcus and ends slightly above the pons, by dividing into two terminal branches, the posterior cerebral arteries. It is always easily recognized, pulsating in the cisterns between the clivus and the ventral aspect of the medulla and the pons. It is also easily depicted by transfontanellar color ultrasonography, on a sagittal midline plane (Fig. 2.10). On the frontal scan, the vertebral arteries, their convergence, the basilar

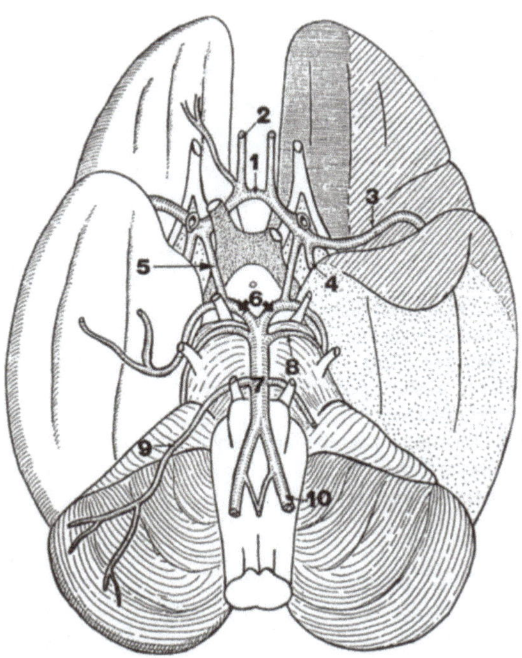

Diagram 2.7. Basilar artery and its branches

 Anterior cerebral artery

 Middle cerebral artery

Posterior cerebral artery

  1 Anterior communicating artery
  2 Anterior cerebral artery
  3 Middle cerebral artery
  4 Anterior choroidal artery
  5 Posterior communicating artery
  6 Posterior cerebral artery
  7 Basilar artery
  8 Superior cerebellar artery
  9 Middle cerebellar artery
10 Vertebral artery

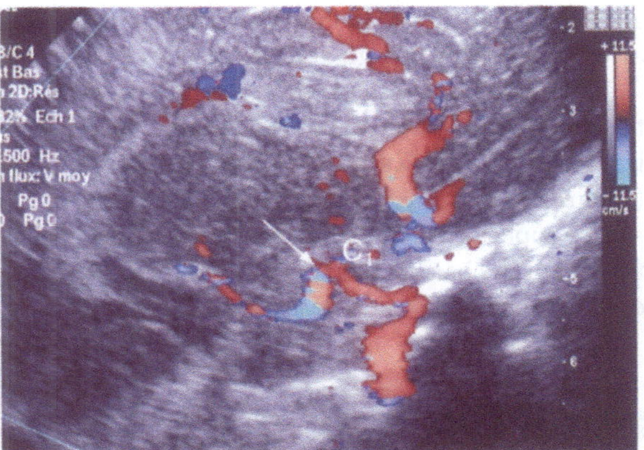

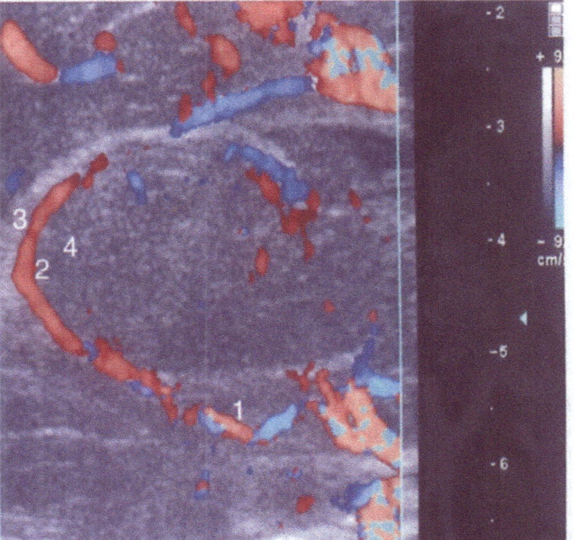

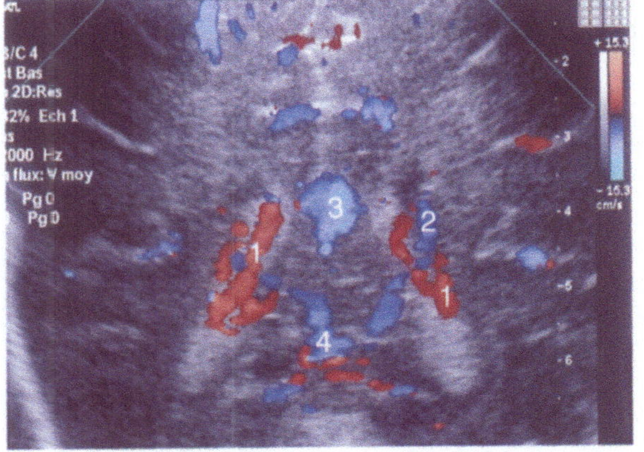

Fig. 2.9a–c. The origin of the anterior choroidal artery (*arrow*) is always individualized (**a**) at the posterior surface of the distal internal carotid artery (C1). On a parasagittal plane (**b**), its whole course is depicted from its proximal cisternal part (*1*) to its distal ventricular part (*2*), which curves, at the level of the choroid plexus glomus (*3*), around the pulvinar (*4*). **c** The two anterior choroidal arteries (*1*) can be recognized on this posteriorly oblique frontal scan. *2* Superior choroidal vein, *3* proximal part of internal cerebral veins, *4* straight sinus

artery, and its division into the posterior cerebral arteries are easily recognized (Fig. 2.11).

The basilar artery sends several tributaries toward the brain stem, but its main branches are the cerebellar arteries (AMARENCO 1980; ICARDO 1982) (Diagram 2.8).
— The superior cerebellar artery arises from the distal part of the basilar artery. It runs anterior then lateral to the peduncle, and describes a superoposterior concavity. It feeds a limited territory of the brain stem, the tegmentum of the pons, and part of the cerebellum (anterior lobules) and of the vermis (central lobule, culmen, declive, folium).

The middle (or anteroinferior) cerebellar artery usually arises from the median third of the basilar artery, and runs laterally and slightly downward to reach the cerebellopontine angle. It supplies the inferior part of the pons, middle cerebellar pedun-

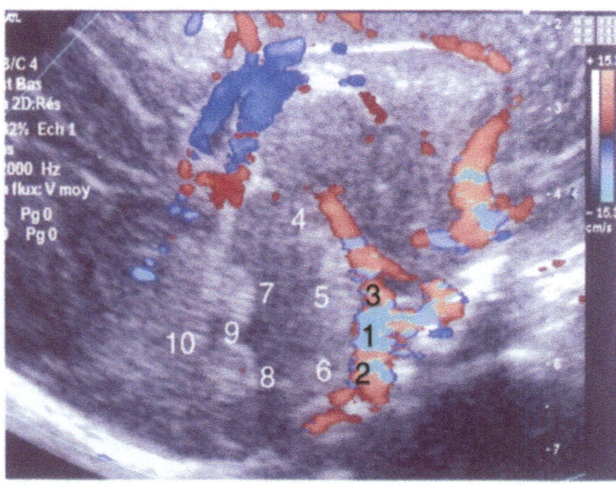

Fig. 2.10. The basilar artery (1) is visualized on a midline sagittal scan. It runs within the subarachnoid spaces: the medullary cistern (2) inferiorly and the pontine cistern (3) superiorly. Its relations are well defined: note the hyperechoic interpeduncular cistern (4) superiorly and the brain stem posteriorly. The brain stem echostructure is characteristic: the basilar ventral part of the pons (5) and medulla (6) is hyperechoic, while the dorsal part of the pons (7) and medulla (8) is hypoechoic. 9 Fourth ventricle, 10 cerebellar vermis

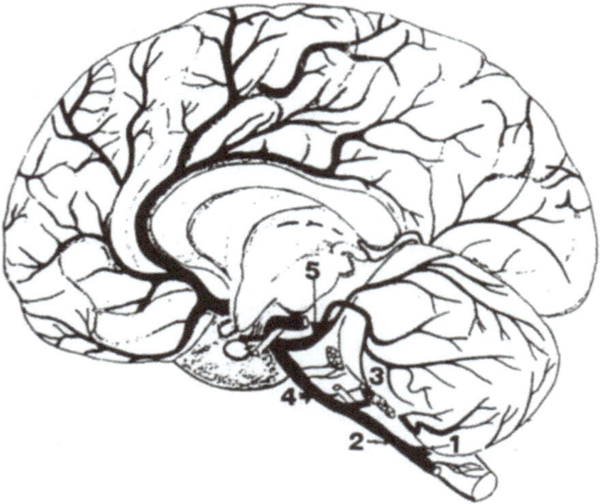

Diagram 2.8. Arterial distribution toward the cerebellum (From SOBOTTA 1985)
   1 Inferior posterior cerebellar artery
   2 Vertebral artery
   3 Inferior anterior cerebellar artery
   4 Basilar artery
   5 Superior cerebellar artery.

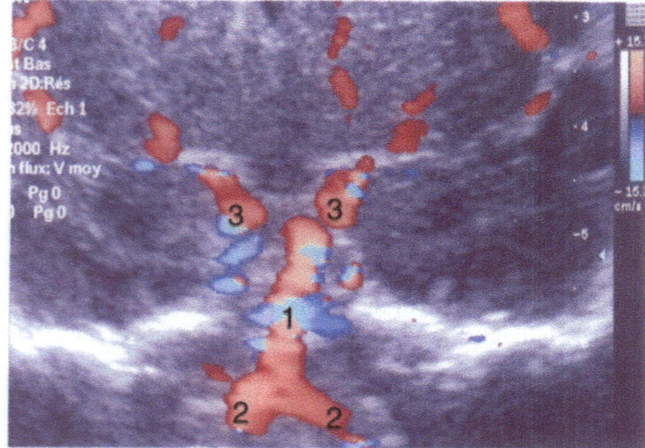

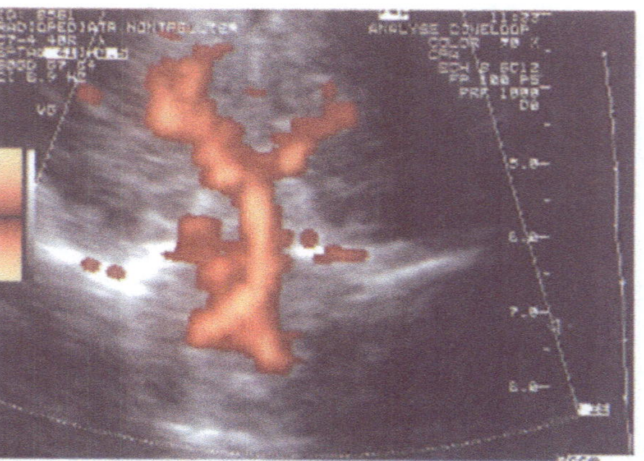

Fig. 2.11a,b. Posterior frontal scan in the axis of the basilar artery. Notice (a) that the basilar artery (1) arises from the junction of the two vertebral arteries (2) and divides in its distal portion into the posterior cerebral arteries (3). The basilar artery is usually median but may exhibit a sinuous, curved (b), slightly eccentric course

cle, flocculus, and adjacent part of the cerebellar lobes.
— The inferior (or posteroinferior) cerebellar artery usually arises from the intracranial portion of the vertebral artery. It irrigates the dorsal medulla, posteroinferior part of the cerebellar hemispheres, and the nodulus, uvula, tuber, and declive in the vermis.

Color imaging provides poor appreciation of the cerebellar arteries. The transfontanellar approach is inappropriate in view of the course and direction of these vessels, deeply located in the posterior fossa. In the best case, the proximal part of the superior cerebellar arteries may be recognized on each side of the basilar artery (Fig. 2.12). The inferior cerebellar arteries are never visible.

2.1.1.3
Circle of Willis

Anatomically, the circle of Willis (Diagram 2.9) is constituted by:
- Anteriorly, the anterior cerebral arteries and anterior communicating arteries, from the carotid system.
- Laterally, the posterior communicating arteries.
- Posteriorly, the posterior cerebral arteries, from the vertebrobasilar system.

MR angiography accurately demonstrates its anatomy (Fig. 2.13).

Since extracorporeal membrane oxygenation (ECMO) has been proposed for treatment of neonatal respiratory distress syndrome (BARTLETT 1985), knowledge of the normal circle of Willis is required to

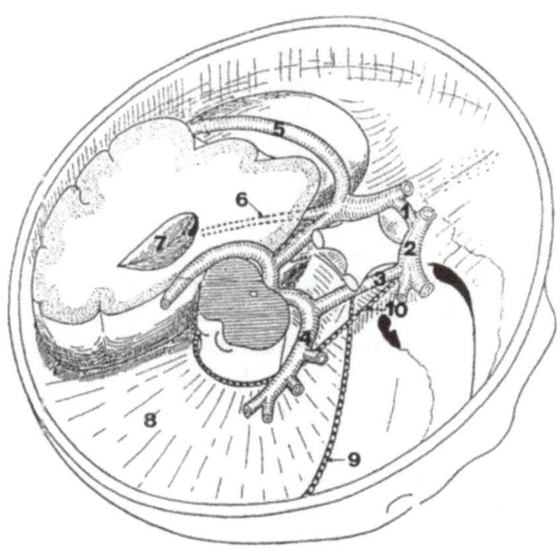

Diagram 2.9. Superior view of the circle of Willis
 1 Anterior communicating artery
 2 Anterior cerebral artery
 3 Posterior communicating artery
 4 Posterior cerebral artery
 5 Middle cerebral artery
 6 Anterior choroidal artery
 7 Lateral ventricle
 8 Tentorium cerebelli
 9 Outer edge of tentorium cerebelli
10 Inner edge of tentorium cerebelli

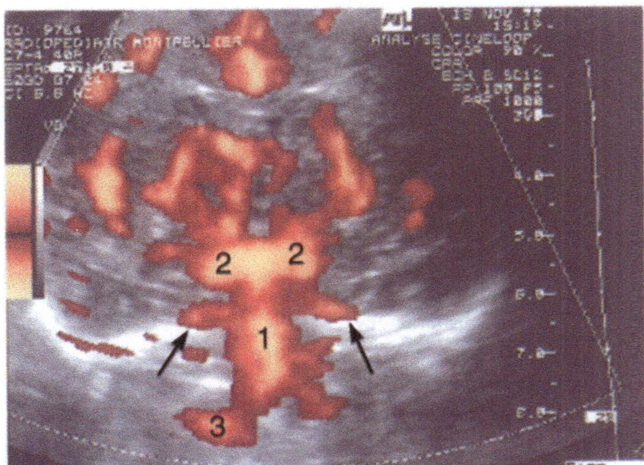

Fig. 2.12. Whatever the plane, clear visualization of the superior cerebellar arteries (*arrow*) is exceptional. *1* Basilar artery, *2* posterior cerebral arteries, *3* vertebral artery

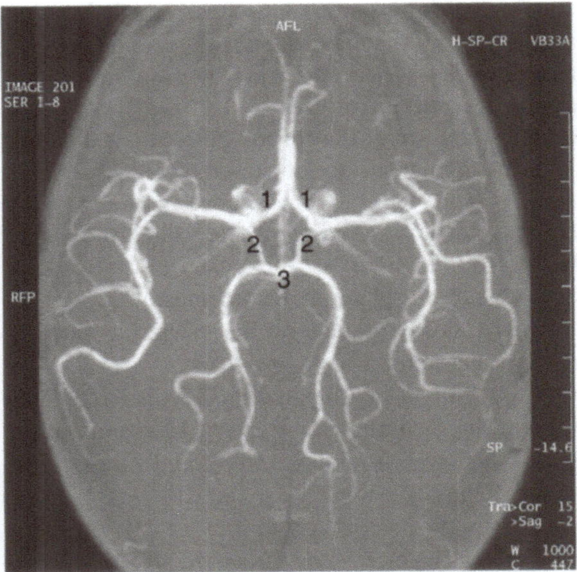

Fig. 2.13. MR angiography. The circle of Willis is constituted by the anterior cerebral arteries (*1*), posterior communicating arteries (*2*), and P_1 segments of the posterior cerebral arteries (*3*). The anterior communicating artery is not seen

maintain the correct perfusion of the right hemisphere after ligation of the right common carotid artery (RAJU 1989). Hemorrhagic and hypoxic-ischemic cerebral complications are frequent after ligation of carotid and jugular vessels (MATAMOROS 1989; MITCHELL 1988; TAYLOR 1992). Twenty-two anatomical variants of the circle of Willis have been described, including duplication, hypoplasia, and agenesis of one or more arterial segments. SEYDEL (1964) reported anatomical variations in 79% of 98 fetal brains. Thus, it is essential to take into account the morphology and, possibly, the hemodynamic pattern of the circle of Willis before ECMO treatment.

The color Doppler technique provides good imaging of the entire circle of Willis. All the arteries, especially the anterior and posterior communicating arteries, may be visualized by a transfontanellar approach, although the transosseous temporal access allows the best depiction of the entire circle (Fig. 2.14).

2.1.1.4
Anterior Cerebral Artery
(BRACARD 1997; DUNKER 1976; GOMEZ 1986; PERLMUTTER 1976, 1978)

The anterior cerebral artery arises from the medial surface of the termination of the carotid in the supra- and laterosellar region. Its diameter is approximately 1.5 mm in the full-term newborn (less than that of the middle cerebral artery).

After an initial supraoptic anteromedial course toward the interhemispheric fissure, it joins the contralateral artery via the anterior communicating artery. It courses forward and curves posteriorly around the genu of the corpus callosum. It then follows the medial surface of the cerebral hemisphere, along the pericallosal gyrus, above the body of the corpus callosum (Diagram 2.10). Finally, it goes backward and ends as the posterior pericallosal artery, near the splenium, before anastomosing with the pericallosal branch of the posterior cerebral artery (Diagram 2.10).

Five segments may be described: A1 is proximal to the anterior communicating artery, A2 ascends to the genu, A3 curves around it, and A4 and A5 run close to the corpus callosum.

● The A1 segment (MARINKOVIC 1986) courses medially, approaching the contralateral artery, until their junction via the anterior communicating artery. This junction is usually located above the optic chiasm, less frequently above the optic nerve

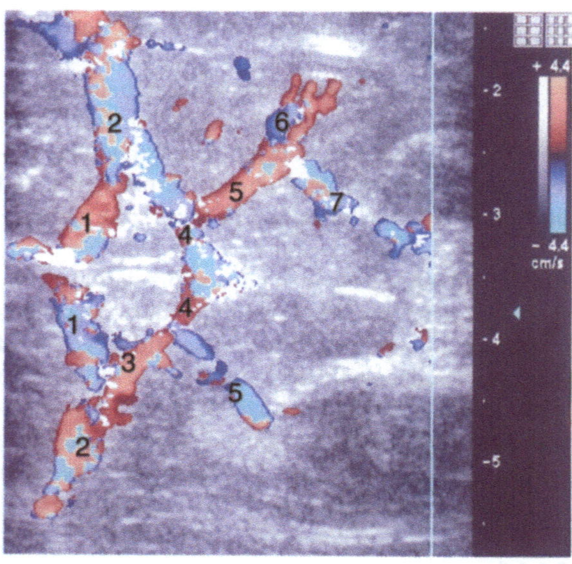

Fig. 2.14. Transcranial temporal axial scan. The circle of Willis is completely visualized. *1* Anterior cerebral artery, *2* middle cerebral artery, *3* posterior communicating artery, *4* P1 segment of posterior cerebral artery, *5* P2 segment of posterior cerebral artery, *6* temporal branches of posterior cerebral artery, *7* P3 segment of posterior cerebral artery

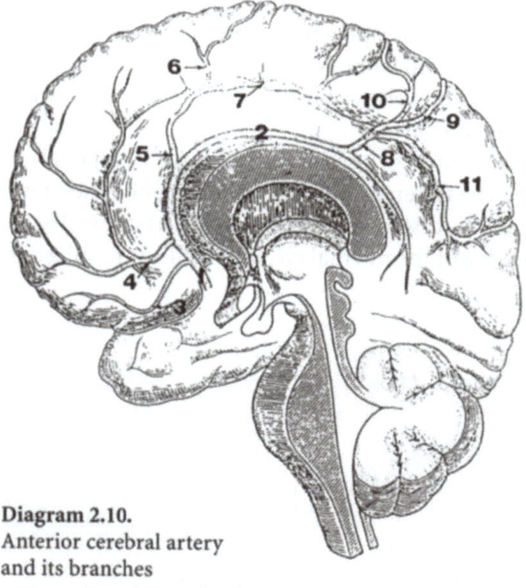

Diagram 2.10.
Anterior cerebral artery
and its branches

    1 Anterior cerebral artery
    2 Pericallosal artery
    3 Orbitofrontal artery
    4 Anterior medial frontal artery
    5 Callosomarginal artery
    6 Middle medial frontal artery
    7 Posterior medial frontal artery
    8 Medial parietal artery
    9 Precuneal artery
  10 Precentral artery
  11 Parieto-occipital artery

(PERLMUTTER 1976). The A1 segment gives off 2–15 arterioles (LAZORTHES 1958) and ends in the anterior perforated space, dorsal surface of the optic chiasm, suprachiasmatic part of the hypothalamus, optic tract, and several other sites such as the inferior surface of the frontal lobe (Diagram 2.11). More distally, it gives rise to a larger artery, the so-called recurrent artery of Heubner, that is of special interest (DUNKER 1976; GOMES 1984; GORCZYCA 1987; PERLMUTTER 1976).

- In the literature, there is a great degree of inconsistency in the description of the origin of this artery. OSTROWSKI (1960) and AHMED (1967) reported that the artery of Heubner emerges just near the anterior communicating artery, but other authors observed several variations: GOMES (1984) and PERLMUTTER (1976) found it arising in the first millimeters of segment A2, in 57% and 78% of brains, respectively. These variations will not be discussed here, but it is important to note, with PERLMUTTER (1976), that this artery arises within 2 mm of the anterior communicating artery in 52% of cases, within 3 mm in 80%, and within 4 mm in 100%.
- The course of this vessel is also variable. GOMES (1984) reported the artery running superior to the A1 segment in 63% of 65 cases, anterior in 34%, and posterior in 3%.
- The artery of Heubner commonly arises from the lateral wall of the A1 segment (Diagram 2.11), but usually remains adherent to A1 by arachnoid strands (GOMES 1984; PERLMUTTER 1976).
- Its point of penetration of the anterior perforated substance may vary since the terminal branches may be single or multiple (ROSNER 1984). These branches run on the anterior perforated substance but are part of the anteromedial and anterolateral groups of lenticulostriate arteries (Diagram 2.12). The artery of Heubner supplies the caudate nucleus head, inferior part of the anterior limb of the internal capsule, and anterior third of the putamen.

● The anterior communicating artery (PERLMUTTER 1976)

This artery joins the two anterior cerebral arteries and closes the circle of Willis anteriorly. It is a short, single, transverse vessel, located anterior and inferior to the anterior part of the chiasm. It sends several arterioles (MARINKOVIC 1990) toward the suprachiasmatic area, dorsal surface of optic chiasm, anterior perforated substance, and frontal lobe. It perfuses the septum lucidum, fornix, and anterior hypothalamus.

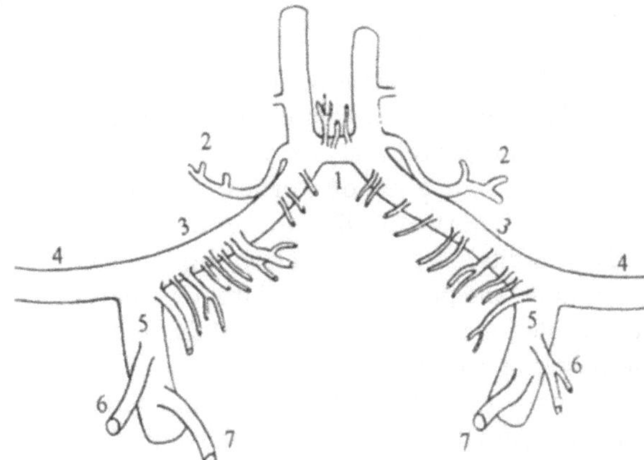

Diagram 2.11. Recurrent artery of Heubner and A1 segment of the anterior cerebral artery (From DUNKER 1976)

1 Anterior communicating artery
2 Artery of Heubner
3 Anterior cerebral artery (A1 segment)
4 Middle cerebral artery
5 Internal carotid artery
6 Anterior choroidal artery
7 Posterior communicating artery

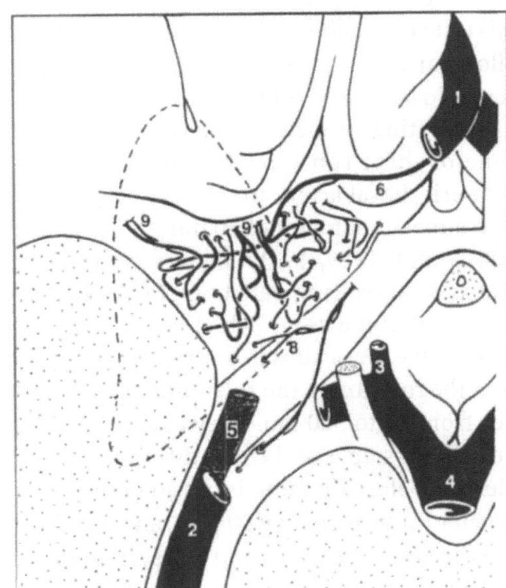

Diagram 2.12. Origin of central arteries at the level of the anterior perforated space (From WOLFRAM-GABEL 1995)

1 Anterior cerebral artery
2 Posterior cerebral artery
3 Posterior communicating artery
4 Basilar artery
5 Basal vein
6 Artery of Heubner
7 Central arteries from internal carotid artery
8 Central arteries from anterior choroidal artery
9 Central arteries from middle cerebral artery

● The distal anterior cerebral artery
(PERLMUTTER 1978):
The distal part begins at the A2 segment of the anterior cerebral artery and runs around the corpus callosum; it is called the pericallosal artery. In this course (segments A2–A5), it gives off cortical branches (FARNARIER 1977; MARINO 1976): the orbitofrontal artery feeds the orbital part of the first frontal gyrus; the anterior, middle, and posterior medial frontal arteries supply the inferior and medial portion of the frontal lobe, the posterior half of the first frontal gyrus, and the medial part of the precentral gyrus; the paracentral artery irrigates the paracentral lobule; while the superior and inferior medial parietal arteries feed the parietal lobules. These cortical branches supply the whole medial frontoparietal cortex and the superior part of frontal and parietal lobes.

There is a great variability in the origin of cortical arteries (Diagram 2.13). They may arise separately from the anterior cerebral and pericallosal artery, but most often they come from common trunks (orbitofrontal and frontopolar, middle and posterior medial frontal, paracentral superior and inferior medial parietal arteries). The orbitofrontal and frontopolar arteries emerge usually from the callosomarginal artery. This last vessel follows the precallosal segment of pericallosal artery in the callosomarginal sulcus.

The pericallosal artery supplies the corpus callosum via perforating branches (KAKOU 1988; TURE 1996). Some of them run directly from the central part of the pericallosal artery toward the corpus callosum, with a mean diameter of 30 µm (in the adult) (WOLFRAM-GABEL 1989, 1991). Others come from the callosal and callosocingulate branches (tributaries of the pericallosal artery), which arise from the lateral wall of the pericallosal artery, all along its course from the rostrum to the splenium; their diameter ranges from 50 to 300 µm. They course laterally within the callosal sulcus and constitute seven or ten arterial clusters before dividing into two branches of equal diameter (approximately 10 µm), an ascending one toward the cingulate gyrus and a descending one toward the corpus callosum.

Finally, the anterior cerebral artery ends by the posterior pericallosal artery, close to the splenium.

● Color imaging
Color imaging provides an accurate, complete assessment of the anterior cerebral artery and its branches. Four questions need to be asked:
- Can the anterior cerebral artery be efficiently evaluated without color Doppler? The answer is: yes and no.

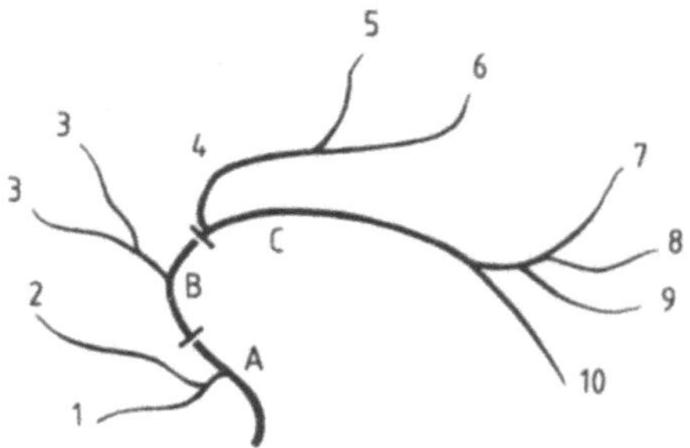

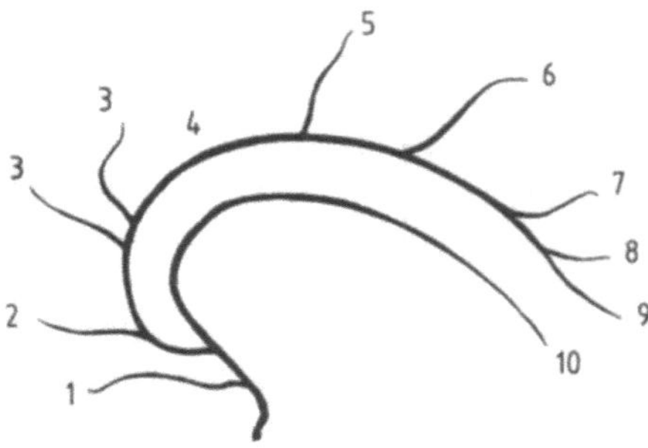

Diagram 2.13. Variable origin of cortical branches of the anterior cerebral artery
   1 Orbitofrontal artery
   2 Frontopolar artery
   3 Anterior medial frontal artery
   4 Callosomarginal artery
   5 Middle medial frontal artery
   6 Posterior medial frontal artery
   7 Paracentral lobule artery
   8 Medial parietal artery (or superomedial parietal artery)
   9 Parieto-occipital (or inferomedial parietal artery)
   10 Posterior pericallosal artery
   A Subcallosal segment
   B Precallosal segment
   C Supracallosal segment

Yes, because the main arterial axis may be recognized by its pulsatile beats; an anterior oblique frontal scan demonstrates the cortical rami of the anterior cerebral artery (orbitofrontal, frontopolar, anterior medial frontal branches); a vertical frontal scan demonstrates the anterior cerebral artery in the subarachnoid spaces, lateral to the suprachiasmatic cistern; a midline sagittal scan shows the pulsatile beats of the pericallosal artery and its branches (Fig. 2.15).
No, because this assessment is incomplete, often obscured by the hyperechoic falx cerebri, and does not allow reliable spectral analysis.
- What can color imaging provide?
This technique shows the anatomy of this vessel almost completely.

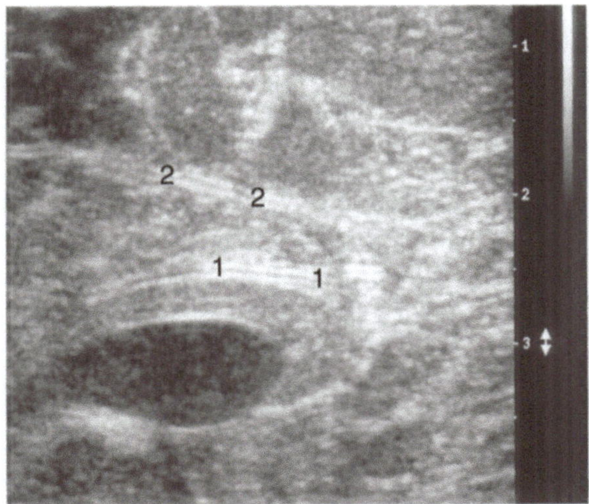

Fig. 2.15. Midline sagittal plane, high-frequency probe. The branches of the anterior cerebral artery are infrequently visualized for any length. On this favorable plane there is excellent visualization of the pericallosal arteries (*1*) and callosomarginal trunk (*2*)

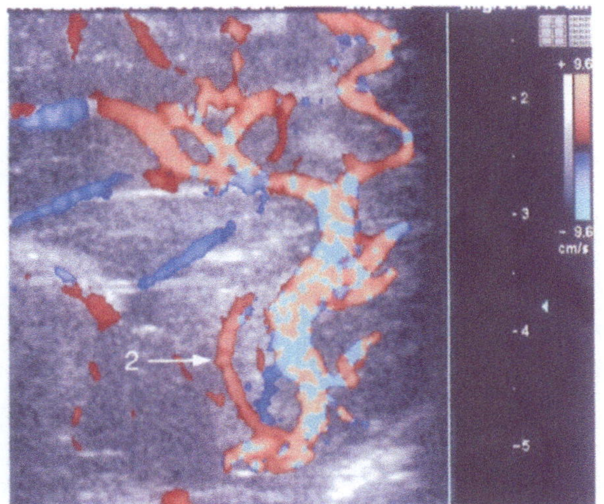

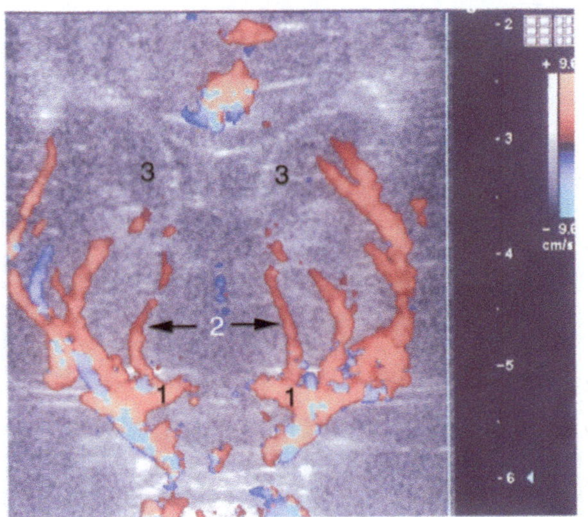

Fig. 2.17a,b. On both planes (**a,b**), the artery of Heubner has a well-depicted course: after arising from the A1 segment of the anterior cerebral artery (*1*), the vessel (*2*) ascends toward the caudate nucleus head (*3*)

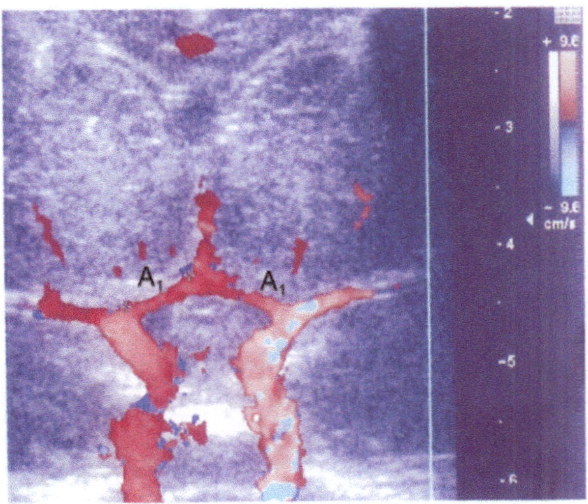

Fig. 2.16. Full-term neonate. Anterior frontal scan demonstrates the orientation of the A1 segments of the two anterior cerebral arteries, superiorly and medially oblique. The right A1 segment measures 6 mm

• On a coronal plane, the A1 segment of the anterior cerebral artery runs superomedially (Fig. 2.16). In a study of 46 full-term newborns, we found it to measure 6–8 mm. The small arterioles are not visualized, but the origin and course of the recurrent artery of Heubner are constantly recognized on sagittal and coronal planes (Fig. 2.17). The anterior communicating artery is not distinguished: it is too short, close to the two anterior cerebral arteries, and obscured by a partial volume effect.

• The course of the anterior cerebral artery from the A2 segment to the posterior pericallosal artery is ideally demonstrated by a midline sagittal plane (Fig. 2.18).

The pericallosal artery runs close to the corpus callosum, and when it moves away the perforating callosal branches may be recognized (Fig. 2.19). It might be valuable to detect them since callosal ischemia is more commonly observed on ultrasonography.

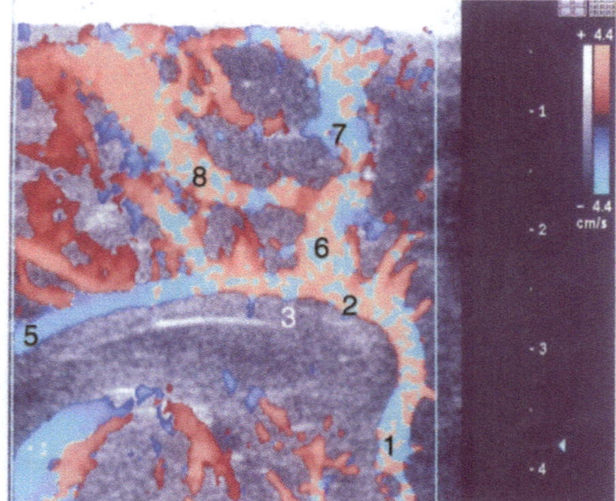

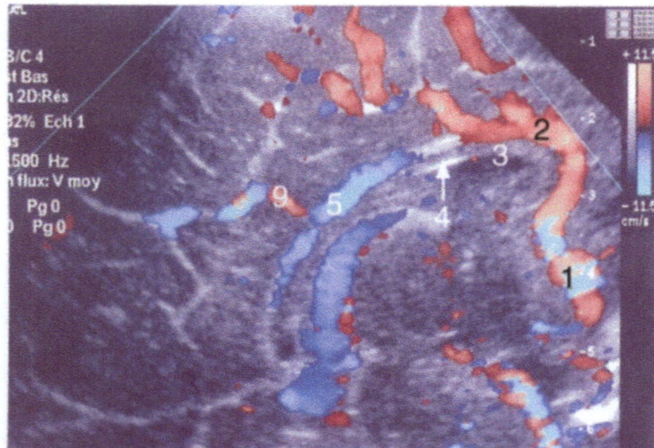

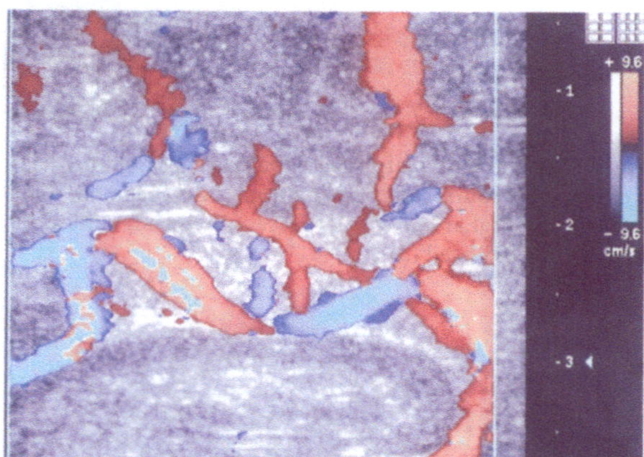

Fig. 2.18a–c. Anterior cerebral artery and pericallosal artery. Midline sagittal scan (**a,b**). Anterior cerebral artery (*1*) and proximal pericallosal artery (*2*) just near the corpus callosum come toward the transducer and are coded *red*. The middle portion (*4*) is not visible since it is perpendicular to the beam axis. The posterior pericallosal artery (*5*) goes away from the transducer and is coded *blue*. Notice that several cortical arteries are shown: the callosomarginal trunk (*6*), middle medial frontal artery (*7*), posterior medial frontal artery (*8*), and medial parietal artery (*9*). **c** Although the usual pattern is close contact between the pericallosal artery and corpus callosum, the arterial course may be different and show a wavy course

This plane is also ideal for depicting cortical branches of the anterior cerebral artery and showing the frequent anatomical variations: separate or common origin (Fig. 2.20), or the presence of a callosomarginal artery (Fig. 2.21).
- Which is to be preferred: standard color Doppler or power Doppler?

Most often, power Doppler is preferred to demonstrate the anterior cerebral artery and its branches (RUBIN 1999). This method, relatively indepen-

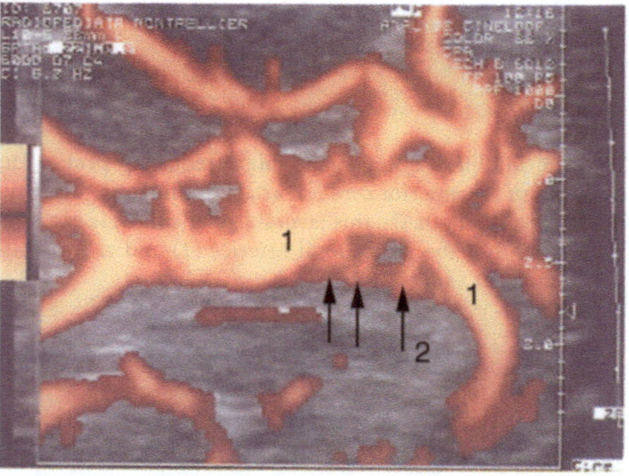

Fig. 2.19. Exceptionally, perforating callosal arteries may be seen. In this preterm newborn, the pericallosal artery (*1*) runs distant from the corpus callosum (*2*) and the perforating vessels may be detected (*arrow*)

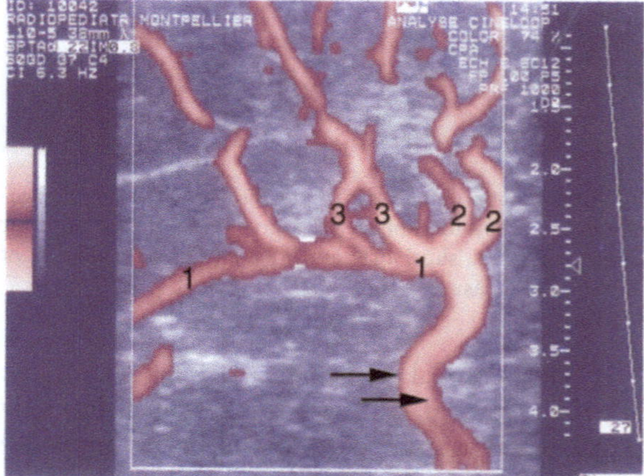

Fig. 2.20. Power Doppler imaging of the pericallosal artery and its branches, showing absence of the callosomarginal trunk. The cortical arteries arise directly from the pericallosal artery. The arrangement of the anterior cerebral arteries is unusual: two separate arteries are observed on a sagittal plane (*arrow*). *1* Pericallosal artery, *2* middle medial frontal arteries, *3* posterior medial frontal arteries

dent of the axis angle, provides a more complete and accurate image (Fig. 2.22). It improves the distinction between the two anterior cerebral arteries, mainly at the level of the pericallosal and callosomarginal vessels (Fig. 2.23). Of course, if the direction of flow has to be assessed (Fig. 2.24), standard color Doppler should be performed.

- Does color imaging allow evaluation of the variations of course, diameter, and origin of the branches of the anterior cerebral artery?

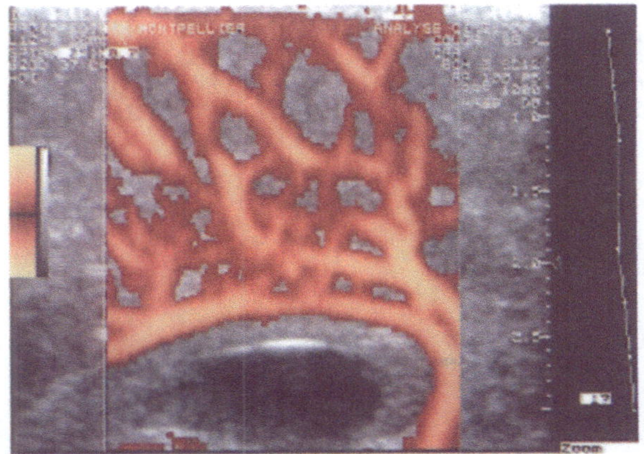

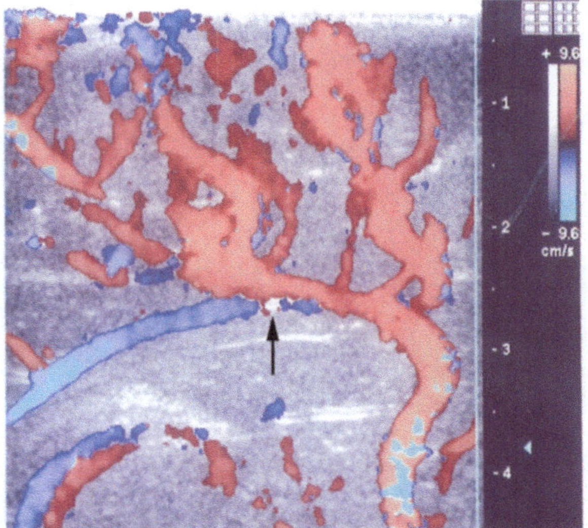

Fig. 2.22a,b. Power Doppler imaging is independent of the beam axis; this explains (a) the excellent visibility of the pericallosal artery and superior sagittal sinus. Standard color Doppler depends on the beam axis; this explains the absence of colored signal where the Doppler axis is perpendicular to the vessel (b). The sensitivity of vessel depiction is very much greater with power Doppler

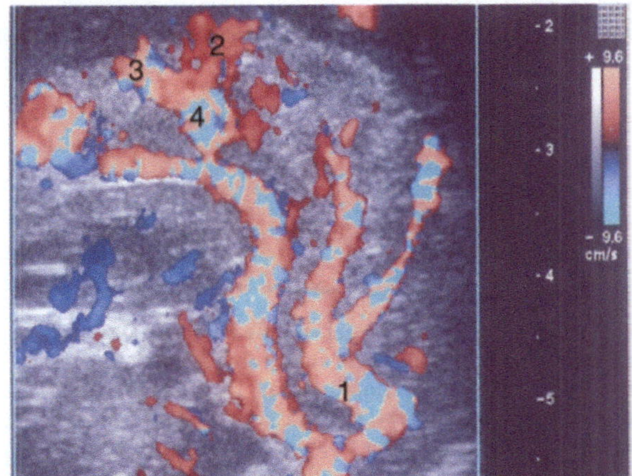

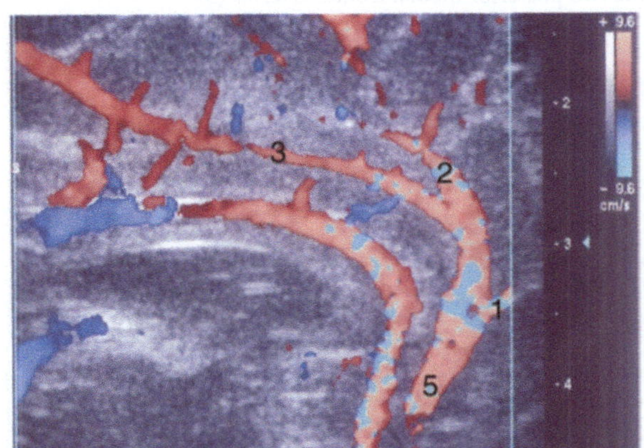

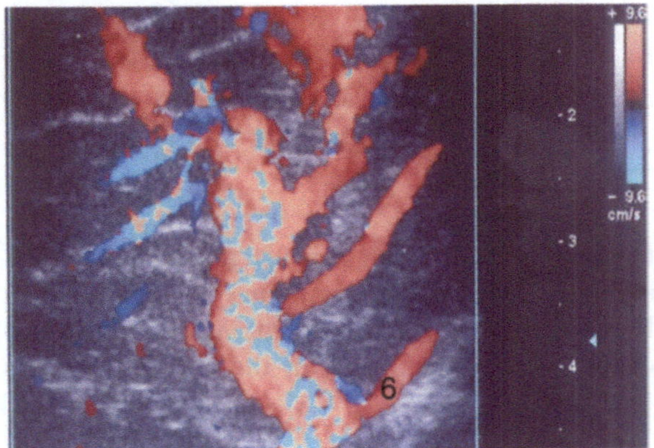

Fig. 2.21a–c. Great variability in the origin of cortical branches of the anterior cerebral artery. a In this example, the anterior medial frontal artery (1) arises and distributes normally, while the middle (2) and posterior (3) medial frontal arteries arise from the callosomarginal trunk (4). b By contrast, in this other example there is a common trunk (5) for the three medial frontal arteries and the callosomarginal trunk does not exist. Notice that the orbitofrontal artery (6), which always arises alone, is difficult to visualize on color Doppler (c): this deeply located artery requires a wide anterior fontanelle to be seen

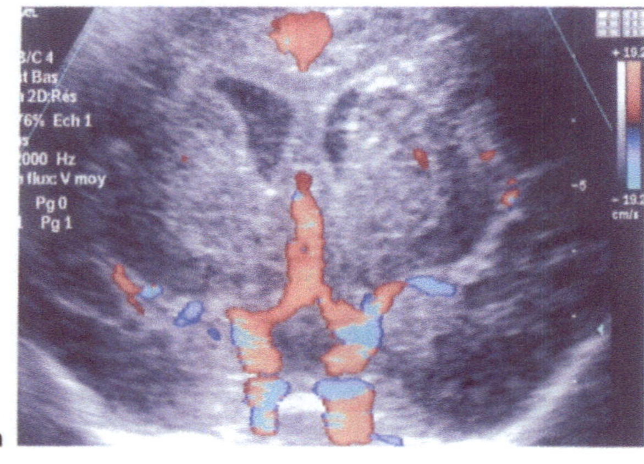

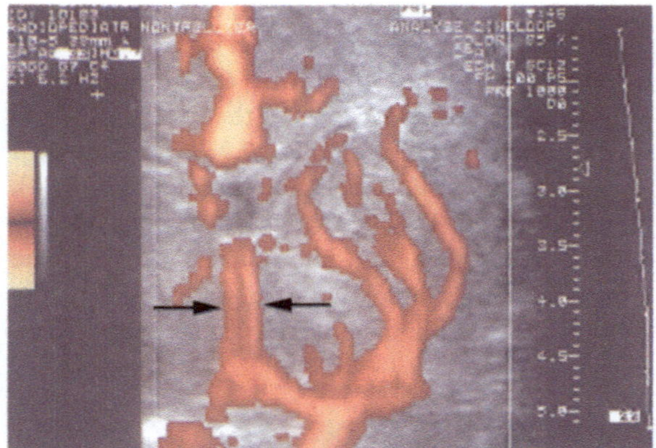

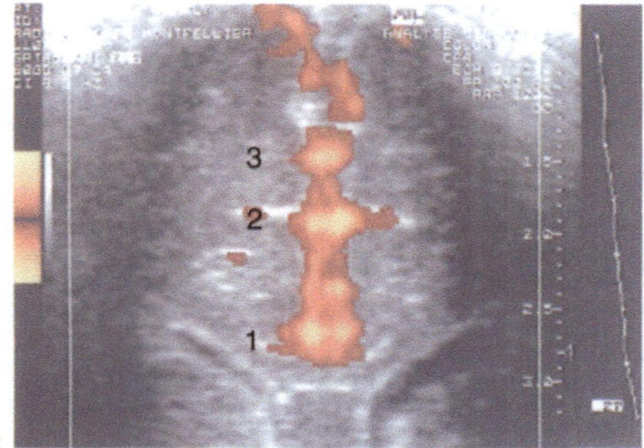

Fig. 2.23a–c. Because of partial volume effect, the two anterior cerebral arteries, which are in close contact, cannot be visualized separately on standard color Doppler imaging (a), whereas with power Doppler this is easy to do (b) (*arrow*). In another example (c), power Doppler distinguishes the two pericallosal arteries (*1*), the two callosomarginal arteries (*2*), and the two posterior medial frontal arteries (*3*)

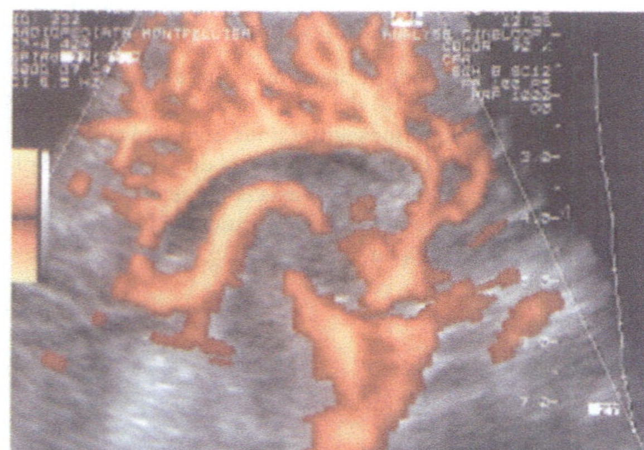

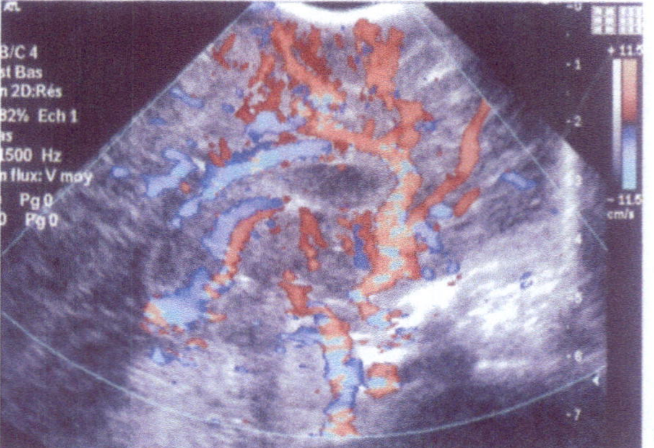

Fig. 2.24a,b. On power Doppler imaging (a) pericallosal artery and internal cerebral vein are coded *red*. Standard color Doppler (b) easily recognizes the direction of flow

The variable origin of cortical branches is easily appreciated, as is the absence or presence of a callosomarginal artery (MIERZWA 1989) (Figs. 2.20, 2.21). Although it is rare for the A1 segment to be absent, it is often asymmetric; when there is true hypoplasia, the equilibrium of the circle of Willis may be disturbed (Fig. 2.25). It can be useful to detect such variations in arterial diameter, since these segmental hypoplasias may correlate with anterior communicating arterial aneurysms in the adult (STEHLENS 1963).

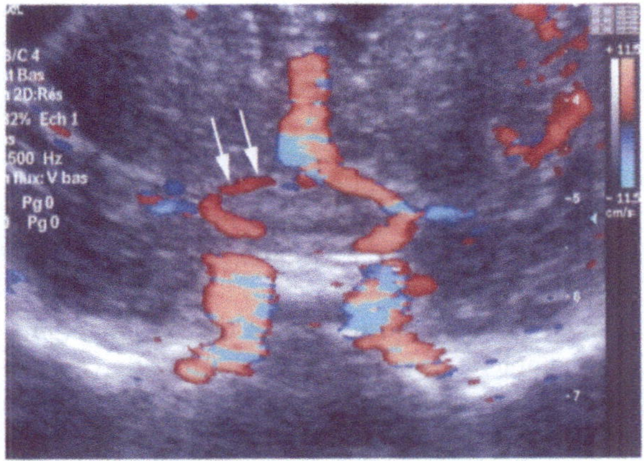

Fig. 2.25. Preterm neonate. The A1 segment of the right anterior cerebral artery (*arrow*) is hypoplastic

2.1.1.5
Middle Cerebral Artery

The middle cerebral artery is the largest (2 mm in the neonate) and the most important terminal branch of the internal carotid artery. Its central branches supply the major part of the basal ganglia and its cortical branches the lateral surface of the cerebral hemispheres. It courses mainly in the fissure of Sylvius and is divided into four segments: sphenoidal (M1), insular (M2), opercular (M3), and cortical (M4) (Diagram 2.14).

2.1.1.5.1
M1 (Sphenoidal) Segment

The M1 segment runs from the origin of the artery to its entrance into the sylvian fissure, near the insula. The middle cerebral artery arises from the end of the carotid artery, lateral to the optic chiasm, posterior to the division of the olfactory tract, below the anterior perforated substance (Diagram 2.15). The segment courses horizontally in the sphenoidal part of the sylvian fissure, parallel to the sphenoid ridge; it turns sharply and runs posterosuperiorly into the fissure at a curve, called the genu, between the sphenoidal and the operculoinsular compartments of the fissure.

The M1 segment divides into a superior and an inferior trunk, proximal to the genu: the postbifurcation part is short and horizontal (GIBO 1981). It gives rise to central or lenticulostriate branches, which have been well described in the literature (DONZELLI 1998; HERMAN 1963; KAPLAN 1965; MARINKOVIC 1985; ROSNER 1984; SALAMON 1966; UMANSKI 1985; VINCENTELLI 1990; WOLFRAM-GABEL 1995, 1997).

The lenticulostriate or perforating arteries arise from the superior wall or, less frequently, the posterior or lateral wall of the middle cerebral artery. In adult brain, their numbers vary from 1 to 21 (mean 10.4) as reported by WOLFRAM-GABEL (1995), from 2 to 13 (mean 7) as reported by VINCENTELLI (1990), and from 5 to 29 (mean 15) as reported by UMANSKI (1985). They also are variable in size, and the lateral ones are usually greater than the medial ones. In the adult, WOLFRAM-GABEL (1995) found a diameter of

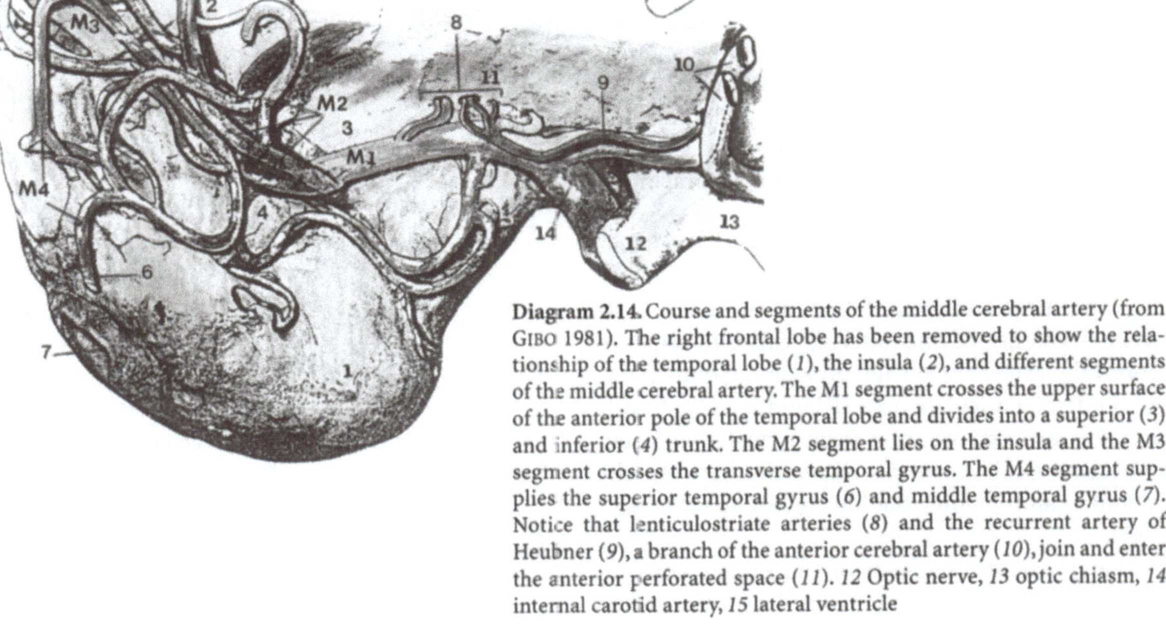

Diagram 2.14. Course and segments of the middle cerebral artery (from GIBO 1981). The right frontal lobe has been removed to show the relationship of the temporal lobe (*1*), the insula (*2*), and different segments of the middle cerebral artery. The M1 segment crosses the upper surface of the anterior pole of the temporal lobe and divides into a superior (*3*) and inferior (*4*) trunk. The M2 segment lies on the insula and the M3 segment crosses the transverse temporal gyrus. The M4 segment supplies the superior temporal gyrus (*6*) and middle temporal gyrus (*7*). Notice that lenticulostriate arteries (*8*) and the recurrent artery of Heubner (*9*), a branch of the anterior cerebral artery (*10*), join and enter the anterior perforated space (*11*). *12* Optic nerve, *13* optic chiasm, *14* internal carotid artery, *15* lateral ventricle

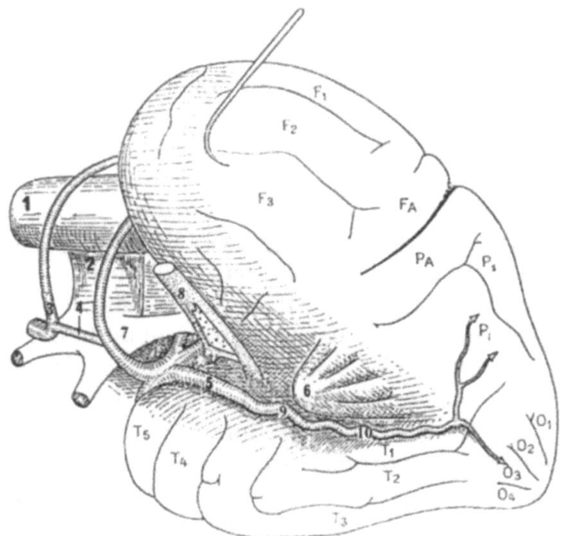

Diagram 2.15. Middle cerebral artery: anterolateral view
 1 Corpus callosum
 2 Supraoptic plate
 3 Anterior cerebral artery
 4 Anterior communicating artery
 5 Middle cerebral artery (M1 segment)
 6 Insula
 7 Optic chiasm
 8 Olfactory tract
 9 Sylvian genu
 10 Middle cerebral artery (M2 segment)

sonography: most authors (MITCHELL 1988; TATSUNO 1989; WONG 1989) report that the anterior fontanelle is an inappropriate approach since the beam axis is perpendicular to the M1 segment; the transcranial temporal access seems more accurate and reliable. According to TATSUNO (1989), the medial and lateral branches of the lenticulostriate arteries were visible in 53% and 87%, respectively, of 15 neonates.

In fact, recent high-resolution US equipment provide complete visualization of the middle cerebral artery and lenticulostriate arteries. The M1 segment is excellently depicted from its origin to the genu, following a horizontal, slightly superior oblique direction, with a superior concavity, deeply located in the subarachnoid spaces, between the frontal and temporal lobes (Fig. 2.26).

High-frequency transducers are required to appreciate the number, size, direction, and end of the lenticulostriate arteries, toward the caudate nucleus, putamen, and globus pallidus; their oblique (lateral branches) or vertical (medial branches) axis is demonstrated (Fig 2.27).

520 μm at their origin, VINCENTELLI (1990) more than 1 mm in 45% of cases, and UMANSKI (1985) from 0.4 mm to 1.8 mm.

In their cisternal portion, the anteromedial arteries arise usually with a 90° angle at their origin, while the anterolateral arteries emerge with an acute angle and follow a recurrent course to reach the anterior perforated substance. This course (Diagram 2.12), is variable, either short and linear, or long, sinuous, and recurrent. These vessels do not anastomose and constitute a dense arterial cluster in the subarachnoid tissues.

Their intracerebral course is ascending, often sinuous. They end near the lateral ventricular floor and supply the head and body of the caudate nucleus, different segments of the internal capsule, centrum semiovale, external capsule, putamen, globus pallidus, and sublenticulate area (Diagram 2.16). At this level, the terminal branches form a cluster with several anastomotic networks, especially between the putamen and globus pallidus (WOLFRAM-GABEL 1995).

The sphenoidal segment of the middle cerebral artery is known as poorly imaged by color ultra-

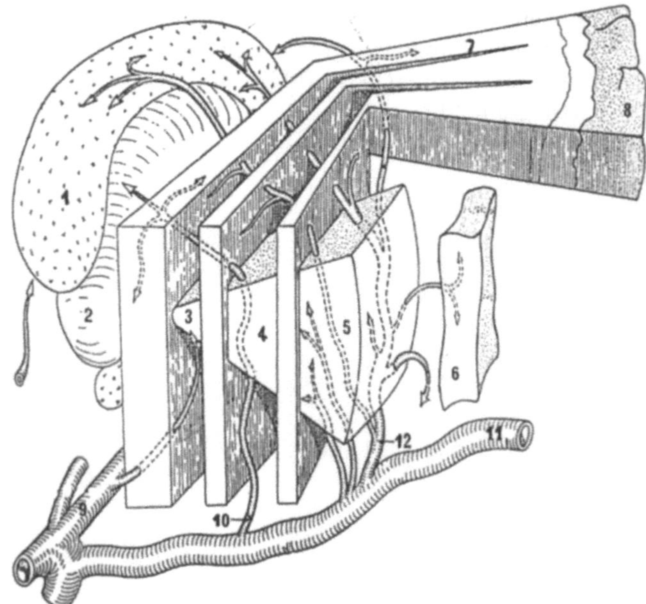

Diagram 2.16. Middle cerebral artery: central branches

1 Caudate nucleus	7 Posterior limb of internal capsule
2 Optic plate	8 Precentral gyrus
3 Internal globus pallidus	9 Anterior choroidal artery
4 External globus pallidus	10 Pallidal artery
5 Putamen	11 Middle cerebral artery
6 Claustrum	12 Lenticulostriate arteries

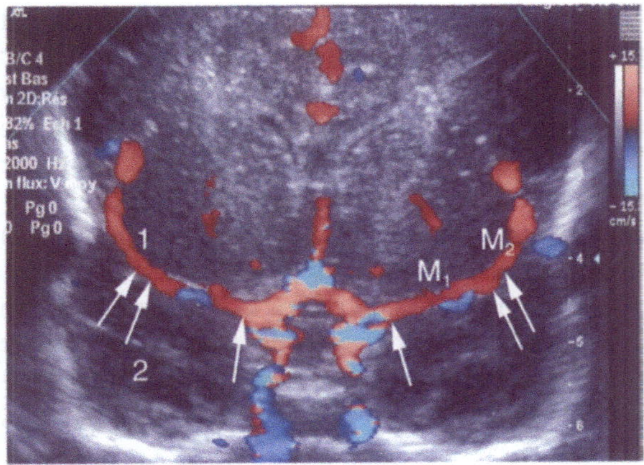

Fig. 2.26. The M1 segment of the middle cerebral artery is totally visualized from its origin (*arrow*) to the sylvian genu (*double arrow*) and M2 segment. Its course is initially horizontal and becomes superiorly oblique with a superior concavity, between the frontal (*1*) and temporal (*2*) parenchymas

2.1.1.5.2
M2 (Insular) Segment to M4 (Cortical) Segment

● Before feeding the frontal, parietal, and temporal cortex, the middle cerebral artery follows a complex course in the sylvian fissure.

The M2 segment begins at the genu, distal to the arterial division into a superior trunk supplying frontal and parietal cortex, and an inferior trunk supplying the temporal cortex. GIBO (1981) reported such bifurcation in 78% of 25 adult brains, and a trifurcation in only 12%.

The M2 insular segment deepens within the sylvian fissure, in a posterior and slightly superior direction. The branches to the anterior cortex (temporal and frontal) cross the anterior part of the insula, over the short gyri, before leaving the insular surface, but the branches to the posterior cortex pass across the short gyri, the central sulcus and the long gyri of the insula, before leaving the insular surface (Diagram 2.17).

The M3 (opercular) segment begins at the circular sulcus of the insula and ends at the surface of the sylvian fissure. The branches forming the M3 segment are close to the frontoparietal and temporal opercula. The cortical branches undergo two 180° turns (Diagram 2.18); the first turn is located where the vessels course upward over the insular surface and pass downward over the medial surface of the frontoparietal operculum. The second turn is located

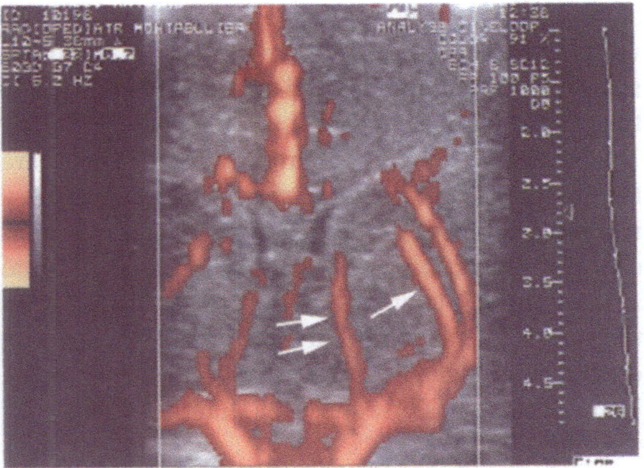

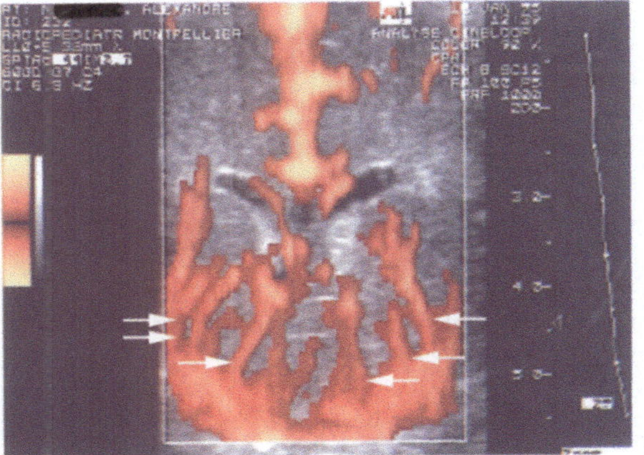

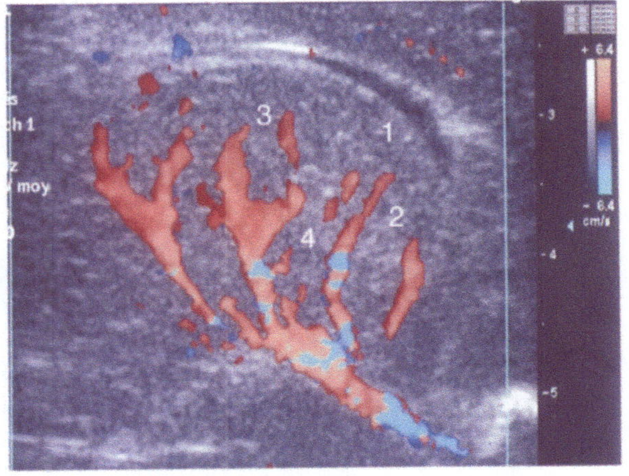

Fig. 2.27a–c. Color Doppler imaging is necessary to appreciate the central rami of the middle cerebral artery. The lenticulostriate arteries (a) arise from the superior aspect of the middle cerebral artery, with a constant ascending course, and end at the level of the lateral ventricular floor. They irrigate the caudate nucleus and putamen. Notice the oblique axis of the lateral arteries (*arrow*), which are larger than medial arteries (*double arrow*), whose axis is more vertical. **b** These arteries are variable in number; they arise from a single trunk (*arrow*) or from a common trunk (*double arrow*). **c** This paramedian plane shows the terminal vascularization of the lenticulostriate arteries toward the caudate nucleus (*1*), the putamen (*2*), the internal capsule (*3*), and the globus pallidus (*4*)

at the external surface of the sylvian fissure where the vessels go around the inferior margin of the frontoparietal operculum, and upward on the lateral surface of the frontal and parietal lobes.

The arteries supplying temporal cortical areas are less tortuous: after reaching the circular sulcus, they run on the temporal operculum without any abrupt change in direction, and upon reaching the external surface of the sylvian fissure they turn downward on the surface of the temporal lobe. Finally, the arterial course simplifies in its posterior part because the insular fissure has disappeared (Diagram 2.18).

The M4 cortical segment begins on the surface of the sylvian fissure and extends over the hemispheric cortex. The more anterior branches course vertically after leaving the fissure (upward or downward), the intermediate branches follow a gradual posterior oblique course, and the posterior branches run parallel to the long axis of the fissure (Diagram 2.19) (KOMIYAMA 1998).

Commonly (but several variations exist), twelve main cortical arteries are described that supply twelve cortical areas: orbitofrontal, prefrontal, precentral, central, anterior parietal, posterior parietal,

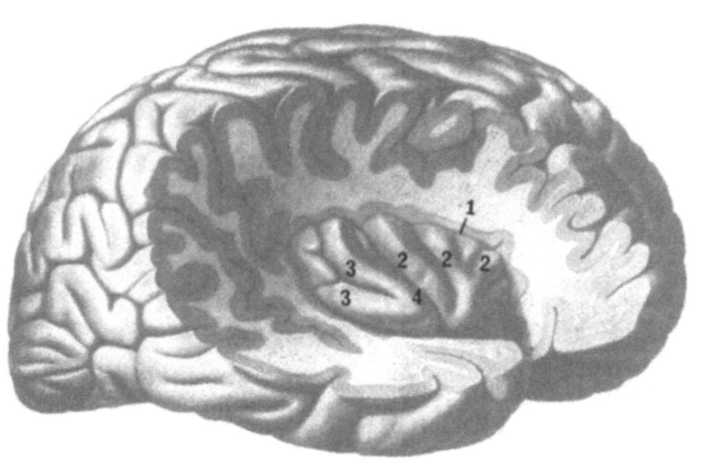

Diagram 2.17. Anatomy of the insula after removal of frontal, frontoparietal, and temporal opercula (From SOBOTTA 1985)
  1 Circular sulcus
  2 Short gyri
  3 Long gyri
  4 Central sulcus

Diagram 2.18 A–D. Vascular anatomy of the operculoinsular compartment (From GIBO 1981)
This schematization of serial frontal scans of the brain (**A–D**) clearly explains the vascular anatomy in the sylvian fissure. **A** The anterior coronal scan demonstrates the course of segment M1 (*1*) of the middle cerebral artery. Segments M2 (*2*) and M3 (*3*) are located in the operculoinsular compartment, which is characterized by a cleft (*5*) between the insula and the temporal and frontoparietal opercula. The cleft is divided into a superior limb (*7*), located medial to the frontoparietal operculum, and an inferior limb (*8*), located medial to the temporal operculum. On this plane, M1 courses in the sphenoidal compartment, M2 on the insula, M3 over the deep surface of the opercula, and M4 (*4*) on the cortical surface. The frontal operculum covers more of the insula than the temporal operculum. **B** Notice that the frontal and temporal opercula are nearly same height. **C** On this posterior coronal scan, the temporal operculum covers more of the insula than the frontoparietal operculum. **D** At the distal portion of the sylvian fissure, only the opercular cleft remains. The insular cleft has disappeared

parieto-occipital (or angular), temporo-occipital, anterior temporal, middle temporal, posterior temporal and temporopolar arteries (Diagram 2.19).

After emerging at the external brain surface the middle cerebral artery ends on the posterior part of Sylvian fissure.

● What part or parts of this complex course of the middle cerebral artery may be shown by color Doppler?

According to the literature the role of color imaging is modest. TATSUNO (1989) and MITCHELL (1988) demonstrated opercular arteries on parasagittal planes. WONG (1989) reported that M1 and M2 segments may be detected on frontal planes. In fact, these results are inconstant and incomplete.

In our experience, the bifurcation of the middle cerebral artery cannot be appreciated, probably because of superposition, but the anatomy of the insular and opercular areas is strikingly demonstrated: the superior trunk is recognized close to the

insula, forms two loops in the insular and opercular fissures, and then lies on the external hemispheric surface (Fig. 2.28). These changes in direction are successively coded red (M2), blue (M3), and red (M4). Diagram 2.18 (GIBO 1981) shows the anatomical pattern of the insula and opercula on different coronal sections; it may be easily reproduced by color imaging of the frontoparietal (superior) and temporal (inferior) branches (Fig. 2.29). In favorable cases, especially on vertical coronal scans, cortical rami may be observed at some length (Fig. 2.30). Finally, parasagittal planes, in the axis of the insula, provide good depiction of cortical branches (Fig. 2.31).

2.1.1.6
Posterior Cerebral Artery

This vessel presents several characteristics:

— The posterior cerebral artery serves the function of vision; it supports a long list of ocular functions, including pupillary reflexes, eye movement, visual memory, and binocular visual spatial integration.

— Unlike the other major cerebral vessels, the posterior cerebral artery is difficult to analyze through a transfontanellar approach, mainly because of its predominantly horizontal course: WONG (1989) reported a study of 24 neonates where this artery was demonstrated in 66% of cases through the anterior fontanelle, in 62% through the posterior fontanelle, and in 68% through the temporal bone. TATSUNO (1990) and MITCHELL (1989) noted that it was better recognized on a transcranial temporal approach.

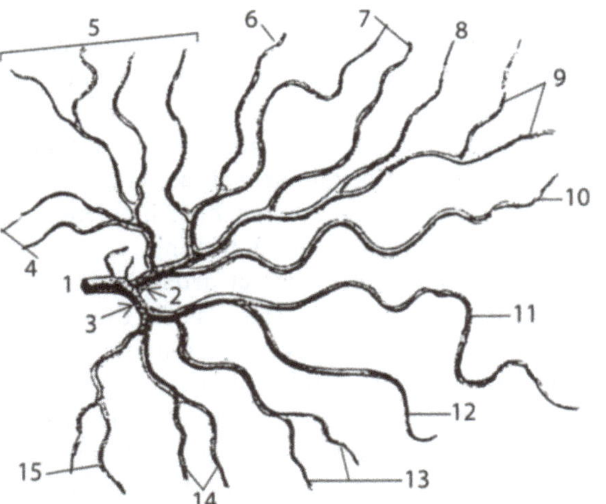

Diagram 2.19. Distribution of cortical branches of the middle cerebral artery
  1 Middle cerebral artery
  2 Superior trunk
  3 Inferior trunk
  4 Orbitofrontal artery
  5 Prefrontal artery
  6 Precentral artery
  7 Central artery
  8 Anterior parietal artery
  9 Posterior parietal artery
  10 Parieto-occipital or angular artery
  11 Temporo-occipital artery
  12 Posterior temporal artery
  13 Middle temporal artery
  14 Anterior temporal artery
  15 Temporopolar artery

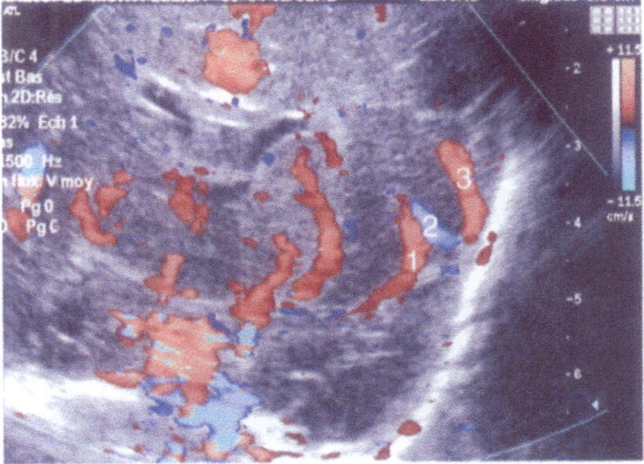

Fig. 2.28. On this frontal scan, the different segments of the middle cerebral artery in the sylvian fissure are excellently shown: M2 segment is coded *red* (*1*) within the insular cleft. The first loop shows the M3 segment, coded *blue* (*2*) that courses in the opercular cleft. The second loop gives rise to the cortical frontal branch, which is coded *red* (*3*)

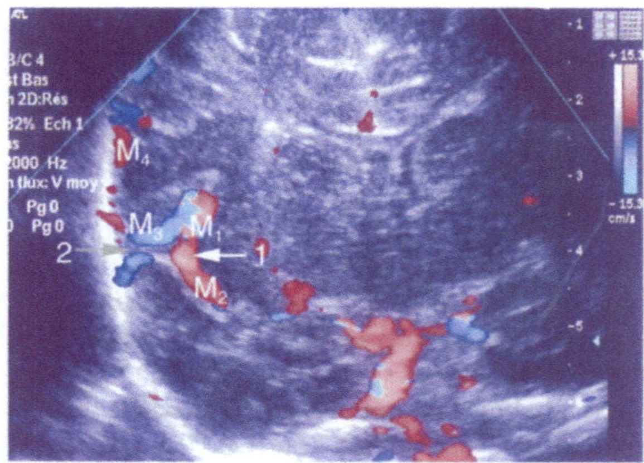

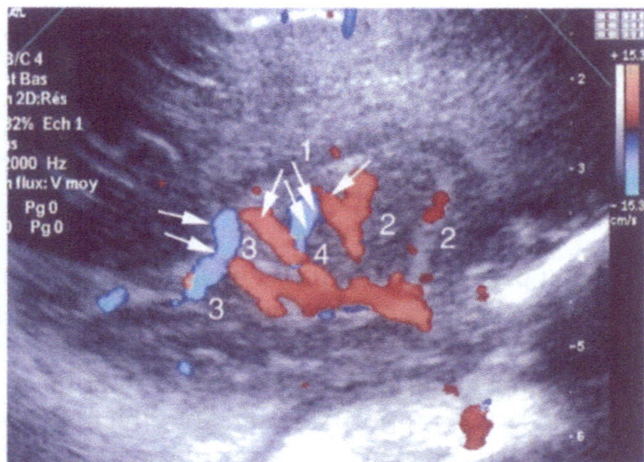

Fig. 2.31. Oblique parasagittal plane in the axis of the insula. The anatomy of the insula (Diagram 2.17) is shown with striking precision: *1* circular sulcus, *2* short gyrus, *3* long gyrus, *4* central sulcus. There is accurate visualization of the cortical rami: at the distal portion of segment M2, these branches have a superior orientation in the deep insula and are coded *red* (*arrow*). They run with a first turn, become segment M3, and course inferiorly at the inferior part of the frontoparietal operculum: they are coded *blue* (*double arrow*)

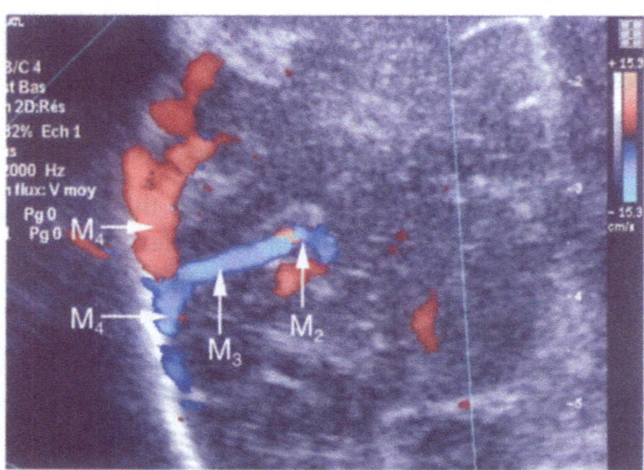

Fig. 2.29. a On this frontal plane (which corresponds to Diagram 2.18B), frontal and temporal opercula demonstrate nearly the same height and symmetrically cover the insula. The arrangement of the insular (*1*) and opercular cleft (*2*) allows segments to be differentiated: M2 (insular) segment, M3 (opercular) segment, and M4 (cortical) segment. **b** On the posterior frontal plane (which corresponds to Diagram 2.18D), at the distal part of the sylvian fissure, the insular cleft has disappeared and only the opercular cleft remains: M2 and M3 are in the same axis, coded *blue*; the opercular loop of segment M3 displays the cortical segment M4, coded *red* for frontal vessels or *blue* for temporal vessels

Color imaging of the distal choroidal and cortical branches of the posterior cerebral artery has not yet been described in the literature.

— Finally, the artery shows considerable variation in its size, course, and origin, as well as its branches (BRACARD 1997). In the adult, a high incidence of hypoplastic posterior communicating artery is reported. The posterior cerebral artery may arise from the internal carotid artery, as in the initial embryological disposition. Variations in number are rare, but unusual origin and/or division is possible: the anterior choroidal artery may come from the posterior communicating artery and the superior cerebellar artery from the posterior cerebral artery.

2.1.1.6.1
Course

● The posterior cerebral artery contributes to the circle of Willis and supplies the temporal and occipital cortex, basal ganglia, and tela choroidea of the third and lateral ventricles. It arises from the bifurcation of the basilar artery on the anterior surface of the pons (Diagram 2.7).

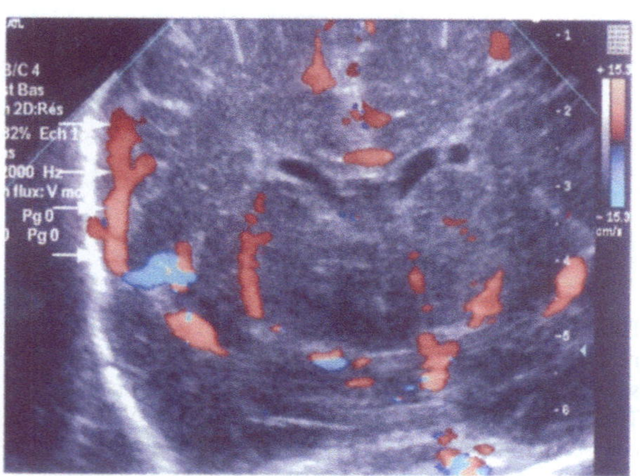

Fig. 2.30. A 32-weeks'-gestation preterm infant with periventricular leukomalacia. Notice the presence of a cortical frontal arterial branch, coded *red* (*arrow*): this is probably a cortical prefrontal or precentral artery

Four segments have been described by FISCHER (1938) and excellently demonstrated by MR angiography (Fig. 2.32):

- The P1 segment runs from the origin to the posterior communicating artery (Diagram 2.9); it runs upward and forward in the interpeduncular cistern, then turns laterally around the cerebral peduncles.
- The P2 segment courses around the mesencephalon, superior to the oculomotor nerve (III), into the interpeduncular and ambient cisterns, then into the lateral part of the quadrigeminal cistern.
- The P3 segment proceeds posteriorly from the pulvinar, into the lateral and posterior aspect of the quadrigeminal cistern, and ends at the anterior limit of the calcarine fissure. It often divides into its major terminal branches, the calcarine and parieto-occipital arteries (Diagram 2.20).

● On color imaging, the posterior cerebral artery cannot be studied by transfontanellar ultrasonography. This acoustic window can only show the initial superolateral course of the two posterior cerebral arteries (Fig. 2.33), on serial sections, perpendicular to the arterial axis.

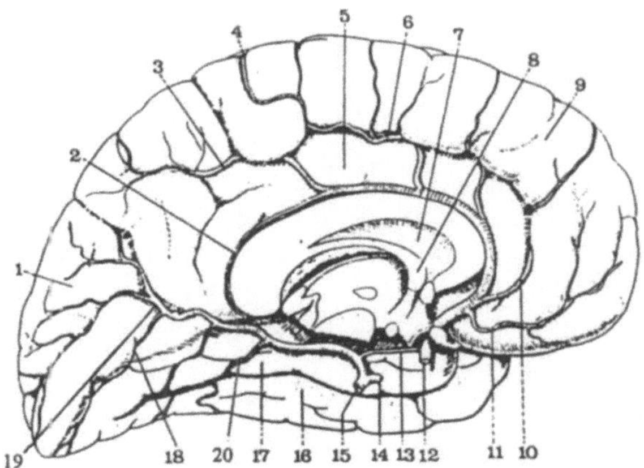

Diagram 2.20. Posterior cerebral artery: medial surface of hemisphere (From BOUCHET-CUILLERET 1983)

 1 Cuneus
 2 Pericallosal artery
 3 Artery of precuneus
 4 Artery of paracentral lobule
 5 Corpus callosum gyrus
 6 Callosomarginal artery
 7 Septum lucidum
 8 Trigone
 9 Frontal lobe
 10 Prefrontal artery
 11 Inferior orbital artery
 12 Anterior cerebral artery
 13 Posterior communicating artery
 14 Posterior cerebral artery
 15 Basilar artery
 16 Fourth temporal gyrus
 17 Fifth temporal gyrus (hippocampus)
 18 Calcarine artery
 19 Parieto-occipital artery
 20 Temporal artery

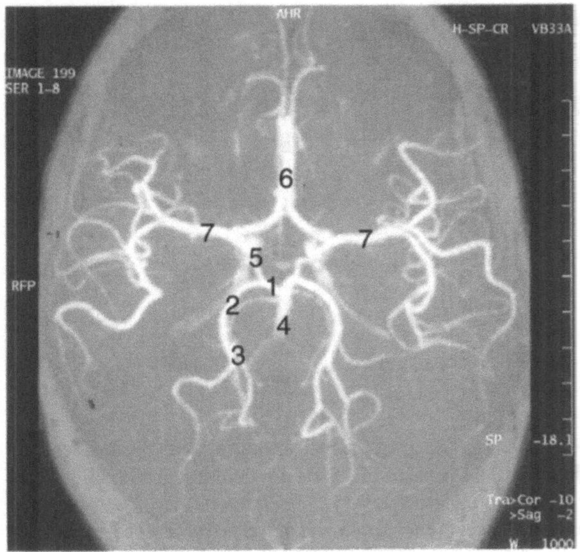

Fig. 2.32. MR angiography, axial transverse scan. The segmentation of the posterior cerebral artery is easily analyzed: segment P1 (*1*), segment P2 (*2*), which encircles the cerebral peduncle, and segment P3 (*3*). The orientation of the posterior cerebral artery is obviously unfavorable to transfontanellar investigation. *4* Basilar artery, *5* posterior communicating artery, *6* anterior cerebral artery, *7* middle cerebral artery

In fact, everything (the direction, course, and axis of the vessel) favors the transcranial temporal approach: this plane easily shows the P1 segment, followed by the P2 and P3 segments in the hyperechoic subarachnoid spaces at the interpeduncular, ambient, and quadrigeminal cisterns (Fig. 2.34).

The terminal part of the vessel is more difficult to assess because of great variations in the arterial distribution and inadequate vascular orientation. Usually, the artery runs close to the medial surface of the temporal lobe, especially the fifth temporal gyrus, gives rise to temporal branches (which cannot be depicted by color Doppler), and ends on the medial surface of the occipital lobe, giving off parieto-occipital and calcarine arteries.

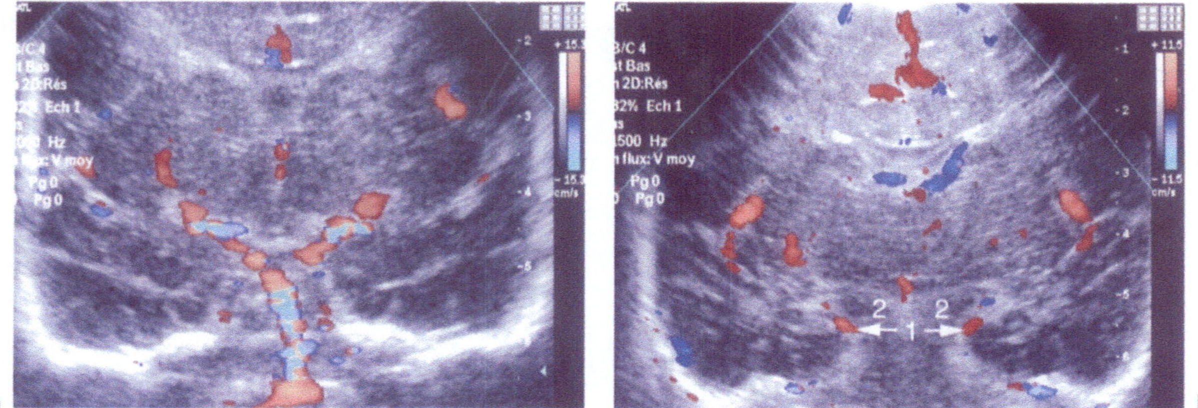

Fig. 2.33. **a** Posterior oblique frontal scan. Correct visualization of P1 segment of the posterior cerebral artery that courses posteriorly in the choroidal fissure. **b** The two posterior cerebral arteries (*1*) encircle the cerebral peduncles (*2*)

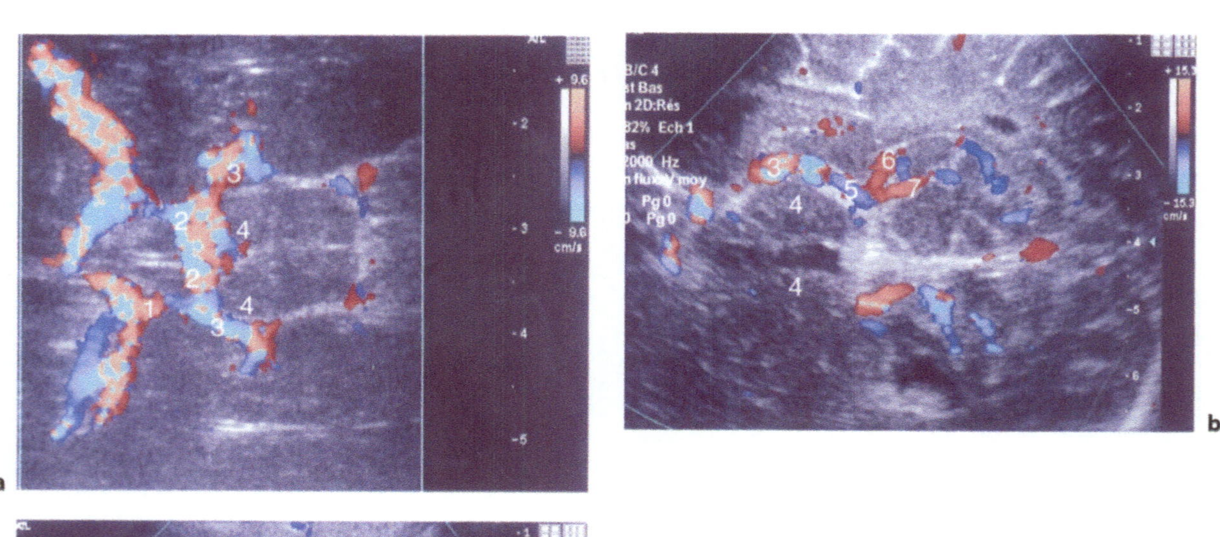

Fig. 2.34a–c. The transcranial temporal scan is the best for defining the course of the posterior cerebral artery. The posterior communicating artery (*1*) separates the P1 segment (*2*) and the P2 segment (*3*), which encircles the cerebral peduncles (*4*) and gives rise to segment P3 (*5*) at the lateral and posterior aspect of the quadrigeminal cistern. In favorable cases, the temporal rami (*6*) and the common trunk (*7*) of the calcarine and parieto-occipital arteries are visualized

2.1.1.6.2
Branches

The posterior cerebral artery gives off multiple branches that support major functions: the central branches distribute to the brain stem and thalamus, the choroidal arteries supply the tela choroidea and walls of the third and lateral ventricles, and the cortical branches feed the temporo-occipital cortex and callosal splenium.

● The central arteries (PEDROSA 1987; SAEKI 1977; ZEAL 1978) arise from the P1 and P2 segments and supply the thalamus, geniculate bodies, colliculi, posterior hypothalamus, median part of the cerebral peduncles, oculomotor nerve nucleus (III), substantia nigra, and red nucleus. They include (HARA 1966; PERCHERON 1976):

- The thalamus perforating arteries, which emerge from the P1 segment or the posterior communicating artery. They enter the brain through the posterior perforated substance, interpeduncular fossa, and cerebral peduncle and feed the ventral thalamic nuclei and posterior portion of the internal capsule.
- The thalamogeniculate arteries, which arise from the posterior communicating artery in the ambient cistern and irrigate the posterior half of the lateral thalamus, posterior limb of the internal capsule, and optic tract.

● The peduncular arteries arise from the P2 segment and supply the cerebral peduncles, substantia nigra, and red nucleus.

The circumflex arteries emerge from the P1 and P2 segments and encircle the midbrain; they are divided into short circumflex arteries that reach the geniculate bodies, and long circumflex arteries that reach the colliculi.

The peduncular and circumflex arteries are not visible on US, probably because of their small size and because none of the US planes is satisfactory. The vasculature of the thalamus and pulvinar, on the other hand, is well depicted by color ultrasonography (Fig. 2.35).

● The choroidal branches of the posterior cerebral artery feed the tela choroidea of the third and lateral ventricular choroid plexus, which is also supplied by the anterior choroidal artery (from the internal carotid artery) and the superior posterior choroidal artery (from the anterior cerebral artery) (Diagram 2.21).

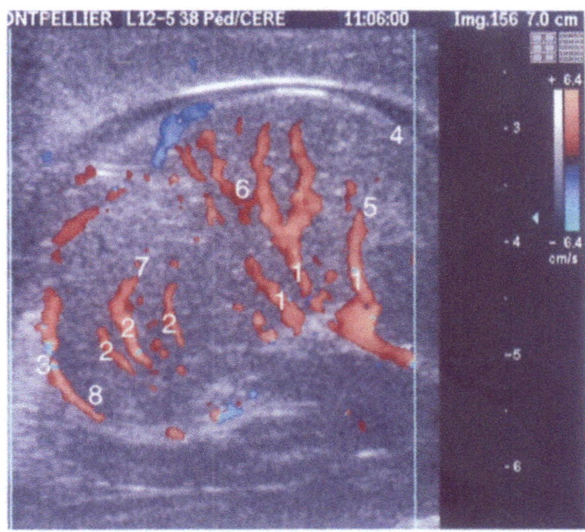

Fig. 2.35. This parasagittal scan of a basal ganglion shows its supply coming from the three main arteries: the lenticulostriate vessels (*1*), which are branches of the middle cerebral artery, thalamic vessels (*2*), arising from segment P1 of the posterior cerebral artery, and anterior choroidal artery (*3*), a branch of the internal carotid artery. *4* Caudate nucleus, *5* putamen, *6* internal capsule and globus pallidus, *7* thalamus, *8* pulvinar

— The tela choroidea of the third ventricle is supplied by posteromedial choroidal branches and a superior posterior choroidal artery, when present. The posteromedial choroidal artery almost always arises from the postcommunicating segment of the posterior cerebral artery (BAUMGARTNER 1981; FUJII 1980; GALLOWAY 1960; WOLFRAM-GABEL 1984). In its mesencephalic portion, it turns backward around the cerebral peduncle and accompanies the basal vein and posterior cerebral arteries. It courses superoposteriorly and reaches the transverse cerebral fissure, where it runs sagittally and forward between the tela choroidea and the internal cerebral veins (Diagram 2.22). It reaches the region of the interventricular foramen and gives off a lateral and a medial branch: the lateral branch, near the superior choroidal wall of the interventricular foramen, curves posterolaterally and anastomoses with a branch from the posterolateral choroidal artery (Diagram 2.6); the medial branch turns posteromedially and divides within the tela choroidea of the third ventricle.

This arterial supply may be completed by the superior posterior choroidal artery, the final ramification of the anterior cerebral artery. This inconstant vessel curves downward and forward around the splenium

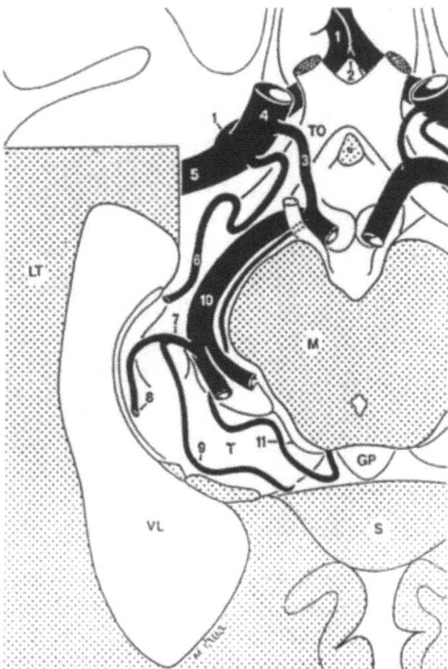

Diagram 2.21. Origin of choroidal arteries (From WOLFRAM-GABEL 1987)
On this inferior view of the brain, after sectioning the mesencephalon (*M*), temporal lobe (*LT*), and splenium of the corpus callosum (*5*), the origin of the choroidal arteries is displayed: the anterior choroidal artery (*6*) supplies the optic tract (*To*) and reaches the anterior part of the inferior horn of the lateral ventricle (*VL*). Posterior and lateral choroidal arteries arise from a common trunk (*7*) and divide into an inferior artery (*8*) that reaches the tela choroidea of the lateral ventricle, and a superior artery (*9*) that curves around the posterior aspect of the thalamus (*T*). The posterior and medial cerebral artery (*11*) encircles the cerebral peduncle, curves around the pulvinar, and reaches the pineal body (*GP*). *1* Anterior cerebral artery, *2* anterior communicating artery, *3* posterior communicating artery, *4* internal carotid artery, *5* middle cerebral artery

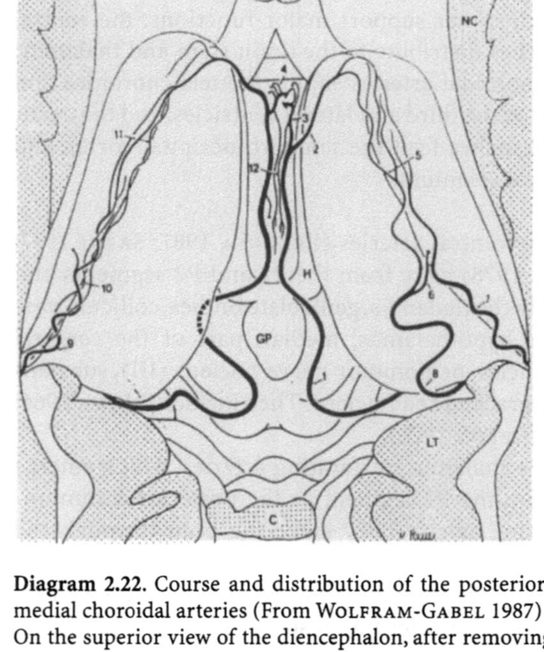

Diagram 2.22. Course and distribution of the posterior and medial choroidal arteries (From WOLFRAM-GABEL 1987)
On the superior view of the diencephalon, after removing the fornix (*F*), caudate nucleus (*NC*), temporal lobe (*LT*), and cerebellum (*c*), the posterior and medial choroidal arteries (*1*), close to the pineal body (*GP*), reach the third ventricular tela choroidea via long (*12*) and short (*4*) branches. Near the interventricular foramen, they divide into lateral (*2*) and medial (*3*) branches. The inferior (*7*) and superior (*8*) branches of the posterior lateral choroidal artery supplies the lateral ventricular tela choroidea and anastomoses (*5*) with the posterior medial choroidal artery, sending out thalamic branches (*6*). The anterior choroidal artery (*9*) supplies the lateral ventricular tela choroidea, the branches of which (*10*) anastomose with those (*11*) of the posterior medial choroidal artery

of the corpus callosum (Diagram 2.23). It runs on the superior surface of the pineal body and reaches the transverse cerebral fissure, where it courses longitudinally. Above the internal cerebral vein, it moves to the anterior extremity of the third ventricular tela choroidea and contributes to its supply. It anastomoses with the posteromedial choroidal artery and reaches the tela choroidea of the lateral ventricle, where it joins with branches of the anterior choroidal artery and posterolateral choroidal artery.

— The tela choroidea of the lateral ventricle is supplied by the anterior choroidal artery, posterolateral choroidal artery, and posteromedial choroidal artery.

The posterolateral choroidal arteries arise from the posterior cerebral artery, either separately or

after a common trunk. In their variable course (MILLEN 1953; PLETS 1974; ZEAL 1978), an inferior and a superior artery may be distinguished. Both emerge in the superior part of the transverse cerebral fissure and run posteriorly under the inferior surface of thalamus (Diagram 2.22). The inferior vessel reaches the tela choroidea of the temporal horn, the superior vessel curves around the pulvinar and reaches the tela choroidea of the ventricular body. They then give rise to thalamic branches before dividing in the region of the interventricular foramen.

— The posteromedial choroidal artery is always shown by color Doppler imaging on the midline sagittal plane: it runs downward and forward upon the internal cerebral vein (Fig. 2.36). and its tributar-

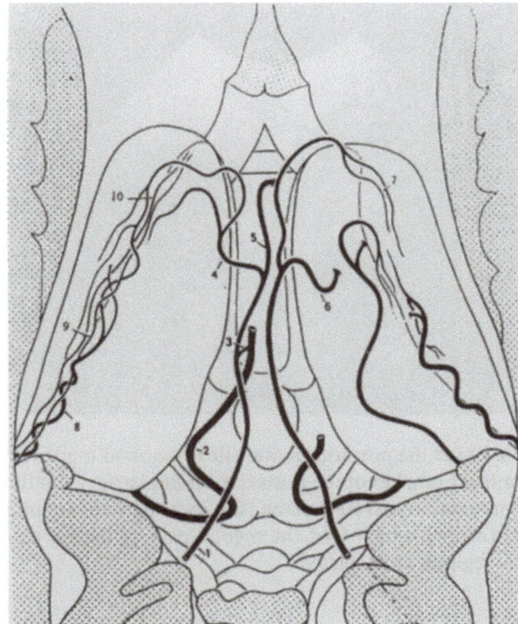

Diagram 2.23. Course and distribution of the posterior and superior choroidal arteries (From WOLFRAM-GABEL 1987) The third ventricular tela choroidea is supplied by posterior superior choroidal arteries (*1*) arising from anterior cerebral arteries, and by posterior medial choroidal arteries (*2*). These two vessels anastomose (*3*), and the posterior superior choroidal artery, which sends out thalamic rami (*6*), divides into medial (*5*) and lateral (*4*) branches whose long tributaries (*7*) supply the lateral ventricle. The anterior choroidal artery (*8*) gives off numerous choroidal arteries (*9*) and anastomoses with the posterior superior choroidal artery (*10*)

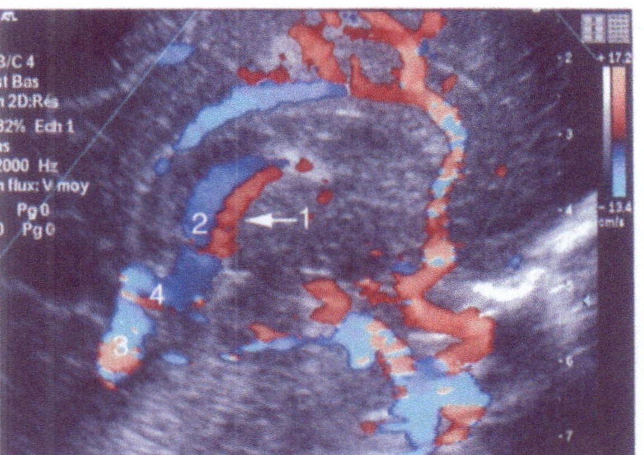

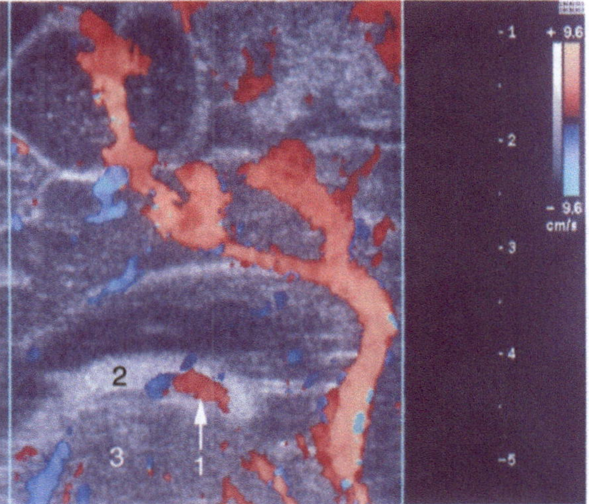

Fig. 2.36. a The posterior medial choroidal artery (*1*) runs close to the internal cerebral vein (*2*). Notice the swirling flow of the straight sinus (*3*), resulting from a change in direction of the vein of Galen (*4*). **b** The medial branch of the posterior medial choroidal artery is constantly visible and supplies the choroid plexus (*2*) of the third ventricle (*3*)

ies may be identified at the level of the third ventricle, especially the medial branch.

The superior posterior choroidal artery is inconstant. When present, it is always seen on high-frequency color imaging, on the midline sagittal scan. The internal cerebral vein acts as the center of the choroidal vasculature, superior to the posteromedial choroidal artery and inferior to the superior posterior choroidal artery (Fig. 2.37).

Finally, posterolateral choroidal arteries are not visualized on color Doppler imaging, because of their complex lateral course.

● The posterior cerebral artery gives rise to three major trunks supplying the cortex of part of the temporal lobe and occipital region, but they show great variability in distribution and division.

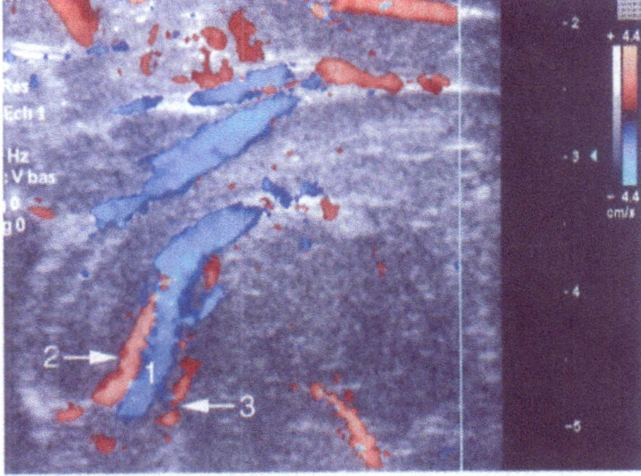

Fig. 2.37. The midline sagittal plane easily displays the internal cerebral vein (*1*) between the posterior superior choroidal artery (*2*) and the posterior medial choroidal artery (*3*)

- The temporal arteries, variable in number, arise from the P2 segment and distribute to the inferior parts of the temporal lobe. The hippocampal branches are thin, invisible on color Doppler, and feed the fourth and fifth temporal gyri. The anterior and middle temporal arteries join in a common trunk and supply the posterior part of the fifth temporal gyrus and middle part of the fourth temporal gyrus. The posterior temporal artery, more frequently identified, feeds the posterior part of the fourth temporal gyrus and lateral parts of the fourth and fifth occipital gyri (Fig. 2.14).
- The parieto-occipital artery arises from the distal P2 segment or from the P3 segment and feeds the medial parieto-occipital region, with a variable extension.
- The calcarine artery, a terminal branch of the posterior cerebral artery, passes into the calcarine fissure and distributes to the occipital cortex. It supplies the visual cortex.
- The splenial (or posterior pericallosal) artery may arise from the posterior cerebral artery or its parieto-occipital branch; it curves around the callosal splenium and anastomoses with the pericallosal branch of the anterior cerebral artery.
- Depiction of these cortical vessels through the anterior fontanelle is obviously difficult, since their course is predominantly horizontal. Only the transcranial temporal planes may show the greater branches: the temporal arteries are commonly visualized (Fig. 2.34), while the parieto-occipital and calcarine arteries are always difficult to assess (Fig. 2.38).

2.1.1.7
Territories of the Cerebral Arteries

The arterial territories have been determined from correlations between angiographic data and clinical manifestations of brain infarction.

- Cortical territories
- The lateral surface of the cerebral hemisphere is supplied by the middle cerebral artery in its central part, on each side of the sylvian fissure, by the anterior cerebral artery in the superior part of the frontal and parietal lobes as far as the lateral parieto-occipital fissure, and by the posterior cerebral artery in the occipital lobe (Diagram 2.24).
- On the medial surface of the cerebral hemisphere, the pericallosal area is fed by the anterior cerebral artery, the cuneus and medial part of temporal lobe by the posterior cerebral artery, and the ante-

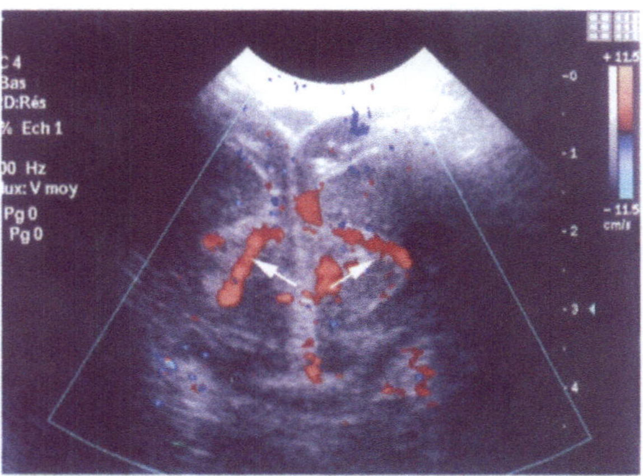

Fig. 2.38. Use of the posterior fontanelle is required to identify the terminal branches of the posterior cerebral artery. On this posterior axial transverse plane, the two parieto-occipital arteries (*arrow*), which feed the medial part of the parieto-occipital regions, are depicted

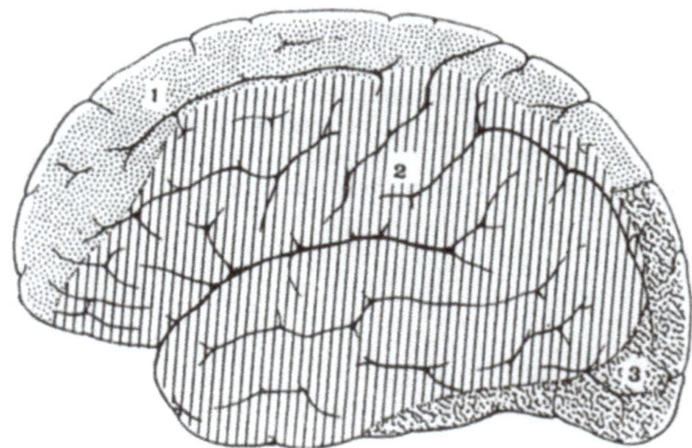

Diagram 2.24. Arterial territories of the brain: lateral view of the hemisphere (From Bouchet-Cuilleret 1983)
  1 Anterior cerebral artery
  2 Middle cerebral artery
  3 Posterior cerebral artery

rior tip of the temporal lobe, especially the hippocampal uncus by the middle cerebral artery (Diagram 2.25).
- On the inferior surface of the cerebral hemisphere, the anterior cerebral artery supplies the orbital lobe and olfactory structures, the middle cerebral artery supplies the lateral half of the orbital and temporal lobes, and the posterior cerebral artery supplies the third and fourth temporal gyri and the occipital lobe (Diagram 2.26).

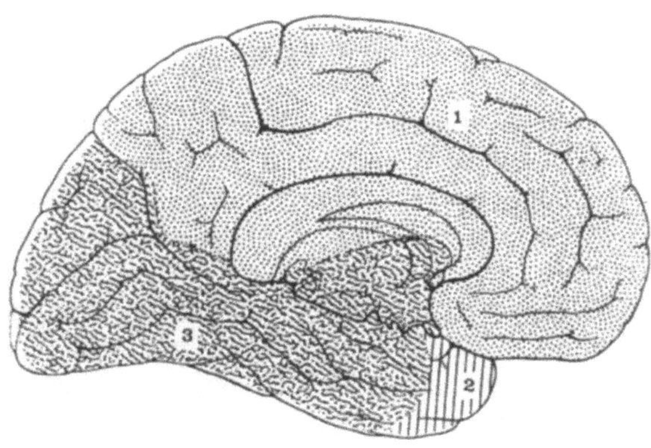

Diagram 2.25. Arterial territories of the brain: medial view of the hemisphere (From BOUCHET-CUILLERET 1983)
  1 Anterior cerebral artery
  2 Middle cerebral artery
  3 Posterior cerebral artery

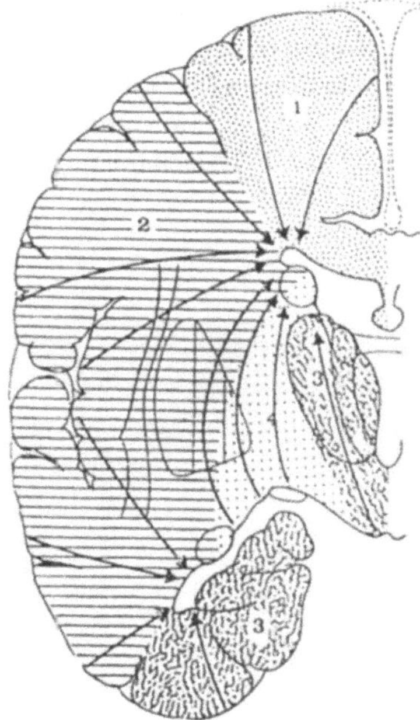

Diagram 2.27 Arterial territories of the brain: frontal plane (From BOUCHET-CUILLERET 1983)
  1 Anterior cerebral artery
  2 Middle cerebral artery
  3 Posterior cerebral artery

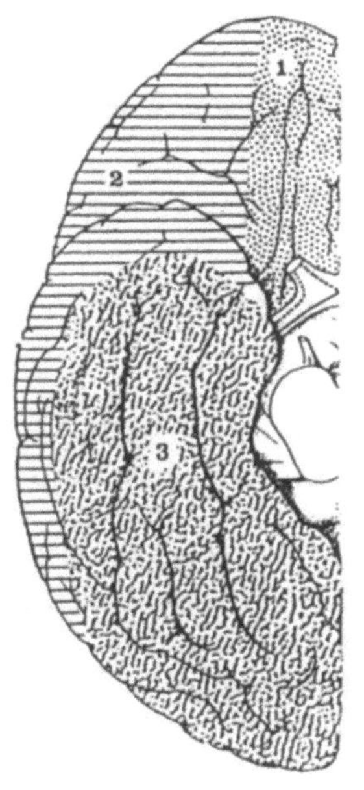

Diagram 2.26. Arterial territories of the brain: inferior view of the hemisphere (From BOUCHET-CUILLERET 1983)
  1 Anterior cerebral artery
  2 Middle cerebral artery
  3 Posterior cerebral artery

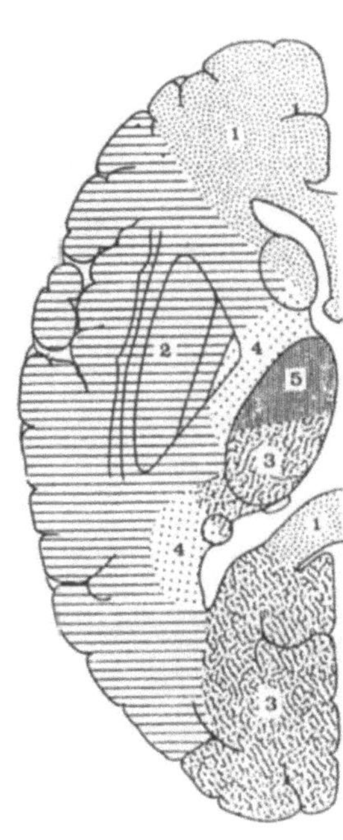

Diagram 2.28. Arterial territories of the brain: axial transverse plane (From BOUCHET-CUILLERET 1983)
  1 Anterior cerebral artery
  2 Middle cerebral artery
  3 Posterior cerebral artery
  4 Anterior choroidal artery
  5 Posterior communicating artery

● Central territories (Diagrams 2.27, 2.28)
– The caudate nucleus is irrigated by the anterior and middle cerebral arteries on its head, and by the middle cerebral artery and anterior choroidal artery on its body and tail.
– The lenticulate nuclei are supplied by the middle cerebral artery and anterior choroidal artery in the globus pallidus, and by the anterior cerebral artery (artery of Heubner) and the middle cerebral artery (lenticulostriate vessels) in the putamen.

– The thalamus is fed by the posterior communicating artery (ventral nucleus) and the posterior cerebral artery (dorsal lateral nuclei).
– Finally, the internal capsule is supplied by the middle cerebral artery (anterior limb, knee, and sublenticulate segment), the anterior choroidal artery (posterior limb), and the posterior cerebral artery (retrolenticulate segment).

Knowledge of these arterial territories is obviously important to locate ischemic damage. Guided by the morphological US examination, color Doppler (for thrombosis) and pulsed Doppler (for abnormal blood flow) help the clinician to approach the physiopathological events (Fig. 2.39).

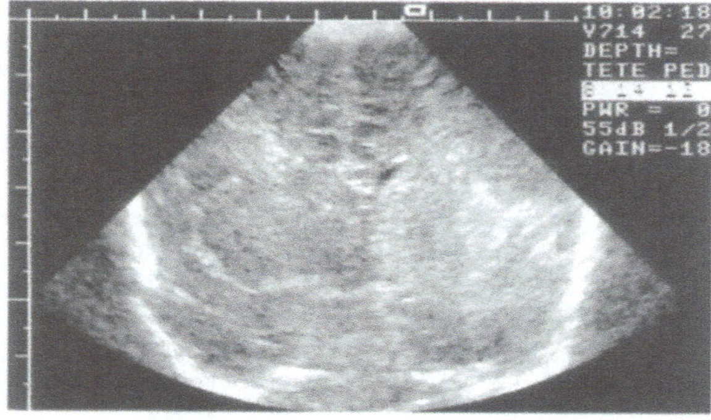

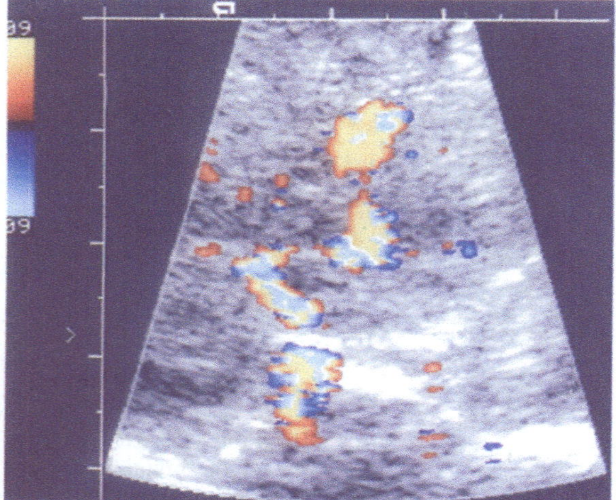

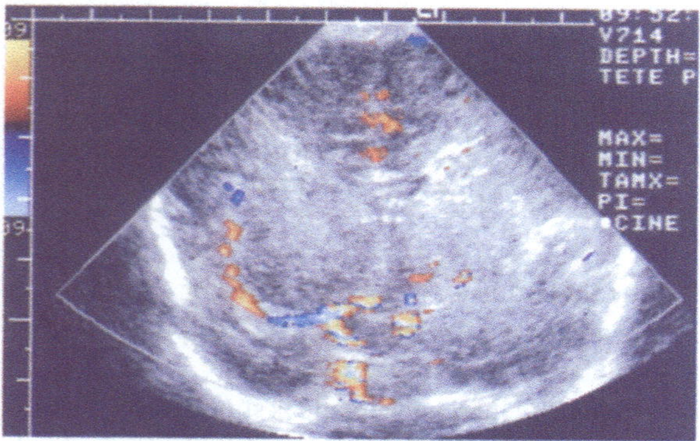

Fig. 2.39. Asymptomatic preterm infant. There is an abnormal hyperechoic area in the superficial and deep territories of the left middle cerebral artery (**a**). Color Doppler demonstrates that the infarction does not result from low blood flow but from an extended thrombosis of the left internal carotid artery (**b**) and anterior cerebral artery (**c**)

2.1.2
Anatomy of the Cerebral Veins

Venous vasculature remains poorly described in the literature, especially in children and infants, and few color Doppler data relate to the venous system (BEZINQUE 1995; DEAN 1995; FENTON 1991; TAYLOR 1992; WINKLER 1989). The lack of parallelism between arterial and venous distribution, and the multiple individual variations in their organization and anastomoses are the reasons why the veins are so difficult to systematize (MEDER 1994).

The venous vasculature consists in a rich network of superficial and deep veins that empty into dural sinuses. The superficial system receives blood from the superficial medullary veins, which begin under the cortex and drain it and part of the underlying white matter toward the peripheral dural sinuses (superior sagittal sinus and transverse sinuses). The deep system receives blood from the deep medullary veins and drain the rest of the hemispheric white matter, the basal ganglia, and the diencephalon before joining the great vein of Galen and straight sinus.

This complex venous anatomy is well demonstrated by MR angiography (Fig. 2.41).

2.1.2.1
Superficial Veins, Superior Sagittal Sinus, and Transverse Sinus

The superficial venous system has been described in the adult by anatomists, neurosurgeons, and neuroradiologists (DELMAS 1950; LAZORTHES 1976; OKA 1985; McCORD 1972; PADGET 1956; PERESE 1960; PIFFER 1980). OKUDERA (1988, 1994) has studied the development of cerebral veins in the fetus.

Veins are present on the lateral, medial, and inferior aspects of each cerebral lobe. On the lateral surface of the hemisphere, centrifugal drainage toward the superior sagittal sinus and transverse sinuses is associated with a lesser one that joins the superficial veins. On the medial surface, there is a predominant centrifugal arrangement and a smaller territory that drains into the deep system. On the inferior surface, centrifugal veins join the superior sagittal sinus anteriorly and the lateral sinus posteriorly, while a small compartment converges toward the deep venous system.

2.1.2.1.1
Superficial Veins and Superior Sagittal Sinus
(Diagrams 2.29, 2.30)

● These veins lie in the pia of the hemispheric surface and accompany their arteries infrequently. They arise from the lateral and medial aspects, cross the subarachnoid space, and empty into the superior sagittal sinus. They drain the frontal, parietal, and occipital lobes (BRACARD 1996).

● Frontal region
- On the lateral surface, the frontopolar, anterior frontal, middle frontal, and posterior frontal veins drain the white matter from the first three frontal gyri. The precentral vein drains the posterior part of the first three frontal gyri and the anterior part of the precentral gyrus. They course upward toward the superior sagittal sinus; the anterior frontal vein runs slightly forward, while the middle frontal vein is vertical, perpendicular to the sinus. The middle and posterior frontal veins often join the precentral vein and the homologous medial ones and form one or more trunks before draining into the sinus.
- On the medial surface, three or four veins (anterior, middle, posterior) drain the medial part of the superior frontal gyrus, the cingulate gyrus; the anterior veins enter the sinus at a right angle while the more posterior ones have a frequent recurrent subdural course.
- On the inferior surface, the anterior orbitofrontal and frontopolar veins drain into the sinus.

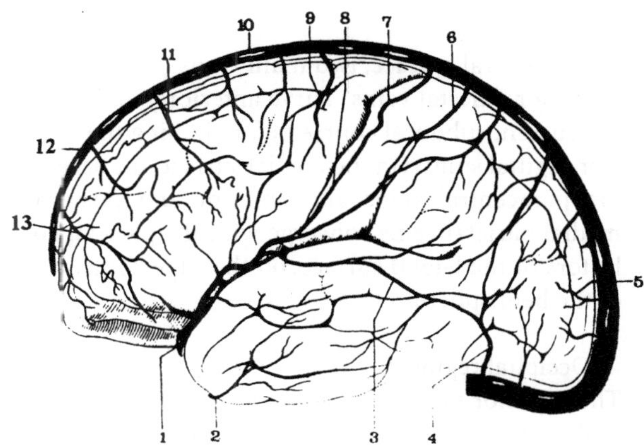

Diagram 2.30. Venous anatomy of the medial surface of the hemisphere (From BOUCHET-CUILLERET 1983)
  1 Superficial middle cerebral vein
  2 Anterior temporal vein
  3 Vein of Labbé
  4 Anastomotic vein of Labbé
  5 Lateral occipital vein
  6 Parietal vein
  7 Postrolandic vein
  8 Vein of Trolard
  9 Rolandic vein
  10 Superior sagittal sinus
  11 Posterior frontal vein
  12 Middle frontal vein
  13 Anterior frontal vein

● Central (or rolandic) region
This area, which is of great functional importance, has a rich venous drainage including three great veins (precentral, central, and postcentral) on the lateral surface. They often curve anteriorly and enter the sinus in a countercurrent fashion. On the medial surface, the central area is drained by paracentral veins.

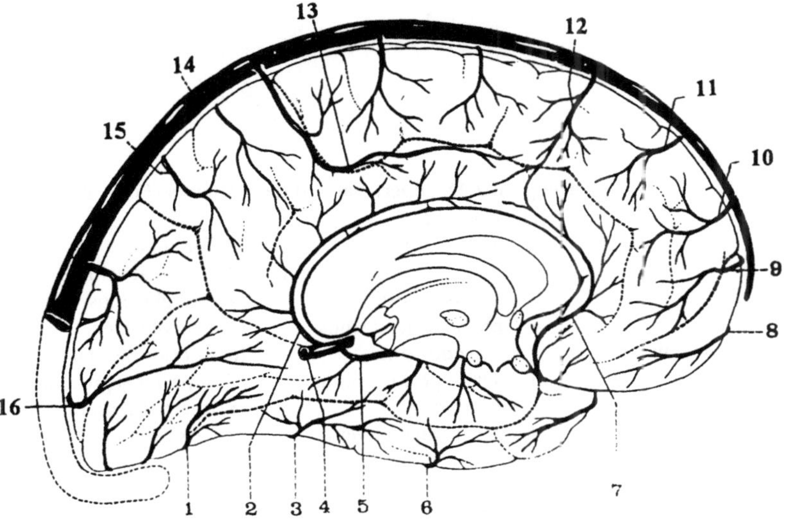

Diagram 2.29. Venous anatomy of the lateral surface of the hemisphere (From BOUCHET-CUILLERET 1983)
  1 Posterior temporal vein
  2 Posterior vein of corpus callosum
  3 Middle temporal vein
  4 Vein of Galen
  5 Basilar vein
  6 Anterior temporal vein
  7 Anterior cerebral vein
  8 Orbital vein
  9 Frontopolar vein
  10 Anterior frontal vein
  11 Middle frontal vein
  12 Posterior frontal vein
  13 Paracentral vein
  14 Superior sagittal sinus
  15 Vein of precuneus
  16 Occipital vein

● Parietal region

On the lateral surface, two main veins (anterior and posterior parietal veins) curve anteriorly and follow a recurrent subdural course before joining the superior sagittal sinus. On the medial surface, the ascending paracentral veins and anterior and posterior medial parietal veins converge with the parietal collectors of the lateral surface, on the superior aspects of the hemisphere.

● Occipital region

The superior sagittal sinus drains the occipital veins of the lateral surface and the posterior calcarine vein of the medial surface.

● In addition, ANDREWS (1989) reported the study of ten human brains from young adults (Diagram 2.31). On the surface of each hemisphere, an average of 6.5 veins drain the anterior frontal region, 3 veins the parietal region, and 1 vein the occipital region; their mean diameter is 0.1–1 mm, but greater diameters may be encountered: 3 mm for anterior frontal and occipital veins, and 3.5 mm for posterior frontal veins. Although they are based on adult brains, these data are important since the anterior fontanelle is a favorable acoustic window for assessing the frontal region.

● The superior sagittal sinus (SCHMIDEK 1985)

The superior sagittal sinus is a midline, poorly contractile sinus running from the frontal region to the torcular (Diagram 2.32). It courses at the deep surface of the sagittal suture, in the outer margin of the falx cerebri, limited by a dural wall with fibrous endothelium. Its size increases progressively as it receives the cortical and subcortical superficial veins. It becomes wider with lakes where granulations of Pacchioni protrude (Diagram 2.33). It drains into the torcular before the occipital protuberance and joins the lateral sinuses.

● Sonographic aspects of the superior sagittal sinus and its afferences:

Morphologic imaging is imperfect for several reasons: veins cannot be detected by pulsation and direct visualization of their lumen is required. This is impossible for the avalvular superficial veins. The superior sagittal sinus may be shown but it is usually

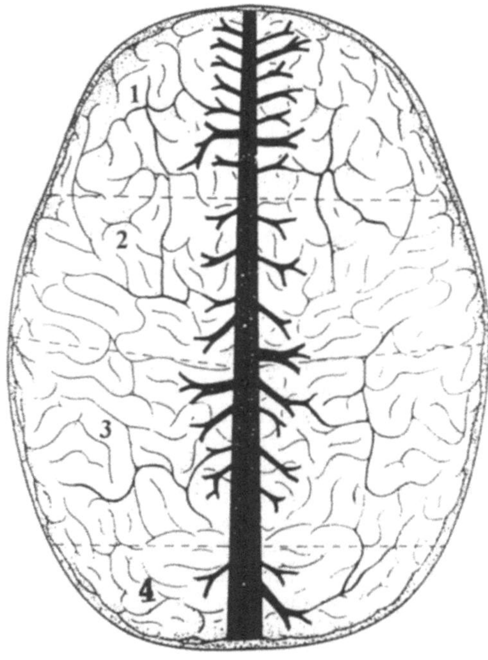

Diagram 2.31. Vertex view of the hemisphere showing the mean number and size of veins draining each region (From ANDREWS 1989)

   1 Anterior frontal region
   2 Posterior frontal region
   3 Parietal region
   4 Occipital region

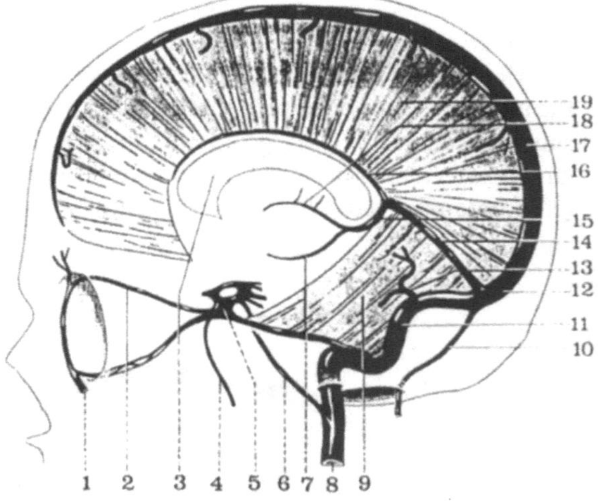

Diagram 2.32. Superficial and deep sinuses (From BOUCHET-CUILLERET 1983)

1	Angular vein	*12*	Torcular
2	Superior ophthalmic vein	*13*	Occipital vein
3	Corpus callosum	*14*	Straight sinus
4	Sphenoparietal sinus	*15*	Vein of Galen
5	Cavernous sinus	*16*	Inferior sagittal sinus
6	Inferior petrosal sinus	*17*	Superior sagittal sinus
7	Basilar vein	*18*	Internal cerebral vein
8	Internal jugular vein	*19*	Falx cerebri
9	Tentorium cerebelli		
10	Posterior occipital sinus		
11	Lateral sinus		

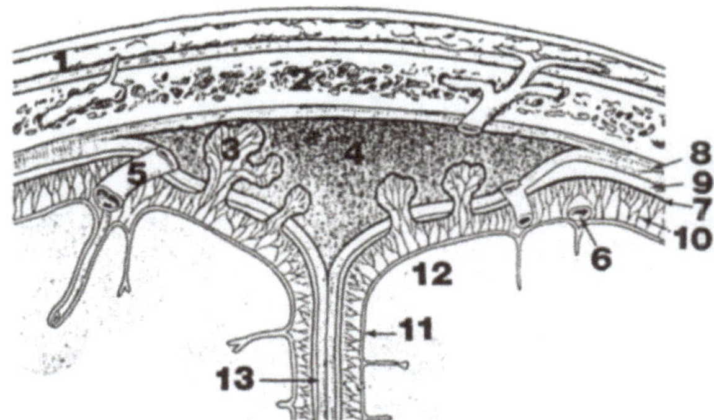

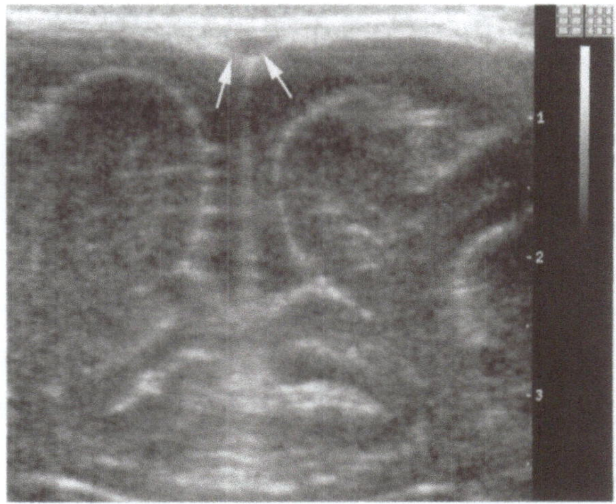

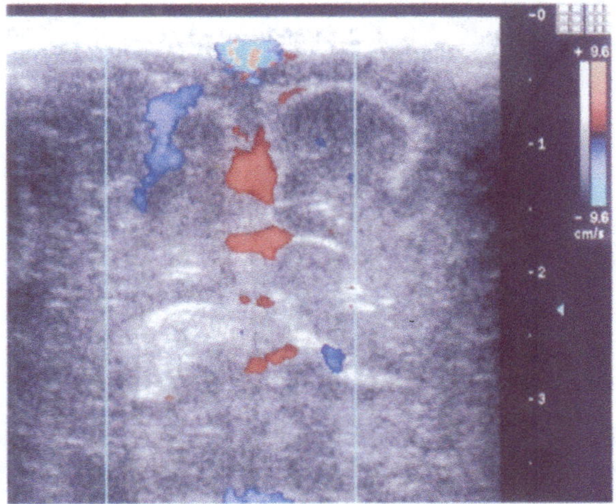

Diagram 2.33. Frontal plane at the level of the superior sagittal sinus (From BOUCHET-CUILLERET 1983)

1 Skin
2 Diploe
3 Granulation of Pacchioni
4 Superior sagittal sinus
5 Cerebral vein
6 Cerebral artery
7 Arachnoid
8 Dura mater
9 Subdural space
10 Subarachnoid space
11 Pia
12 Cerebral cortex
13 Falx cerebri

Fig. 2.40. a This 2-month-old infant is crying, and the superior sagittal sinus (*arrow*) appears as a triangular anechoic image. It is also easily shown by the color Doppler technique (**b**)

small in size or collapsed in the quiet newborn; when the infant moves or cries, the lumen of the sinus widens and may be detected by high-frequency probes (Fig. 2.40).

In fact, accurate analysis of the superior sagittal sinus requires a color Doppler investigation (DEAN 1995; MITCHELL 1988; TATSUNO 1989; TAYLOR 1992; VAN BEL 1993; WINKLER 1989; WONG 1989):

- Whatever the size of the anterior fontanelle, the superior sagittal sinus is always demonstrated by the color Doppler technique (either standard or power). BEZINQUE (1995) reported that, out of 95 neonates and infants, the sinus was identified in 94; in the remaining 2, the absence of colored flow suggested a venous thrombosis that was subsequently confirmed by CT. Thus, the use of high-frequency probes (10–12 MHz) on the fontanellar acoustic window is ideal for visualizing this superficial sinus.
- From a technical point of view, power Doppler, which is relatively independent of the angle axis, is to be preferred.
- On a frontal plane, the sinus appears triangular with a superior base. On a sagittal plane, it appears tubular and usually gradually increases in size (Fig. 2.41); less frequently it widens abruptly: from

1.5 mm or less in the frontal region to more than 4 mm in the parietal region. The length of sinus that is visualized depends on the size of the anterior fontanelle; usually, the thin anterior part and the posterior parietal part are not seen. By contrast, its distal portion, near the convergence with the torcular, is often depicted (Fig. 2.42).
- Obviously, lateral and medial superficial veins are incompletely shown. The anterior fontanelle is usually located over the posterior frontal region and the anterior frontal and posterior parietal veins are rarely demonstrated, but the number, size, and mode of drainage of the veins that are visualized are well displayed (Fig. 2.43).
The larger medial veins are observed in the posterior frontal region (Fig. 2.44); they may converge with lateral veins into a common trunk.

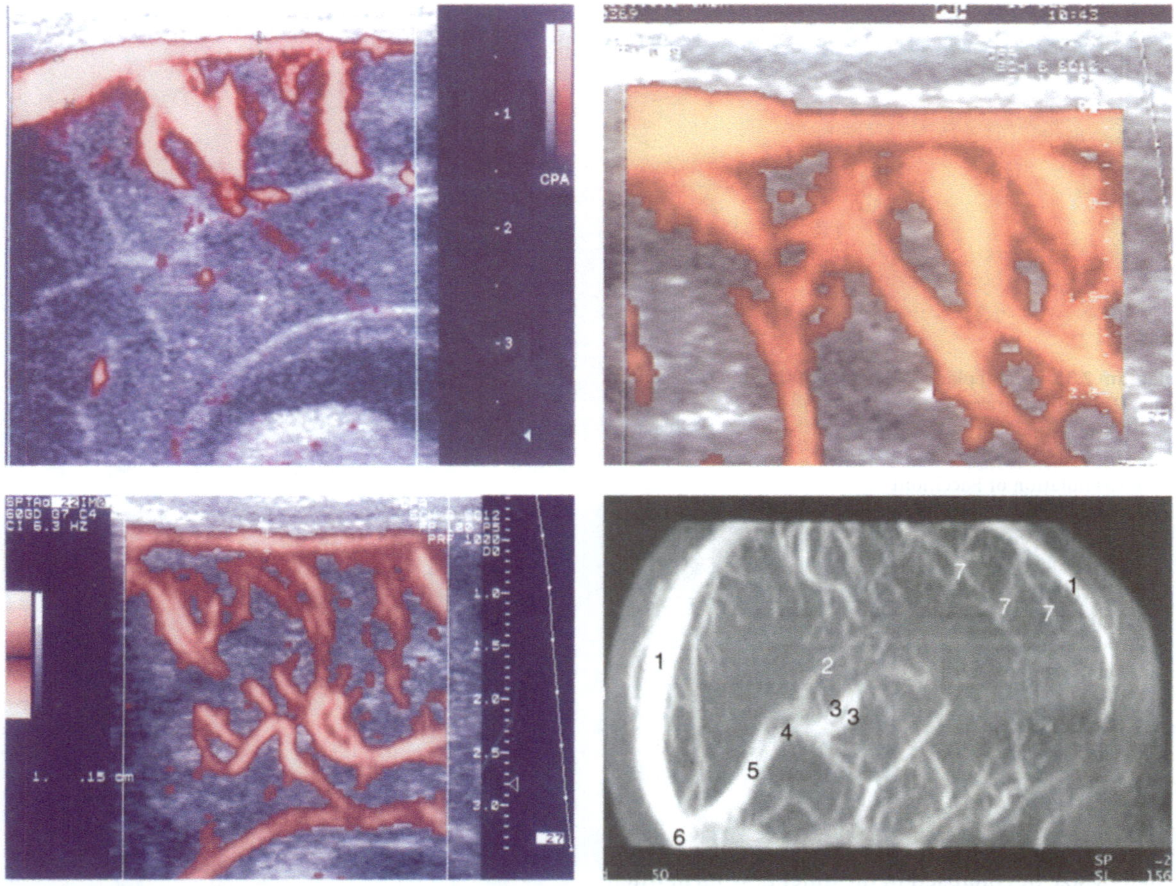

Fig. 2.41. a Usually, as in this preterm infant, the size of the superior sagittal sinus increases gradually: this one is 1.6 mm anteriorly and 4.3 mm posteriorly. **b** Infrequently, it increases abruptly. **c** Exceptionally, its diameter is uniform. **d** Venous MR angiography. The gradual increase in size of the superior sagittal sinus *1*, fed by the medial and lateral superficial veins, is well shown. The deep venous system is identified, *2* inferior sagittal sinus, *3* internal cerebral veins, *4* vein of Galen, *5* straight sinus, *6* torcular, *7* superficial veins

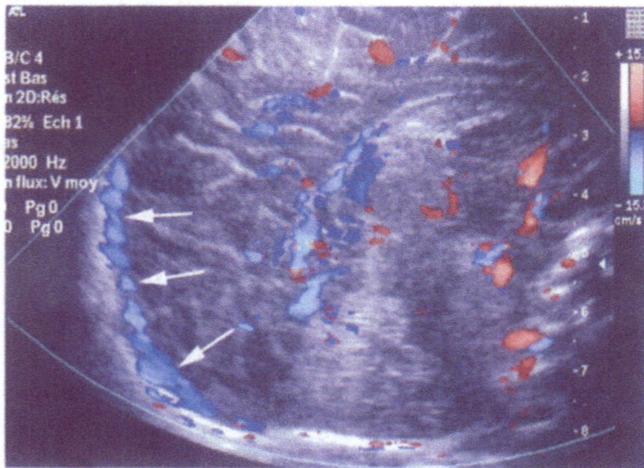

Fig. 2.42. Sagittal scan showing the distal portion of the superior sagittal sinus (*arrow*)

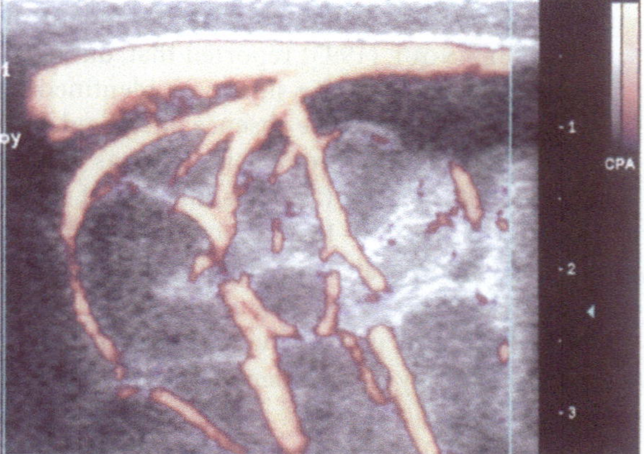

Fig. 2.43. In this case, the superficial medial veins have a long course in the subarachnoid and subdural spaces before draining into the superior sagittal sinus

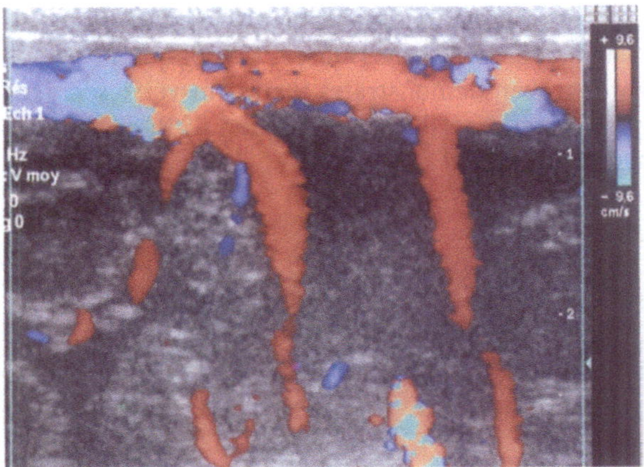

Fig. 2.44. Sagittal scan showing the posterior frontal part of the superior sagittal sinus. In this region, the superficial medial veins are always wide

The medial veins are easier to show than the lateral ones: a pericerebral effusion helps in their detection. An anterograde or retrograde course may be visualized before they enter the sinus (Fig. 2.45). On standard color Doppler imaging, the cortical veins and cortical branches of the anterior cerebral artery course in the same direction and are both coded red. Pulsed Doppler is required to distinguish between them (Fig. 2.46).

- It is important to define the anatomy of the superior sagittal sinus, because color Doppler ultrasonography is essential for a good-quality hemodynamic assessment, especially since reliable spectral analysis of this sinus requires an angle correction.

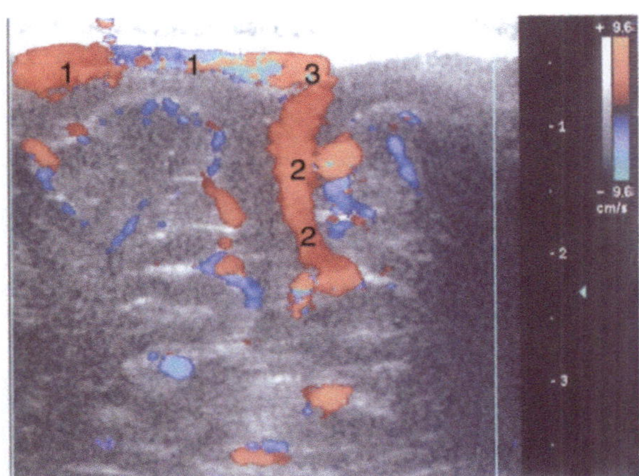
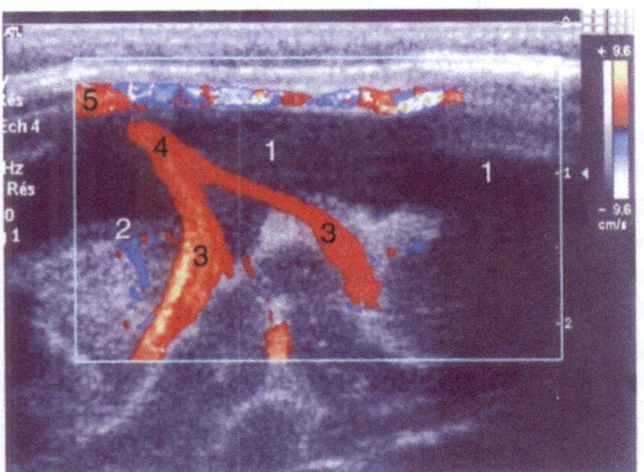

Fig. 2.45a,b. The pericerebral collection improves visualization of the superficial medial and lateral veins. a The lateral veins are difficult to depict because their course is perpendicular to the beam axis. In this 1-month-old infant with a pericerebral collection, a lateral (*1*) and a medial vein (*2*) are seen draining into the superior sagittal sinus (*3*). b In this infant with macrocrania, subdural hygroma (*1*), and minimal subarachnoid collection (*2*) are seen. There is excellent visualization of the subdural course of two medial veins (*3*) that converge in a common stem (*4*) and drain into the superior sagittal sinus (*5*)

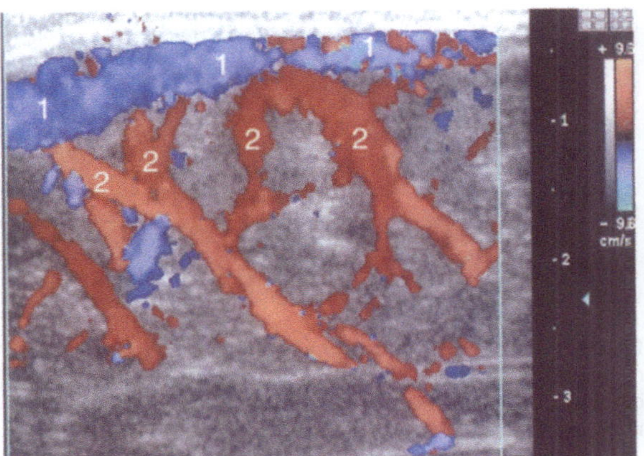
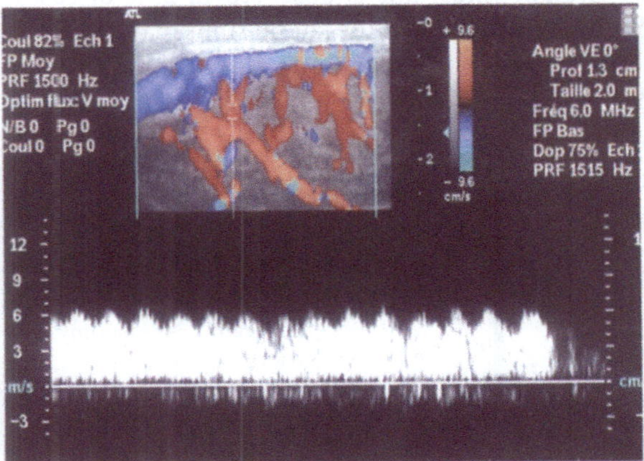

Fig. 2.46a,b. Multiple vessels (*2*) coded *red* (a) drain into the superior sagittal sinus (*1*). Pulsed Doppler is required to identify the vessel; it shows a sinusoidal flow that indicates a medial cortical vein (b)

2.1.2.1.2
Superficial Cerebral Veins and Lateral Sinuses

● The lateral sinus receives the cortical and subcortical veins from the temporal region. On the lateral surface, three temporal veins drain the second and third temporal gyri: the posterior temporal vein for their posterior thirds, the middle temporal vein (inconstant) for their median thirds, and the anterior temporal vein for their anterior thirds. They run on the surface of the temporal lobe, turn onto the medial surface, and join the lateral sinus.

On the inferior surface, the inferior temporal veins drain the median part of the third and fourth temporal gyri.

On the inferior surface of the occipital lobe, the inferior occipital veins connect in a common stem that links with the inferior temporal veins and converges to the sinus.

● The lateral sinuses arise from the division of the superior sagittal sinus (Diagram 2.34) and course on each side of the internal occipital protuberance toward the jugular foramen. They are called transverse sinuses in their initial horizontal segment and run on a bony rim of the occipital bone, on the outer tentorial margin. Then they curve medially on the petrous bone and reach the jugular foramen, anterolaterally; in this portion they are called sigmoid sinuses.

The diameter of the lateral sinuses is large, ranging from 8 to 10 mm (SINDOU 1996), which is why they are easily depicted in the fetus by color Doppler imaging (LAURICHESSE-DELMAS 1999).

The two lateral sinuses are most frequently asymmetric (80% of cases). One lateral sinus may even drain the whole superior sagittal sinus and the other the straight sinus; this is observed in 25% of cases (SINDOU 1996). Finally, the lateral sinus may be hypoplastic or even absent on one side (BISARIA 1985, 1993).

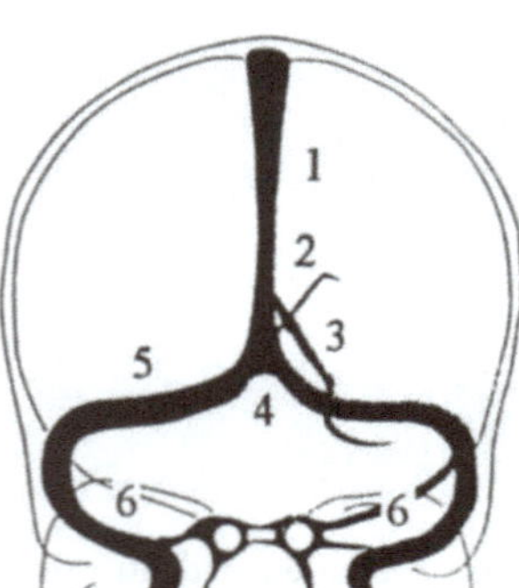

Diagram 2.34. Anatomy of lateral sinuses
  1 Superior sagittal sinus
  2 Internal cerebral vein
  3 Basal vein
  4 Torcular
  5 Transverse sinus
  6 Sigmoid sinus

● The anterior fontanelle seems inappropriate for visualizing the lateral sinuses. An oblique posterior coronal scan demonstrates their transverse segment and, sometimes, the distal portion of their sigmoid segment (Fig. 2.47).

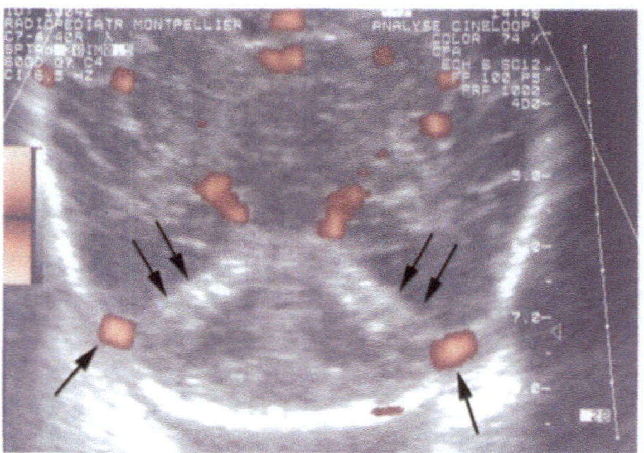

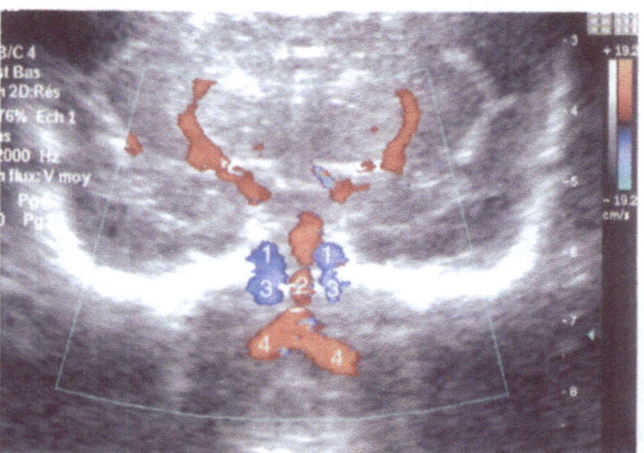

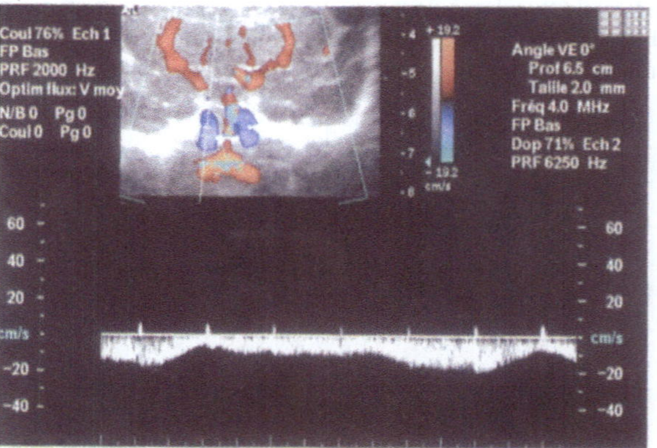

Fig. 2.47. a Posterior oblique frontal scan. The transverse portion of the lateral sinuses is always visible (*arrow*) at the level of the outer tentorial margin (*double arrow*). **b** At the level of the foramen magnum, the distal portions of the two sigmoid sinuses (*1*) run on each side of the basilar artery (*2*) and continue in the two jugular veins (*3*) through the jugular foramen. (*4*) Vertebral arteries. Note the characteristic respiratory modulation of the internal jugular vein on pulsed Doppler imaging (**c**)

A temporal transcranial scan, by contrast, shows their course (Fig. 2.48). Color imaging confirms the great variability in the anatomy of the lateral sinuses; failure to detect one sinus (Fig. 2.49) may indicate sinusal agenesis as well as asymptomatic venous thrombosis.

Finally, superficial temporal veins cannot be depicted by color Doppler.

2.1.2.2
Deep Venous System (HASSLER 1966)

The deep venous system drains the white matter, basal ganglia, and part of the medial temporal cortex, via multiple venules and veins that converge toward the internal cerebral veins. These last veins join with the basilar veins and form the great vein of Galen that is followed by the straight sinus toward the torcular.

Among these vessels that form a midline deep venous confluence, the vein of Galen is obviously the most important.

2.1.2.2.1
Great Vein of Galen (VELUT 1987)

This vein results from the convergence of the two internal cerebral veins; following their anteroinferior curve, it runs under the splenium of the corpus callosum with a posterosuperior concavity and joins the straight sinus (GHALI 1989) at an angle open inferomedially.

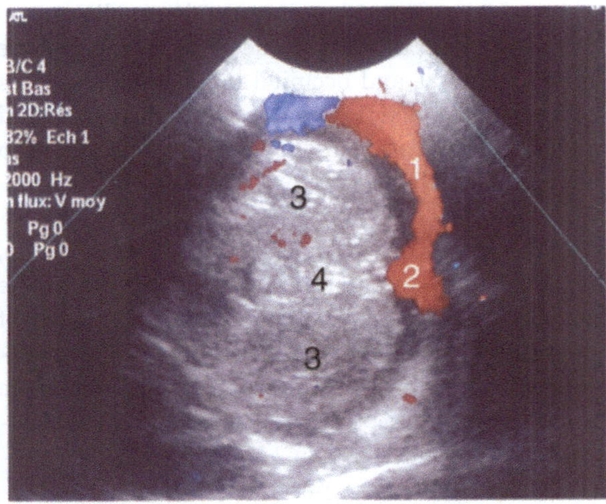

Fig. 2.48. Transcranial scan at the level of posterior fossa. This plane is ideal for assessing the lateral sinuses. Note the large diameter (5 mm) of the right lateral sinus (*1*). *2* Torcular, *3* cerebellar hemispheres, *4* vermis

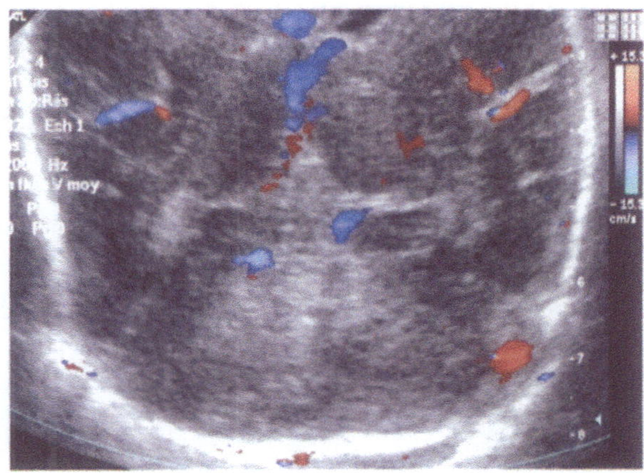

Fig. 2.49. Preterm infant. Routine neonatal screening showing normal US morphology. The right lateral sinus is not depicted. Clinical evolution was normal. Follow-up ultrasonography at two month of age still failed to depict the right lateral sinus, suggesting agenesis

Inferiorly, it locates over the quadrigeminal cistern; superiorly, it is covered by the splenial pia; anteriorly it is connected to the two internal cerebral veins junction; laterally, it lies close to the anteromedial surface of the occipital lobes and to the cingulate gyrus.

Besides the internal cerebral veins and the basilar veins that empty into its proximal segment in half of the cases (YAMAMOTO 1981), the great vein of Galen receives multiple afferences: the pericallosal posterior veins, from the superior part of the corpus callosum, the medial veins, from the ventricular walls, the medial occipital vein, from the calcarine area, the medial atrial vein, from the periventricular white matter, and the thalamocaudate vein, near the end of internal cerebral veins.

Thus, the vein of Galen is a major venous confluence. Moreover, it is close to several great arteries (posteromedial choroidal artery, posterolateral choroidal artery, terminal branches of posterior pericallosal artery, calcarine artery, parieto-occipital artery, posterior temporal artery), which explains the great anatomical variability of galenic aneurysms.

On color Doppler ultrasonography, the vein of Galen is easily visualized (DEAN 1995): it was seen in 95% of 20 healthy neonates (TAYLOR 1992). In our experience, it is always depicted. It presents a short superior curve with a swirling flow in the downstream proximal part of the straight sinus (Fig. 2.50). The internal cerebral veins and terminal part of basilar veins are easily displayed (Fig. 2.53), unlike the other afferent veins, which are not detected.

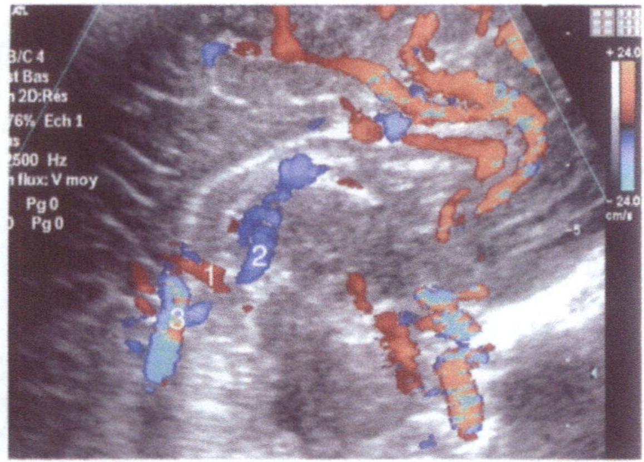

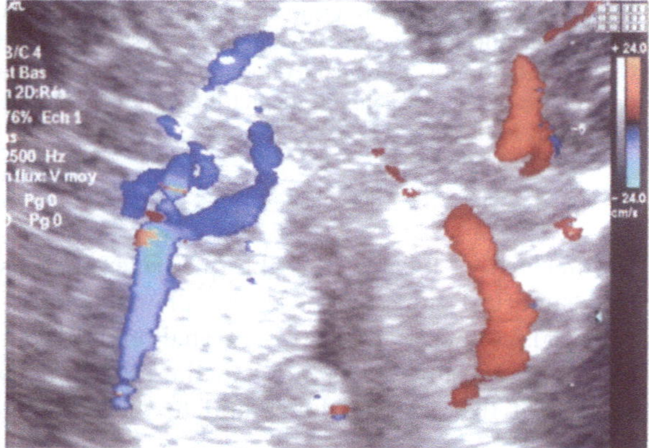

Fig. 2.50a,b. The great vein of Galen (*1*) is intensely angulated with the distal internal cerebral veins (*2*) and the proximal straight sinus (*3*): the vein of Galen is coded *red* and the downstream flow is turbulent (**a**). Sometimes angulations are less marked (**b**), and the downstream flow is stable

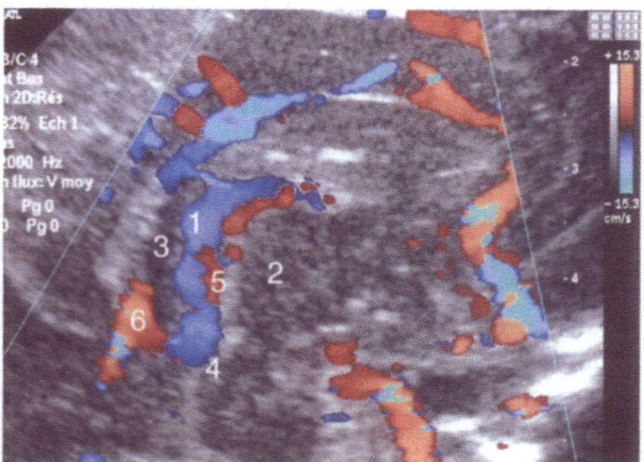

Fig. 2.51. The relations of the internal cerebral vein (*1*) are well assessed by a midline sagittal plane: anteriorly, third ventricle (*2*); posteriorly, splenium of the corpus callosum (*3*); inferiorly, tectum (*4*). There is close contact with the posterior medial choroidal artery (*5*). The acute angle between the internal cerebral vein (*1*) and the vein of Galen (*6*) explains why it is coded *red*

2.1.2.2.2
Internal Cerebral Veins

Each internal cerebral vein arises near the foramen of Monro, from the junction of the anterior septal vein, thalamostriate vein, and superior choroidal vein (Diagram 2.35). The vein runs between the two leaves of the third ventricular tela choroidea, close to the posterior choroidal artery. At this level, the two internal cerebral veins lie beneath the trigone; they diverge under the fornix and pass along the splenium of corpus callosum, where they join to form the great vein of Galen. They course on the superior surface of third ventricle.

All authors (DEAN 1995; MITCHELL 1988; TAYLOR 1992; TATSUNO 1989; WONG 1989) agree that the internal cerebral veins are always demonstrated by color imaging. On a sagittal scan, they are coded blue, with an inferior curve (Fig. 2.51). They are close to the superior posterior choroidal artery superiorly and to the posteromedial choroidal artery inferiorly (Fig. 2.37). They are also well displayed by a posterior oblique coronal scan: the two vessels, which are close together, are more easily identified by power Doppler (Fig. 2.52) than by standard color imaging, because of the partial volume effect. Finally, this plane is appropriate for showing important draining vessels such as the superior choroidal vein and the basal veins (Fig. 2.53).

The internal cerebral vein receives multiple afferences: the subependymal ventricular veins, thalamic veins, and choroidal veins:

◆ The subependymal veins run along the ependyma of the lateral ventricles and are divided into two groups (ONO 1984; WOLF 1964). The medial group drains almost exclusively the deep white matter of the frontal, parietal, and occipital lobes and the corpus callosum. The lateral group drains the superolateral portion of the basal ganglia, together with the deep white matter. They include:

● *The veins of the frontal horn.* The medial group, represented by the anterior septal veins, drains the genu of the corpus callosum and the white matter of the frontal pole; these veins converge on the antero-superolateral surface of the frontal horn, in a single trunk toward the septum, and contribute to the internal cerebral vein (Diagram 2.35).

The lateral group, represented by the anterior caudate veins, runs on the anterosuperolateral surface of the frontal horn; the veins converge on the caudate head, form an inferior caudate vein, and end in the thalamostriate vein (Diagram 2.35).

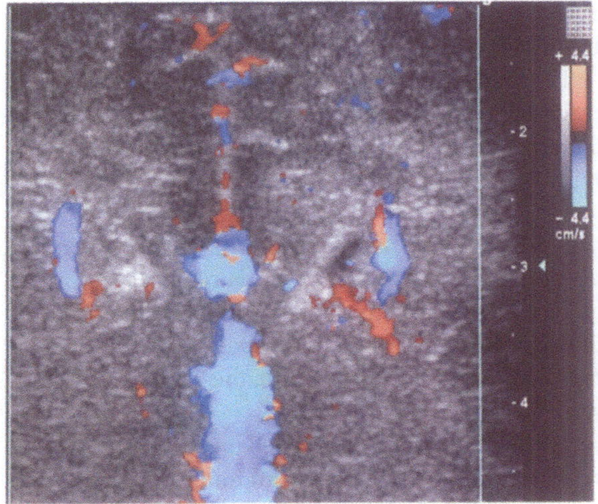

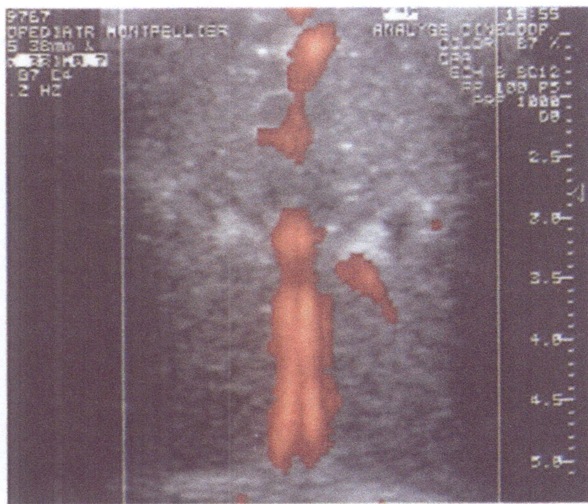

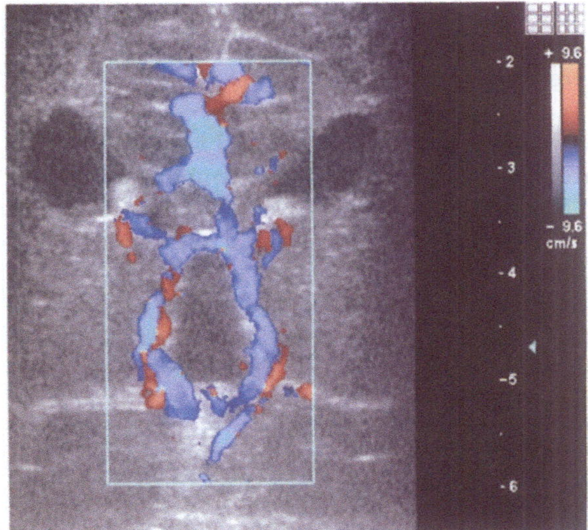

Fig. 2.52a,b. The internal cerebral veins appear as a false common trunk on standard color Doppler imaging (**a**), whereas they are well distinguished on power Doppler (**b**). If the third ventricle is dilated, as in this infant with myelomeningocele (**c**), the two internal cerebral veins and choroidal arteries are more distant and are easier to identify

● *Veins of the ventricular body* (GOLDSTEIN 1986). The medial group, formed by one or two posterior septal veins, runs on the ventricular roof, goes downward along the septum, enters the trigonoseptal junction, and ends in the internal cerebral vein; it drains the corpus callosum and frontal white matter. The lateral group is formed by the thalamostriate, thalamocaudate, and posterior caudate veins.

The thalamostriate vein arises from the venules of the caudate nucleus and courses forward to pass under the choroid plexus and along the posterior edge of the foramen of Monro; it enters the tela choroidea and empties into the internal cerebral vein. It drains the frontal and parietal white matter, the internal capsule, and caudate nucleus. When absent, the thalamostriate vein gives place to the thalamocaudate vein that runs on the medial surface of the caudate nucleus and thalamus. It passes through the

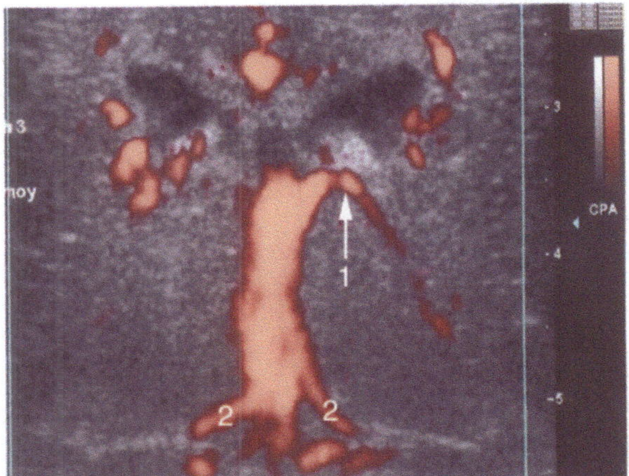

Fig. 2.53. Several draining vessels are visualized: the left superior choroidal vein (*1*) and the two basilar veins (*2*). Note that the two internal cerebral veins are not distinct despite the use of power Doppler technique

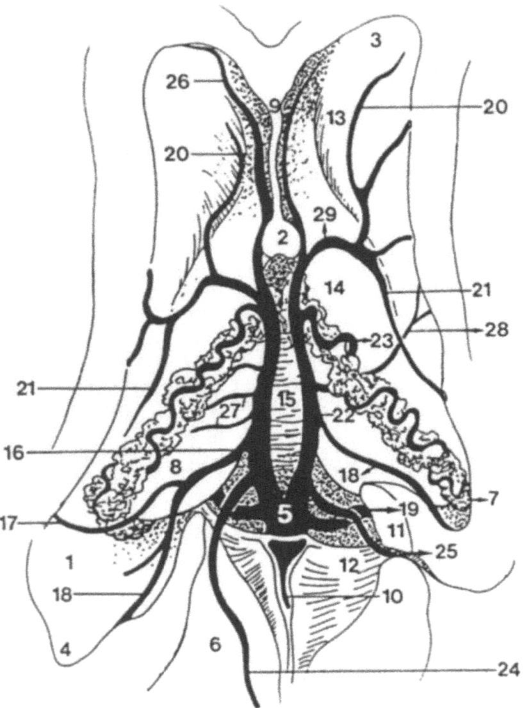

Diagram 2.35. Anatomy of internal cerebral veins: superior view of the lateral ventricles (From Bracard 1996)

 1 Lateral ventricular atrium
 2 Fornix
 3 Frontal horn
 4 Occipital horn
 5 Vein of Galen
 6 Occipital lobe
 7 Choroid plexus
 8 Pulvinar
 9 Septum pellucidum
 10 Straight sinus
 11 Splenium of the corpus callosum
 12 Tentorium cerebelli
 13 Caudate head
 14 Thalamus
 15 Superior tela choroidea
 16 Common atrial vein
 17 Lateral atrial vein
 18 Medial lateral vein
 19 Basilar vein
 20 Anterior caudate vein
 21 Posterior caudate vein
 22 Internal cerebral vein
 23 Superior choroidal vein
 24 Medial occipital vein
 25 Posterior pericallosal vein
 26 Anterior septal vein
 27 Superficial posterior thalamic veins
 28 Thalamocaudate vein
 29 Thalamostriate vein

choroidal fissure, far behind the foramen of Monro, and empties into the internal cerebral vein.

The posterior caudate vein arises at the superolateral angle of the ventricular body, runs downward on the caudate body, and empties into the thalamostriate vein.

● *Veins of the posterior (occipital) horn and ventricular atrium.* The medial group is represented by the medial atrial veins that follow the medial surface of the posterior horn and atrium, pass through the choroidal fissure and empty into the internal cerebral vein.

The lateral group is formed by the lateral atrial veins that drain the lateral and anterior walls of the atrium and the lateral wall of the posterior horn. They cross the caudate tail and the pulvinar, pass through the choroidal fissure, and join the internal cerebral vein (Ono 1984).

● *Veins of the inferior (temporal) horn.* The medial group lies on the floor of the temporal horn, and the lateral group on its roof. The medial group includes the tonsillar vein and the hippocampal transverse veins that run medially, reach the transverse fissure, and join the basilar vein or the internal cerebral vein. The lateral group is represented by the inferior ventricular vein that empties into the basilar vein.

◆ The thalamic veins (Guidicelli 1970). The superior thalamic vein appears at the anterior part of the superomedial surface of thalamus and drains backward into the internal cerebral vein. The anterior thalamic vein, the inferior thalamic vein and the posterior thalamostriate veins are small vessels that empty into several veins: the internal cerebral vein, the anterior septal vein, the thalamostriate vein, and the anterior caudate or basilar vein.

◆ The choroidal veins drain the prosencephalic tela choroidea (Guidicelli 1970; Takahashi 1972; Wolf 1964) and Wolfram-Gabel (1987) distinguishes three groups (Diagram 2.36):
– The superior choroidal vein arises from the confluence of several choroidal venules at the level of the glomus; it constitutes the main drainage of the choroid plexus and of the tela choroidea of the lateral ventricles. It runs anteriorly on the tela, toward the interventricular foramen roof, and ends in the internal cerebral vein by joining with the thalamostriate vein and the anterior septal vein.

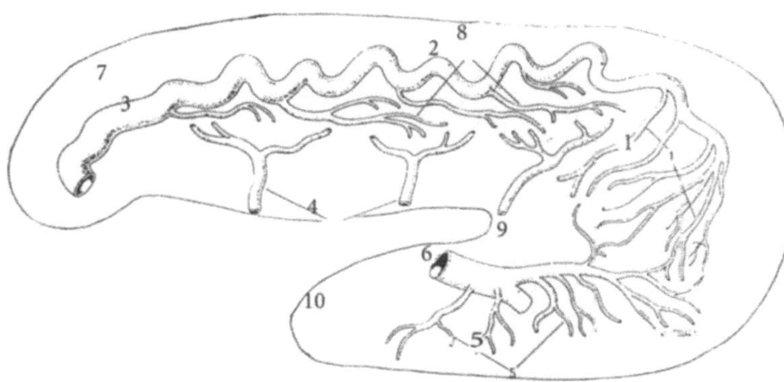

Diagram 2.36. Venous drainage of the tela choroidea of the lateral ventricles (From Wolfram-Gabel 1989)
The posterior (*1*) and superior (*2*) choroidal venules drain upward and converge to form the superior choroidal vein (*3*). The middle choroidal venules (*4*) drain medially into the internal cerebral vein. The inferior choroidal venules (*5*) are tributaries of the choroidoventricular vein (*6*). *7* Frontal horn, *8* foramen of Monro, *9* choroid glomus, *10* temporal horn

– The medial choroidal veins drain directly the tela choroidea and the choroid plexus of the central part of the lateral ventricle, into the internal cerebral vein.

– The inferior choroidal vein drains the tela choroidea and choroid plexus of the inferior ventricular horn toward the basal vein via the inferior choroidoventricular vein (Diagram 2.36). It arises at the ventricular atrium from the convergence of several choroidal venules (Diagram 2.36). It appears on the inferior surface of the pulvinar and runs toward the anterior extremity of the inferior ventricular horn.

◆ In reality, the deep venous drainage is more complex than suggested by anatomical studies (Bracard 1996; Ono 1984; Wolf 1964). Volpe (1997) has shown that the anterior septal, thalamostriate, and superior choroidal veins, as well as several medullary veins that drain the deep white matter, converge into a common terminal vein before emptying into the internal cerebral vein (Diagram 2.37).

◆ Imaging data (morphology and color Doppler) are scarce in the literature. Goldstein (1986) reported that the walls of septal veins may appear as thin linear structures on morphological ultrasonography, but this finding remains infrequent (Fig. 2.54). Color imaging provides much more information: in the reports of Taylor (1992) and Dean (1995), the subependymal terminal veins were always detected by color Doppler in the region of the caudate head.

Using standard color Doppler technique, Taylor (1992) depicted these veins and their drainage in 90% of 20 healthy newborns. Our experience confirms these observations: on color Doppler, these veins lie lateral and inferior to the lateral ventricle floor, close to the germinal matrix, and run downward and medi-

ally (Fig. 2.55) to drain posteriorly into the internal cerebral vein (Fig. 2.56).

The abilities of color Doppler to image the tributaries of the deep venous system are unequal: the ventricular veins are rarely detected except, in some favorable cases, the very small septal veins (Fig. 2.57). The thalamic veins are not depicted. On the other hand, the superior choroidal vein, which is the main mode of drainage of the tela choroidea, is always easily imaged; it may drain directly into the internal cerebral vein (Fig. 2.53) and its relations with the glomus are accurately shown (Fig. 2.58).

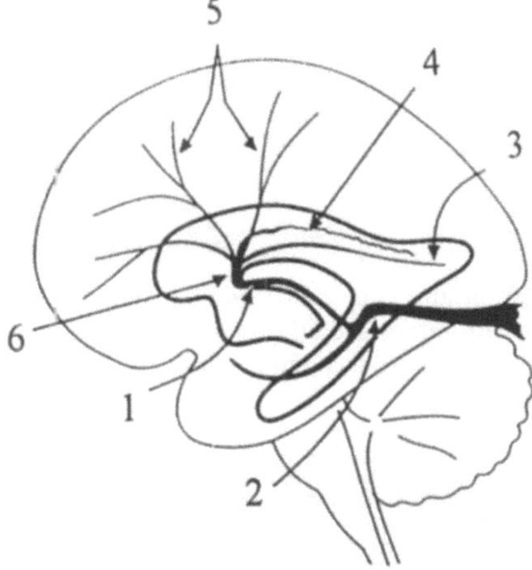

Diagram 2.37. Anatomy of the terminal vein (From Volpe 1995) Note that the thalamostriate, septal, choroidal, and medullary veins come to a point of confluence to form the terminal vein

  1 Internal cerebral vein
  2 Vein of Galen
  3 Thalamostriate vein
  4 Choroidal vein
  5 Medullary veins
  6 Terminal vein

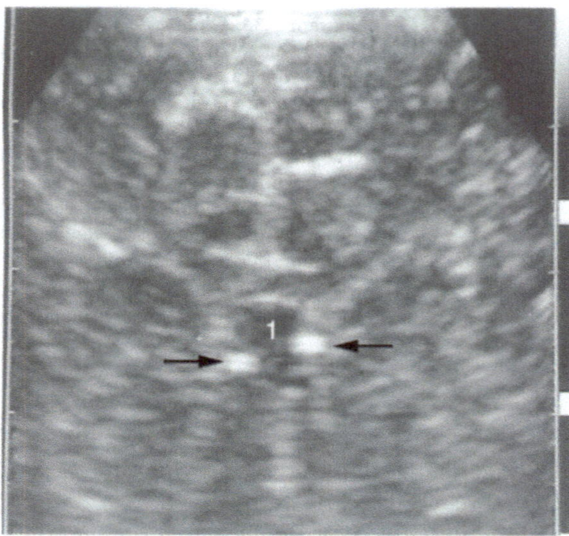

Fig. 2.54. The septal veins appear as two hyperechoic structures (*arrow*) in the walls of the cavity of septum pellucidum

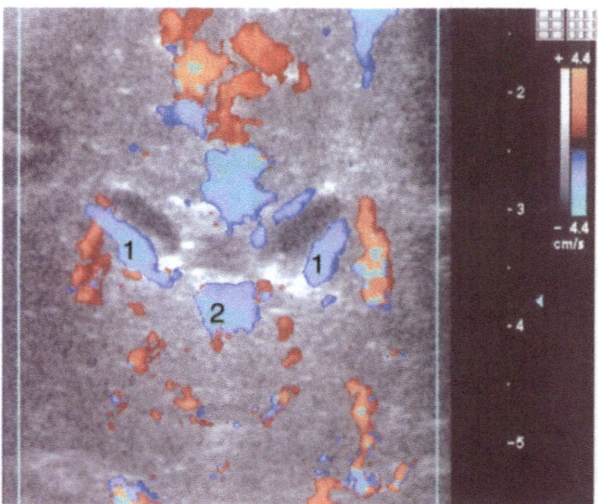

Fig. 2.55. The situation and course of terminal veins (*1*) are characteristic; they run inferomedially, under the lateral ventricle, and drain into the internal cerebral veins (*2*)

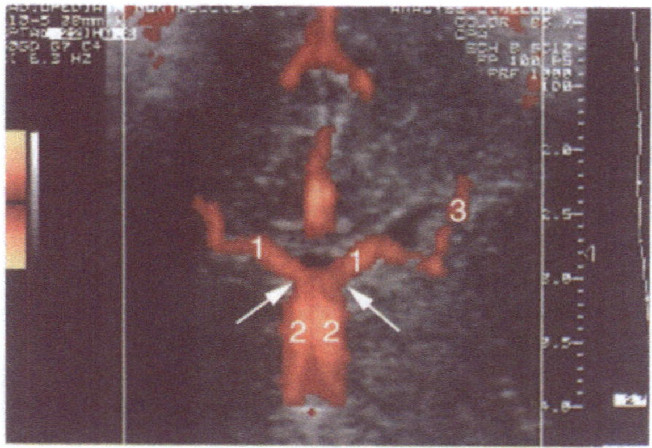

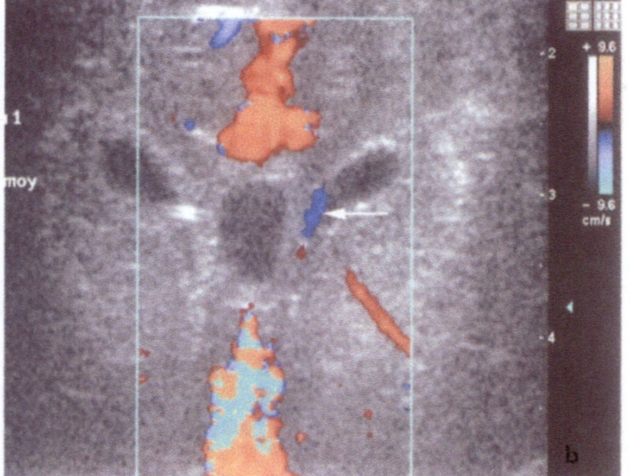

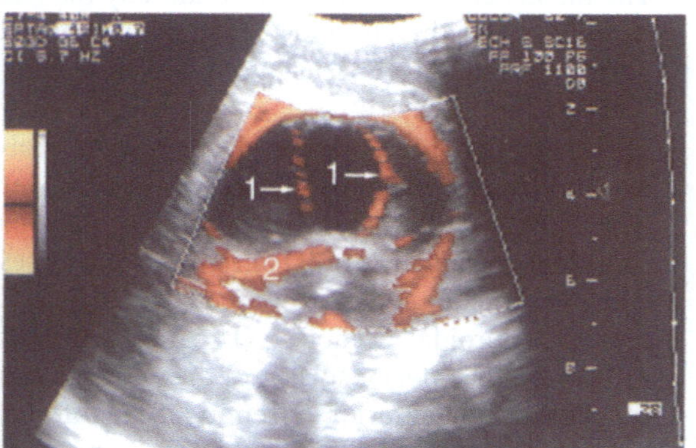

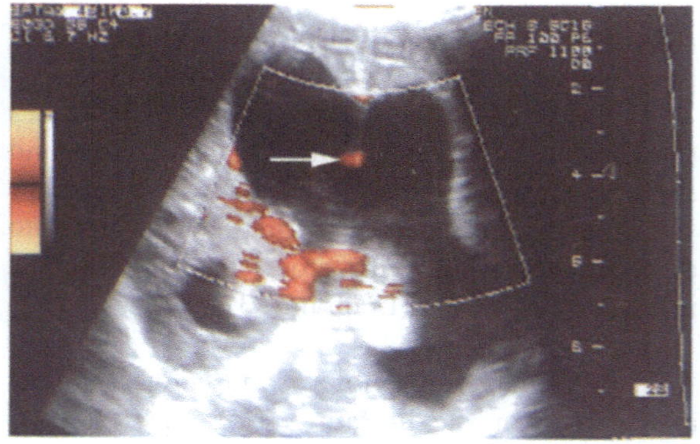

Fig. 2.57. a In this 32-weeks' gestation preterm neonate, the septal vein (*arrow*) is difficult to depict because of its very small size. **b** A 1-month-old infant with posthemorrhagic hydrocephalus. On the sagittal scan, two thin septal veins (*1*) run toward the internal cerebral vein (*2*). The frontal scan (**c**) confirms that these veins are located within the interventricular septum (*arrow*)

Fig. 2.56. On a coronal scan, slightly angulated posteriorly, the drainage (*arrow*) of terminal veins (*1*) into internal cerebral veins (*2*) is well depicted. Note the left medullary vein (*3*) that drains the periventricular white matter and empties into the terminal vein

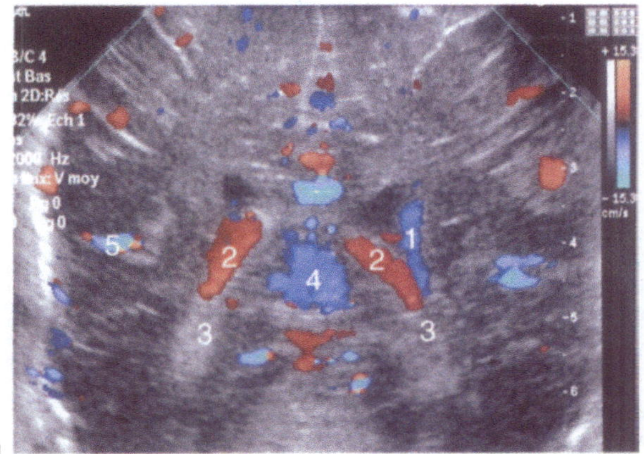

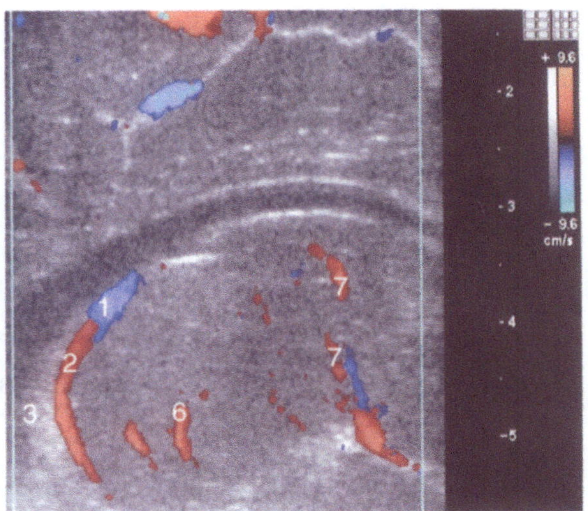

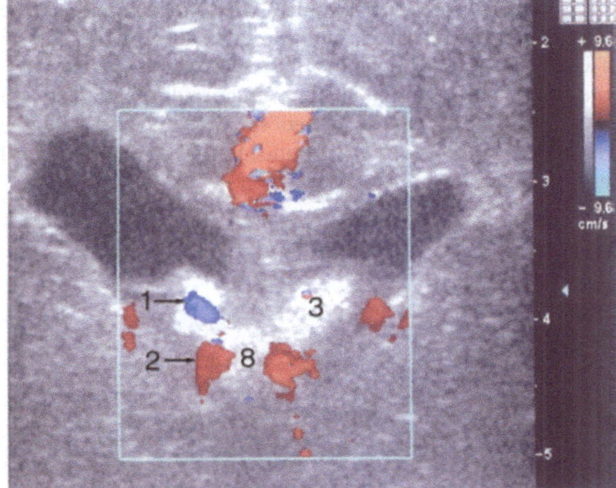

Fig. 2.58a–c. The left superior choroidal vein (*1*) is close to the anterior choroidal artery (*2*), a branch of the internal carotid artery, in the choroid plexus (*3*). *4* Internal cerebral vein, *5* opercular branch of the middle cerebral artery, *6* thalamic artery, *7* lenticulostriate artery. The anatomical location of the choroidal vessels is accurately assessed by a frontal plane (c): the superior choroidal vein (*1*) runs in the choroid plexus of the lateral ventricle (*3*), the anterior choroidal arteries (*2*) encircle inferiorly the choroid plexus of the third ventricle (*8*)

2.1.2.2.3
Basal Vein

This vein (also designated as the basal vein of Rosenthal) (Diagram 2.38), arises at the level of the anterior perforated space, from the confluence of the olfactory vein, the orbitofrontal vein, the anterior cerebral vein, the deep middle cerebral vein, and the anterior and posterior hypothalamic veins.

It presents an anterior segment that turns around the uncus of the fifth temporal gyrus, a middle segment that encircles the cerebral peduncle, and a posterior segment that curves around the pulvinar to join the vein of Galen or the internal cerebral vein (YAMAMOTO 1981). In this course, it receives several tributaries: in its middle segment, it drains the temporal, uncal, hippocampal and lateral mesencephalic veins; in its posterior segment it drains the thalamic, pineal, tectal, posterior pericallosal, subependymal, and anterior calcarine veins.

Transfontanellar color Doppler imaging is not appropriate for visualizing the basal veins, except where they end in the internal cerebral veins (Fig. 2.53) or the vein of Galen. Using the transcranial access, WINKLER (1989) has well described its course around the cerebral peduncle (Fig. 2.59).

2.1.2.2.4
Straight Sinus (BROWDER 1976; SAXENA 1974)

The straight sinus runs backward on the tentorium cerebelli, with a posteroinferior direction, from the vein of Galen to the torcular. The convergence of the straight sinus, lateral sinuses, and occipital sinuses is located at the level of the superior sagittal occipital ridge. However, variations are multiple and the sinusal confluence is most often incomplete (BISARIA 1985; GOTO 1976).

At its proximal part, the straight sinus drains the inferior sagittal sinus, which runs along the posterior two-thirds of the inferior edge of the falx cerebri, close to the splenium of corpus callosum, and receives small veins from the corpus callosum and superficial vessels from the medial surface of the cerebral hemispheres and falx (McCORD 1972).

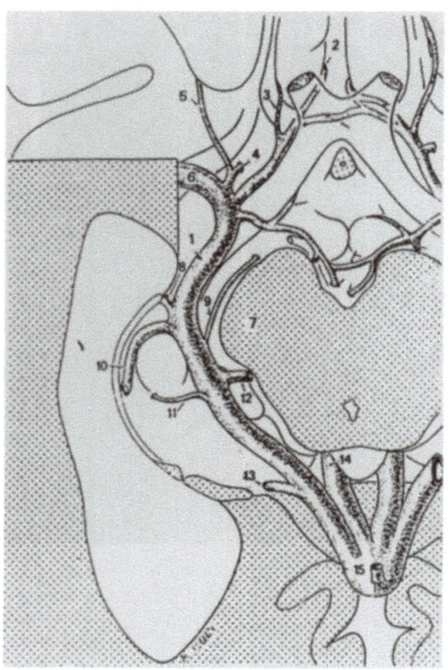

Diagram 2.38. Anatomy of the basal vein: inferior view of the brain
(From Wolfram-Gabel 1989)
The basal vein (*1*) arises at the anterior perforated substance from the confluence of several vessels: the anterior cerebral vein (*2*), the olfactory vein (*3*), the striate vein (*4*), the inferior frontal vein (*5*), and the wide deep middle cerebral vein (*6*). It curves around the cerebral peduncle (*7*), receives the inferior ventricular vein (*8*), the peduncular vein (*9*), the inferior choroidoventricular vein (*10*), the geniculate vein (*11*), the lateral mesencephalic vein (*12*), and the medial occipital vein (*13*). It ends by joining with the internal cerebral vein (*14*) and forms the vein of Galen (*15*)

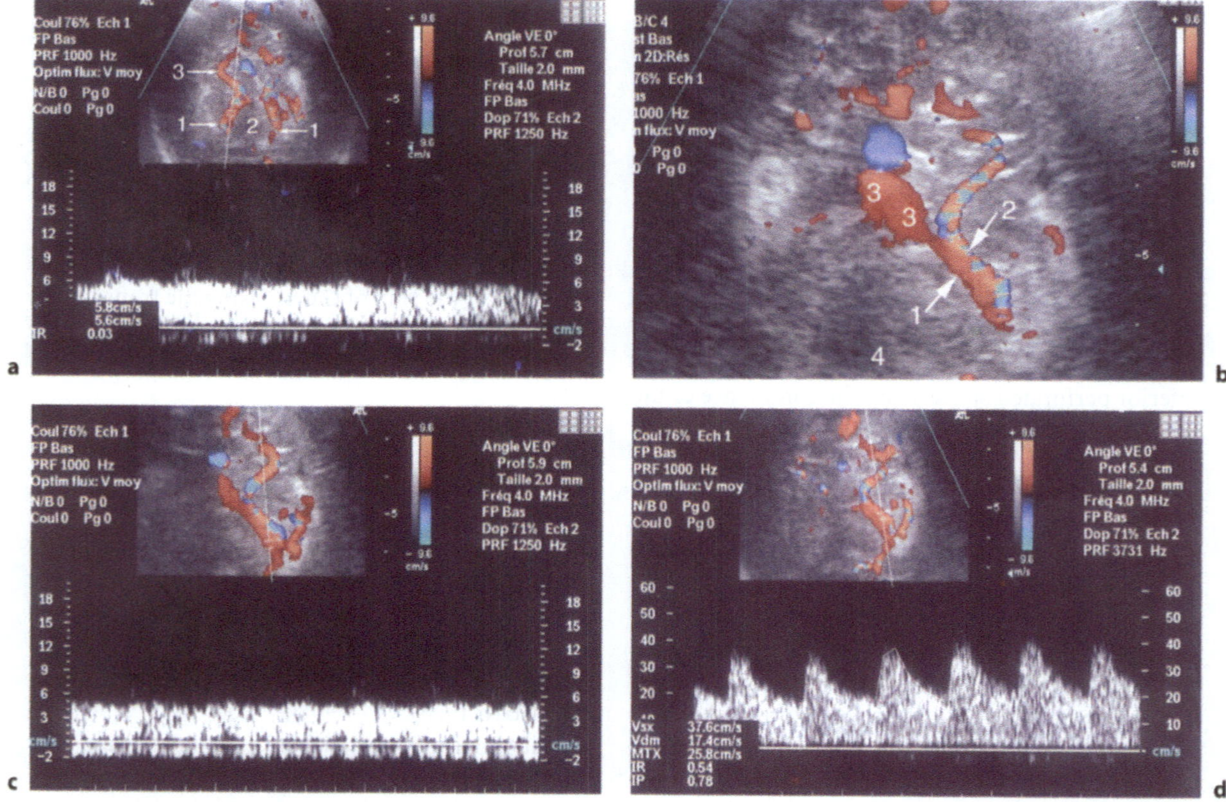

Fig. 2.59a–d. Doppler imaging of basal veins requires a transverse scan through the posterior fontanelle (Winkler 1989). In this example (**a**) the two basilar veins (*1*) curve around the brain stem (*2*). Posteriorly, the distal part of the posterior cerebral artery (*3*) may be seen. The mean velocity in the right basilar vein is 5.7 cm/s. In another case (**b**), the left basilar vein (*1*) and the P3 segment of the left posterior cerebral artery (*2*) are close; pulsed Doppler is required to distinguish the two vessels (**c,d**). *3* Internal cerebral veins, *4* brain stem

In the neonate, color imaging always displays the straight sinus behind the cerebellar vermis, and often shows a swirling flow, because the vein of Galen changes direction (Fig. 2.60). Its deep location is the reason why its peripheral course and its confluence with the torcular are rarely detected by color Doppler, and why it is often not insonated after 3 months of age.

The inferior sagittal sinus is not always visible. When observed, it appears as a small-sized sinus that drains in the vein of Galen (Fig. 2.61) or the straight sinus. Pulsed Doppler imaging is required to differentiate the inferior sagittal sinus from the distal part of the pericallosal artery (Fig. 2.62).

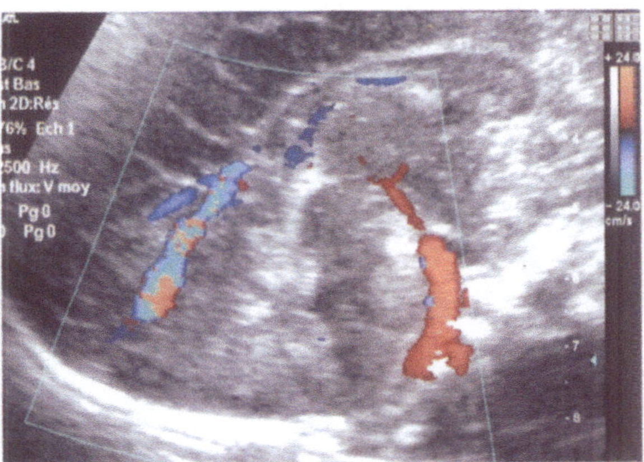

Fig. 2.60. Characteristic swirling flow in the straight sinus

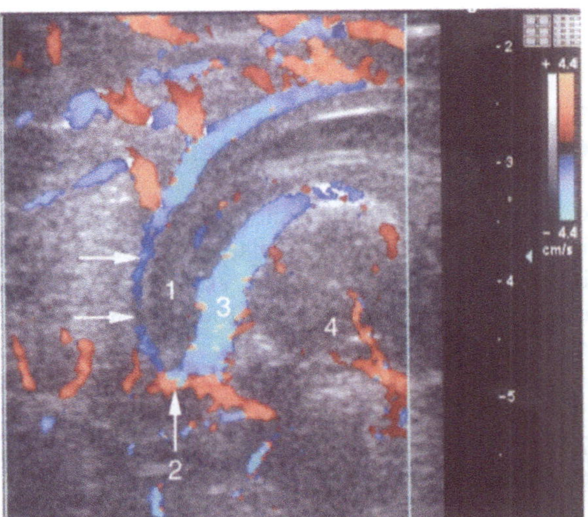

Fig. 2.61. The inferior sagittal sinus appears extremely thin (*arrow*) in contact with the splenium of corpus callosum (*1*) and drains into the vein of Galen (*2*). *3* Internal cerebral vein, *4* third ventricle

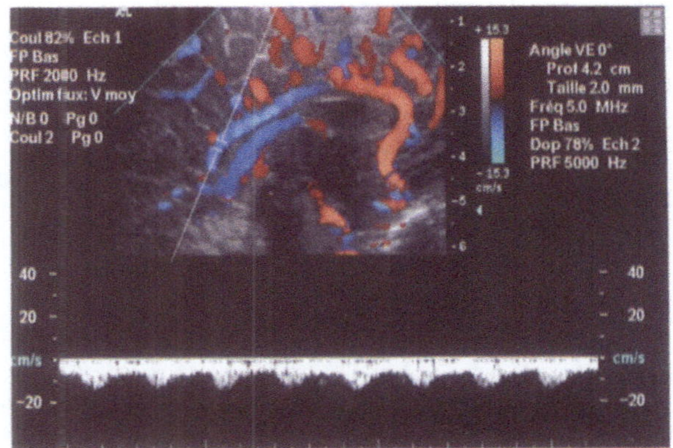

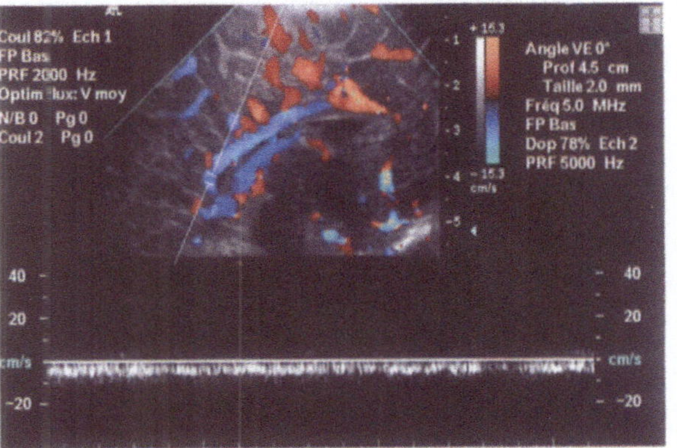

Fig. 2.62a,b. Color Doppler cannot differentiate between the inferior sagittal sinus and the posterior pericallosal artery: both vessels have the same course along the splenium, their flow is away from the transducer and is coded *blue*. Only pulsed Doppler can identify them. **a** Spectral analysis of the posterior pericallosal artery. **b** Spectral analysis of the inferior sagittal sinus

2.1.2.3
Venous Anastomoses

From a functional point of view, the superficial and the deep venous systems are not completely separate. Indeed, angiographic investigations have demonstrated that cerebral veins tend to anastomose (BRACARD 1997) and create an extended network.

In addition to their connection with the meningeal and extracranial veins, the superficial cerebral veins are widely anastomosed with each other. On the lateral surface of each cerebral hemisphere, two main channels are described (Diagram 2.30): the vein of Trolard links the veins of the lateral sulcus and the superior sagittal sinus (DI CHIRO 1972; OKA 1985); the vein of Labbé (BIGELOW 1993) links the veins of the lateral sulcus and the transverse sinus. The superficial middle cerebral vein, which receives the fronto-sylvian, parietosylvian, and temporosylvian veins, drains into the cavernous sinus after crossing the subarachnoid spaces.

According to MEDER (1994), the superficial veins may be divided into three groups: the dorsomedial group toward the superior sagittal sinus, the ventrolateral group toward the lateral sinus, and the anterior group (superficial middle cerebral vein) toward the cavernous sinus.

Usually, each group interconnects with the others via regional anastomoses, which are frequent in the rolandic and sylvian regions.

Multiple anastomoses connect the deep cerebral veins with the other venous systems (GILLOT 1966; McCORD 1972). For example, HASSLER (1966) shows that contrast injection into the vein of Galen promptly opacifies the transverse and superior sagittal sinuses via transcerebral veins.

This demonstrates how the notion of venous territory is relative, even if described by MEDER (1994) (Diagrams 2.39, 2.40); it is easy to understand why a venous thrombosis has less consequences than an arterial one. In our experience there has been no case of parenchymal ischemia following isolated thrombosis of the superior sagittal sinus.

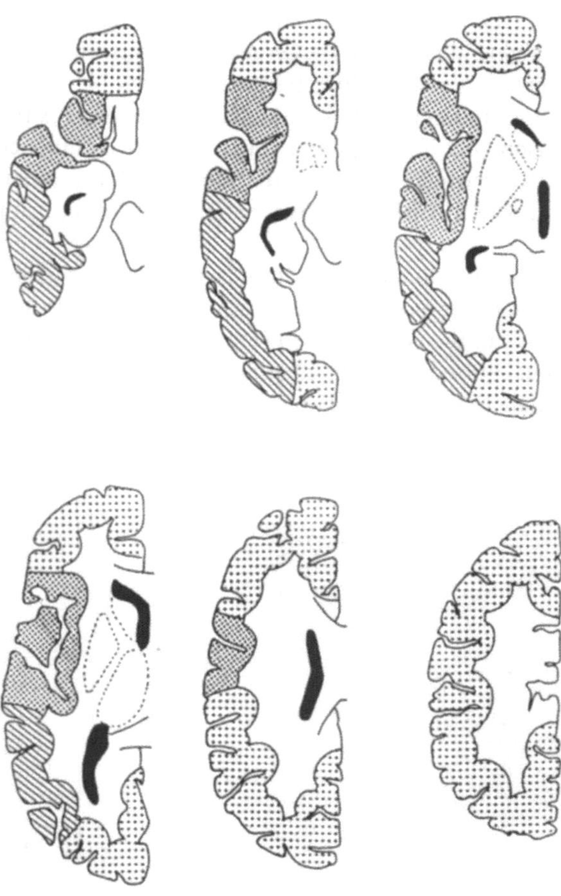

Diagram 2.40. Cerebral venous territories: horizontal sections (From MEDER 1994)

	Sagittal sinus		Lateral sinus
	Cavernous sinus		Vein of Galen

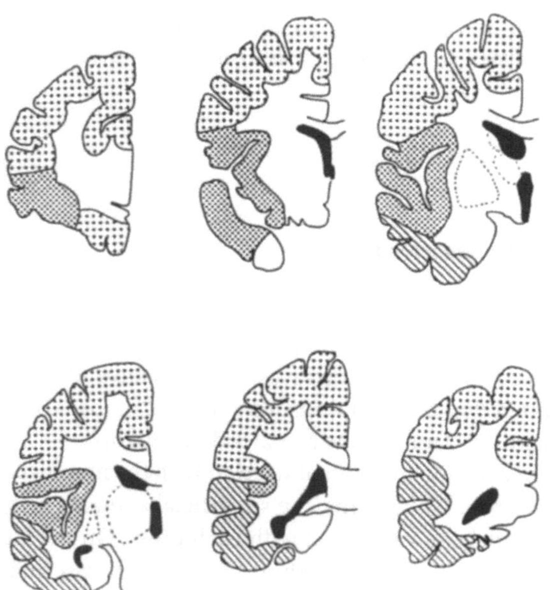

Diagram 2.39. Cerebral venous territories: frontal sections (From MEDER 1994)

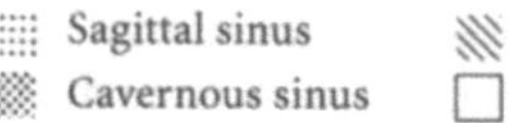 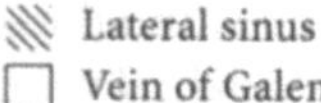

	Sagittal sinus		Lateral sinus
	Cavernous sinus		Vein of Galen

2.2
Cerebral Hemodynamics: Pulsed Doppler

Color and pulsed Doppler should not be dissociated in the study of cerebral vascularization. Color imaging improves the diagnosis of a cerebral vascular disease while pulsed Doppler improves the prognostic evaluation (COUTURE 1994).

2.2.1
Cerebral Blood Flow

The cerebral blood flow (CBF) represents an extremely complex problem. Its regulation depends on multiple factors; total and regional CBF changes significantly with maturation in the fetus (LAUGIER

1986), and intense physiological variations in CBF occur during the first 3 days of life, partly resulting from the ductal closure (MAESEL 1994; SONESSON 1997; WINBERG 1990). All these data should be known and taken into account in the analysis of a hemodynamic investigation.

2.2.1.1
Fetal and Neonatal Cerebral Vascularization

Several characteristics are to be noted:

● The neonatal brain represents 10% of body weight, compared with 2% in the adult (SANN 1985). During the first year of life, brain weight doubles, and cell proliferation continues until the sixth month of life as shown by the evolution of DNA amount as correlated with increase in head circumference. The amount of RNA and protein follow a linear increase later than 6 months of age, corresponding to cell maturation and myelination. This intense metabolic activity is coupled with CBF that represents 22%–25% of cardiac output in the neonate, compared with 15% in the adult.

● A knowledge of the development of arterial vasculature in the fetal brain is important for an understanding of the regional distribution of blood flow and the consequences of changes in this distribution.

In the fetus, the cerebral arterial supply has a double origin, with ventriculopetal cortical arteries and ventriculofugal basal arteries (LAUGIER 1986). Anastomoses are rare and the border and end zones are most susceptible to a fall in blood flow and perfusion pressure (Diagram 2.41).

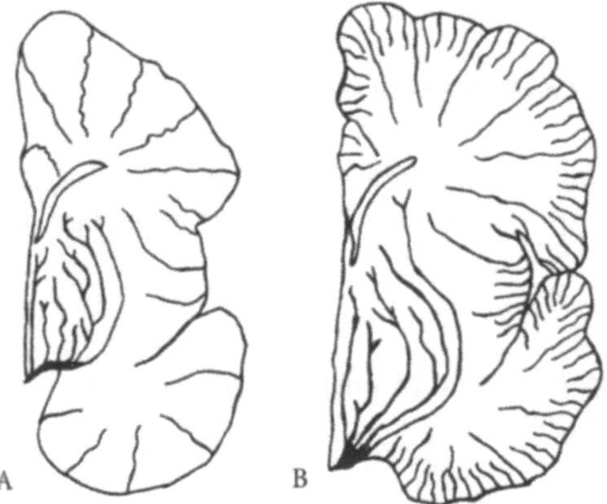

Diagram 2.41. Arterial architecture of the premature brain
A At the age of 24 weeks' gestation
B At the age of 34 weeks' gestation

Up to the 24th week of gestation, the basal arteries that feed the brain stem and basal ganglia are well developed, while the thin cortical arteries reach the periventricular region, which receives high blood flow.

From 28 to 32 weeks, blood flow increases in the cerebral cortex from the cortical arteries; long penetrators develop and supply the deep white matter and short penetrators feed the gray matter and subcortical white matter (VOLPE 1997). At 32 weeks, the ratio of blood flow is inverted.

These changes correlate with the metabolic activity of the different cerebral regions: after the phase of cell proliferation in the subependymal area, neuronal migration toward the cortex ends between 28 and 32 weeks and glial multiplication and dendritic development take place in the cortex, explaining the inverted distribution of blood flow.

Hemodynamic assessment of fetal cerebral arteries is developing at present (CONNORS 1992; MAESEL 1994; MARI 1995; NOORDAM 1994; VEILLE 1993; WLADIMIROFF 1987). Pulsed Doppler recording of fetal vessels, guided by color Doppler (FORTUNATO 1996; POOH 1996), seems to be easy for trained examiners.

2.2.1.2
Cerebral Autoregulation

Cerebral blood flow is regulated through an autonomous system that maintains a constant blood flow and avoids transmitting changes in systemic blood pressure to the brain; such changes are especially intense during the perinatal period. This constancy of CBF results from arteriolar vasoconstriction in response to increased perfusion pressure and vasodilatation in response to decreased perfusion pressure. In the human neonate, this mechanism of autoregulation is operative (PANERAI 1996) and easy to demonstrate. The response of a healthy newborn to arousal maneuvers such as skin stimulation includes an increased heart rate and changes in CBF: the diastolic and mean velocities increase immediately, while the systolic component remains unchanged. As a consequence, the RI decreases, more gradually. After the end of stimulation, diastolic and mean velocities return to normal values (Fig. 2.63).

Thus, in the normal newborn, there is a prompt hemodynamic adaptation to any stimulation. In a routine pulsed Doppler investigation, these changes are often observed, for example in the presence of bradycardia (Fig. 2.64).

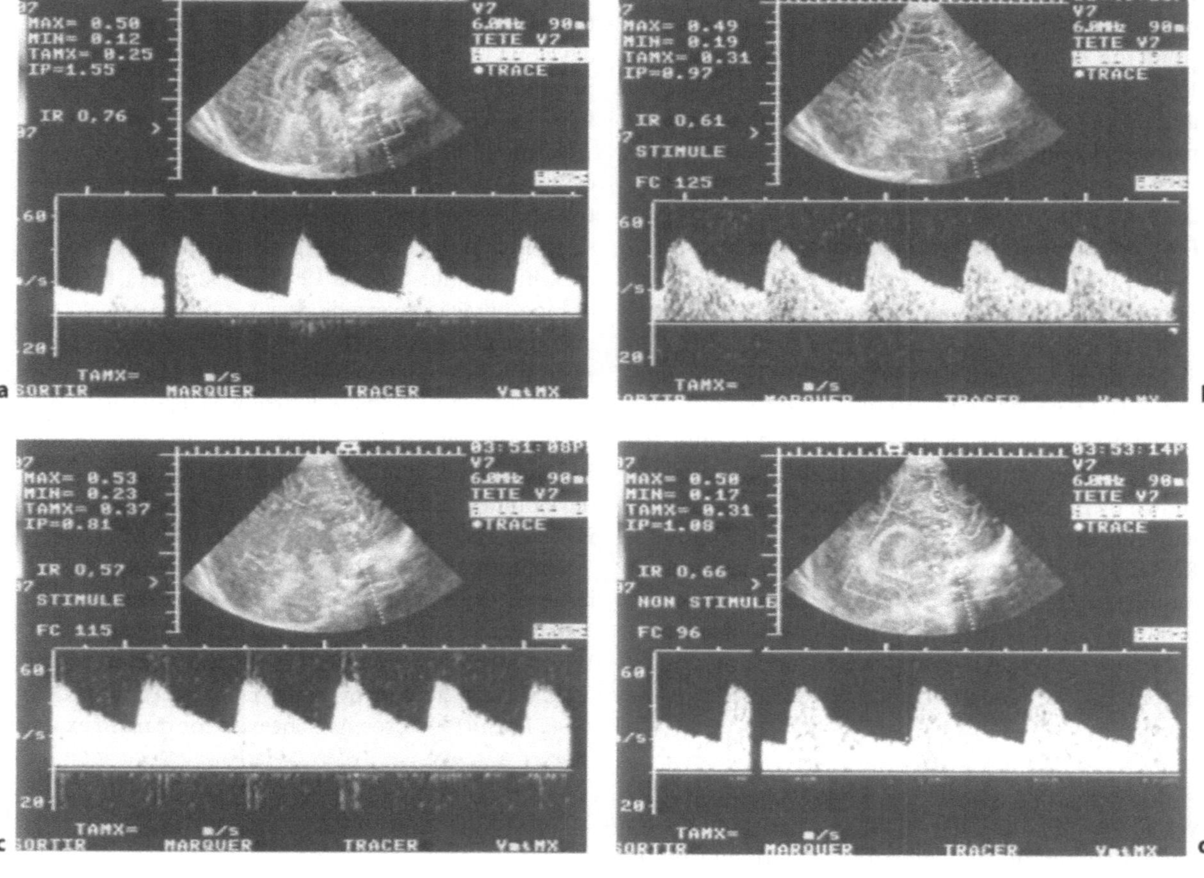

Fig. 2.63a–d. Twin gestation. A 7-day-old infant with normal brain ultrasonography. **a** Initial velocities (To) are normal: PSV=50 cm/s, EDV=12 cm/s, TAV=25 cm/s, RI=0.76. **b,c** After cutaneous stimulation, diastolic flow velocity significantly increases and RI decreases: at T1, EDV=19 cm/s, RI=0.61, and at T2, EDV=23 cm/s, RI=0.57. **d** After the end of stimulation (T3), velocities return to initial values: PSV=50 cm/s, EDV=17 cm/s, TAV=31 cm/s, RI=0.66. This course is characteristic of normal autoregulation. In parallel, heart rate increases from 100 (To) to 125 (T1) and 115 (T2) and normalizes at T3 (96)

These mechanisms of autoregulation appear to be fragile in the premature neonate. Experimental animal studies (HERNANDEZ 1979; PAPILE 1985) show that autoregulation is operative over a narrow range of arterial blood pressure. In the preterm lamb (PAPILE 1985), CBF remains unchanged, with mean carotid artery blood pressure ranging from 45 to 80 mmHg. Below and above these levels, CBF changes linearly with the arterial blood pressure, as a pressure-passive system. Knowledge of the clinical condition is essential during a pulsed Doppler investigation, since several clinical and biological circumstances may disturb this mechanism of regulation: ischemic or/and hemorrhagic damage is associated with hypotension or hypertension, hypoxia, or hypercapnia. A 20-min exposure to hypoxia impairs autoregulation, which does not recover until 7 h after restoration of normoxia (LOU 1979).

Assessment of cerebral autoregulation is important since this mechanism permits prompt adjustment of the CBF to perinatal injury (Fig. 2.65).

2.2.1.3
Changes in Cerebral Blood Flow

In the neonate, CBF follows several physiological changes (COUGHTREY 1997) that are important to consider.

2.2.1.3.1
Circulatory Adaptation from Fetus to Newborn
(MEERMAN 1990)

● Plethysmographic techniques have shown a sharp decrease in CBF in the first hours after delivery (COOKE 1979): in 3 h, CBF falls from 59 to 32 ml/min per 100 g (mean values). This has been widely con-

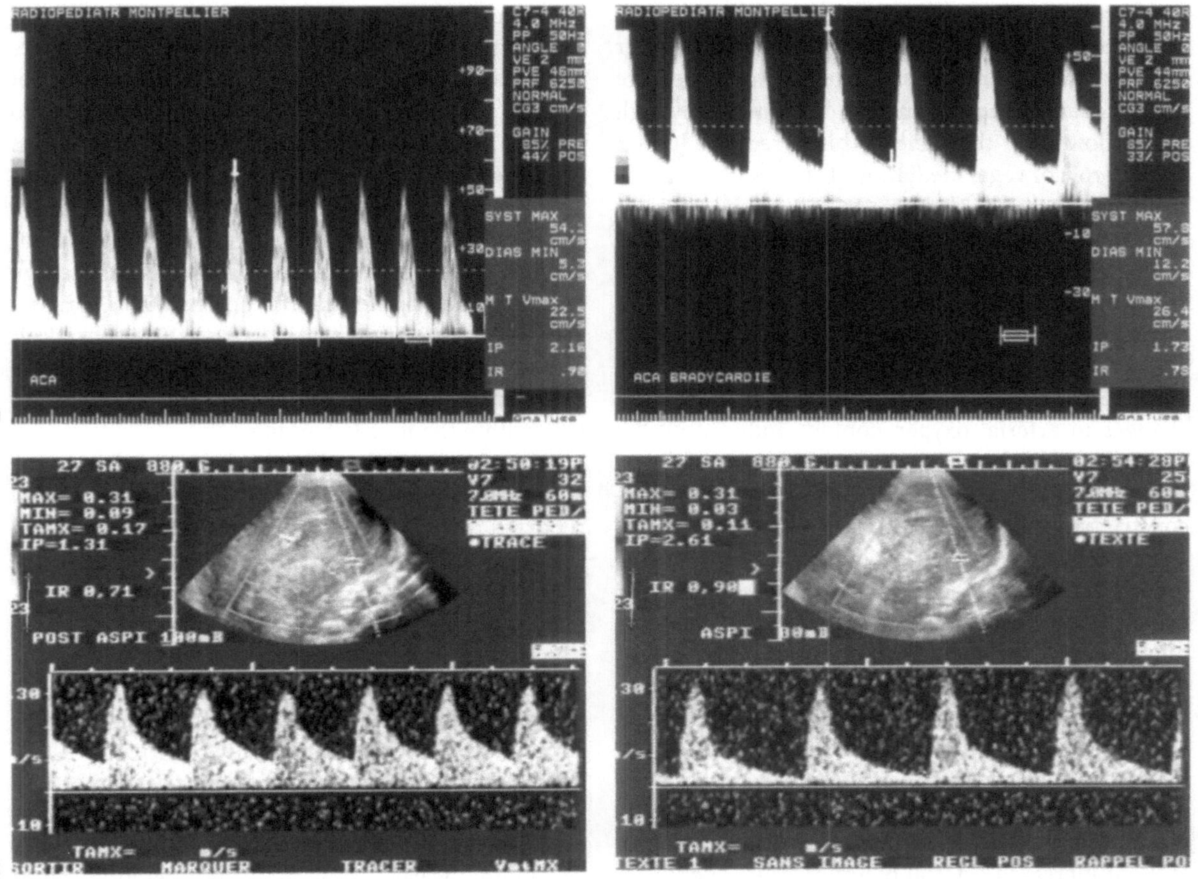

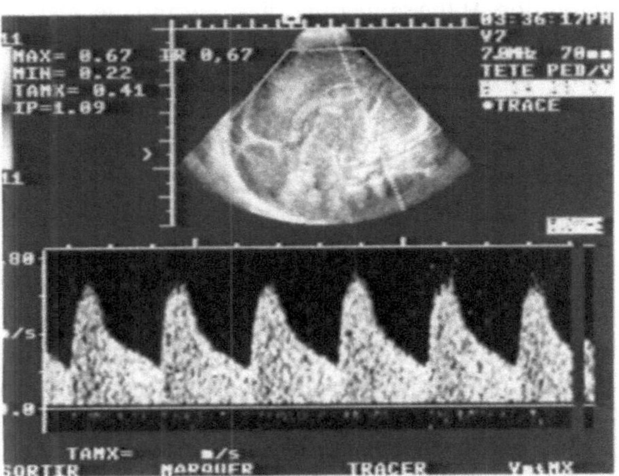

Fig. 2.64. a,b A 32-weeks' gestation infant. Normal spectrum in the anterior cerebral artery (a). Bradycardia occurred, prompting efficient hemodynamic adaptation with increase in the diastolic component (b). c,d A preterm infant with severe neurological distress and ischemic parenchymal lesion. Normal spectrum in the anterior cerebral artery (c). Bradycardia occurred during tracheal suctioning. The decrease in the diastolic component (EDV: 3 cm/s) shows loss of autoregulation (d)

firmed by neonatal pulsed Doppler investigations (CONNORS 1992; IPSIROGLU 1993; JORCH 1993; KEMPLEY 1996; MAESEL 1994; SONESSON 1987; WINBERG 1990). JORCH (1993) recorded blood flow velocity in the anterior cerebral artery in 16 nonasphyxiated, ventilated, very immature infants at five time intervals up to 20 min after birth and reported a transitory increase in both systolic and end-diastolic velocities (from 29 to 35 and from 1 to 10 cm/s respectively) during the first 5 min after birth.

MAESEL (1994) observed high systolic (67.2±13 cm/s), diastolic (26.3±10 cm/s), and mean (44±10 cm/s) velocities, and a low pulsatility index (1.06) immediately after birth, in the full-term newborn. During the first hour, vascular resistance rose significantly (pulsatility index increased from 1.06 to 1.52).

These publications confirm the previous demonstration by SONESSON (1987), who assessed intracranial blood flow velocity in 20 healthy term

Fig. 2.65. A preterm infant: abrupt desaturation with stable arterial blood pressure. Doppler examination was performed 10 s later and showed vasodilatation (EDV=22 cm/s, RI=0.67). The vascular response of the brain to hypoxia is immediate. The Doppler spectrum returned to normal after 2 min

newborns, using an undisclosed methodology. Arterial velocities decreased during the first 30 min after birth, whereas heart rate and arterial blood pressure did not change. The explanation of the relatively high blood flow near the time of birth remains under debate [role of vagal mediation (PURVES 1969), moderate increase in arterial PCO_2 levels], but it represents a striking adaptive mechanism to extrauterine life: the high flow may provide a margin of safety for cerebral metabolic needs during the period of adaptation to birth (GRAY 1983; VAN BEL 1989). The gradual increase in vascular resistance (LEY 1992; MAESEL 1994; SONESSON 1987) may result from changes in arterial oxygen content, induced by the first breaths of the newborn. Increased arterial PO_2 and decreased arterial PCO_2 explain cerebral vasoconstriction (LUCAS 1970; PARKER 1966).

From 30 min to 2 h of life, SONESSON (1987) reported that systolic velocity increase, diastolic velocity decrease, and mean velocity remains unchanged; simultaneously, heart rate and mean and diastolic arterial blood pressure decrease. Patent ductus arteriosus is known to reduce diastolic cerebral velocity, probably by ductal vascular steal. The stability of the mean velocity suggests a compensatory diminution of intracranial vascular resistance or cardiac output volume, while increased systolic velocity without increased arterial blood pressure suggests a decrease in downstream cerebral vascular resistances.

From 2 to 72 h of life, mean velocity does not change, while systolic and end-diastolic velocities change in opposite directions: there is decreased peak-systolic amplitude and increased end-diastolic amplitude. At the same time, diastolic and mean arterial blood pressure (and, to a lesser degree, systolic blood pressure) increase. This may be due to the decreased ductal shunt, as suggested by the rise in cerebral end-diastolic velocity and diastolic blood pressure (SONESSON 1987).

After the third day of life, all authors (BATTON 1992; DEEG 1989; HAYASCHI 1992; HORGAN 1989; KOJO 1996; KUBOTA 1991; LOW 1993; MINARIK 1993; YOSHIDA 1991) observed a gradual increase in systolic and diastolic velocities. These hemodynamic changes depend on multiple factors and are not completely clear; the increase in arterial blood pressure, ductal closure, and increase in cerebral metabolism and blood flow probably play a large role.

These works demonstrate that a full-term newborn, after a period of adjustment of cerebral perfusion during the neonatal phase of circulatory transition, is able to maintain a constant CBF.

● Radioactive xenon clearance (GREISEN 1984) and plethysmographic techniques (COOKE 1979; LEAHY 1979) have been used to determine normal values of CBF. In the full-term newborn, it ranges from 40 to 60 ml/100g per minute, but in the preterm newborn it is lower, ranging from 10 to 20 ml/100 g per minute. This suggests gradual maturation of CBF regulation (ARCHER 1985; BORGH 1998; CALVERT 1988). Moreover, CBF in neonates who are small for gestational age is significantly higher than in infants with appropriate intrauterine growth (BAENZIGER 1994; LEY 1992; YOSHIDA 1991). Probably, the prolonged intrauterine stress with chronic hypoxia leads to an increase in CBF within the first 36 h of life.

Several factors or events, such as sex, sleep state, and feeding, also affect CBF. BAENZIGER (1994) reported that CBF in girls is significantly lower than in boys (11.5 ± 2.8 ml/100 mg per minute versus 14 ± 4.1 ml/100 mg per minute). A possible mechanism is related to differences in hormone concentrations between the two sexes.

Plethysmographic methods have been widely used to demonstrate the increase in CBF during active sleep (MUKTHAR 1982; REHAN 1996; RAHILLY 1980). FERRARRI (1993) described cyclical variations of CBF velocities during sleep (2–6 cycles/min), which have a greater amplitude during quiet sleep, and relate to vasomotor waves resulting from cerebral autoregulation.

NELLE (1997) showed in 14 neonates that bolus tube feeding can decrease cerebral perfusion (mean velocity changes from 37 cm/s before feeding to 33 cm/s after feeding), despite unchanged blood pressure and oxygen saturation.

Finally, COWAN (1985) has shown interference between CBF and head position. Great variations in superior sagittal sinus velocity correlated with rotation of the head (ANTHONY 1993, 1991).

2.2.1.3.2
Dependence of Regulation on Blood Gas Concentration

One of the strongest regulators of CBF is arterial PCO_2 (GREISEN 1987; LOU 1978; PRYDS 1989, 1990; YAMASHITA 1991), with hypercapnia resulting in cerebral vasodilatation. Marked hypercapnia may induce a pressure-passive state with CBF in linear correlation to systemic blood pressure. GREISEN (1985) observed an increase in CBF of 8.6% per 1 mmHg increase in $PaCO_2$.

Hypoxemia is also a strong vasodilator (Fig. 2.66), while an increase in oxygen tension correlates with decreased CBF velocities, especially in preterm

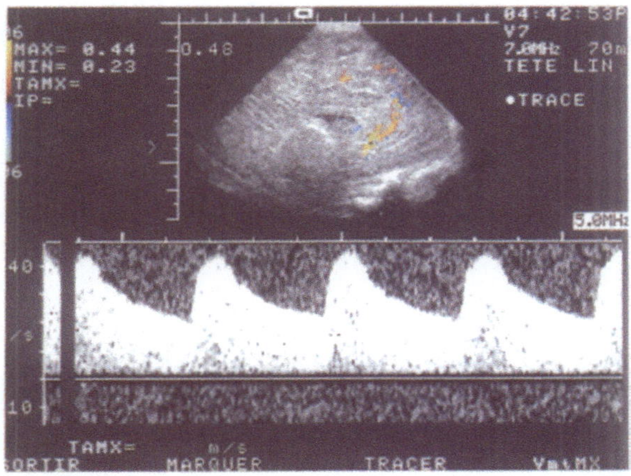

Fig. 2.66. A 34-weeks' preterm infant with persistent hypoxia. Vasodilatation with EDV=23 cm/s, RI=0.48. Rapid death ensued

infants (MOCHALOVA 1983; NIJIMA 1988). The magnitude of the vasodilatory response varies in brain regions, proportionally to their metabolic levels, which decrease from the brain stem to the cerebellum to the cerebral hemispheres (YOUNKIN 1988).

All these factors (arterial blood pressure, blood gas concentration) influence CBF through local mediators (BERNE 1982). More than arterial pH, extracellular pH seems to be an important factor. In the same way, the vasodilating effect of carbon dioxide probably relates to the increase in perivascular hydrogen ion concentration (LOU 1978). Adenosine is currently considered a main regulator of CBF, since it is released in cases where CBF is increased, showing coupling of blood flow and metabolic activity.

Finally, the role of the autonomous neurological system remains unclear: we know only that stimulation of the sympathetic system, which induces vasoconstriction and decreased CBF, plays a protective role against blood pressure changes and hypercapnia.

2.2.1.3.3
Possible Effect of Several Pharmacologic Agents on Cerebral Resistive Index and Blood Flow Velocities

Doppler techniques have demonstrated that several treatments currently used in neonatal intensive care units affect CBF.

- The potential danger of intravenously administered indomethacin has been reported (AUSTIN 1992; CABANAS 1997; EDWARDS 1990; HAMMERMAN 1995; MOSCA 1997; VARVARIGOU 1996; YANOWITZ 1998): it induces a significant reduction in CBF, ranging from 25% to 60% during the first 2 h after infusion. Pulsed Doppler imaging shows

well this cerebral vasoconstriction after administration of indomethacin, probably caused by increased downstream vascular resistance. It is important to know this before interpreting a spectral analysis curve. This medication should be used with caution in very-low-birth-weight premature babies with patent ductus arteriosus (KRESCH 1988; TAMMELLA 1999). This is leading to replacement of indomethacin by ibuprofen (VARVARIGOU 1996), which appears to be devoid of cerebral vascular effects.

- Vasoconstriction is known to be induced by aminophylline, frequently used in preterm infants with apneic spells (GOVAN 1995; McDONNELL 1992; PRYDS 1991).

- The beneficial effect of pancuronium has been demonstrated (CHEMTOB 1987; PERLMAN 1985) in the premature infant with a fluctuating spectral analysis curve: curarization prevents the risk of intraventricular hemorrhage by regularizing blood pressure and CBF velocities (PERLMAN 1985; VEYRAC 1994).

- Intravenous injection of thiopental is followed by a prompt moderate decrease in the middle cerebral artery velocity (DE BRAY 1993), while caffeine seems not to affect blood flow velocity in the premature infant (SALIBA 1989).

- Several other procedures may influence CBF, such as neonatal transfusion, exogenous surfactant administration, phototherapy, and mechanical ventilation.

Pulsed Doppler imaging, performed in 11 preterm infants with anemia, showed that flow velocities decrease significantly after transfusion because of increased cerebral vascular resistance and blood viscosity (RAMAEKERS 1988, 1992; ROSENKRANZ 1982).

Administration of surfactant (SCHIPPER 1997) induces a significant drop in mean arterial blood pressure and CBF.

BENDERS (1998) reported a significant increase in mean CBF velocities after phototherapy in 22 preterm infants.

Finally, BAENZIGER (1994) observed, in 60 preterm newborns, that CBF in those requiring mechanical ventilation was significantly lower than in those who were spontaneously breathing (11.5 ±3.7 ml/ 100 g per minute, versus 14.2±3.1 ml/100 g per minute).

2.2.1.3.4
Conclusion

Clinical history and findings, biological parameters, and therapeutic procedures should be known for a reliable interpretation of any hemodynamic cerebral investigation. Several criteria should be checked before judging an examination as normal:

- Normal stable arterial blood pressure
- Normal biological parameters (pH, PaO_2, $PaCO_2$)
- Appropriate cerebral autoregulation
- Known gestational and postnatal ages
- Normal heart function and closed ductus arteriosus
- Finally, any treatment that might change CBF should be noted.

If these conditions are respected, the interpretation of a spectral analysis curve is reliable and of maximum value. If not, an abnormal Doppler recording provides dubious information.

2.2.2
Doppler Technology: How to Use It

In the absence of color Doppler, pulsed Doppler is always difficult to analyze, due to the small size of brain arteries and veins. In all anatomical (Fig. 2.67) and radiological (Fig. 2.68) studies, brain arteries are less than 2 mm in diameter. In the fetus, it is impossible to recognize cerebral vessels without color Doppler.

The morphological examination may only detect pulsatile beats in real-time ultrasonography since the arterial lumen cannot be seen. The circle of Willis, and anterior cerebral, pericallosal, middle cerebral, posterior cerebral, and basilar arteries (Fig. 2.15) may be located. Other vessels, such as the lenticu-

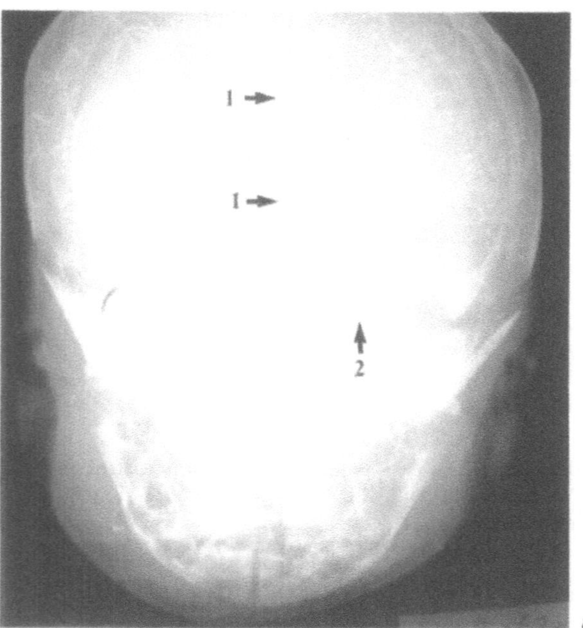

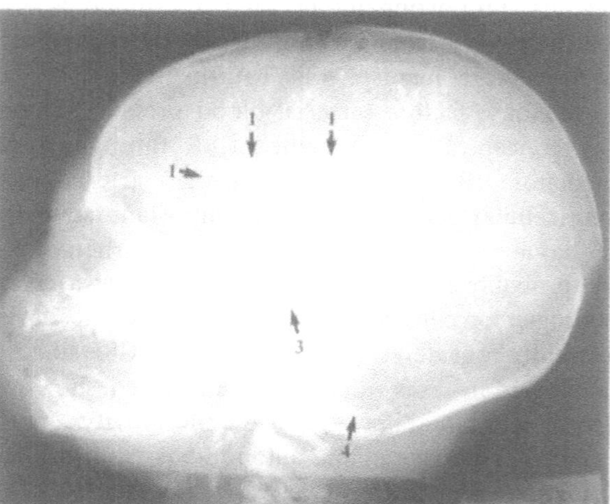

Fig. 2.68a,b. Postmortem skull X-rays in a term newborn after injection of mixed gelatin, barium, and colored mineral powder. The carotid system, circle of Willis, and facial arteries were injected. The thinness of the cerebral vessels is obvious: anterior cerebral artery (*1*), middle cerebral artery (*2*), posterior cerebral artery (*3*), middle cerebellar artery (*4*). Secondary and tertiary arteries constitute a hairy network. Note the excellent visualization of the lingual and ophtalmic arteries

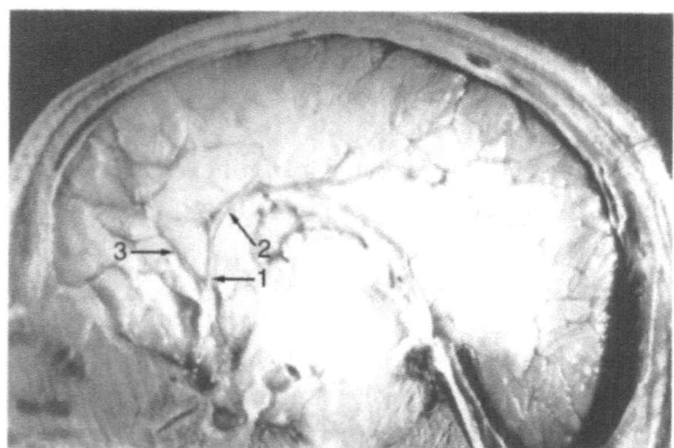

Fig. 2.67. Postmortem sagittal plane of the brain in a term newborn, after injection of mixed gelatin, barium, and colored mineral powder. Visualization of the anterior cerebral artery (1), the pericallosal artery (2), and the callosomarginal artery (3). These vessels are obviously difficult to locate and assess by pulsed Doppler since they do not exceed 1 or 2 mm in size

lostriate and choroidal arteries, cannot be depicted despite their great functional importance. The venous system is impossible to assess, because it is nonpulsating and too small, except for the superior sagittal sinus.

All this emphasizes the importance of color Doppler imaging, which alone enables a reliable, accurate hemodynamic investigation (MITCHELL 1989; OHLSSON 1991; TATSUNO 1990; TAYLOR 1990; WONG 1989).

Although determination of the resistive and pulsatility indices and velocities is technically easy, there are two conditions:

● Measurement of a cerebral flow velocity requires the use of color imaging (DEEG 1989; WINKLER 1989, 1990). The probe is placed with an ideal angle axis, on the anterior cerebral artery before the third ventricle, on the basilar artery before the brain stem, or on the internal carotid artery above the sella turcica (Fig. 2.69).

The veins of the deep venous system also have a favorable orientation, especially the straight sinus and internal cerebral veins (Fig. 2.70).

For these vessels the angle axis is near zero and may be ignored.

The best approach may be chosen. Basilar artery, anterior cerebral artery, internal carotid artery, inter-

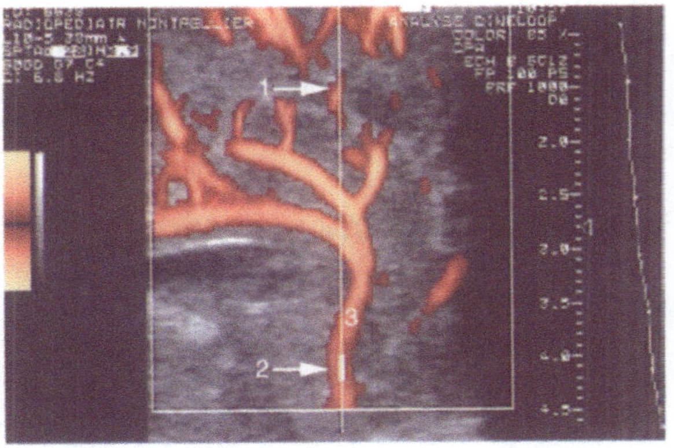

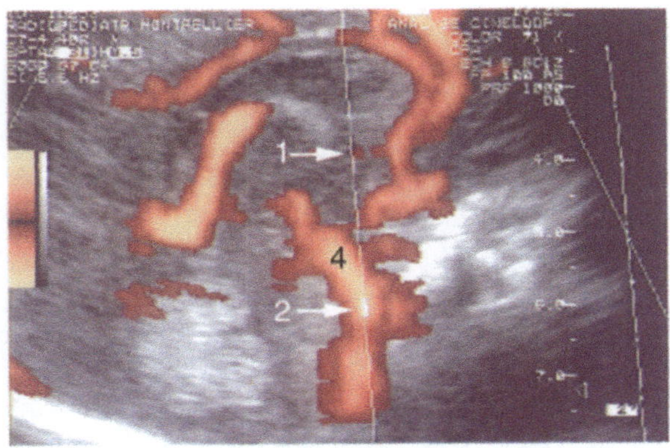

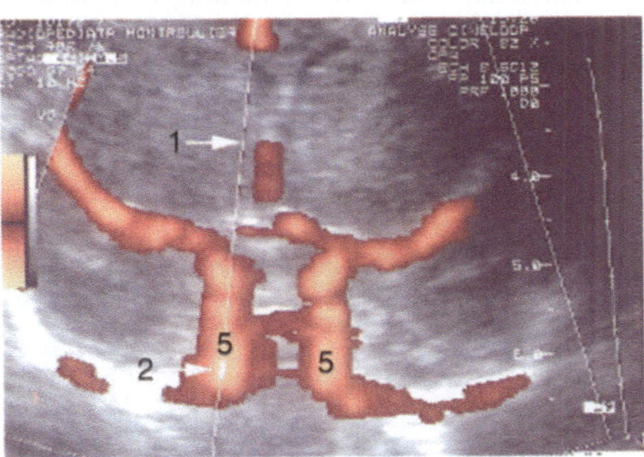

Fig. 2.69. Color Doppler location of the anterior cerebral artery (a), basilar artery (b), and internal carotid artery (c). For these three vessels, the Doppler axis (1) and sample volume (2) are ideally positioned in the vessel. An angle correction is useless and the recorded velocities are absolute velocities. 3 Anterior cerebral artery, 4 basilar artery, 5 internal carotid artery

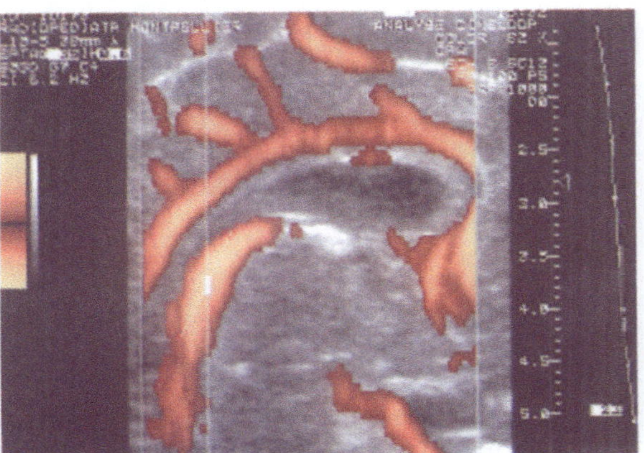

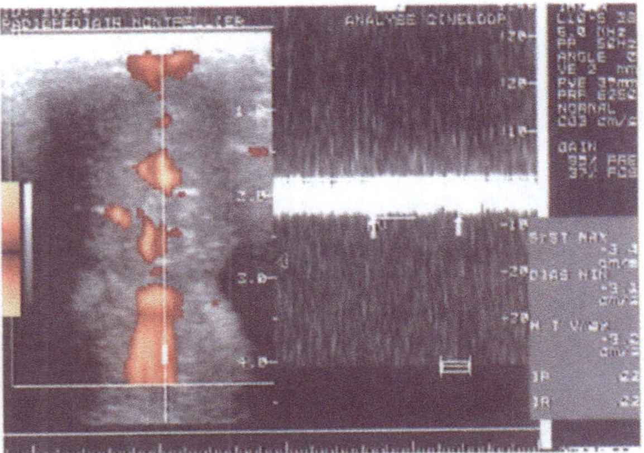

Fig. 2.70. a Doppler recording of the internal cerebral vein in a 34-weeks' gestation infant. The angle axis is 20° and may be ignored: mean velocity is 7 cm/s without angle correction and 7.2 cm/s with correction: the difference is minimal. b The angle axis may be avoided with a posterior oblique frontal plane: mean velocity is 8 cm/s

nal cerebral vein, and straight sinus are well depicted through the anterior fontanelle. Middle cerebral artery, posterior cerebral artery, cerebellar artery, and basilar vein are better insonated through the transcranial access (Fig. 2.71).

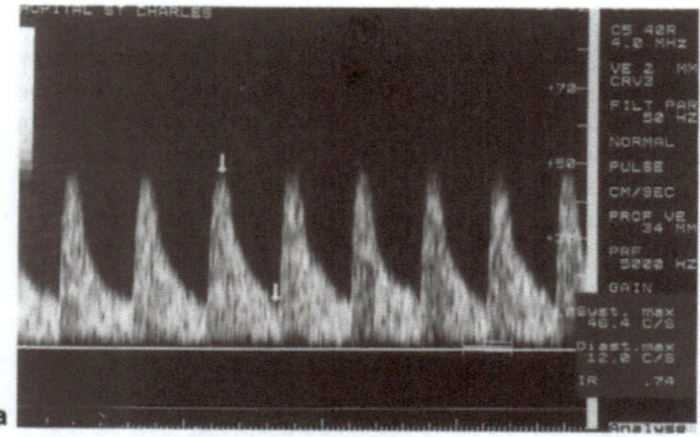

Fig. 2.71. Pulsed Doppler evaluation of the middle cerebral artery requires a transtemporal approach: the beam axis and vessel axis are the same

● Velocities should be calculated after angle correction. If the angle axis is near the ideal (less than 30°) the error is mild (Fig. 2.72).
If it is far from the ideal, the error is major and angle correction should be remembered, as is the case for the superior sagittal sinus (Fig. 2.73). This is shown by the multiple mistakes encountered in several publications (HORGAN 1989). A cerebral blood flow velocity cannot be validated if the angle axis or angle correction is not noted and if it is not measured on color Doppler.

In conclusion, optimal technical conditions are required to obtain reliable values of flow velocities.

2.2.2.1
Pulsed Doppler: Material and Methods

Validation of normal values is required prior to any interpretation. In our department, we carried out measurements in 491 infants, divided into age groups until fontanellar closure: 72 neonates were less than 3 days old; of the remaining 419, 218 were preterm infants (from 32 weeks' gestation), 201 were full-term newborns and infants up to 8 months old (Table 2.1).

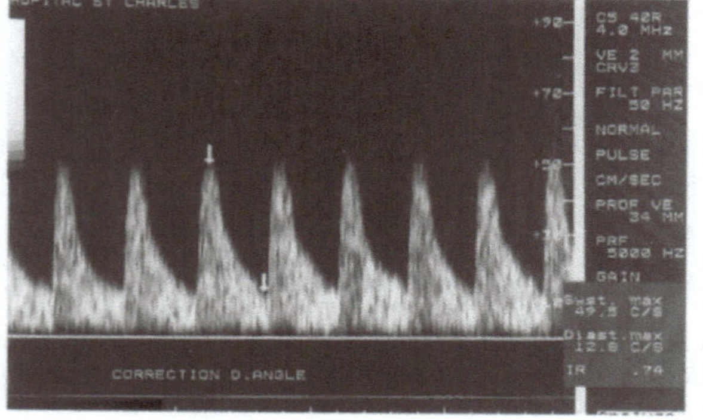

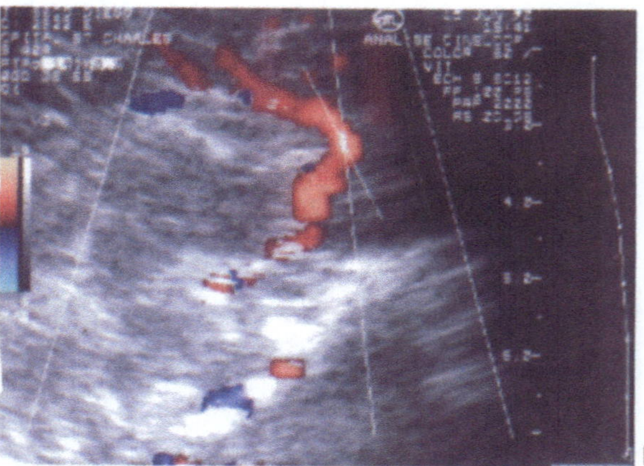

Fig. 2.72a–c. Measurement of velocities of the pericallosal artery. a Without angle correction: PSV=46.4 cm/s, EDV=12 cm/s, RI=0.74. b,c After angle correction (21°): PSV=49.5 cm/s, EDV=12.6 cm/s, RI=0.74. When the angle axis is less than 30°, recorded velocities are not very different from absolute velocities

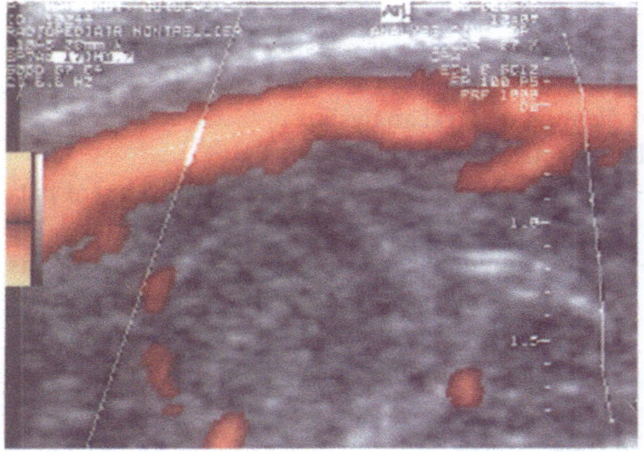

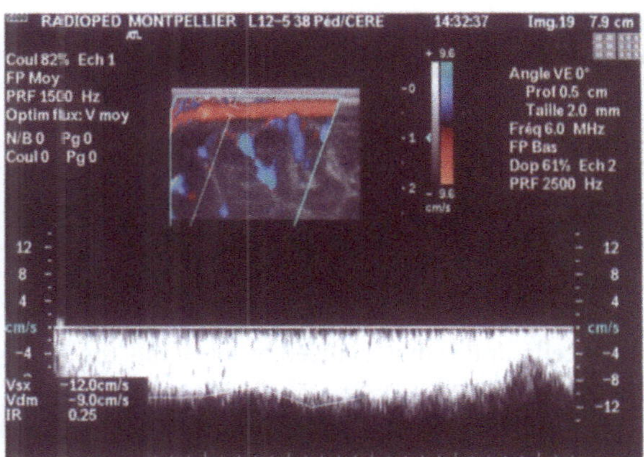

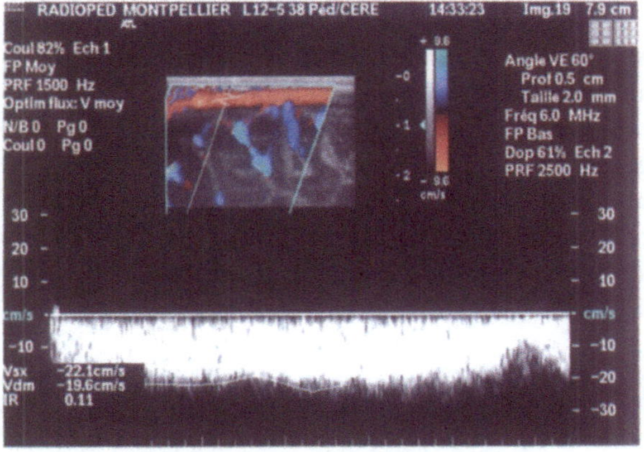

Fig. 2.73a–c. Measurement of velocities of the superior sagittal sinus. **a** Whatever the technique of examination, the angle axis is always great (60°). **b** Without correction, mean velocity is 10.5 cm/s. **c** After correction, the velocity is 21 cm/s. The difference is major: when the angle axis is great, any measure of blood velocity requires an angle correction

Table 2.1. 419 infants

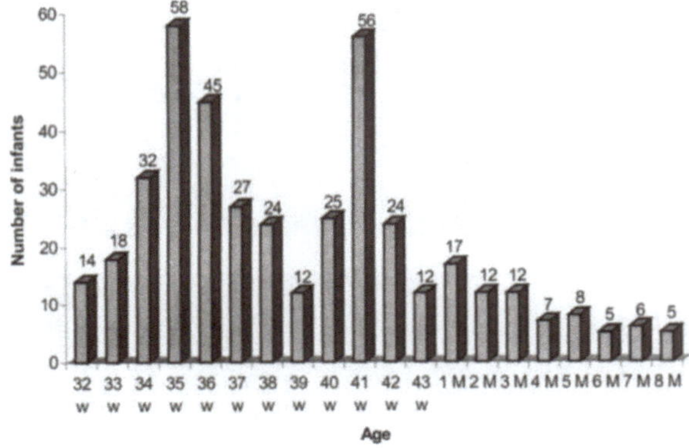

The selection criteria were:
- Gestational age must be determined.
- Clinical examination and heart function must be normal.
- There must be no treatment that might affect cerebral hemodynamics.
- Arterial blood pressure must be normal.
- Biological parameters must be normal, especially $PaCO_2$, PaO_2, and pH.

Four different equipments were used, with color and pulsed Doppler: Acuson, ATL UM9HDI, ATL 3000, ATL 5000.

The investigation protocol was standardized in the 491 infants:
- For each patient, anterior cerebral artery, basilar artery, internal carotid artery, lenticulostriate artery, internal cerebral vein, straight sinus, and superior sagittal sinus were depicted.
- Each vessel was first located on color imaging; a correct beam axis and sample volume were placed and a spectral analysis was obtained. All the examinations were performed through the anterior fontanelle and angle correction was always done when required.
- On the Doppler spectrum the following were measured: peak-systolic velocity (PSV), end-diastolic velocity (EDV), time-average velocity (TAV), resistive index (RI), and pulsatility index (PI) on the arteries, time-average velocity on the veins.

2.2.2.2
Pulsed Doppler: Results

2.2.2.2.1
Spectral Analysis Curves

Doppler velocimetry is based on the retrodiffusion of sound waves from moving red blood cells that induce a frequency shift – the Doppler effect. This differential in frequency is proportional to the velocity of the blood cells, and is materialized by a tracing, the spectral analysis curve.

● Arterial spectral analysis
The shape of an arterial tracing depends on the distal vascular resistance. In normal brain, this resistance is low enough to ensure a forward diastolic flow in cerebral arteries. With stable arterial blood pressure, the amplitude of the diastolic component relates to the amplitude of distal circulatory resistances (BEJAR 1982).

The spectral analysis provides information on the distribution of velocities within the vessel; the Doppler spectrum shows a rapid ascending wave up to the peak-systolic frequency followed by a gentle slope down to the end-diastolic frequency (Fig. 2.74).

This pattern characterizes all the cerebral arteries. However, some physiological variations are observed, depending on:
- What patient is studied: a preterm newborn, a neonate with intrauterine growth retardation, a full-term newborn, or an infant (RAJU 1989; VAN DE BOR 1990).
- The baby's age: velocities vary intensely during the adaptive phase of the first 3 days of life (SONESSON 1987).

- What artery is assessed: lenticulostriate arteries demonstrate a lower resistive index.

● Venous spectral analysis
The spectrum is often uniform:
- A continuous frequency is the most frequent pattern in the entire venous system (Fig. 2.75).
- Less frequent is a sinusoidal pattern, synchronous to arterial pulsations; this appearance may also be observed when artery and vein are included in the same sample volume (Fig. 2.76).

2.2.2.2.2
Arterial Velocities and Indices

● There is a progressive increase in peak-systolic and end-diastolic velocities from 32 weeks of gestation to 8 months of age, which evolves in parallel with gestational age and infant age. This augmentation is uniform and linear, but more pronounced in the anterior cerebral artery, internal carotid artery, and basilar artery from 43 weeks to 1 month of age. This is

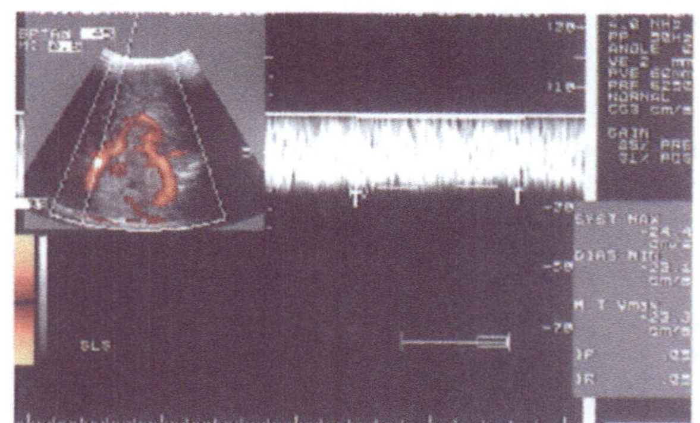

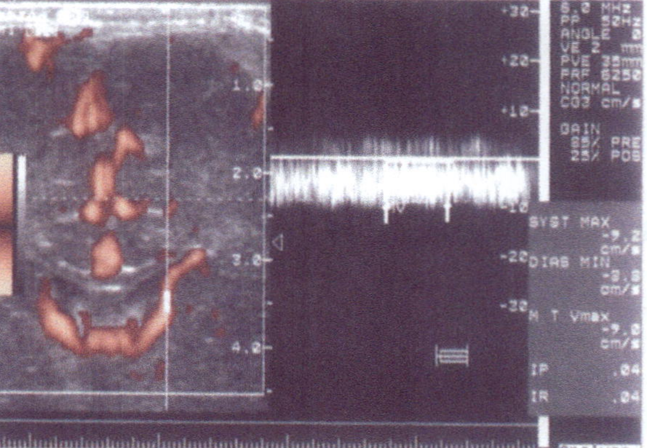

Fig. 2.75a,b. Doppler spectrum of the straight sinus (a) and terminal vein (b): continuous band-like aspect

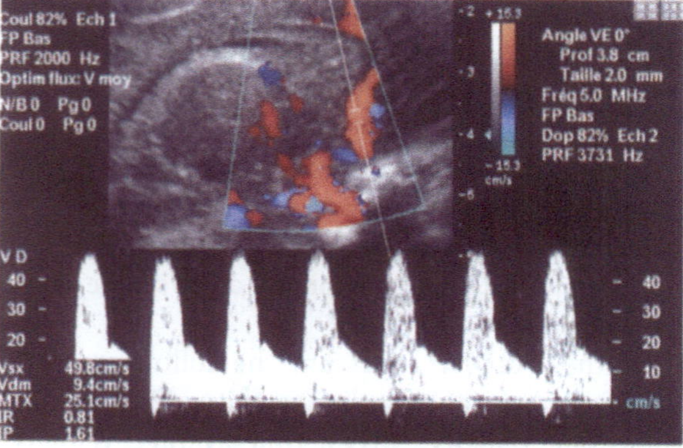

Fig. 2.74. Preterm infant, 5 days old. Characteristic waveform of the anterior cerebral artery. PSV=49.8 cm/s, EDV=9.4 cm/s, TAV=25.1 cm/s, RI=0.81, PI=1.61

well demonstrated by the mean results in each age group; for example, anterior cerebral artery velocities are: PSV=43.1 cm/s, EDV=9.8 cm/s, TAV=21.9 cm/s at 32 weeks gestation; they are moderately increased at 40 weeks' gestation and markedly higher at 6 months of age (Table 2.2)

- Velocities have different normal values according to the artery. The maximum peak-systolic velocity is observed in the internal carotid artery (Diagram 2.42), whereas the anterior cerebral artery (Diagram 2.43) and basilar artery (Diagram 2.44) show the same peak-systolic velocity. There is no difference in diastolic velocities between these three great arteries.
- Lenticulostriate arteries were studied in 147 infants from 32 weeks of gestation to 6 months of age. The waveform is characteristic: velocities are

lower than in the great cerebral arteries but the diastolic component is proportionally higher (Diagram 2.45).

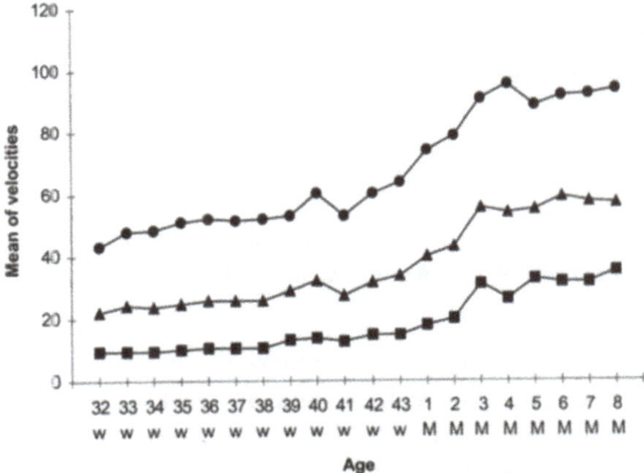

Diagram 2.42. Arterial velocities: internal carotid artery (419 infants). ●—● Peaksystolic velocity (PSV), ▲—▲ time-average velocity (TAV), ■—■ end-diastolic velocity (EDV). *w* Weeks, *M* months

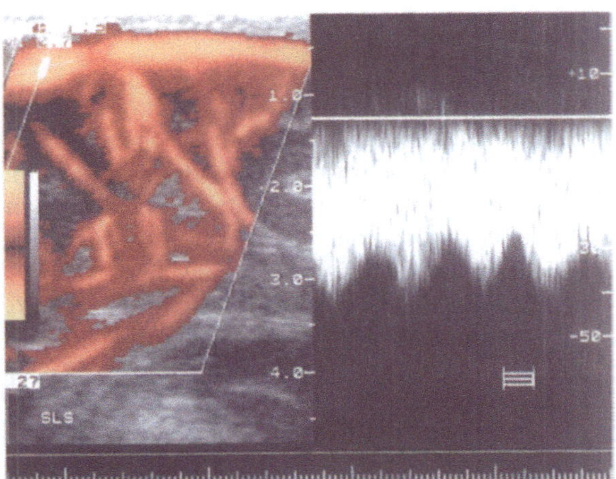

Fig. 2.76. A 1-month-old infant, showing characteristic sinusoidal pattern of the superior sagittal sinus. After angle correction, mean velocity is 31 cm/s

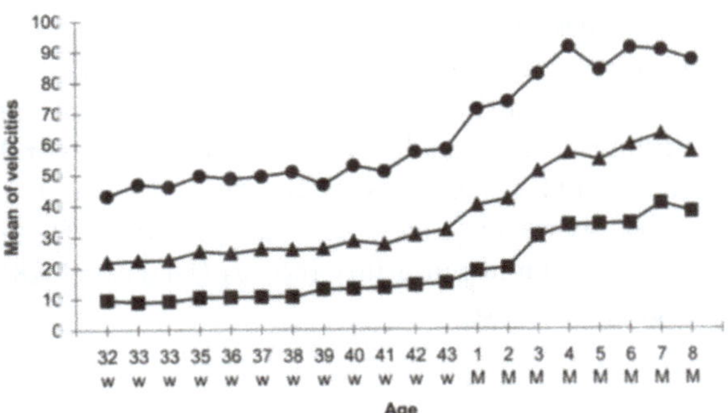

Diagram 2.43. Arterial velocities: anterior cerebral artery (419 infants). ●—● PSV, ▲—▲ TAV, ■—■ EDV

Table 2.2. Arterial velocities: increases in velocities evolve in parallel with the age of the infant

	Velocities	32 weeks	40 weeks	6 months
Anterior cerebral artery	PSV	43.1	52.9	91.2
	EDV	9.6	13.2	34.2
	TAV	21.9	28.7	59.7
Basilar artery	PSV	37.6	54.2	84.3
	EDV	8.2	13.0	31.3
	TAV	19.6	28.9	52.5
Internal carotid artery	PSV	43.3	60.2	92.1
	EDV	9.7	13.7	31.6
	TAV	22.2	31.9	59.2

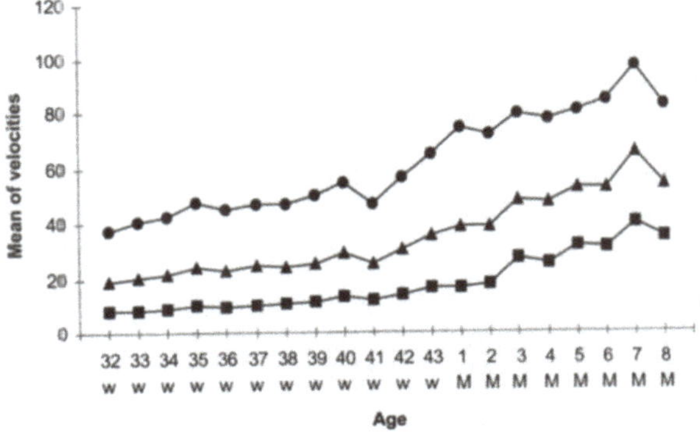

Diagram 2.44. Arterial velocities: basilar artery (419 infants). ●—● PSV, ▲—▲ TAV, ■—■ EDV

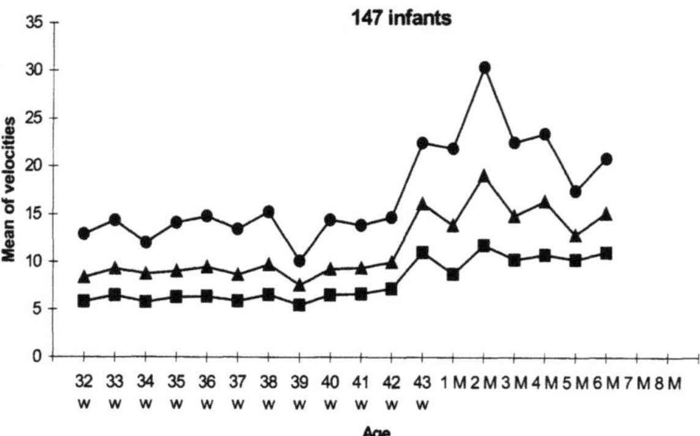

Diagram 2.45. Arterial velocities: lenticulostriate artery (147 infants). ●—● PSV, ▲—▲ TAV, ■—■ EDV

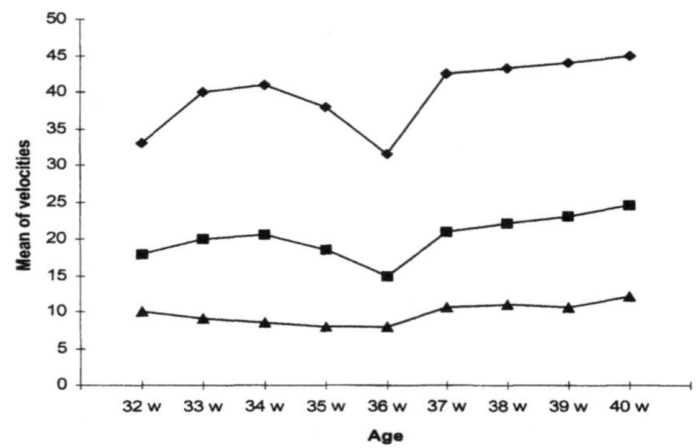

Diagram 2.46. Evolution of arterial velocities (72 newborns 3 days old or less). ◆—◆ PSV, ■—■ TAV, ▲—▲ EDV

- Finally, velocities were markedly lower in the 72 neonates (between 32 and 40 weeks' gestation) who were investigated during the first 3 days of life than in older infants (Diagram 2.46). This was observed in all cerebral arteries (Table 2.3).
- Resistive and pulsatility indices are obviously less informative than are velocities. From 32 to 43 weeks' gestation, their normal values remain unchanged. For example, in the internal carotid artery, resistive index is 0.77 at 32 weeks and 0.76 at 43 weeks, while the velocities are: PSV=43 cm/s, EDV=9.6 cm/s at 32 weeks and PSV=63.8 cm/s, EDV=14.5 cm/s at 43 weeks (Table 2.4). The same findings were made in the anterior cerebral (Diagram 2.47) and basilar arteries.
- After 43 weeks (Table 2.5), the resistive (Diagram 2.47) and pulsatility indices (Diagram 2.48) markedly decrease.

- Resistive and pulsatility indices are lower in the lenticulostriate arteries (0.60 and 0.60–1 respectively) because of their high diastolic component (Diagrams 2.47, 2.48).

2.2.2.2.3
Venous Velocities

- From a hemodynamic point of view, the most representative vessel is the internal cerebral vein. Velocities gradually moderately increase from 32 weeks' gestation to 8 months of age (Diagram 2.49). Mean values evolve from 7.2 cm/s at 32 weeks, to 9.8 cm/s at 40 weeks and 15.9 cm/s at 8 months of age. Before 3 days of life are reached, venous velocities are lower (Diagram 2.50).

Table 2.3. Internal carotid artery velocities; 72 newborns (3 days old or less)

	Velocities	32 weeks	34 weeks	38 weeks	40 weeks
Internal carotid artery	PSV	33.1	41.1	43.6	45.2
	EDV	10.4	9.4	11.5	11.9
	TAV	18	20.4	22.2	24.3
Anterior cerebral artery	PSV	30.8	37.5	39	39.5
	EDV	10.5	9.3	10.8	11.4
	TAV	16.9	20	20.8	21.4
Basilar artery	PSV	27.1	33.7	40.7	42
	EDV	8.2	8.3	12.9	11.4
	TAV	15.3	16.9	22.4	22.6
Lenticulostriate artery	PSV	11.5	11.6	13.8	11.9
	EDV	5.8	5.7	7.3	6.5
	TAV	8.2	7.9	9.8	8.5

Table 2.4. Resistive index and velocities in the internal cerebral artery

	32 weeks	43 weeks
Resistive index	0.77	0.76
Velocities		
PSV	43.1	63.8
EDV	9.6	14.5
TAV	21.9	33.4

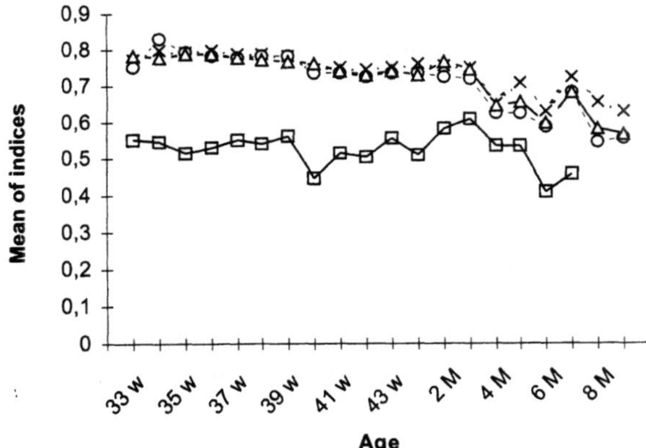

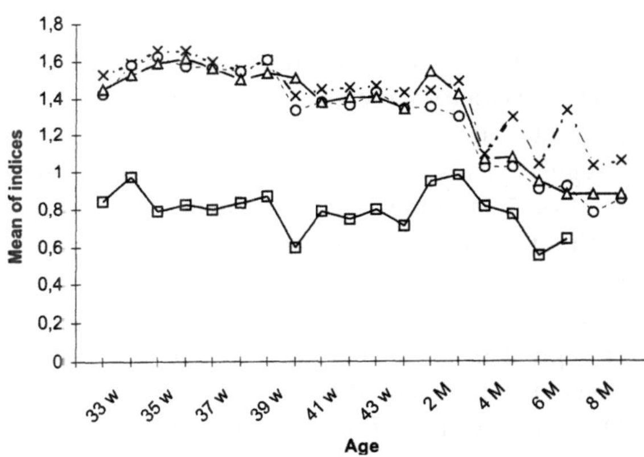

Diagram 2.47. Resistive index (419 infants). **X—X** Internal carotid artery, ○—○ anterior cerebral artery, △—△ basilar artery, □—□ Lenticulostriate artery

Diagram 2.48. Pulsatility index (419 infants). **X—X** Internal carotid artery, ○—○ anterior cerebral artery, △—△ basilar artery, □—□ Lenticulostriate artery

Table 2.5. Resistive index and pulsatility index: evolution with age

		32 weeks	40 weeks	43 weeks	7 months
Resistive index	Internal carotid artery	0.77	0.74	0.76	0.66
	Basilar artery	0.78	0.76	0.74	0.58
	Anterior cerebral artery	0.75	0.74	0.74	0.55
	Lenticulostriate artery	0.55	0.51	0.51	0.46
Pulsatility index	Internal carotid artery	1.53	1.41	1.46	1.04
	Basilar artery	1.44	1.38	1.34	0.87
	Anterior cerebral artery	1.42	1.38	1.34	0.78
	Lenticulostriate artery	0.84	0.79	0.71	0.64

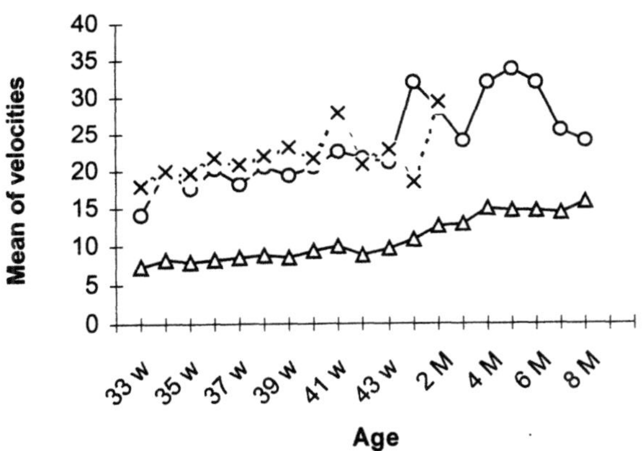

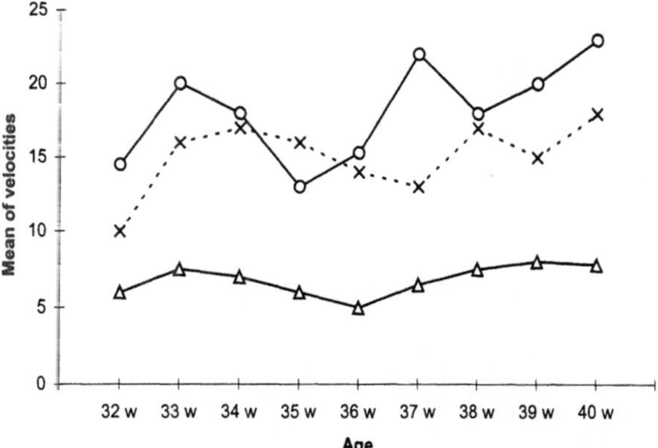

Diagram 2.49. Cerebral veins and sinuses (419 infants). △—△ Internal cerebral vein, ○—○ superior sagittal sinus, **X—X** straight sinus

Diagram 2.50. Evolution of venous velocities (72 newborns, 3 days old or less). ○—○ Superior sagittal sinus, **X—X** straight sinus, △—△ internal cerebral veins

– These results contrast with those in the straight sinus and superior sagittal sinus. In the 419 infants, velocities increased with gestational and postnatal age. However, the mean values show irregular peaks, since velocities may be multiplied by 2 or 3 in some normal neonates and infants without any obvious explanation (resting infants, sitting in same posture as others); they often gradually return to normal if the examination is long enough (Fig. 2.77). There may exist cyclical variations in sinusal velocities.

Moreover, straight sinus may often not be investigated later than at 1 month of life, because it is only exceptionally visualized by color imaging after this age.

In the 72 patients less than 3 days old, velocities were obviously lower (Diagram 2.50).

2.2.2.3
Pulsed Doppler: Discussion

Which measure should be preferred: resistive index or blood velocities?

The value of the pulsatility and resistive indices have been known for many years, as have as their inadequacies; the determination of velocities offers multiple potentialities but is relatively recent.

2.2.2.3.1
Resistive Index

● The resistive index was the first available information obtained by cerebral Doppler US. Its reproducibility and advantages have been demonstrated, as has as its usefulness in several perinatal events (BADA 1979, 1984; BEJAR 1982; BURNS 1985; GRANT 1987; GREISEN 1984; OZEK 1995; PERLMAN 1985; SEIBERT 1989; VAN BEL 1989; VOLPE 1982).

Pourcelot's resistive index is a ratio given by the formula: peak-systolic frequency minus end-diastolic frequency divided by peak-systolic frequency. The pulsatility index of GOSLING (1971) is defined by: peak-systolic frequency minus end-diastolic frequency divided by mean frequency. These indices are strongly correlated with distal cerebrovascular resistances.

The resistive index has several advantages: it is easy to measure; its value is not affected by changes in probe angle (peak-systolic and end-diastolic velocities are similarly changed). It appears valuable to

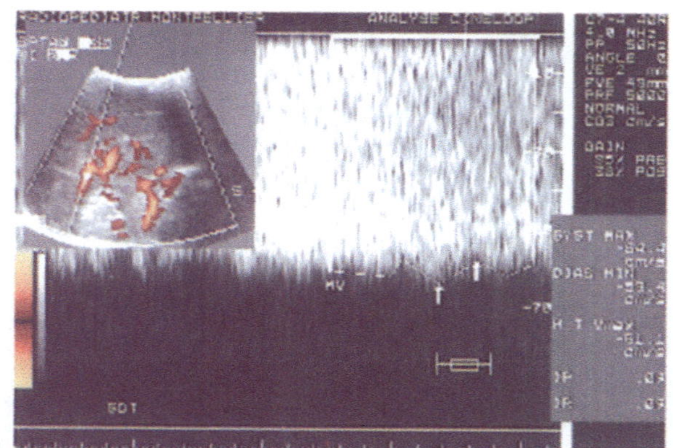

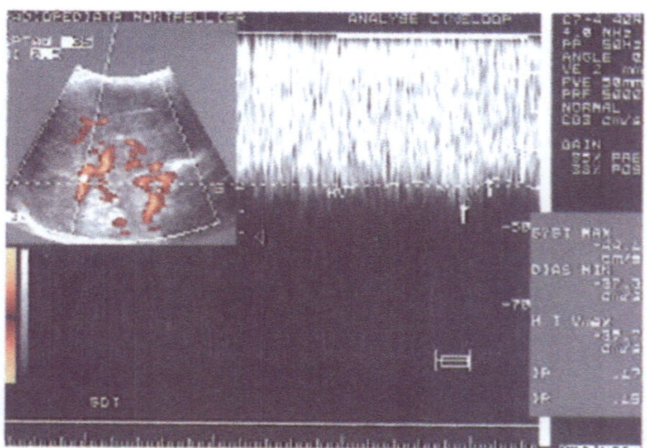

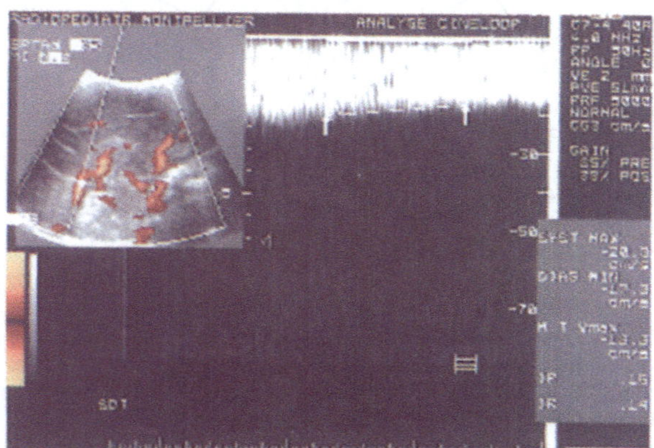

Fig. 2.77a–c. A 34-weeks' gestation infant, 8 days old: resting newborn after feeding, spectrum of the superior sagittal sinus. a The first measured velocity is 61 cm/s. b Continuous recording shows the velocity to be 39.7 cm/s, 1 min later. c After 4 min, the velocity has a normal value: 18.6 cm/s

compare serial determinations of blood flow velocities. The two indices are especially altered when the hemodynamic disturbances affect preferentially either the systolic or the diastolic velocity. In most clinical events, major changes occur in diastolic flow velocity (WRIGHT 1988): patent ductus arteriosus (Fig. 2.78), pneumothorax, seizures, hydrocephalus, tracheal suctioning, and anoxic–ischemic injury (Fig. 2.79).

In these clinical circumstances, the resistive index represents an accurate reliable marker of the CBF changes. Nevertheless, several limitations should be known:

- The adaptation to postnatal life is characterized by intense variations in CBF velocities that are poorly reflected by the resistive and pulsatility indices. Some changes have been reported. MAESEL (1994) described a significant decrease in the pulsatility

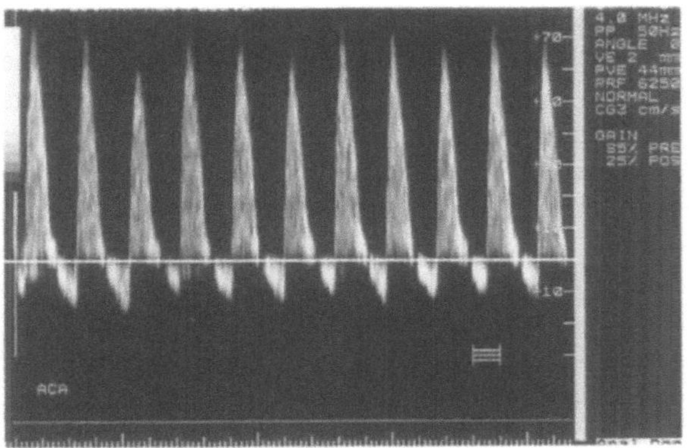

Fig. 2.78. A 28-weeks' gestation infant with patent ductus arteriosus. The spectral analysis curve, combined with clinical findings (left subclavicular murmur) is suggestive: reversed diastolic flow and RI=1.16

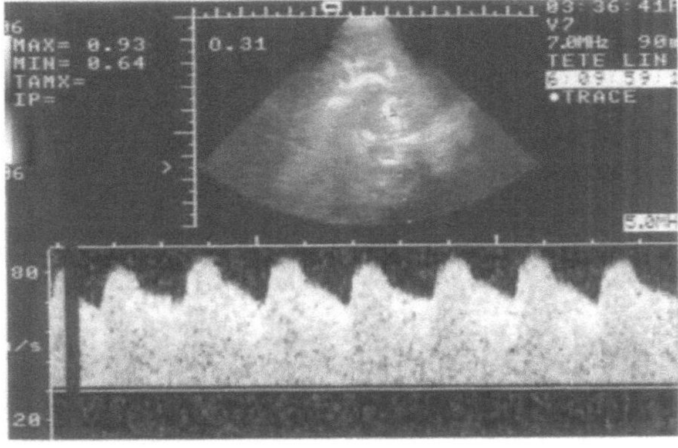

Fig. 2.79. Term newborn with seizures and cortico-subcortical ischemic lesions. Luxury perfusion with PSV=93 cm/s, EDV=64 cm/s, RI=0.31. Death occurred on day 4

index compared with fetal values, indicating normal postnatal adaptation and resulting from ductal closure. YOSHIDA (1991) and AKSEL'ROD (1991) reported a marked increase in resistive and pulsatility indices by the second hour of life, which is probably related to the first respiration and increased blood O_2 concentration, and parallels the reduction in arterial blood pressure. This increase affects the internal carotid, anterior cerebral, and middle cerebral arteries, but is not noticeable in basilar and posterior cerebral arteries.

Thus, during this neonatal hemodynamic storm (arterial blood pressure fluctuations, ductus arteriosus closure, increase in cerebral metabolism, consistent changes in vascular resistance), the indices seem unable to provide information concerning physiological changes in cerebral vascularization.

- PERLMAN (1985) observed that the pulsatility index does not correlate perfectly with CBF (measured by radioactive xenon clearance) in the human newborn brain. The dissociation between increased blood flow and unchanged pulsatility index is explained by a simultaneous parallel rise in systolic and diastolic velocities. Thus, a normal resistive index may falsely reassure in what is actually a severe situation, such as low blood flow. PERLMAN (1985) preferred measuring the area under the velocity waveform.

Determination of the indices is insufficient for a hemodynamic investigation in the first months of life. Following 121 newborns up to 1.5 months in age, DEEG (1989) reported that velocities gradually increase in the internal carotid artery, basilar artery, and anterior cerebral artery, although the resistive index does not significantly change: RI=0.77±0.08, 0.72±0.09, and 0.73±0.08 respectively.

After 1 month of age, diastolic velocities increase more than systolic ones, and the resistive index decreases, but during the first month most authors have found it of little value (DEEG 1989; TATSUNO 1990; TSAI 1990). Moreover, the results of NISHIMAKI (1991) were contradictory: he showed a decreased resistive index from day 1 to day 5, followed by an increase up to day 15. Finally, the resistive index is not significantly different between term, preterm, and very-low-birth-weight infants (KUBOTA 1991).

In conclusion, the indices seem to correctly reflect the distal vascular resistance that mainly affects the diastolic velocity. However, vascular resistance may be influenced by heart rate, arterial blood pressure (systemic and focal), blood viscosity, and vascular elasticity (Raju 1991).

Finally, Taylor (1990) pointed out that indices correlate poorly with values for CBF since equivalent changes in systolic and diastolic velocities can be present without affecting the resistive index (Hansen 1983).

– These literature data correspond very well to our personal experience: the resistive index (Diagram 2.47) and pulsatility index (Diagram 2.48) change only slightly in the first month of life, unlike arterial velocities (Fig. 2.80).

After 1 month of age, they have a greater value because of the predominant increase in the diastolic component. The poor discriminatory value of indices is also reported in children and adults studied by transcranial Doppler. Schoning (1996) investigated 94 healthy children and adolescents between 3 and 18 years of age and observed changes in arterial velocities from early childhood to adulthood, but unchanged RI values. As an example, in the middle cerebral artery, RI is constant before and after 10 years of age (0.56), whereas velocities are: PSV=141 cm/s, EDV=62 cm/s before age 10 years, PSV=128 cm/s, EDV=56 cm/s after age 10 years. Indices remain constant since velocities vary in parallel.

These limitations in the interpretation of the resistive index value emphasize the importance of measuring absolute velocities.

2.2.2.3.2
Blood Flow Velocities

The literature concerning quantification of cerebral blood flow velocities is poor. However, first publications demonstrate well that it permits an accurate approach to neonatal hemodynamic events.

● Arterial velocities

Few publications report normal values in the neonate (Bode 1988; Deeg 1989; Horgan 1989; Low 1993; Maesel 1994; Yoshida 1991). In those that do, despite the different methods used, the results are similar (Table 2.6).

Deeg (1989) determined mean values in the full-term newborn: peak-systolic velocities are 58 cm/s, 54 cm/s, and 47 cm/s in the internal carotid artery, anterior cerebral artery, and basilar artery, respectively, while end-diastolic velocities do not differ between the three arteries. Bode (1988) noted lower mean values: PSV=35 cm/s, EDV=11 cm/s, TAV=18 cm/s in the internal carotid artery, PSV=32 cm/s, EDV=11 cm/s, TAV=17 cm/s in the anterior cerebral artery – but his cohort of 25 infants included a great number of prematures.

Velocities in the middle cerebral artery have been measured: Yoshida (1991) reported peak-systolic velocities of 44 cm/s in 19 newborns (age range: 39–42 weeks gestation); Maesel (1994) finds the same values in 18 cases (PSV=44.2±7 cm/s, EDV=15.6±5 cm/s, TAV=26.7±6 cm/s) as Bode at day 15 and 45 cm/s at day 45. In parallel to this, EDV increases from 5 or 6 cm/s at day 1 to 10 cm/s at day 45 in the three arteries.

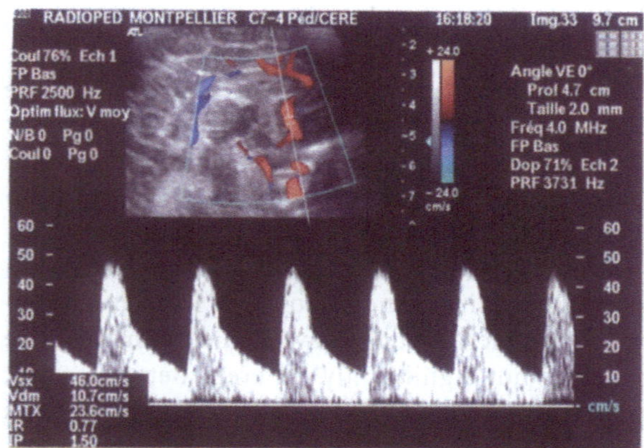

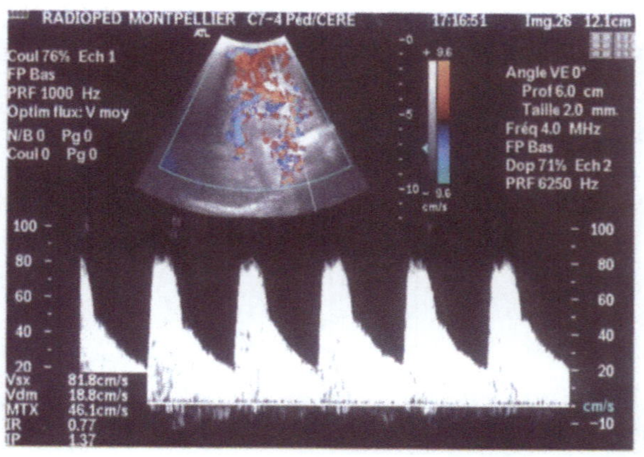

Fig. 2.80 a,b. Resistive index is similar in these two patients, RI=0.77. Velocities, however, are obviously quite different: in this 34-weeks' gestation newborn (**a**) PSV=46 cm/s, EDV=10.7 cm/s, and TAV=23.5 cm/s, whereas in this 2-month-old infant (**b**) PSV=81.8 cm/s, EDV=18.8 cm/s, and TAV=23.5 cm/s

Table 2.6. Arterial velocities in the literature

	Technique	Age	Velocities			
			Artery	PSV	EDV	TAV
Deeg (1989)	TF	Neonate	ACA	54	13	25
		40 weeks	BA	47	11	23
			ICA	58	12	26
Maesel (1994) 18 cases	TC	D1 Term	MCA	44.2±7	15.6±5	26.7±6
Yoshida (1991) 19 cases	TC	39-42 Weeks D1	MCA	44		
Bode (1988) 25 cases	TC	Preterm, full term	MCA	43	13	22
		D1	ICA	35	11	18
			ACA	32	11	17
			MCA	54	15	26
		D5	ICA	44	12	22
			ACA	42	13	21
			MCA	61	16	30
		D10	ICA	51	14	27
			ACA	44	13	23
Low (1993) 95 cases	TF	Term H1		43.2	9.3	
		Preterm		31.8	3.3	
Horgan (1989)	TC	Neonate	MCA	55	12	
		40 weeks	PCA	37	10	
Schoning (1996)	TC	< 10 Years, 45 cases	MCA	141	62	95
			ACA	116	50	78
			PCA	91	40	63
			BA	97	45	68
		> 10 Years, 49 cases	MCA	128	56	82
			ACA	103	43	66
			PCA	84	36	54
			BA	84	40	58
		Adult, 48 cases	MCA	108	48	67
			ACA	91	40	58
			PCA	70	33	46
			BA	67	33	46

TF Transfontanellar	*ACA* Anterior cerebral artery	*MCA* Middle cerebral artery	
TC Transcranial	*PCA* Posterior cerebral artery	*ICA* Internal carotid artery	
BA Basilar artery			

The age dependence of arterial velocities has been observed by all authors (Deeg 1989; Evans 1988; Hayashi 1992; Horgan 1991; Kubota 1991; Kurmanavichiu 1991; Tsai 1990; Winberg 1990), and is confirmed by our experience (Fig. 2.81).

For Bode (1988) the mean increase of blood velocities per day is about 1.5 cm/s for PSV, 0.4 cm/s for EDV, 0.8 cm/s for TAV.

Most authors have not found significant differences of velocities for various birth weights (Bode 1988; Low 1993). Others have reported contradictory results: Kubota (1991) observed, among 59 newborns, higher velocities in neonates of higher birth weight; in contrast to this, Cheung (1994) and Ley (1992) noted higher velocities in newborns with intrauterine growth retardation, while Yoshida

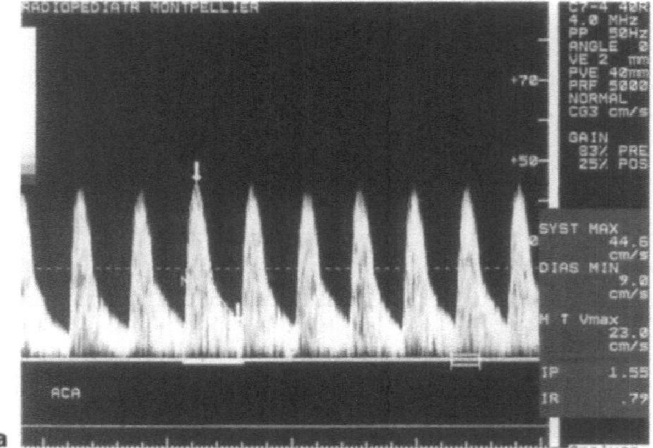

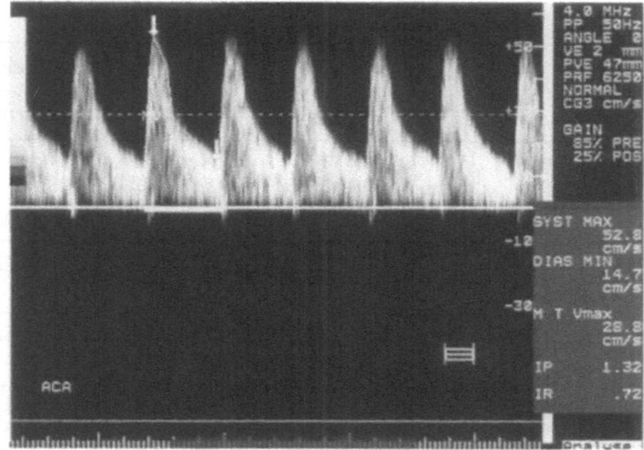

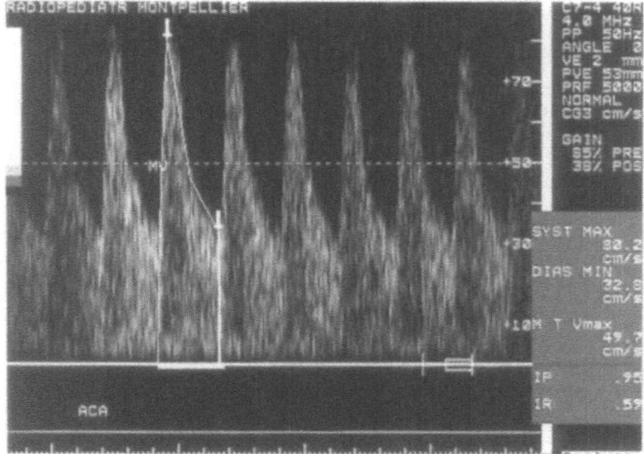

Fig. 2.81a–c. Evolution of the Doppler spectra with the infant age. **a** A 30-weeks' gestation infant, day 10. **b** Full-term newborn, day 7. **c** A 5-month-old infant. Progressive augmentation of flow velocities, especially the diastolic component, which increases from 9 to 14 and then 32 cm/s. Resistive index decreases from 0.79 to 0.59

(1991) investigated 62 neonates and reported that velocities increased more rapidly in small-for-date neonates (69.1±9.7 cm/s) than in normal infants (48.2±8.5 cm/s) for the first 10 days of life. The reason for this is known: chronic hypoxemia induces increased CBF.

In our cohort, we did not confirm the birth-weight dependence but we found a relationship between postnatal age and blood velocities: comparison of newborns of the same gestational age showed higher velocities in the older one (Fig. 2.82).

Small arteries may demonstrate a specific spectral pattern, such as the lenticulostriate arteries: a low vascular resistance is commonly observed with a relatively high diastolic component and low resistive index (less than 0.60) (Fig. 2.83).

This is interesting since lenticulostriate arteries participate in the arterial supply of the periventricular regions, and detection of hemodynamic disturbances in these vessels might help one to anticipate the formation of periventricular leukomalacia. This hypothesis prompts investigation of other small cerebral arteries of great functional importance (Fig. 2.84) such as the cortical, cerebellar, and choroidal arteries and branches of the middle cerebral artery.

We know that arterial velocities are influenced by transducer-induced pressure on the anterior fontanelle. TAYLOR (1992) proposed fontanellar compression to identify infants with abnormal intracranial compliance; he defined a ratio (ΔRI) that determines the elevation of baseline RI: RI with compression minus baseline RI divided by baseline RI.

In the healthy neonate, fontanellar compression induces a moderate increase in RI and moderate reduction in mean velocity. In our experience of 125 infants, aged 31 weeks to 4 months (Diagram 2.51), ΔRI was less than 18%, EDV fell significantly, and PSV decreased to a lesser degree (Fig. 2.84). It is important to know this, since elevation of intracranial pressure correlates with alteration of cerebral compliance. Thus, if ΔRI is less than 20%, cerebral compliance may be considered as normal; whereas intracranial hypertension is ascertained if ΔRI is more than 30% (Fig. 2.85).

Any interpretation of a cerebral Doppler spectrum should be careful: every result should be compared with validated normal values, every evaluation

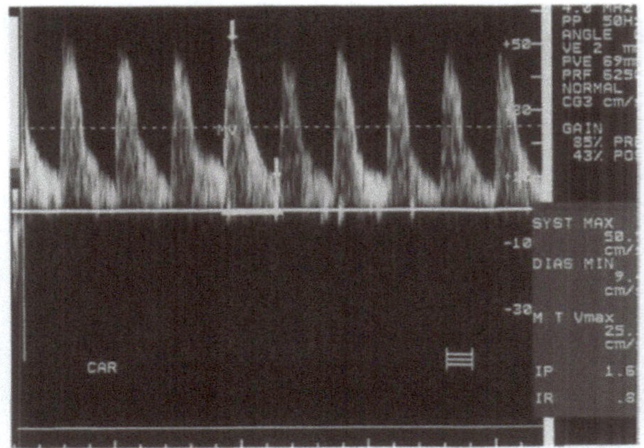 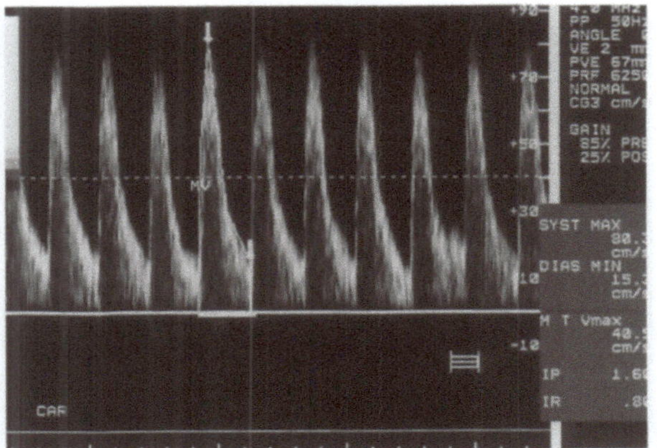

Fig. 2.82. a A 35-weeks' gestation infant, 5 days old. Hemodynamic evaluation is normal: PSV=51 cm/s, EDV=9.4 cm/s, TAV=25 cm/s. **b** In this other 35-weeks' gestation newborn, velocities are markedly higher: PSV=80 cm/s, EDV=15.3 cm/s, TAV=40 cm/s. In fact, this investigation was performed 2 months after birth in a baby that was a 27-weeks' gestation infant

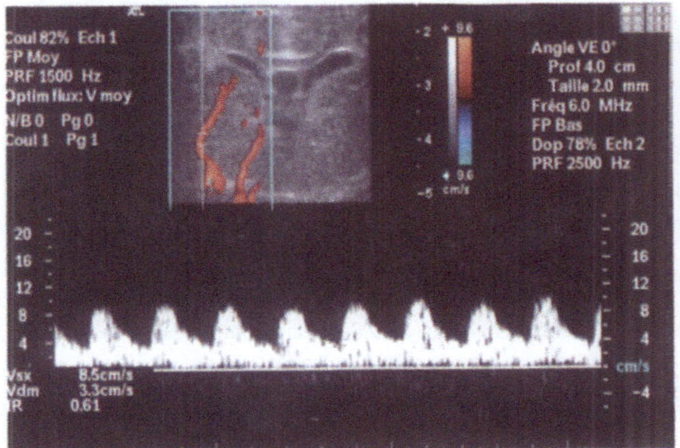 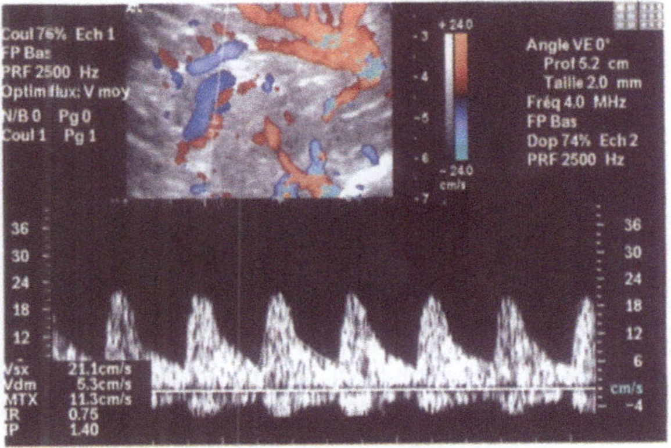

Fig. 2.83. A 27-weeks' gestation newborn, 8 days old. Doppler assessment of a lenticulostriate artery: PSV=8.5 cm/s, EDV=3.3 cm/s. RI is characteristic at 0.61

Fig. 2.84. Full-term infant, 8 days old. Doppler assessment of the posterior medial choroidal artery: PSV=21.1 cm/s, ED=5.3 cm/s, TAV=11.3 cm/s, RI=0.75, PI=1.40

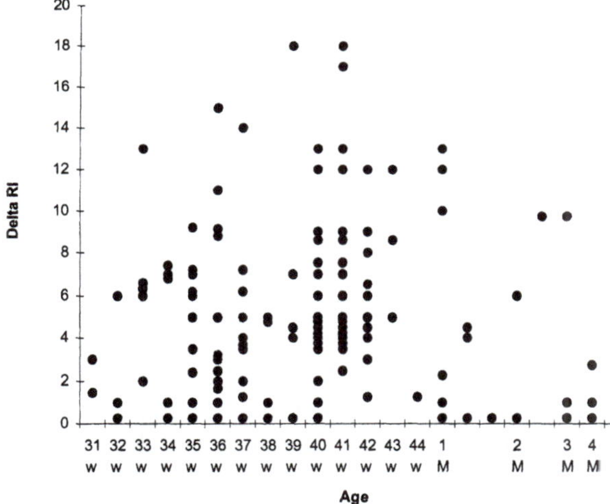

Diagram 2.51. ΔRI in 125 infants

should require investigation of several vessels; in each evaluation the regional velocities should be carefully studied.

– Finally, the potentialities of Doppler evaluation seem to be most interesting for the immediate neonatal period, since complex changes occur during the phase of cardiorespiratory transition (SONESSON 1987): reduced velocities during the first 30 min, increased systolic and decreased diastolic velocities from 30 min to 2 h, and decreased systolic and increased diastolic velocities from 2 h to 72 h. This confirms the main role of the ductus arteriosus with accentuation of the left-to-right shunt in the first postnatal hours, followed by a reduction in the ductal shunt at about 24 h of life (Moss 1963). The first 3 days represent a period of adaptation and adjustment in order to maintain a constant CBF. This is why it is important to measure arterial velocities.

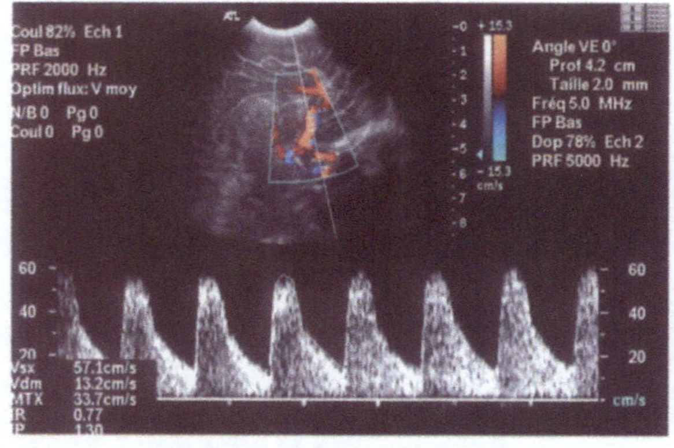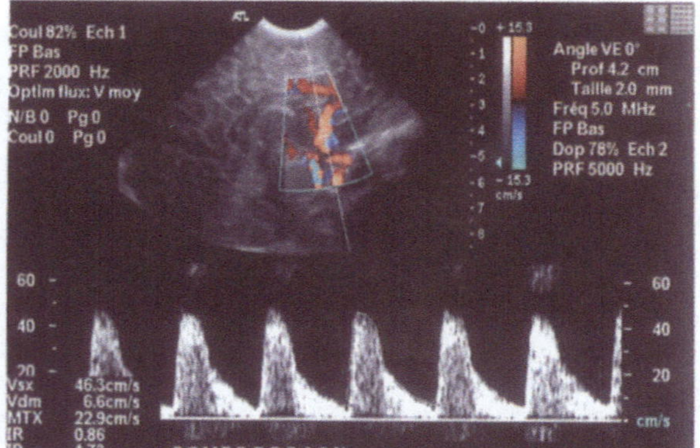

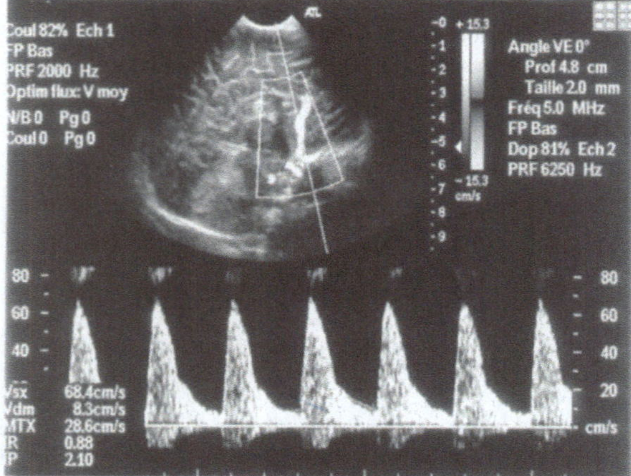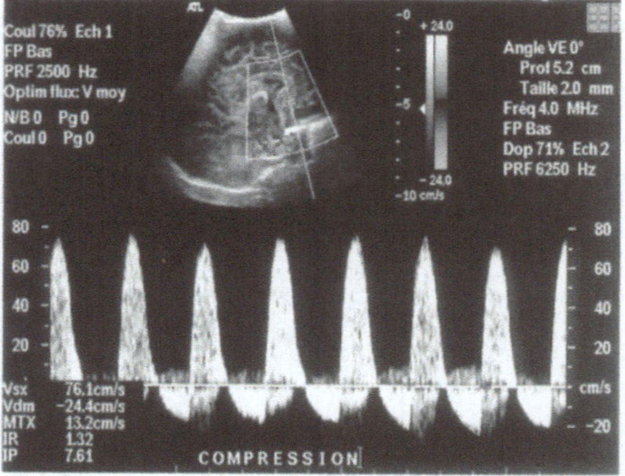

Fig. 2.85a–d. a,b Preterm birth. Routine Doppler ultrasonography at 1 month of age. Normal findings in the anterior cerebral artery with RI=0.77 (a). After fontanellar pressure, RI=0.86, ΔRI=12% (normal). Note that decrease in velocity predominates in the diastolic flow (b). c,d One-month-old infant with myelomeningocele. Increased intracranial pressure correlates with disturbance of cerebral compliance: before fontanellar pressure, RI=0.88 (c), whereas after pressure it reaches 1.32; ΔRI=50%

● Venous Velocities

WINKLER (1989) was the first to report duplex scanning of the deep venous drainage in 49 healthy infants: the mean values of peak-velocities were 13.2 cm/s for the straight sinus, 5.6 cm/s for the vein of Galen, and 5.9 cm/s and 5.6 cm/s for the basilar veins. Other authors (FENTON 1991; GRANT 1987; PFANNSCHMIDT 1989; TAYLOR 1992) have also brought their personal experiences (Table 2.7). TAYLOR (1992) proposed a detailed hemodynamic map of the deep veins (subependymal veins, internal cerebral veins, vein of Galen, straight sinus, inferior sagittal sinus) in 20 healthy full-term infants: velocities ranged from 3 cm/s in the subependymal veins to 5.9 cm/s in the straight sinus.

Few works exist concerning the superficial venous drainage, especially the superior sagittal sinus. TAYLOR (1992) found a velocity of about 9.2 cm/s in this sinus, while BEZINQUE (1995) obtained variable values ranging from 3 to 107 cm/s.

Our experience is based on 419 newborns and infants and provides higher values than literature.

The internal cerebral vein shows the lowest variability between infants of the same age group; its flow velocity is about 3.3 cm/s according to TAYLOR (1992), 5.5 cm/s according to PFANNSCHMIDT (1989), and was 9.8 cm/s in our cohort. PFANNSCHMIDT (1989) reported homogeneous results in the internal jugular vein, internal cerebral vein, and straight sinus, but a high variability from time to time and from child to child. For BEZINQUE (1995), velocities of superior sagittal sinus ranged from 3 cm/s to 107 cm/s. Besides the progressive increase of velocities with age, we also observed great variations in superior sagittal sinus and straight sinus velocities (Diagram 2.49) in each age group (Fig. 2.86).

The flow velocities of superficial and deep venous drainage are probably regulated in a complex manner that remains poorly understood. In an infant (especially preterm), velocities may change sharply

Table 2.7. Venous velocities in the literature

	TECHNIQUE	AGE	VEINS	VELOCITIES cm/s
Grant (1987)	TF	Neonate	Vein of Galen	2-8
Winkler (1989)	TF	Preterm neonate 30-42 weeks	Vein of Galen Straight sinus Basilar vein	5.6 13.2 5.8
Pfannschmidt (1989)	TF	Neonate	Internal jugular vein Internal cerebral vein Straight sinus	8.4±4.7 5.5±1.6 12.6±7.8
Fenton (1991)	TF	22 Neonates	Vein of Galen	2.3-9.5
Taylor (1992)	TF	20 Neonates	Subependymal vein Internal cerebral vein Inferior sagittal sinus Vein of Galen Straight sinus Superior sagittal sinus	3 3.3 3.5 4.3 5.9 9.3
Bezinque (1995)		96 cases Neonate infant	Superior sagittal sinus	3-107

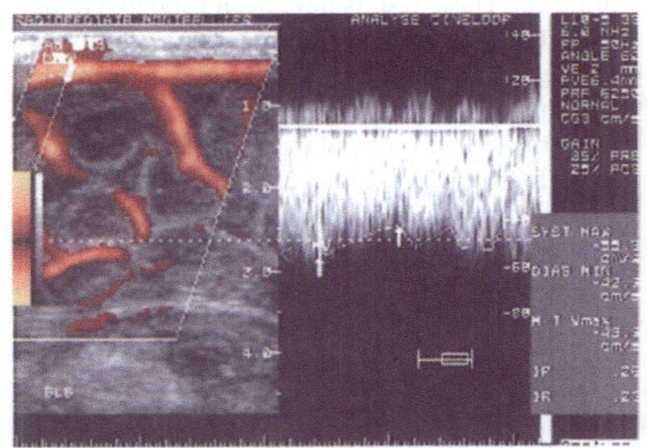

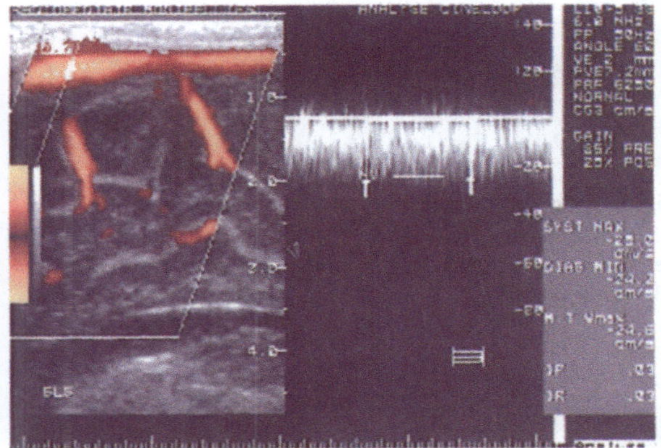

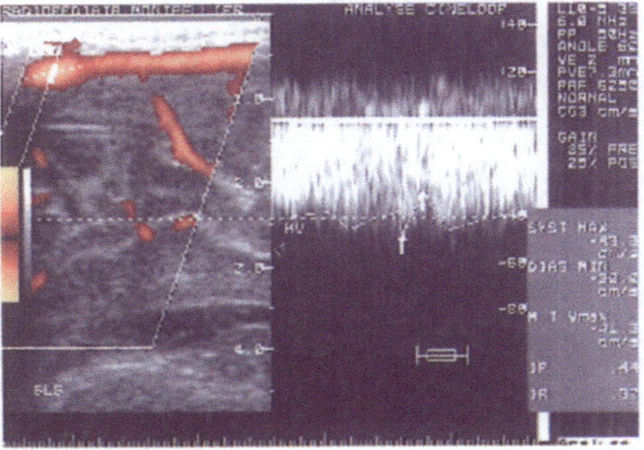

Fig. 2.86a–c. A 36-weeks' infant, 15 days old. a Resting newborn. High mean velocity in the superior sagittal sinus: 48 cm/s (with angle correction). b After 2 min, the baby is asleep and mean velocity shows normal value: 24 cm/s. c Four minutes later the baby is still asleep, but mean velocity has jumped to 41 cm/s

without any obvious explanation: in a resting or sleeping baby, without fontanellar compression. They often return to normal when the Doppler recording continues (Fig. 2.77), but alternating high and low values may be observed in the same recording (Fig. 2.86).

These data have not been described in the literature, and remain unexplained. Cowan (1985) reported that considerable changes in superior sagittal sinus velocities can occur with head rotation, neck flexion, and external pressure on the fontanel.

Fenton (1991) noted that light bilateral jugular compression in 17 term neonates produced a fall of up to 63% in venous velocities in 12 infants. The fluctuations that we have observed in our practice may result from unexpected neck flexion, since most of these examinations are performed in a baby chair.

Fontanellar pressure induces marked changes in venous velocimetry. Bezinque (1995) reported that 55 out of 96 patients increased their superior sagittal sinus velocity with compression, while 36 decreased it, and 5 did not change. We have made similar observations (Fig. 2.87).

The physiology of the intracerebral venous system remains poorly known, but several facts have been established:

– The two internal cerebral veins and their tributaries (subependymal, terminal, basilar veins) represent reliable markers of the venous hemodynamics. The normal values of velocities of the internal cerebral vein have been validated and our initial experience shows encouraging reproducible results on the deep venous system. In each age group, blood velocity in terminal veins and the superior choroidal veins shows low variability (Fig. 2.88). When great variations occur in the superior sagittal sinus, with velocity reaching 60–90 cm/s in a neonate, decrease of fontanellar pressure and correction of a pronounced flexion of the neck may normalize this velocity.

– With increasing age, there is a linear increase in venous velocities, especially in the internal cerebral vein. These results have been validated in our cohort of 419 infants: the internal cerebral vein showed a mean velocity of 7.2 cm/s at 32 weeks, 9.8 cm/s at 40 weeks, 13 cm/s at 2 months, and 14.8 cm/s at 6 months of age, with low deviations in each group (Diagram 2.52). This vessel, a main vascular crossroad, is the reference of the deep venous system.

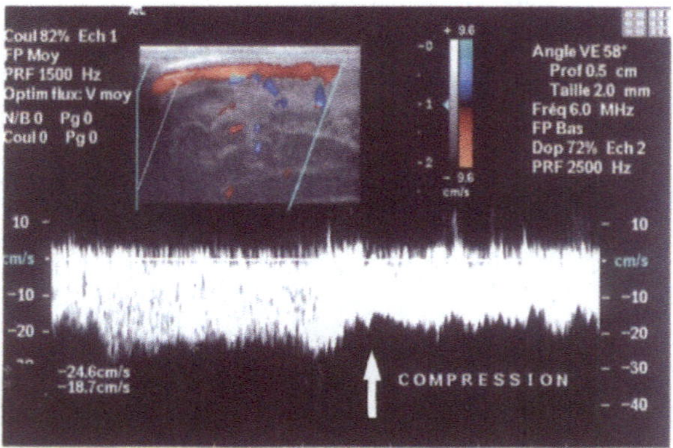

Fig. 2.87. Spectral analysis of the superior sagittal sinus in a 34 weeks' gestation infant. With angle correction, mean velocity is 24.6 cm/s. After fontanellar pressure, it decreases to 18.7 cm/s

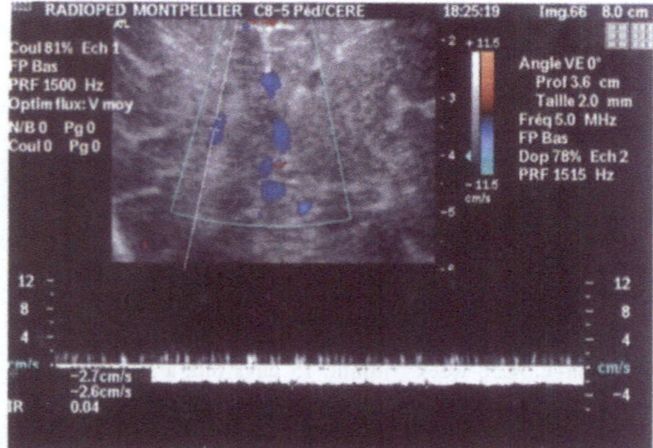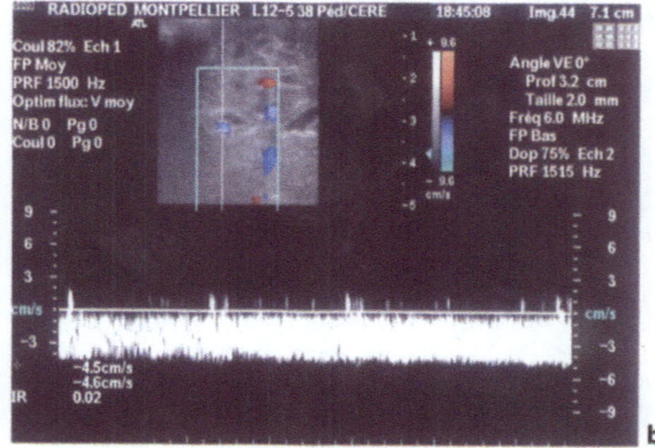

Fig. 2.88. A 36-weeks' gestation newborn. a Spectral analysis of the superior choroidal vein; mean velocity is 2.7 cm/s. b Spectral analysis of the terminal vein; mean velocity is 4.6 cm/s

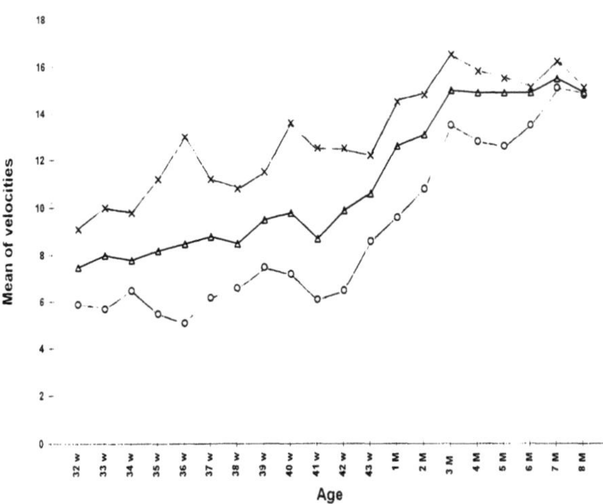

Diagram 2.52. Venous systems (419 infants). Maximal mean and minimal velocities of the internal cerebral vein, in each group: **X—X** maximal values △—△ mean velocities, ○—○ minimal velocities

2.2.2.3.3
Pulsed Doppler: The Last Step

Color Doppler identifies a cerebral vessel while pulsed Doppler determines whether it is an artery or a vein.

Standard color Doppler demonstrates the direction of flow, but is insufficient to differentiate an artery from a vein; pulsed Doppler resolves the problem. For example, it allows one to distinguish the posterior pericallosal artery from the inferior sagittal sinus (Fig. 2.62), the superficial medial veins from the peripheral branches of the pericallosal artery (Fig. 2.46), the basal vein from the posterior cerebral artery (Fig. 2.59), and the anterior choroidal artery from the superior choroidal vein.

Quantitation of velocities should obviously be preferred. Their assessment helps us to understand the complex mechanisms of regulation during the first days of life and to appreciate their progressive evolution with age. From our experience and the literature reports, normal values have now been validated for arteries and veins. This gives a basis for discussion in a pathological clinical condition. Finally, it is important to argue not from a single measurement but from the assessment of several vessels, in order to support the concept of regional vascularization. The resistive index remains useful but gives only rough information on the cerebral hemodynamics, especially in the neonatal period and first month of life.

2.2.3
Pulsed Doppler: Limitations and Pitfalls

Cerebral Doppler investigation is very valuable but has several limitations:

● Quantitative evaluation of cerebral blood flow remains impossible: the course and small size of neonatal cerebral arteries prevent accurate measurement of their cross-sectional area.

● The complex relationship between blood flow velocity and cerebral blood flow has been documented. Blood flow is calculated as the product of blood velocity and cross-sectional area. Provided measurements are reliable and reproducible, recorded changes in blood velocity reflect parallel changes in cerebral blood flow. However some factors remain unknown:
- Despite the absence of enough studies, most authors assume that cerebral vessels do not change significantly in caliber. However, if they do, the correlation between velocity and blood flow could disappear (DRAYTON 1987); for example, when velocity increases, blood flow may remain unchanged because of vasoconstriction.
- Experimental studies (HANSEN 1983) in the newborn piglet show a poor correlation between blood velocity (measured by pulsed Doppler) and blood flow when CBF increases, resulting from simultaneous changes in the systolic and telediastolic velocities.
- Cerebral perfusion is a dynamic process. Even repeated noninvasive Doppler investigations give only a brief view of cerebral circulation. A serial follow-up using special probes might be proposed, but a permanent insonation might produce deleterious biological effects in the neonatal brain.

● Despite their obvious contribution to neonatal care, Doppler techniques expose those who use them to pitfalls and errors of analysis, calculation, and/or interpretation that have been outstandingly reported by WINKLER (1990). Major pitfalls may result from inadequate consideration of the physics of sound waves and Doppler instruments:
- One of the first errors of an investigator is to conclude that "absence of Doppler signal means absence of flow." This highlights the importance of Doppler technology, the use of software able to detect low blood velocity (approximately 1 cm/s), low wall filter settings (between 30 and 50 Hz), and high-frequency transducers.

– Potential errors are due to the partial volume effect: inadequate separation between two adjacent vessels with the same flow direction, or erroneous projection of colored signals in a nonvascular structure. The use of high-frequency probes and focus on the area of interest may avoid these errors. Distinguishing the two pericallosal arteries (as also the two anterior cerebral arteries and the two internal cerebral veins) now seems to be possible with the new equipment and/or power Doppler.
– The examination technique may be a source of error in itself. Moderate fontanellar compression induces a decrease in arterial velocities, especially in small premature babies; determination of absolute flow velocities requires angle correction if the angle of incidence is more than 30°; some vessels (such as the middle cerebral artery) should be studied by transcranial Doppler; and the vascular anatomy may result in unreliable measurements of blood velocity, as for the internal carotid artery. For these reasons, WINKLER (1990) proposes the term "velocity estimate" rather than "absolute velocity."

2.3
Fetal Evaluation

Sonographers have been interested in the cerebral vascularization of the fetus for many years. Detection of arterial vasodilatation in the hypoxemic fetus is the reason behind this enthusiasm (CHANDRAN 1993; DEGANI 1994; MARI 1992; NOORDAM 1994; UERPAIROJKIT 1996; WLADIMIROFF 1987). A progressive chronic insult to the fetus induces hypoxemia, acidosis, and hypercapnia that lead to a compensatory cerebral vasodilatation: the increase in diastolic flow and reduction of cerebrovascular resistance divert part of the fetal blood toward the brain in order to maintain the O_2 content in cerebral parenchyma: this is the brain-sparing effect.

Pulsed Doppler detects a decreased resistive index (DUBIEL 1997); increase in diastolic velocity in the anterior and middle cerebral arteries seems to be the more accurate parameter for detecting fetal growth retardation (MARI 1992; NOORDAM 1994).

Nowadays assessment of fetal circulation is required in the case of chronic insult to the fetus:

– Cerebral index and cerebroplacental ratio (ARBEILLE 1987) represent reliable markers of fetal hypoxia.
– Abnormal end-diastolic velocity and resistive index in cerebral vessels indicate a poor prognosis, especially when combined with abnormal umbilical or uterine index: alteration of fetal heart rate or even fetal death may occur.

These important observations have led to the progressive description of fetal cerebral vessels by color imaging and the development of hemodynamic investigations in the fetal brain.

2.3.1
Vascular Anatomy: Color Doppler

The quality of vascular imaging in the fetus is due to advances in US technology and to the characteristics of the fetal head (the bone does not prevent sound-wave progression). VAN DEN WIJNGAARD (1989) reported that a pulsatile beat may be recognized in the internal carotid artery, anterior cerebral artery, middle cerebral artery, and posterior cerebral artery in 89%, 64%, 91%, and 58% respectively. Color imaging has greatly improved these results (NOORDAM 1994): internal carotid artery, anterior cerebral artery, middle cerebral artery, and posterior cerebral artery may be depicted in 100%, 98%, 100%, and 88% respectively. This highlights the fact that color Doppler constitutes the first step of hemodynamic evaluation in both fetus and the neonate.

The multiplicity of scanning planes enables good vascular mapping:
– Axial transverse planes show the circle of Willis (Fig. 2.89), posterior cerebral artery, transverse

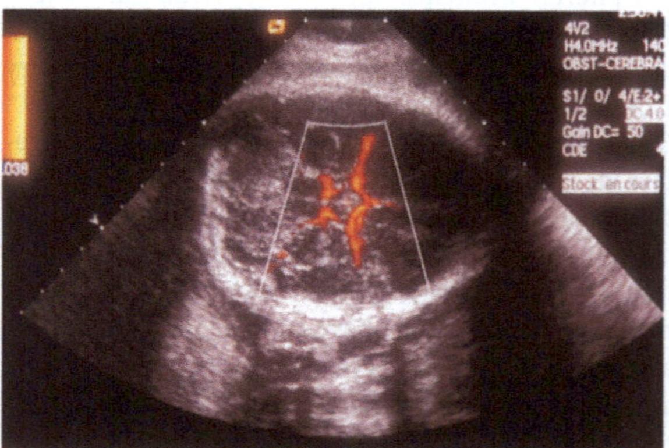

Fig. 2.89. Power Doppler imaging: axial transverse plane of the fetal skull, showing the characteristic appearance of the circle of Willis. (From Dr. Bernard, Paris)

sinuses (Fig. 2.90) (Laurichesse-Delmas 1999), and superior cerebellar arteries (Uerpairojkit 1996).

– The midline sagittal plane (transfontanellar equivalent) allows easy identification of the anterior cerebral artery, pericallosal artery and its branches (Fig. 2.91), superior sagittal sinus, and the whole deep venous drainage (inferior sagittal sinus, internal cerebral vein, vein of Galen, straight sinus) (Fig. 2.92).

As in the neonate, power Doppler (Fortunato 1996; Konje 2000; Pooh 1996) seems to be more sensitive and more accurate than standard color Doppler (Arbeille 1989).

The difference between fetus and newborn in visualization of cerebral vessels is progressively disappearing. In the future, some vessels that have been

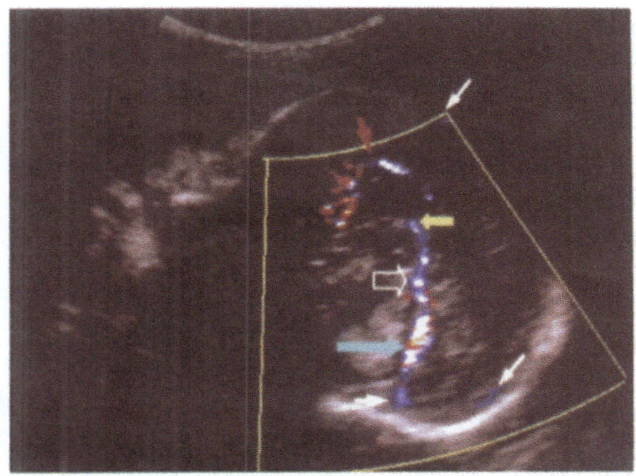

Fig. 2.92. Standard color Doppler: midline "transfontanellar" sagittal plane. The deep venous system is depicted: the inferior sagittal sinus (*yellow arrow*) joins the internal cerebral vein (*thick unfilled arrow*) toward the vein of Galen and straight sinus (*turquoise arrow*) before ending at the torcular (*thick white arrow*). Note partial visualization of the distal part of the superior sagittal sinus (*thin white arrow*). (From Drs. Laurichesse-Delmas and Ville, Paris)

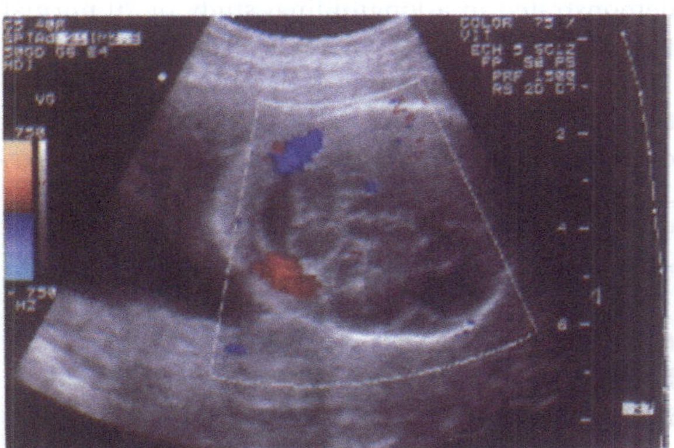

Fig. 2.90. A 24-weeks' fetus. Easy visualization of the lateral sinuses on each side of the cisterna magna

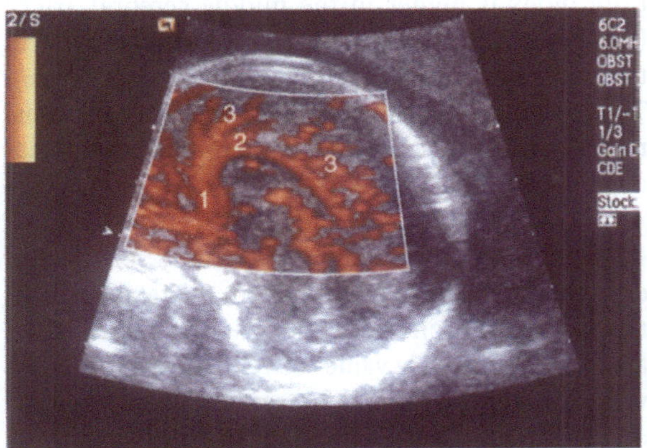

Fig. 2.91. Power Doppler imaging: midline "transfontanellar" sagittal plane, with depiction of the anterior cerebral artery (*1*), pericallosal artery (*2*), and cortical branches (*3*). (From Dr. Morice, Montpellier)

recently depicted in the neonate (ophthalmic artery, artery of Heubner, lenticulostriate arteries, choroidal arteries, calcarine arteries, parieto-occipital arteries, medial and lateral superficial veins, terminal veins) will surely be visualized in the fetus. Even today, the anterior choroidal artery is already frequently shown (Kurjak 1994).

2.3.2
Fetal Cerebral Hemodynamics: Pulsed Doppler

2.3.2.1
Problems

The fetal vascular physiology remains incompletely known.

● The arterial vasculature follows a complex development. Up to the 24th week of gestation, the basal arteries, which supply the brain stem and basal ganglia, are well developed, while the cortical arteries are extremely thin. From 28 to 32 weeks, the ratio of regional flows inverts, with increased flow in the cortex (Volpe 1997).

● There is one main difference between fetus and infant: as fetal systemic blood pressure is low whereas cardiac output and heart rate are high, cardiac output in the fetus changes only with heart rate. The regulation of fetal circulation depends on catecholamines, the renin-angiotensin system, prostaglandins, and central autonomic mechanisms. Fetal regulation of CBF is poorly known. After fetal anoxia there is a two-fold increase in CBF and a three-fold increase in myocardial blood flow, while total cardiac outflow remains unchanged; that shows a redistribution of blood volume toward preferential regions in the brain and the heart. However, many questions remain: does cerebral autoregulation exist? At what time does it appear (it is present in the 30-weeks' gestation preterm infant)? Are there intrauterine changes in arterial blood pressure that can induce protective cerebral mechanisms?

● Several physiological variations of CBF occur as in the neonate. There is an inverse correlation between the heart rate and the pulsatility index of the middle cerebral artery (MARI 1991). High-amplitude breathing movements produce fluctuations in the resistive and pulsatility indices (BURGHOUWT 1992; WLADIMIROFF 1987). Maternal hyperglycemia correlates with increased cerebrovascular resistance (DEGANI 1991; GILLIS 1992). Compression of the fetal head (due to transducer pressure (VYAS 1990)), oligoamnios (VAN DEN WIJNGAARD 1988), or intrapartum uterine contractions (MAESEL 1990) are associated with increased resistive index in the middle cerebral artery.

Finally, some medications may influence CBF. Infusion of retrodine (for treatment of preterm labor) induces a decrease in middle cerebral artery resistive index (MARI 1991). During magnesium sulfate administration, diastolic blood flow decreases in the middle cerebral artery (FACCHINETTI 1992; KEELEY 1993). Within 48 h after indomethacin treatment, 11 of 13 fetuses show constriction of the ductus arteriosus (MARI 1989). Finally, animal experiments show that repeated nicotine injection induces fetal cerebral vasoconstriction (ARBEILLE 1992).

2.3.2.2
Current Data

Doppler investigation of normal human fetuses leads to several conclusions:

● As in the newborn, most authors use only the resistive and pulsatility indices to quantify CBF (HATA 1991; KURMANAVICIUS 1997; LEWINSKY 1991; MARI 1994; SATOH 1988; UERPAIROJKIT 1996; VAN DEN WIJNGAARD 1989; VAN EYCK 1987; WOO 1987). In the

opinion of all of them, these indices are poorly discriminating from 27 to 36 weeks' gestation. SATOH (1988) reported that resistive and pulsatility indices remain unchanged between 27 and 35 weeks and decrease between 36 and 41 weeks. HATA (1991) confirmed that resistive index does not change from 28 weeks to term, while pulsatility index is unchanged from 28 to 33 weeks, and decreases at 34 weeks. Finally, VAN DEN WIJNGAARD (1989) observes significantly reduced indices in the last 2 weeks of gestation; that relates to all cerebral arteries. This late decrease results from an increased diastolic component and represents the main characteristic of fetal brain hemodynamics.

● Studies of arterial velocities in the fetal brain, although they remain extremely rare (KONJE 2000; MEERMAN 1990; NOORDAM 1994; VEILLE 1993), provide very interesting information. VEILLE (1993) demonstrated in a longitudinal study of 20 normal fetuses that blood flow increases from 23 ml/min at 19 weeks to 133 ml/min at 37 weeks; systolic velocities in the middle cerebral artery increase significantly with gestational age: 23 cm/s at 19 weeks, 32 cm/s at 24 weeks, and 43 cm/s at 29 weeks, 47 cm/s at 32 weeks, and 54 cm/s at 37 weeks; in parallel, resistive and pulsatility indices do not change.

The same conclusions were drawn by MEERMAN (1990), who reported, in 40 normal pregnancies, a linear increase in arterial velocities and unchanged indices.

NOORDAM (1994) observed, in 28 normal fetuses between 24 and 38 weeks' gestation, higher velocities in the middle cerebral artery and lower velocities in the posterior cerebral artery. This observation highlights the concept of regional distribution: the pulsatility index is higher in the middle cerebral artery (LEWINSKY 1991), while its lowest value is found in the superior cerebellar artery (UERPAIROJKIT 1996). Thus, the cerebral velocity values appear as the most reliable marker of the hemodynamic changes that occur in the fetus (Fig. 2.93).

● In the literature, only one study of quality describes the venous circulation in the fetal brain. In this work, LAURICHESSE-DELMAS (1999) determined the normal reference values of velocities in the transverse sinus in 126 normal fetuses from 20 to 42 weeks of gestation. Flow velocities linearly increased while resistive and pulsatility indices decrease throughout gestation. The waveform is triphasic, with a forward systolic flow during ventricular systole, a forward early diastolic component during passive ventricular

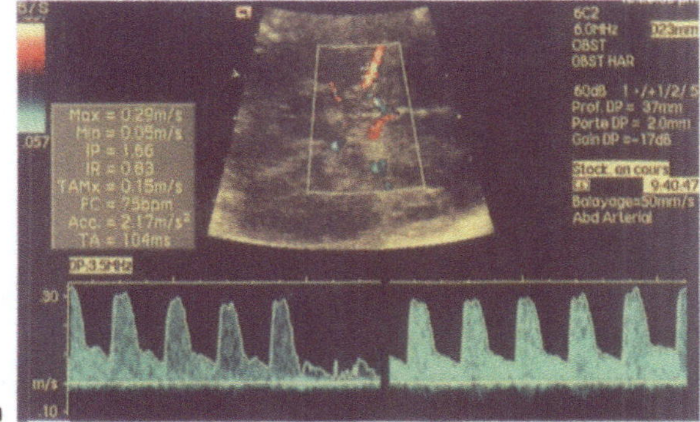

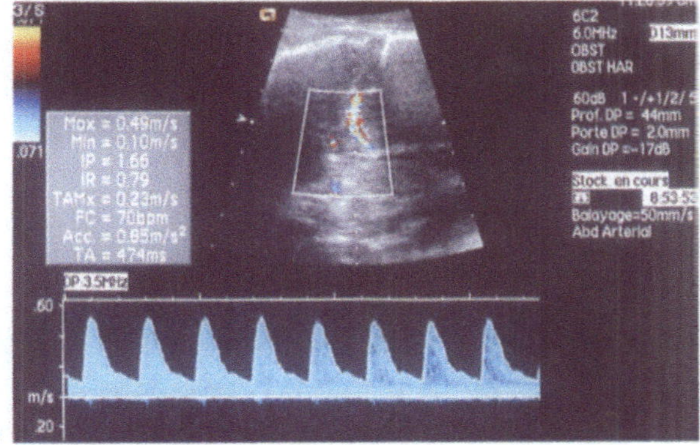

Fig. 2.93 a,b. In the fetus, spectral analysis demonstrates the value of quantifying the arterial velocities. The indices are not very different between these two fetuses aged 27 and 32 weeks respectively: at 27 weeks RI=0.83, PI=1.66; at 32 weeks RI=0.79, PI=1.66. In contrast, arterial velocities markedly increase from 27 to 32 weeks: at 27 weeks TAV=15 cm/s (**a**), while at 32 weeks TAV=23 cm/s (**b**). (From Dr. Morice, Montpellier)

filling, and a lower forward late diastolic component during atrial contraction. A longitudinal study of 37 cases suggests that the spectrum can evolve with pregnancy: a reverse flow during atrial contraction is commonly seen before 23 weeks but not after 30 weeks (Fig. 2.94).

During the last month of gestation, the waveform tends to be less pulsatile and shows the same pattern as in the neonate.

A continuous band-like aspect is common in the vein of Galen, straight sinus, and basal vein (LAU-RICHESSE-DELMAS 1999).

The marked pulsatility of the transverse sinus until the second half of the third trimester and the changes toward a sinusoidal appearance late in pregnancy may be supported by two hypotheses:

- The short distance between the heart and the brain reflects the difference in pressure between the heart and the cerebral vessels during the cardiac cycle; this distance increases with gestation and the transmission of cardiac pulsatility to these ves-

sels decreases progressively. However, it seems difficult to understand the presence of a pulsatile waveform in the deep inferior sagittal sinus while a flat or sinusoidal waveform exists in the basal veins and straight sinus.

- Progressive maturation of muscular components occurs in the vessel wall that would induce an increase in vascular compliance.

● In sum, resistive and pulsatility indices evolve similarly in arteries and veins: they increase up to 28–30 weeks, stabilize, and increase again near term. This is supported by the physiological decrease in placental resistance and the increase in cardiac output toward the cerebral vessels (DE SMEDT 1987). It also explains the progressive increase in arterial and venous velocities with pregnancy.

2.4
Conclusion

Pulsed and color Doppler evaluation of the healthy infant from birth to 8 months of age and of the fetus leads to several conclusions.

● Accurate description of the vascular anatomy requires quality equipment. Only high-level technology allows us to advance our understanding of vascular physiology. This is obvious.

Neonatal and fetal vascular imaging has already progressed, but undoubtedly in future cerebral hemodynamics will be better known and vascular mapping more accurate, especially with the use of contrast medium injections when they are available for use in children (BURNS 1994; TAYLOR 2000).

● In the field of color Doppler, depiction of the great arteries and venous sinuses alone cannot be sufficient. The goal of color imaging is to routinely show their branches and obtain regional mapping of smaller vessels. Visualization of the lenticulostriate arteries and cortical branches of the middle cerebral artery is required, since thromboses in this territory are frequent. Knowledge of the vascular supply of the tela choroidea permits an understanding of the pathology of a galenic aneurysm. To depict the terminal veins is essential to explain the occurrence of a periventricular hemorrhagic infarction (Fig. 2.95). Thus, as complete as possible an assessment of the cerebral vasculature will improve the diagnosis of multiple vascular disease in the neonatal period: arte-

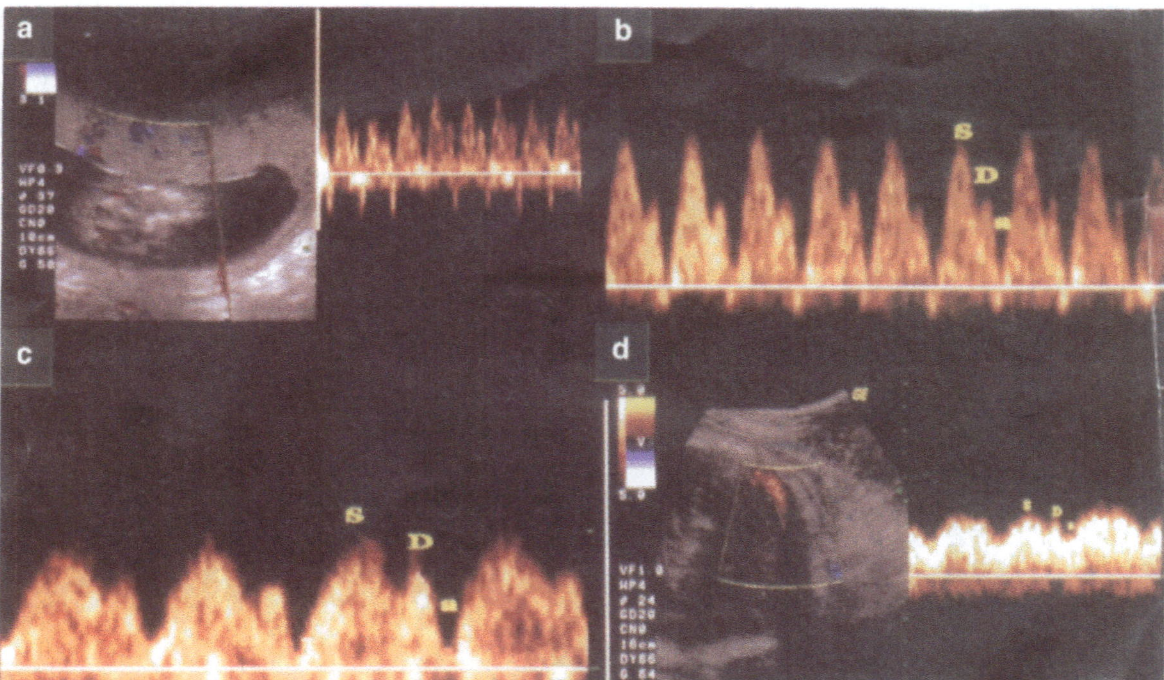

Fig. 2.94a–d. Transverse sinus flow velocity at 14 weeks (**a**), 23 weeks (**b**), 30 weeks (**c**), and 41 weeks (**d**). S Peak systole, D peak diastole, a atrial contraction. Note the common reverse flow before 22 weeks (**a**), which disappears at 30 weeks. Progressive decrease of the pulsatility index (**d**). (From Dr. Laurichesse-Delmas, Paris)

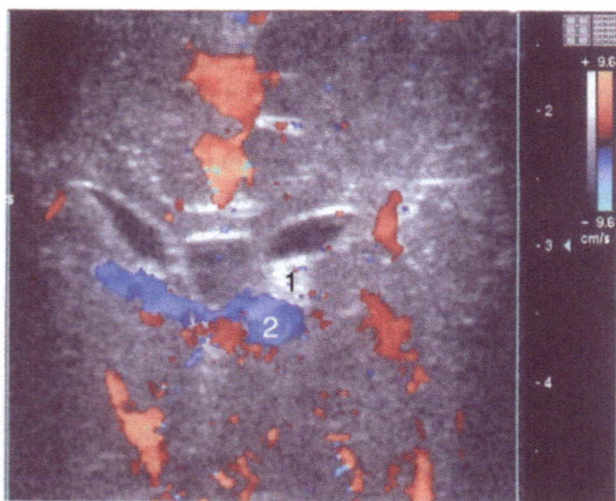

Fig. 2.95. A 32-weeks infant with a small hyperechoic left germinal matrix hemorrhage (*1*) compressing and displacing the underlying terminal vein (*2*). When subependymal hemorrhage is larger and/or associated with intraventricular hemorrhage, the danger of terminal vein obstruction and secondary periventricular hemorrhagic infarction is great

rial or venous thrombosis, ischemic damage from low blood flow or vascular compression, subarachnoid or subdural location of a pericerebral collection, hemorrhagic damage, or vascular malformation.

● To recognize a vessel is the first step; to determine whether its Doppler spectrum is normal or not is the second:

– Diagnosis of a hemodynamic alteration requires knowledge of the normal values in each age group. These have now been validated for the great vessels but not yet for the small arteries and veins.
– Assessment of blood velocities should be constantly preferred; at birth and during the first month of life, resistive index alone is of poor value and may be the source of severe errors. For example, only measurement of velocities will identify a low blood flow, which is most often associated with normal resistive index (Fig. 2.96).

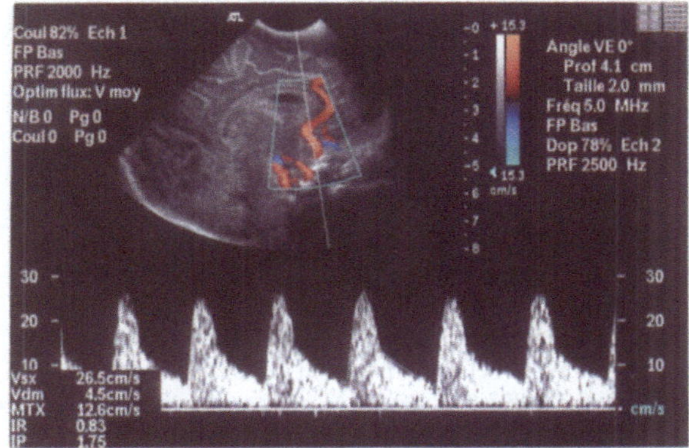
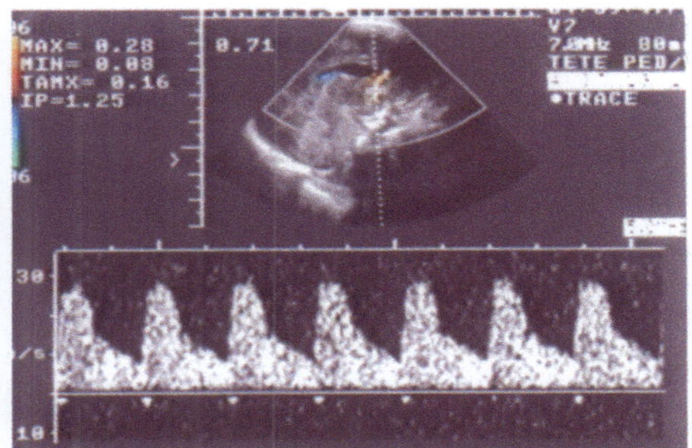

Fig. 2.96a,b. These two cases highlight the importance of measuring flow velocities and correlating them with clinical history and findings. **a** RI=0.83, PSV=26.5 cm/s, EDV=4.5 cm/s, TAV=12.5 cm/s. These are normal values since the patient is a 26-weeks' gestation preterm newborn. **b** RI=0.71, PSV=28 cm/s, EDV=8 cm/s, TAV=16 cm/s. These are low values since the patient is a full-term infant, 5 days old, with neurological distress. The spectral analysis shows a low blood flow. Rapid death ensued

– Although the value of vascular mapping is mainly diagnostic, pulsed Doppler and spectral analysis are of prognostic value: they may demonstrate a low blood flow, show the hemodynamic consequences of a galenic aneurysm, detect postischemic luxury perfusion, confirm intracranial hypertension, etc.

● The anterior fontanelle is the most appropriate window for evaluating cerebral vessels in the neonate, but for complete assessment of the vasculature it must be combined with transcranial Doppler.

● Multiple limitations remain obvious in the depiction of the neonatal cerebral circulation. The great arteries are always demonstrated on color imaging, but other vessels are inconstantly seen, and some are never visualized (Tables 2.8, 2.9).This is mainly owing to anatomical characteristics (small and/or low-flow vessels, and arteries deeply located in the posterior fossa).

● In the fetus, the potentialities of Doppler investigation are evident. Nowadays, color depiction of arteries and veins is becoming as easy as it is in the newborn. The hemodynamic data are still too rare to permit an overall view; quantitation of blood velocities is the most valuable parameter, but many questions remain. Are some spectral waveforms specific to the fetus? Does fetal cerebral autoregulation exist?

More longitudinal studies are required, and the comparison with neonatal velocimetry will be especially interesting.

Table 2.8. Constancy of visualization of cerebral arteries on color Doppler imaging

	Always seen	Inconstantly seen	Never seen
Internal carotid artery	+		
– Intracavernous branches			+
– Supracavernous branches			+
– Ophthalmic artery	+		
– Anterior choroidal artery	+		
– Posterior communicating artery	+		
Basilar artery	+		
– Superior cerebellar artery		+	
– Middle cerebellar artery			+
Anterior cerebral artery	+		
– Anterior communicating artery		+	
– Artery of Heubner		+	
– Pericallosal artery	+		
– Callosomarginal artery	+		
– Artery of the corpus callosum		+	
– Orbitofrontal artery		+	
– Medial frontal artery	+		
– Paracentral artery		+	
– Medial parietal arteries		+	
Middle cerebral artery	+		
- Lenticulostriate arteries	+		
- Operculoinsular arteries	+		
- Cortical arteries		+	
Posterior cerebral artery	+		
- Thalamic arteries	+		
- Peduncular arteries			+
- Circumflex arteries			+
- Temporal branches		+	
- Choroidal artery	+		
- Calcarine artery		+	
- Parieto-occipital arteries		+	
- Splenial artery			+

Table 2.8. Constancy of visualization of cerebral veins on color Doppler imaging

	Always seen	Inconstantly seen	Never seen
Superior sagittal sinus	+		
- Medial superficial veins	+		
- Lateral superficial veins		+	
Lateral sinuses	+		
- Superficial veins		+	
Vein of Galen	+		
- Venous afferences			+
Internal cerebral vein	+		
- Terminal veins	+		
- Septal veins		+	
- Choroidal veins		+	
- Thalamic veins			+
Straight sinus		+	
Torcular		+	
Basilar veins	+		
– Venous afferences			+
Subtentorial veins			+

References

Ahmed DS, Ahmed RH (1967) The recurrent branch of the anterior cerebral artery. Anat Rec 157:699-700

Aksel'rod VG, Gavriushov VV, Aleksandrova NK, Vasilenko LD (1991) Cerebral blood flow in healthy newborn infants in the early neonatal period. Akush Ginekol 8:53-55

Amarenco P, Hauw JJ (1989) Anatomie des artères cérébelleuses. Rev Neurol 145:267-276

Andrews BT, Dujovny M, Mirchandani HG, Ausman JI (1989) Microsurgical anatomy of the venous drainage into the superior sagittal sinus. Neurosurgery 24:514-520

Anthony MY, Evans DH, Levene MI (1991) Cyclical variations in cerebral blood flow velocity. Arch Dis Child 66:12-16

Anthony MY, Evans DH, Levene MI (1993) Neonatal cerebral blood flow velocity responses to changes in posture. Arch Dis Child 69:304-308

Arbeille Ph, Roncin A, Berson M, Patat F, Pourcelot L (1987) Exploration of the fetal cerebral blood flow by duplex Doppler linear array system in normal and pathological pregnancies. Ultrasound Med Biol 13:329-337

Arbeille Ph, Tranquart F, Berson M, Roncin A, Saliba E, Pourcelot (1989) Visualization of the fetal circle of Willis and intracerebral arteries by color-coded Doppler. Eur J Obstet Gynecol Reprod Biol 32:195-198

Arbeille P, Bose M, Vaillant MC, Tranquart F (1992) Nicotine induced changes in the cerebral circulation in ovine fetuses. Am J Perinatol 9:270-274

Archer LN, Evans DH, Levene MI (1985) Doppler ultrasound examination of the anterior cerebral arteries of normal newborn infants: the effect of postnatal age. Early Hum Dev 10:255-260

Austin NC, Pairaudeau PW, Hames TK, Hall MA (1992) Regional cerebral blood flow velocity changes after indomethacin infusion in preterm infants. Arch Dis Child 67:851-854

Baenziger O, Jaggi JL, Mueller AC, Morales CG, Lipp HP, Lipp AE, Duc G, Bucher HU (1994) Cerebral blood flow in preterm infants affected by sex, mechanical ventilation and intrauterine growth. Pediatr Neurol 11:319-324

Barker JN (1966) Fetal and neonatal cerebral blood flow. Am J Physiol 210:897-902

Bartlett RH, Roloff DW, Cornell RG, Andrews AF, Dillon PW, Zwischenberger JB (1985) Extracorporeal circulation in neonatal respiratory failure: a prospective randomized study. Pediatrics 76:479-487

Batton DG, Riordan S, Riggs T (1992) Cerebral blood flow velocity in normal, full-term newborns is not related to ductal closure. Am J Dis Child 146:737-740

Baumgartner J, Tournade A, Plas JY (1981) Etude anatomochirurgicale de la voie d'abord de la toile choroidienne supérieure du 3ème ventricule. A propos d'un anévrysme artérioveineux choroidien postérieur. J. Neurochir 27:97-102

Baumgartner RW, Nirkko AC, Muri RM, Gonner F (1997) Transoccipital power-based color coded duplex sonography of cerebral sinuses and veins. Stroke 28:1319-1323

Bejar R, Merritt TA, Coen RW, Mannino F, Gluck L (1982) Pulsatility index, patent ductus arteriosus and brain damage. Pediatrics 69:818-822

Benders MJ, Van Bel F, Van de Bor M (1998) The effect of phototherapy on cerebral blood flow velocity in preterm infants. Acta Paediatr 87:786-791

Berne RM, Winn HR, Rubio R (1982) La régulation locale du flux sanguin cérébral. Acquisitions nouvelles en pathologie cardio-vasculaire. Presse Méd 24:323-345

Bezinque SL, Slovis TL, Touchette AS, Schave DM, Jarski RW, Bedard MP, Martino AM (1995) Characterization of superior sagittal sinus blood flow velocity using color flow Doppler in neonates and infants. Pediatr Radiol 25:175-179

Bigelow DC, Hoffer ME, Schlakman B (1993) Angiographic assessment of the transverse sinus and vein of Labbé to avoid complications in skull base surgery. Skull Base Surgery 3:217-222

Bisaria KK (1985) Anatomic variations of venous sinuses in the region of the torcular Herophili. J Neurosurg 62:90-95

Bode H, Wais U (1988) Age dependence of flow velocities in basal cerebral arteries. Arch Dis Child 63:606-611

Borch K, Greisen G (1998) Blood flow distribution in the normal human preterm brain. Pediatr Res 43 :28-33

Bouchet A, Cuilleret J (1983) Anatomie topographique, descriptive et fonctionnelle. Tome 1. Le système nerveux central. Ed Simep Lyon-Villeurbane/Paris

Bouthillier A, Van Loveren HR, Keller JT (1996) Segments of the internal carotid artery: a new classification. Neurosurgery 38:425-433

Bracard S, Braun M, Meder JF, Velut S (1996) Anatomie et radioanatomie du système veineux intracranien (à l'exclusion des sinus duraux). Neurochirurgie 42:11-44

Bracard S, Anxionnat R, Braun M, Meder JF, Roland J, Picard L (1997) Vascularisation cérébrale: anatomie-radioanatomie. EMC Radiodiagnostic - Squelette normal. 30-861-1-10:1-31

Browder J, Kaplan HA, Krieger AJ (1976) Anatomical features of the straight sinus and its tributaries. J Neurosurg 44:55-61

Burghouwt M, Wladimiroff JW (1992) Modulation of middle cerebral artery flow velocity waveforms by breathing movements in the normal term fetus. Ultrasound Med Biol 18:821-825

Burns PN, Powers JE, Simpson DH, Brezina A, Kolin A, Chin CT, Uhlendorf V, Fritzsch T (1994) Harmonic power mode Doppler using microbubble contrast agents. An improved method for small vessels flow imaging. JEMU 16:132-142

Cabanas F, Pellicer A, Garcia-alix A, Quero J, Stiris TA (1997) Effect of dexamethasone therapy on cerebral and ocular blood flow velocity in premature infants studied by colour Doppler flow imaging. Eur J Pediatr 156:41-46

Calvert A, Ohlsson A, Hosking MC (1988) Serial measurements of cerebral blood flow velocity in preterm infants during the first 72 hours of life. Acta Paediatr Scand 77:625-631

Chandran R (1993) Fetal cerebral Doppler in the recognition of fetal compromise. Br J Obstet Gynecol 100:139-144

Chemtob S, Laudignon N, Aranda JV (1987) Drug therapy in hypoxic ischemic cerebral insults and intraventricular hemorrhage of the newborn. Clin Perinatal 14:817-842

Cheung YF, Lam PK, Yeung CY (1994) Early postnatal cerebral Doppler changes in relation to birth weight. Early Hum Dev 37:57-66

Cohen HL, Haller JO (1994) Advances in perinatal neurosonography. AJR 163:801-810

Connors G, Hunse C, Gagnon R, Richardson B, Han V, Rosenberg H (1992) Perinatal assessment of cerebral flow velocity wave forms in the human fetus and neonate. Pediatr Res 31:649-652

Cooke RWL, Rolfe P, Howat P (1979) Apparent cerebral blood flow in newborns with respiratory disease. Dev Med Child Neurol 21:154-157

Coughtrey H, Rennie JM, Evans DH (1997) Variability in cerebral blood flow velocity: observations over one minute in preterm babies. Early Hum Dev 47:63-70

Couture A, Veyrac C, Baud C (1994) Echographie cérébrale: du foetus au nouveau-né. Imagerie et hémodynamique. Sauramps Medical Ed. Montpellier. France

Cowan F, Thoresen M (1985) Changes in superior sagittal sinus blood velocities due to postural alterations and pressure on the head of the newborn infant. Pediatrics 75:1038-1047

Czerwinski F, Michalczyk K, Mierzwa A (1996) Types of terminal division of the posterior cerebral artery in man. Folia Morpho 55:161-165

Dean LM, Taylor GA (1995) The intracranial venous system in infants: normal and abnormal findings on duplex and color Doppler sonography. AJR 164:151-156

De Bray JM, Granry JC, Monrigal JP, Leftheriotis G, Saumet JL (1993) Effects of thiopental on middle cerebral artery blood velocities: a transcranial Doppler study in children. Child s Nerv Syst 9 :220-223

Deeg KH, Rupprecht TH (1989) Pulsed Doppler sonography measurement of normal values for the flow velocities in the intracranial arteries of healthy newborns. Pediatr Radiol 19:71-78

Degani S, Paltiely Y, Gonen R, Sharf M (1991) Fetal internal carotid artery pulsed Doppler velocity waveforms and heart rate pattern in the human fetus. Obstet Gynecol 7:379-381

Delmas A, Chifflet J (1950) Le sinus longitudinal superieur et les voies de drainage de la convexité cérébrale. Sem Hop Paris 26:488-492

De Smedt MC, Visser GH, Meijboom EJ (1987) Fetal cardiac output estimated by Doppler echocardiography during mid and late gestation. Am J Cardiol 60:338-342

Donzelli R, Marinkovic S, Brigante L, De Divitiis O, Nikodijevic I, Schonauer C, Maiuri F (1998) Territories of the perforating (lenticulostriate) branches of the middle cerebral artery. Surg Radiol Anat 20:393-398

Drayton MR, Skidmore R (1987) Vasoactivity of the major intracranial arteries in newborn infants. Arch Dis Child 62:236-240

Dubiel M, Gudmundsson S, Gunnarsson G, Marsal K (1997) Middle cerebral artery velocimetry as a predictor of hypoxemia in fetuses with increased resistance to blood flow in the umbilical artery. Early Hum Dev 47:177-184

Dunker Ro, Harris AB (1976) Surgical anatomy of the proximal anterior cerebral artery. J Neurosurg 44:359-367

Edwards AD, Wyatt JS, Richardson C, Potter A, Cope M, Delpy DT, Reynolds EO (1990) Effects of Indomethacin on cerebral haemodynamics in very preterm infants. Lancet 335:1491-1495

Evans DH, Levene MI, Shortland DB, Archer LN (1988) Resistance index, blood flow velocity, and resistance-area product in the cerebral arteries of very low birth weight infants during the first week of life. Ultrasound Med Biol 14:103-110

Facchinetti F, Battaglia C, Benatti R, Borella P, Genazzani AR (1992) Oral magnesium supplementation improves fetal circulation. Magnes Res 5:179-181

Farnarier P, Michotey P, Moscow N, Salamon G (1977) An anatomical and radiological study of the cortical branches of the anterior cerebral artery. Ann Radiol 20:203-221

Fenton AC, Papathoma E, Evans DH, Levene MI (1991) Neonatal cerebral venous flow velocity measurement using a color flow Doppler system. J Clin Ultrasound 19:69-72

Ferrarri F, Kelsall AW, Rennie JM, Evans DH (1994) The relationship between cerebral blood flow velocity fluctuations and sleep state in normal newborns. Pediatr Res 35:50-54

Fischer E (1938) Die Lageabweichungen der vorderen hinarterce in gefa. Bild Zbl Neurochi 3:300-313

Fortunato SJ (1996) The use of power Doppler and color power angiography in fetal imaging. Am J Obstet Gynecol 174:1828-1831

Fujii K, Lenkey C, Rhoton AL (1980) Microsurgical anatomy of the choroidal arteries: lateral and third ventricles. J Neurosurg 52:165-168

Galloway JR, Greitz T (1960) The medial and lateral choroid arteries: an anatomic and roentgenographic study. Acta Radiol 53:352-366

Gibo H, Carver C, Rhoton AL, Lenkey C, Mitchell RJ (1981) Microsurgical anatomy of the middle cerebral artery. J Neurosurg 54:151-169

Gibo H, Lenkey C, Rhoton AL (1981) Microsurgical anatomy of the supraclinoid portion of the internal carotid artery. J Neurosurg 55:560-574

Ghali WH, Rafla MF, Ekladious EY, Ibrahim KA (1989) A study of the junction between the straight sinus and the great cerebral vein. J Anat 164:49-54

Gillis S, Connors G, Potts P, Hunse C, Richardson B (1992) The effect of glucose on Doppler flow velocity waveforms and heart rate pattern in the human fetus. Early Hum Dev 30:1-10

Goldstein MD, Filly RA, Toi A (1986) Septal veins: a normal finding on neonatal cranial sonography. Radiology 161:623-624

Gomes FB, Dujovny M, Umansky F, Berman SK, Diaz FG, Ausman JI, Mirchandani HG, Ray WJ (1986) Microanatomy of the anterior cerebral artery. Surg Neurol 26:129-141

Gomez F, Dujovny M, Umansky F, Ausman J, Diaz FG, Ray WJ, Mirchandani HG (1984) Microsurgical anatomy of the recurrent artery of Heubner. J Neurosurg 60:130-139

Gorczyca W, Mohr G (1987) Microvascular anatomy of Heubner's recurrent artery. Neurol Res 9:259-264

Goto K, Takahashi M, Tamakawa Y (1976) Duplication of the straight sinus. An angiographic study. Radiology 120:117-119

Govan JJ, Ohlsson A, Ryan ML, Myhr T, Fong K (1995) Aminophylline and Doppler time averaged mean velocity in the middle cerebral artery in preterm neonates. J Pediatr 31:461-464

Grand W, Hopkins LN (1977) The microsurgical anatomy of the basilar artery bifurcation. Neurosurgery 1:128-131

Grand W (1980) Microsurgical anatomy of the proximal middle cerebral artery and the internal carotid artery bifurcation. Neurosurgery 7:215-218

Grant EG, White EM, Schellinger D, Choyke PL, Sarcone AL (1987) Cranial duplex sonography of the infant. Radiology 163:177-185

Gray PH, Griffin EA, Drumm JE, Fitzgerald DE, Duignan NM (1983) Continuous wave Doppler ultrasound in evaluation of cerebral blood flow in neonates. Arch Dis Child 58:677-681

Greisen G, Hellstroem-vestas L, Lou H, Rosen I, Svenningen J (1985) Sleep-waking shifts and cerebral blood flow in stable preterm infants. Pediatr Res 19:1156-1159

Greisen G, Johansen K, Ellinson PH, Frederiksen PS, Mai J, Friis-Hansen G (1984) Cerebral blood flow in the newborn infant: comparison of Doppler ultrasound and 133 Xenon clearance. J Pediatr 104:411-417

Greisen G, Trojaborg W (1987) Cerebral blood flow, PaCO2 changes and visual evoked potentials in mechanically ventilated, preterm infants. Acta Paediatr Scand 76:394-400

Guidicelli G, Salamon G (1970) The veins of the thalamus. Neuroradiology 1:92-98

Hammerman C, Glaser J, Schimmel MS, Ferber B, Kaplan M, Eidelman AI (1995) Continuous versus multiple rapid infusions of indomethacin: effects on cerebral blood flow velocity. Pediatrics 95:244-248

Hansen NB, Stonestreet BS, Rosenkrantz TS, Oh W (1983) Validity of Doppler measurement of anterior cerebral artery blood flow velocity: correlation with brain blood flow in piglets. Pediatrics 72:526-531

Hara K, Fujino Y (1966) The thalamoperforate artery. Acta Radiol 5:192-200

Hassler G (1966) Deep cerebral venous sytem in man: a microangiographic study on its areas of drainage and its anastomoses with superficial cerebral veins. Neurology 16:505-511

Hata K, Hata T, Makihara K, Aoki S, Takamiya O (1991) Fetal intracranial arterial hemodynamics assessed by color and pulsed Doppler ultrasound. Int J Gynecol Obstet 35:139-145

Hayashi T, Ichiyama T, Uchida M, Tashiro N, Tanaka H (1992) Evaluation by colour Doppler and pulsed Doppler sonography of blood flow velocities in intracranial arteries during the early neonatal period. Eur J Pediatr 151:461-465

Herman LH, Ostrowski ES, Gurdjian ES (1963) Perforating branches of the middle cerebral artery; an anatomical study. Arch Neurol 8:32-34

Hernandez MJ, Brennan RW, Bowman GS, Vanucci RC (1979) Autoregulation of cerebral blood flow in the newborn dog. Ann Neurol 6:177-181

Horgan JG, Rumack cm, Hay T, Manco-johnson ML, Merenstein GB, Esola C (1989) Absolute intracranial blood-flow velocities evaluated by duplex Doppler sonography in asymptomatic preterm and term neonates. AJR 152:1059-1064

Icardo JM, Ojeda JL, Garcia-Porrero JA, Hurle JM (1982) The cerebellar arteries: cortical patterns and vascularization of the cerebellar nuclei. Acta Anat 113:108-116

Ipsiroglu OS, Stockler S, Hausler MC, Kainer F, Rosegger H, Weiss PA, Winter R (1993) Cerebral blood flow velocities in the first minutes of life. Eur J Pediatr 152:269-270

Jorch G, Rabe H, Michel E, Engels M, Schulz V, Hentschel R, Koch HG, Hultsch E (1993) Resuscitation of the very immature infant: cerebral Doppler flow velocities in the first 20 minutes of life. Biol Neonate 64:215-220

Kakou M, Velut S, Destrieux C (1998) Vascularisation artérielle et veineuse du corps calleux. Neurochirurgie 44:31-37

Kaplan HA (1965) The lateral perforating branches of the anterior and middle cerebral artery. J Neurosurg 23:305-310

Keeley MM, Wade RV, Laurent SL, Hamann VD (1993) Alterations in maternal fetal Doppler flow velocity waveforms in preterm labor patients undergoing magnesium sulfate tocolysis. Obstet Gynecol 81:191-194

Kempley ST, Vyas S, Bower S, Nicolaides KH, Gamsu H (1996) Cerebral and renal artery blood flow velocity before and after birth. Early Hum Dev 46:165-174

Knosp E, Muller G, Perneczky A (1988) The paraclinoid carotid artery: anatomical aspects of a microneurosurgical approach. Neurosurgery 22:896-901

Kojo M, Ogawa T. Yamada K (1996) Normal developmental changes in carotid arterial blood flow measured by Doppler flowmetry in children. Pediatr Neurol 14:313-316

Komiyama M, Nakajima H, Nischikawa M, Yasui T (1998) Middle cerebral artery variations: duplicated and accessory arteries. AJNR 19:45-49

Konje JC, Abrams K, Bell SC, De Chazal RC, Taylor DL (2000) The application of color power angiography to the longitudinal quantification of blood flow volume in the fetal middle cerebral arteries, ascending aorta, descending aorta and renal arteries during gestation. Am J Obstet Gynecol 182:393-400

Kresch MJ, Moya FR, Ascuitto RJ, Ross-Ascuitto NT, Heusser F (1988) Late closure of the ductus arteriosus using indomethacin in the preterm infant. Clin Pediatr 27:140-143

Kubota T, Tatsuno M (1991) A longitudinal study of blood flow velocities in the anterior cerebral artery and the internal cerebral vein in the neonatal period. No To Hattatsu 23:44-49

Kurjak A, Schulman H, Predanic A, Predanic M, Kupesics, Zalud I (1994) Fetal choroid plexus vascularization assessed by color flow ultrasonography. J Ultrasound Med 13:841-844

Kurmanavicius J, Florio I, Wisser J, Hebish G, Zimmermann R, Muller R, Huch R, Huch A (1997) Reference resistance indices of the umbilical, fetal middle cerebral and uterine arteries at 24-42 weeks of gestation. Ultrasound Obstet Gynecol 10:112-120

Kurmanavichius J, Karrer G, Hebisch G, Huch R, Huch A (1991) Fetal and preterm newborn cerebral blood flow velocity. Early Hum Dev 26:113-120

Lasjaunias P, Moret J, Mink J (1977) The anatomy of the infero-lateral trunk of the internal carotid artery. Neuroradiology 13:215-220

Laugier J, Sahla E, Bloc D, Gold F (1986) Physiologie de la circulation cerebrale. In: Progrés en Neonatalogie. Relier JP Ed. Karger:38-52

Laurichesse-delmas H, Grimaud O, Moscovo G, Ville Y (1999) Color Doppler study of the venous circulation in the fetal brain and hemodynamic study of the cerebral transverse sinus. Ultrasound Obstet Gynecol 13:34-42

Lazorthes G, Gaubert J, Poulhes J (1958) La distribution centrale et corticale de l'artère cérébrale antérieure. Etude anatomique et incidences neurochirurgicales. Neurochirurgie 2:237-253

Lazorthes G, Gouaze A, Salamon G (1976) Vascularisation et circulation de l'encéphale. Les veines de l'encéphale. Masson Ed. Tome I:236-263

Leahy FA, Sankaran K, Cates D (1979) Quantitative noninvasive method to measure cerebral blood flow in newborn infants. Pediatrics 64:277-284

Lewinsky RM, Farine D, Ritchie JW (1991) Transvaginal Doppler assessment of the fetal cerebral circulation. Obstet Gynecol 78:637-640

Ley D, Marsal K (1992) Doppler velocimetry in cerebral vessels of small for gestational age infants. Early Hum Dev 31:171-180

Lou HC, Lassen NA, Friis-Hansen B (1979) Impaired autoregulation of cerebral blood flow in the distressed newborn. J Pediatr 96:606-609

Lou HC, Lassen NA, Friis-Hansen B (1978) Decreased cerebral blood flow after administration of sodium bicarbonate in the distressed newborn infant. Acta Neurol Scand 57:239-247

Low JA, Froese AB, Galbraith RS, Smith JT, Karchmar EJ (1993) Middle cerebral artery blood flow velocity in the newborn following delivery. Clin Invest Med 16:29-37

Lucas W, Kirschbaum T, Assali NS (1966) Cephalic circulation and oxygen consumption before and after birth. Am J Physiol 210:287-292

Maesel A, Lingman G, Marsal K (1990) Cerebral blood flow during labor in the human fetus. Acta Obstet Gynecol Scand 69:493-495

Maesel A, Sladkevicius P, Valentin L, Marsal K (1994) Fetal cerebral blood flow velocity during labor and the early neonatal period. Ultrasound Obstet Gynecol 4:372-376

Mari G, Moise KJ, Deter RL, Kirshon B, Huhta JC, Carpenter RJ, Cotten DB (1989) Doppler assessment of the pulsatility index of the middle cerebral artery during constriction of the fetal ductus arteriosus after indomethacin therapy. Am J Obstet Gynecol 161:1528-1531

Mari G, Moise K, Deter R, Carpenter RJ (1991) Fetal heart rate influence in the pulsatility index in the middle cerebral artery. J Clin Ultrasound 19:149-153

Mari G, Deter RL (1992) Middle cerebral artery flow velocity waveforms in normal and small for gestational age fetuses. Am J Obstet Gynecol 166:1262-1270

Mari G (1994) Regional cerebral flow velocity waveforms in the human fetus. J Ultrasound Med 13:343-346

Mari G, Abuhamad A, Uerpairojkit B, Martinez E, Copel J (1995) Blood flow velocity waveforms of the abdominal arteries in appropriate and small for gestational age fetuses. Ultrasound obstet Gynecol 6:15-18

Marinkovic SV, Milisavljevic M, Kovacevic M, Stevic ZD (1985) Perforating branches of the middle cerebral artery. Microanatomy and clinical significance of their intracerebral segments. Stroke 16:1022-1029

Marinkovic SV, Kovacevic M, Marinkovic JM (1985) Perforating branches of the middle cerebral artery: microsurgical anatomy of their extracerebral segments. J Neurosurg 63:266-271.

Marinkovic SV, Milisavljevic M, Kovacevic M (1986) Anatomical bases for surgical approach to the initial segment of the anterior cerebral artery. Surg Radiol Anat 8:7-18

Marinkovic SV, Milisavljevic M, Marinkovic Z (1990) Branches of the anterior communicating artery. Microsurgical anatomy. Acta Neurochir 106:78-85

Marino R (1976) The anterior cerebral artery. I. Anatomo-radiological study of its cortical territories. Surg Neurol 5; 81-87

Matamoros A, Anderson JC, McConnel J, Bolan DL (1989) Neurosonographic findings in infants treated by extracorporeal membrane oxygenation (ECMO). J Child Neurol 4:52-61

McCord GM, Goree JA, Jimenez JP (1972) Venous drainage to the inferior sagittal sinus. Radiology 105:583-589

McDonnell M, Ives NK, Hope PL (1992) Intravenous aminophylline and cerebral blood flow in preterm infants. Arch Dis Child 67:416-418

Meder JF, Chiras J, Roland J, Guinet P, Bracard S, Bargy F (1994) Territoires veineux de l'encéphale. J Neuroradiol 21:118-133

Meerman RJ, Van Bel F, Van Zwieten PH, Oepkes D, Den Ouden L (1990) Fetal and neonatal cerebral blood velocity in the normal fetus and neonate: a longitudinal Doppler ultrasound study. Early Hum Dev 24:209-217

Mierzwa A (1989) Variability of the course of the anterior cerebral artery and its branches in humans. Ann Acad Med Stetin 35:37-56

Millen JW, Woolam DH (1953) Vascular patterns in the choroid plexus. J Anat 87:114-121

Minarik M, Strechova Z, Hlaucova E, Pivkova K (1993) Cerebrovascular blood flow velocity in a healthy neonate in the first days of life. Cesk Pediatr 48:530-534

Mitchell DG, Merton D, Needleman L, Kurtz AB, Goldberg BB, Levy D, Rifkin MD, Pennel RG, Vilaro M, Baltarowich O, Dahnert W, Graziani L, Desai H (1988) Neonatal brain: color Doppler imaging. Part I. Technique and vascular anatomy. Radiology 167:303-308

Mitchell DG, Merton D, Desai H, Needleman L, Kurtz AB, Goldberg BB, Graziani L, Wolfson P (1988) Neonatal brain: color Doppler imaging. Part II. Altered flow patterns from extracorporeal membrane oxygenation. Radiology 167:307-310

Mitchell D, Merton D, Mirsky P, Needleman L (1989) Circle of Willis in newborns: color Doppler imaging of 53 healthy full term infants. Radiology 172:201-205

Mochalova LD, Khodov DA, Zhukova TP (1983) Cerebral circulation control in healthy full term neonates. Acta Paediatr Scand 311:20-22

Morris PP, Cha IS (1996) Cerebral vascular anatomy. Neuroimaging Clin N Am 6:547-560

Mosca F, Bray M, Lattanzio M, Fumagalli M, Tosetto C (1997) Comparative evaluation of the effects of indomethacin and ibuprofen on cerebral perfusion and oxygenation in preterm infants with patent ductus arteriosus. J Pediatr 131:549-554

Moss AJ, Emmanouilides G, Duffie ER (1963) Closure of the ductus arteriosus in the newborn infant. Pediatrics 32:25-30

Mukhtar AI, Cowan FM, Stothers JL (1982) Cranial blood flow and blood pressure changes during sleep in the human neonate. Early Hum Dev 6:59-63

Nelle M, Hoecker C, Linderkamp O (1997) Effects of bolus tube feeding on cerebral blood flow velocity in neonates. Arch Dis Child Fetal Neonatal Ed. 76:54-56

Nijima S, Shortland DB, Levene M, Evans DH (1988) Transient hyperoxia and cerebral blood flow velocity in infants born prematurely and at full term. Arch Dis Child 63:1126-1130

Nischimaki S, Kawakami T, Akamatsu H, Iwasaki Y (1991) Cerebral blood flow velocities in the anterior cerebral arteries and basilar artery. I. Investigation in term infants. No To Hattatsu 23:247-251

Noordam MJ, Heydanus R, Hop WC, Hoekstra FM, Wladimiroff JW (1994) Doppler colour flow imaging of fetal intracerebral arteries and umbilical artery in the small for gestational age fetus. Br J Obstet Gynecol 101:504-508

Oka K, Rhoton AL, Barry M, Rodriguez R (1985) Microsurgical anatomy of the superficial veins of the cerebrum. Neurosurgery 17:711-748

Okudera T, Huang YP, Ohta T, Yokota A, Nakamura Y, Maehara F, Utsunomiya H, Uemura K, Fukasawa H (1994) Development of posterior fossa dural sinuses, emissary veins, and jugular bulb: morphological and radiologic study. AJNR 15:1871-1883

Okudera T, Ohta T, Huang YP, Yokota (1988) Etude anatomique et radiologique du developpement des vaisseaux superficiels de la convexité chez le foetus humain. J Neuroradiol 15:205-224

Ohlsson A, Fong K, Ryan ML; Yap L, Smith JD, Shennan AT, Glanc P (1991) Cerebral blood flow velocity measurements in neonates: technique and interobserver reliability. Pediatr Radiol 21:395-397

Ono M, Rhoton AL, Peace D, Rodriguez RJ (1984) Microsurgical anatomy of the deep venous system of the brain. Neurosurgery 15:621-657

Ostrowski AZ, Webster JE, Gurdjian ES (1960) The proximal anterior cerebral artery: an anatomic study. Arch Neurol 3:661-664

Ozek E, Koroglu TF, Karakoc F, Kich T, Tangoren M, Pamir N, Basaran M, Bekiroglu N (1995) Transcranial Doppler assessment of cerebral blood flow velocity in term newborns. Eur J Pediatr 154:60-63

Padget DH (1956) The cranial venous system in man in reference to development, adult configuration and relation to the arteries. Am J Anat 98:307-355

Panerai RB, Kelsall AW, Rennie JM, Evans DH (1996) Analysis of cerebral blood flow autoregulation in neonates. IEEE Trans Biomed Eng 43:779-788

Papile LA, Rudolph AM, Heymann MA (1985) Autoregulation of cerebral blood flow in the preterm fetal lamb. Pediatr Res 19:159-164

Pedrosa A, Dujovny M, Artero JC, Umansky F, Berman SK, Diaz FG (1987) Microanatomy of the posterior communicating artery. Neurosurgery 20:228-235

Percheron G (1976) Les artères du thalamus humain. I. Artère et territoire thalamiques polaires de l'artère communicante postérieure. Rev Neurol 132:297-307

Perese DM (1960) Superficial veins of the brain from a surgical point of view. J Neurosurg 17:402-412

Perlmutter D, Rhoton AL (1976) Microsurgical anatomy of the anterior cerebral, anterior communicating, recurrent artery complex. J Neurosurg 45:259-272

Perlmutter D, Rhoton AL (1978) Microsurgical anatomy of the distal anterior cerebral artery. J Neurosurg 49:204-228

Perlman JM (1985) Neonatal cerebral blood flow velocity measurement. Clin Perinatol 12:179-193

Pfannschmidt J, Jorch G (1989) Transfontanelle pulsed Doppler measurement of blood flow velocity in the internal jugular vein, straight sinus, and internal cerebral vein in preterm and term neonates. Ultrasound Med Biol 15:9-12

Piffer CR, Horn Y, Hureau J, Meininger V (1980) Etude anatomique des veines cérébrales supérieures. Anat Anr 160:271-283

Plets C, Van Den Bergh R (1974) Contribution des artères choroïdiennes dans la vascularisation du thalamus humain. C R Ass Anat 58:1009-1019

Pooh R, Aono T (1996) Transvaginal power Doppler angiography of the fetal brain. Ultrasound Obstet Gynecol 8:417-421

Pryds O, Greisen G (1989) Effect of PaCO2 and haemoglobin concentration on day to day variation of CBF in preterm neonates. Acta Paediatr Scan Suppl 360:33-36

Pryds O, Greisen G, Skov L (1990) Carbon dioxide related changes in cerebral blood volume and cerebral blood flow in mechanically ventilated preterm neonates: compared of near infrared spectrophotometry and 133 xenon clearance. Pediatr Res 27:445-449

Pryds O, Schneider S (1991) Aminophylline reduces cerebral blood flow in stable, preterm infants without affecting the visual evoked potential. Eur J Pediatr 150:366-369

Purves MJ, James IM (1969) Observations of the control of cerebral blood flow in the sheep fetus and newborn lamb. Cir Res 25:651-654

Rahilly PM (1980) Effects of sleep state and feeding on cranial blood flow of the human neonate. Arch Dis Child 55:265-270

Raju TN, Kim SY (1989) Cerebral artery flow velocity acceleration and deceleration characteristics in newborn infants. Pediatr Res 26:588-592

Raju TN (1991) Cerebral Doppler studies in the fetus and newborn infant. J Pediatr 119:165-174

Ramaekers V, Casaer P, Marchal G, Smet M, Gooseens W (1988) The effect of blood transfusion on cerebral blood flow in preterm infants: a Doppler study. Dev Med Child Neurol 30:334-341

Ramaekers V, Casaer P, Daniels H, Marchal G (1992) The influence of blood transfusion on brain blood flow autoregulation among stable preterm infants. Early Hum Dev 30:217-220

Rehan VK, Fajardo CA, Haider AZ, Alvaro RE, Cates DB, Kwiatkowski K, Nowaczyk B, Rigatto H (1996) Influence of sleep state and respiratory pattern on cyclical fluctuations of cerebral blood flow velocity in healthy preterm infants. Biol Neonate 69:357-367

Rhoton AL, Fujii K, Fradd B (1979) Microsurgical anatomy of the anterior choroidal artery. Surg. Neurol 12:171-187

Rosenkrantz TS, Oh W (1982) Cerebral blood flow velocity in infants with polycythemia and hyperviscosity: effects of partial exchange transfusion with plasmanate. J Pediatr 101:94-98

Rosenberg AA, Narayanan V, Jones (1985) Comparison of anterior cerebral artery blood flow velocity and cerebral blood flow during hypoxia. Pediatr Res 19:67-70

Rosner SS, Rhoton AL, Ono M, Barry M (1984) Microsurgical anatomy of the anterior perforating arteries. J Neurosurg 61:468-485

Rubin JM (1999) Power Doppler. Eur Radiol 5318-5322

Saeki N, Rhoton AL (1977) Microsurgical anatomy of the upper basilar artery and the posterior circle of Willis. J Neurosurg 46:653-578

Salamon G, Boudouresques J, Combalbert A (1966) Les artères lenticulostriées. Etude artériographique. Leur intérêt dans le diagnostic des hématomes intra-cérébraux. Rev Neurol 114:361-373

Saliba E, Autret E, Gold F, Bloc D, Pourcelot L, Laugier J (1989) Effect of cafeine on cerebral blood flow velocity in preterm infants. Biol Neonate 56:198-203

Sann L, Simonnet C (1985) Données récentes sur la circulation cérébrale et le métabolisme du cerveau du nouveau-né. Presse Méd 14:1465-1469

Satoh S, Kojanagi T, Hara K, Shimokawa H, Nakamo J (1988) Developmental characteristics of blood flow in the middle cerebral artery in the human fetus in utero, assessed using the linear array-pulsed Doppler method. Early Hum Dev 17:195-203

Saxena RC, Beg MA, Das AC (1974) The straight sinus. J Neurosurg 41:724-727

Schipper JA, Mohammad GI, Van Straaten HL, Koppe JG (1997) The impact of surfactant replacement therapy on cerebral and systemic circulation and lung function. Eur J Pediatr 156:224-227

Schmidek HH, Auer LM, Kapp JP (1985) The cerebral venous system. Neurosurgery 17:663-677

Schöning M, Niemann G, Hartig B (1996) Transcranial color duplex sonography of basal cerebral arteries: reference data of flow velocities from childhood to adulthood. Neuropediatrics 27:249-255

Seydel HG (1964) The diameter of cerebral arteries in human fetus. Anat Rec 150:79-86

Sindou M, Alaywan M, Hallacq P (1996) Chirurgie des grands sinus veineux duraux intracraniens. Neurochirurgie 42:45-87

Sobotta J (1985) Atlas d'anatomie humaine. 1. Tête, cou, membres, thorax. Ed by H Ferner and J Staubesan. Munich, Vienne, Baltimore: Urban and Schwarzenberg. Paris. Ed Medicales Internat

Sonesson SE, Winberg P, Lundell BP (1987) Early postnatal changes in intracranial arterial blood flow velocities in term infants. Pediatr Res 22:461-464

Stehbens WE (1963) Aneurysms and anatomical variation of cerebral arteries. Arch Pathol 75:45-64

Takahashi M, Okudera T (1972) The choroid plexus and the choroid vein of the lateral ventricle. Radiology 103:113-120

Tammela O, Ojala R, Iivainen T, Lautamatti V, Pokela ML, Janas M, Koivisto M, Ikonen S (1999) Short versus prolonged indomethacin therapy for patent ductus arteriosus in preterm infants. J Pediatr 134:552-557

Taptas JN (1981) The intracranial course of the internal carotid artery. Anatomical features-clinical implications. J Chir 118:719-723

Tatsuno M, Furusho J, Ohno H, Okuyama K (1990) Cerebral blood flow in infants: comparaison of carotid blood flow and cerebral blood velocity. No To Hattatsu 22:336-340

Taylor GA, Short BL, Walker LK, Traystman RJ (1990) Intracranial blood flow: quantification with duplex Doppler and color Doppler flow US. Radiology 176:231-234

Taylor GA, Walker LK (1992) Intracranial venous system in newborns treated with extracorporeal membrane oxygenation: Doppler US evaluation after ligation of the right jugular vein. Radiology 183:453-456

Taylor GA (1992) Intracranial venous system in the newborn: evaluation of normal anatomy and flow characteristics with color Doppler US. Radiology 183:449-452

Taylor G (1992) Effects of scanning pressure on intracranial hemodynamics during transfontanellar duplex US. Radiology 185:763-766

Taylor GA (2000) Potential pediatric applications for US contrast agents: lessons from the laboratory. Pediatr Radiol 30:101-109

Theron J, Newton TH (1976) Artère choroïdienne antérieure. J Neuroradiol 3:6-51

Tsai ML, Hung Kl, Lin FK (1990) The evaluation of cerebral blood flow velocities in normal newborns and infants. Chung Hua Min Kuo Hsiao Erh Ko I Hsueh Hui Tsa Chin 31:343-349

Ture U, Yasargil MG, Krisht AF (1996) The arteries of the corpus callosum: a microsurgical anatomic study. Neurosurgery 39:1075-1084

Uerpairojkit B, Chan L, Reece AE, Martinez E, Mari G (1996) Cerebellar Doppler velocimetry in the appropriate and small for gestational age fetus. Obstet Gynecol 87: 989-993

Umansky F, Gomes FB, Dujovny M, Diaz FG, Ausman JI, Mirchandani HG, Berman SK (1985) The perforating branches of the middle cerebral artery. A microanatomical study. J Neurosurg 62:261-268

Van Bel F, Ouden LD, Van de Bor M, Stijnen T, Baan J, Ruys JH (1989) Cerebral blood flow velocity during the first week of life of preterm infants and neurodevelopment at two years. Dev Med Child Neurol 31:320-328

Van Bel F, Schipper J, Guilt GL, Visser MO (1993) The contribution of color Doppler flow imaging to the study of cerebral haemodynamics in the neonate. Neuroradiology 35:300-306

Van De Bor M, Walther FJ, Sims ME (1990) Acceleration time in cerebral arteries of preterm and term infants. J Clin Ultrasound 18:167-171

Van Den Wijngaard JA, Wladimiroff JW, Reuss A, Stewart PA (1988) Oligohydramnios and fetal cerebral blood flow. Br J Obstet Gynaecol 95:1309-1311

Van Den Wijngaard JA, Groenenberg IA, Wladimiroff JW, Hop WC (1989) Cerebral Doppler ultrasound of the human fetus. Br J Obstet Gynaecol 96:845-849

Van Eyck J, Wladimiroff JW, Van Den Wijngaard JA, Noordam MJ, Prechtl HF (1987) The blood flow velocity waveform in the fetal internal carotid and umbilical artery: its relation to fetal behaviour in normal pregnancy at 37-38 weeks. Br J Obstet Gynecol 94:736-741

Van der Zwan A, Hillen B, Tulleken CA, Dujovny M, Dragovic L (1992) Variability of the territories of the major cerebral arteries. J Neurosurg 77:927-940

Varvarigou N, Bardin CL, Beharry K, Chemtob S, Papageorgiou A, Aranda JV (1996) Early ibuprofen administration to prevent patent ductus arteriosus in premature infants. JAMA 275:539-544

Veille JC, Hanson R, Tatum K (1993) Longitudinal quantification of middle cerebral artery blood flow in normal human fetuses. Am J Obstet Gynecol 169:1393-1398

Velut S, Santini JJ (1987) Anatomie microchirurgicale de l'ampoule de Galien. Neurochirurgie 33:264-271

Vicentelli F, Caruso G, Andriamamonjy C, Rabehanta P, Graziani N, Grisoli F, Gouaze A, Vigouroux RP (1990) Microanatomy of collateral perforating branches of the middle cerebral artery. Neurochirurgie 36:3-14

Volpe JJ (1997) Brain injury in the premature infant. Neuropathology, clinical aspects, pathogenesis and prevention. Clin Perinatol 24:567-587

Vyas S, Campbell S, Bower S, Nicolaides KH (1990) Maternal abdominal pressure alters fetal cerebral blood flow. Br J Obstet Gynaecol 97:740-742

Winberg P, Sonesson SE, Lundell PN (1990) Postnatal changes in intracranial blood flow velocity in preterm infants. Acta Pediatr Scand 79:1150-1155

Winkler P, Helmke K (1989) Duplex-scanning of the deep venous drainage in the evaluation of blood flow velocity of the cerebral vascular system in infants. Pediatr Radiol 19:79-80

Winkler P, Helmke K (1990) Major pitfalls in Doppler investigations with particular reference to the cerebral vascular system. Part I. Sources of error resulting pitfalls and measures to prevent errors. Pediatr Radiol 20:219-228

Winkler P, Helmke K, Mahl M (1990) Major pitfalls in Doppler investigations. Part II. Low flow velocities and color Doppler applications. Pediatr Radiol 20:304-310

Wladimiroff JW, Wijngaard JA, Degani S, Noordam MJ, Eyck J, Tonge HM (1987) Cerebral and umbilical arterial blood flow velocity waveforms in normal and growth retarded pregnancies. Obstet Gynecol 69:705-710

Wladimiroff JW, Van Bel F (1987) Fetal and neonatal cerebral blood flow. Semin Perinatol 11:335-346

Wolf B, Huang YP (1964) The subependymal veins of the lateral ventricle. Am J Roentgenol 91:406-426

Wolfram-Gabel R, Maillot Cl, Koritke JG (1987) La vascularisation de la toile choroïdienne du prosencéphale chez l'homme. J Neuroradiology 14:10-26

Wolfram-Gabel R, Maillot Cl, Koritke JG, Laude M (1984) La vascularisation de la toile choroïdienne du troisième ventricule chez l'homme. Arch Anat Hist Embr Norm Exp 67:3-42

Wolfram-Gabel R, Maillot Cl, Koritke JG (1989) Vascularisation artérielle du corps calleux chez l'homme. Arch Anat Histol Embryol 72:43-55

Wolfram-Gabel R, Maillot Cl, Koritke JG (1991) Systématisation de l'angioarchitectonie du corps calleux chez l'homme. Acta Anat 141:46-50

Wolfram-Gabel R, Maillot Cl (1992) The venous vascularisation of the corpus callosum in man. Surg Radiol Anat 14:17-21

Wolfram-Gabel R, Maillot Cl (1995) La vascularisation artérielle du noyau lenticulaire. J Neuroradiol 22:1-11

Wolfram-Gabel R, Maillot Cl (1997) Architecture vasculaire du noyau caudé. J Neuroradiol 24:23-29

Wong WS, Tsuruda JS, Liberman RL, Chirino A, Vogt JF, Gangitano E (1989) Color Doppler imaging of intracranial vessels in the neonate. AJNR 10:425-430

Woo JK, Liang ST, Lo RS, Chang FY (1987) Middle cerebral artery Doppler flow velocity waveforms. Obstet Gynecol 70:613-616

Wright LL, Baker KR, Hollander DI, Wright JN, Nagey DA (1988) Cerebral blood flow velocity in term newborn infants: changes associated with ductal flow. J Pediatr 112:768-773

Yamashita N, Kamiya K, Nagai H (1991) CO2 reactivity and autoregulation in fetal brain. Child's Nerv Syst 7:327-331

Yamamoto I, Rhoton AL, Peace D (1981) Microsurgery of the third ventricle. Neurosurgery 8:334-373

Yanowitz TD, Yao AC, Werner JC, Pettigrew KD, OH W, Stonestreet B (1998) Effects of prophylactic low-dose indomethacin on hemodynamics in very low birth weight infants. J Pediatr 132:28-34

Yoshida H, Yasuhara A, Kobayashi Y (1991) Transcranial Doppler sonographic studies of cerebral blood flow velocity in neonates. Pediatr Neurol 7:105-110

Younkin D, Delivora-Papadopoulos M, Reivich M, Jaggi J, Obrist W (1988) Regional variations in human newborn cerebral blood flow. J Pediatr 112:104-108

Zeal AA, Rhoton AL (1978) Microsurgical anatomy of the posterior cerebral artery. J Neurosurg 48:534-559

3 Germinal Matrix and/or Intraventricular Hemorrhage in the Preterm Infant

CORINNE VEYRAC

CONTENTS

Germinal matrix and/or intraventricular hemorrhage (IVH) represents a major disease in the premature neonate, carrying both a high mortality rate and the possibility of developing hydrocephalus which may require a shunting procedure, and severe neuromotor sequelae that may appear subsequently.

The spectrum of the disease has altered over the last 10 years:
- The physiopathogenic mechanisms that lead to IVH are better known.
- The multiplication of diagnostic imaging methods allows reliable diagnosis in the postnatal and sometimes even the prenatal period.
- Improvements in resuscitation techniques have reduced the incidence of hemorrhagic injury.
- On the other hand, the greater number of very-low-birth-weight neonates tends to increase the incidence of intracranial hemorrhage.
- Some therapeutic interventions using medications either after birth or in utero (producing some degree of fetal maturation) may be proposed.

C. VEYRAC, MD
Department of Pediatric Radiology, Hôpital Arnaud de Villeneuve, 371 Av. Doyen Gaston Giraud, 34295 Montpellier Cédex 5, France

The overall incidence of IVH varies from one series to another depending on the group of patients being studied. The following rates have been cited:
- 5.5% of infants weighing less than 2250 g (SHETH 1998), but 12% of infants less than 1500 g and 21% of infants less than 1000 g
- 47% of infants of 28 weeks' gestation or less (CLARIS 1996)
- 43% of infants weighing less than 1500 g (MORALES 1986)
- 18% of infants weighing less than 1500 g (ROLAND 1997)

Moreover, among these patients, the incidence of high-grade hemorrhage (grade III or IV (PAPILE 1978)) has also reduced : 23% for SHETH (1998), 6% for BOSCHE (1996).

Despite the decrease in the incidence of IVH, these data demonstrate the magnitude of the problem.

With the appearance and wide use of Doppler ultrasonographic techniques that may be performed at the bedside, several applications may be described:
- Color imaging may help the diagnosis of intraventricular hemorrhage and the understanding and prediction of an ischemo-hemorrhagic infarct.
- Pulsed Doppler may demonstrate some conditions at risk of hemorrhage, and hemodynamic changes occurring with IVH.

3.1 Color Doppler Imaging

3.1.1 Germinal Matrix Hemorrhage

In the opinion of all authors (LARROCHE 1964; VOLPE 1995), the site of origin of IVH is the germinal matrix, located under the ependyma of the lateral ventricle, at the level of the caudate nucleus head. Like any germinative structure, it is a highly vascular region, but with a particular architectural arrangement: germinal matrix vessels have a larger diameter, thinner walls along greater portions of their circumference, a less defined basement membrane, and less perivascular support than other brain regions (GOULD 1988; MENT 1995; SOTREL 1989; TROMMER 1987).

The vascularization of the germinal matrix has been well studied (HAMBLETON 1976). Arterioles arise from the recurrent artery of Heubner, from terminal branches of the lateral striate arteries and callosal penetrating arterioles. They course to supply a continuous capillary network and join a venule. At the superolateral angle of the lateral ventricle, the venules converge into periventricular veins and connect with transcerebral medullary veins. Venous blood drains either centripetally through terminal veins to the great vein of Galen, or centrifugally to the leptomeningeal veins at the brain surface. The direction of blood flow changes in a peculiar U-turn.

Some authors have reported arteriolar-to-venous shunts or arteriolar-to-arteriolar anastomoses (NAKAMURA 1991; PAPE 1979), while others (GHAZI-BIRRY 1997) found only conventional arteriolar-to-capillary-to-vein connections.

Analysis of germinal matrix hemorrhage (GHAZI-BIRRY 1997) demonstrates that most hemorrhagic foci are closely linked to the venous vessels. After post-mortem intravenous and intra-arterial angiography, only material injected via veins leaked into the hemorrhage (NAKAMURA 1990). From this rupture point in the venous wall, blood may spread along the perivenous space, giving rise to a dissecting distension of this space that may cause stretching, tearing, and rupture of smaller venous tributaries. This may explain the secondary extension of a germinal matrix hemorrhage. Blood may subsequently rupture through the ventricular wall and spread into the ventricular lumen. Finally, the hemorrhagic component may compress the terminal veins, causing obstruction of venous return, and, in consequence, an ischemohemorrhagic infarction within the periventricular white matter.

The sequence of events might be: prior rupture of a venule, diffusion of blood into the perivenous spaces of the germinal matrix, increased tissue pressure, venous congestion, venous stasis and thrombosis, distorsion of tissue architecture with stretching of venous tributaries and additional rupture points, tissue congestion that compresses afferent vessels and obstructs arteriolar flow resulting in vessel ischemia and hypoxia, destruction of arteriolar wall, and secondary arteriolar hemorrhage.

On *color Doppler* imaging, terminal veins are easily depicted on coronal planes (Fig. 3.1a).

When a germinal matrix hemorrhage occurs, and appears either hyperechogenic in the acute phase (Fig. 3.1b) or cystic in the secondary phase (Fig. 3.1c), the subependymal veins are displaced downward beneath the lesion. This pattern cannot differentiate a posthemorrhagic cyst from a postinfectious germinolysis, which have same location, but it helps to distinguish these from caudate nucleus lesions. The nonvisualization of any flow within the subependymal veins suggests their thrombosis and that a periventricular ischemic-hemorrhagic infarct may subsequently develop (TAYLOR 1995).

3.1.2
Diagnosis of Intraventricular Hemorrhage

Sonographic diagnosis of IVH is based on morphological imaging: the bleeding first appears as a highly echogenic image, located in the ventricular lumen. In most cases, the amount of blood is large enough and morphological diagnosis is easy. However, when intraluminal hemorrhage is minimal, the diagnosis is uncertain, either because the blood clot is close to the germinal matrix and may be confused with a large germinal matrix hemorrhage, or because it is close to the choroid plexus and may be confused with a dysmorphic choroid plexus (VEYRAC 1994).

Follow-up imaging will confirm the IVH by showing the characteristic evolution of the clot, but *color Doppler* may allow the diagnosis at the first examination. Indeed, several authors have demonstrated a relationship between the presence of small particles in the CSF and Doppler detection of a colored signal in the CSF pathways (TATSUNO 1992; WINKLER 1992a). In vitro studies (WINKLER 1992c) have shown that the lowest concentration of particles required for CSF flow motion detection is of the order of 300 cells/µl or more. This cannot be validated in clinical practice since it would need repeated intraventricular punctures.

The colored CSF flow is characteristic with respect to its aspect and location (Fig. 3.2): it appears as a signal that is alternatively red and blue and fills the sylvian aqueduct and fourth ventricle, with a jet-like pulsatile flow within the lumen of the third ventricle, in the axis of the aqueduct. It may also be observed in the foramina of Monro and at the outlet of the fourth ventricle (rather via a transcranial approach). The most sensitive area is the narrowest portion of the aqueduct of Sylvius. Recognition of the anatomy of

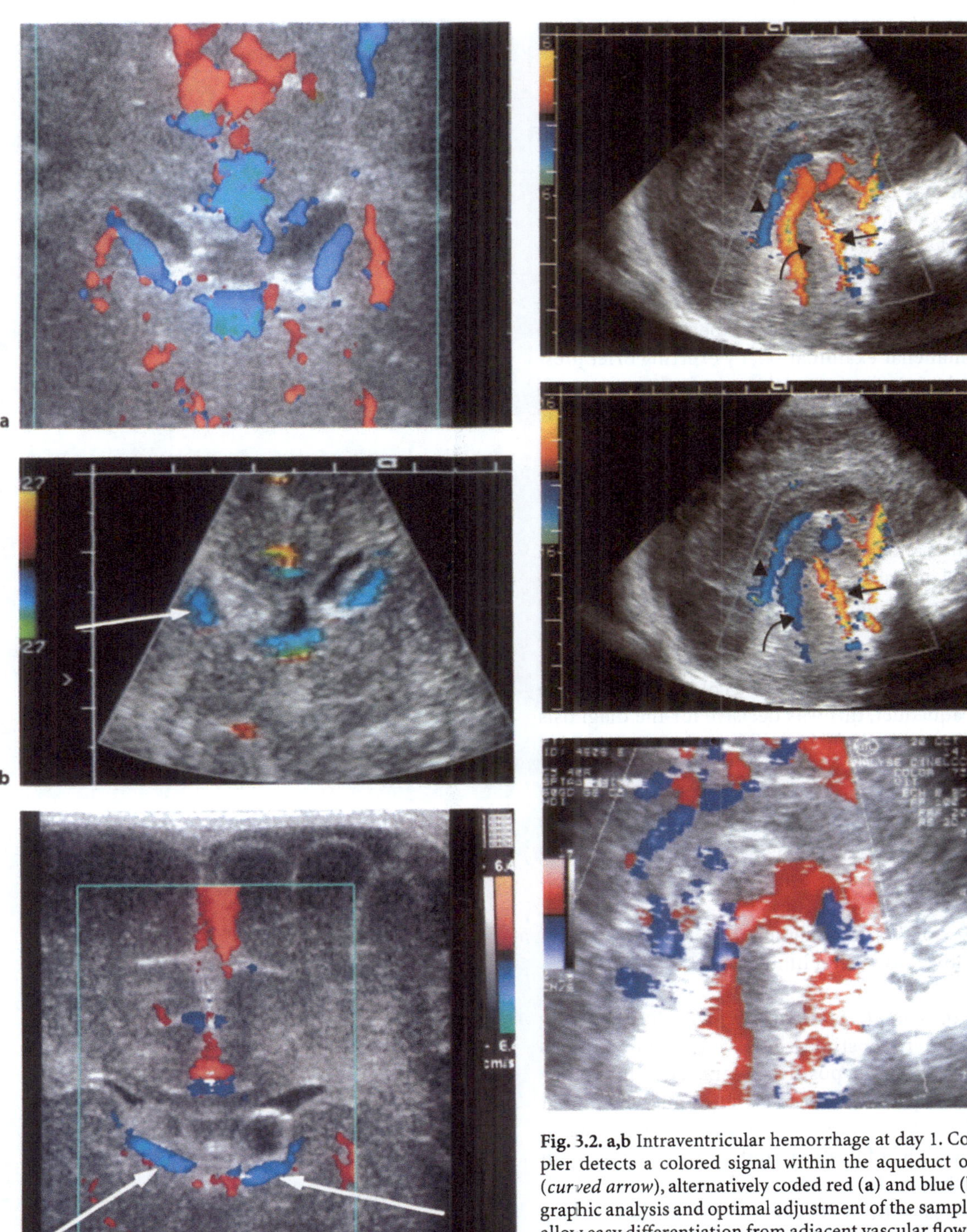

Fig. 3.1. a Normal ultrasonography. Terminal veins are easily visualized (*arrows*), close to the floor of the lateral ventricles. **b** Right hyperechogenic germinal matrix hemorrhage. Downward and lateral displacement of the right terminal vein (*arrow*) that remains patent. **c** A 32 weeks' gestation infant; maternofetal sepsis, first day of life. Germinal matrix cyst displacing the terminal veins (*arrows*), which remain patent

Fig. 3.2. a,b Intraventricular hemorrhage at day 1. Color Doppler detects a colored signal within the aqueduct of Sylvius (*curved arrow*), alternatively coded red (**a**) and blue (**b**). Topographic analysis and optimal adjustment of the sample volume allow easy differentiation from adjacent vascular flows [basilar artery (*straight arrow*), internal cerebral vein (*arrowhead*)]. Notice the jet-like colored signal in the third ventricular lumen. **c** In this other infant, colored CSF flow completely fills the characteristic triangular-shaped fourth ventricle

CSF flow makes it easy to exclude signals arising from adjacent vessels, and spectral analysis provides a confirmation of the diagnosis.

Colored CSF flow may be detected spontaneously, but more commonly it appears only with activity of the child: sucking, crying, hiccuping, or leg movements. It may be produced by some maneuvers that are easy to perform in clinical practice, especially in ventilated sedated newborns: abdominal palpation induces a ventriculopetal CSF motion followed by a ventriculofugal flow when the palpation is lifted. The second method is even easier to perform during the transfontanellar examination; by exerting brief pressure on the anterior fontanel, a ventriculofugal flow is obtained that becomes ventriculopetal when the pressure is removed.

Detection of a colored CSF flow may precede direct visualization of abnormal intraventricular echoes; a 2-day delay has been reported.

On the same way, color Doppler may confirm a suspected diagnosis when tiny echoes are close to the ventricular wall and difficult to assess as intraluminal bleeding. In our experience, among 40 preterm infants with IVH in whom color Doppler has been performed and has discovered a colored signal in the sylvian aqueduct, this was decisive for the diagnosis in 5 patients (doubtful hemorrhage in 3 and normal morphological examination in 2); in these 5 cases follow-up ultrasonography has confirmed the IVH (Fig. 3.3). The duration of visibility of colored CSF flows is quite variable; we have observed this finding for up to 15 days, but we did not perform routine follow-ups.

The use of this new diagnostic tool in clinical practice is subject to several limitations:

- First, the complete lack of specificity. It is currently observed in postinfectious ventriculitis, and is very useful in the positive diagnosis of this condition (Chap. 4); we have also encountered colored CSF flow in an infant with congenital leukemia and blastic CSF infiltration, and in two infants with chylothorax. In our personal experience (which disagrees with WINKLER 1992b) we have never detected such colored signals in clinical conditions with normal CSF.
- Secondly, the timing of intra-ventricular bleeding: if the examination is performed too late, with clots already organized, these flows may not be detected.
- So far, no study has been able to assess the accuracy of this Doppler sign in the positive diagnosis of IVH.

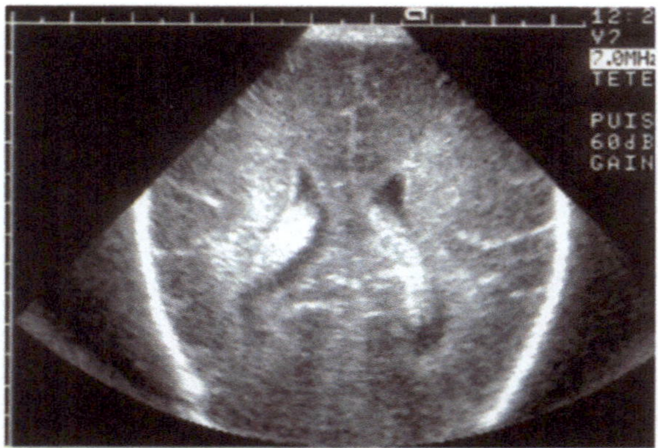

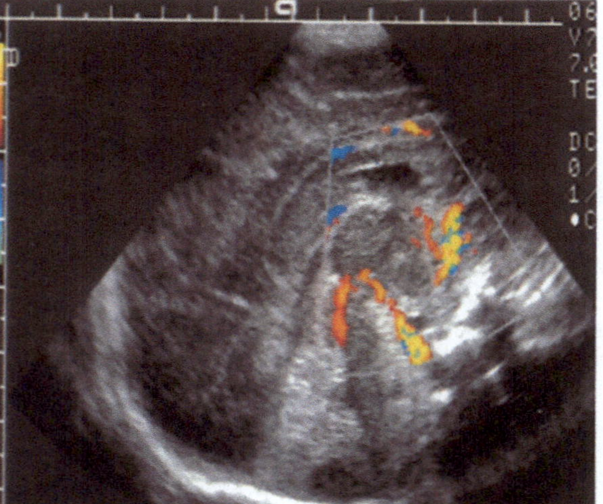

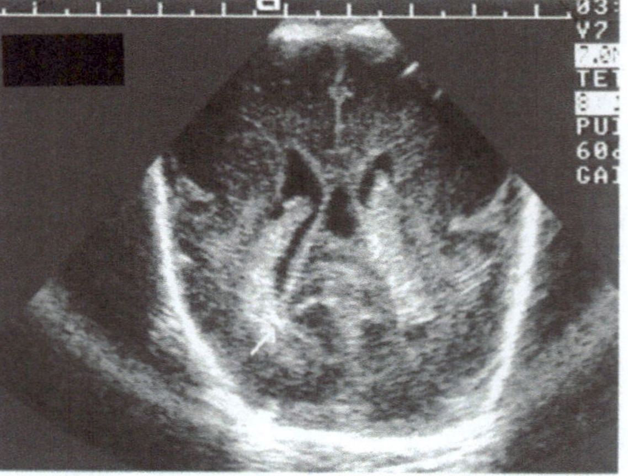

Fig. 3.3a–c. A 29 weeks' gestation preterm infant; preeclampsia, cesarian delivery. (a,b) Day 2: the ventricular lumen is anechoic (a), but Doppler ultrasonography detected a colored signal in the sylvian aqueduct (b). Intraventricular hemorrhage (IVH) is diagnosed. (c) Day 12: confirmation of a right intraventricular small clot (*arrow*)

Finally, WINKLER (1994) has analyzed the CSF pulse wave velocity. He has shown that during pulsed Doppler recording, CSF flow exhibits fluctuations that are most often synchronized with respiration or ventilation, less often with the cardiac cycle. This is not in complete contradiction with the results of MRI studies that investigated only arterial CSF pulsatility. During spontaneous breathing, CSF flows into the ventricular system at inspiration, followed by outflow at expiration. This may be explained by the predominant abdominal component of respiration: at inspiration, the abdominal pressure increases rapidly, initiating a venous volume-pressure pulse that is transferred to the spinal epidural veins and subarachnoid CSF; from there, the pulse travels to the base of the brain and forces CSF into the ventricular system as a result of the pressure differential. During mechanical ventilation, the CSF motion is commonly reversed, and this is more difficult to explain.

WINKLER performed 140 examinations in 35 infants and divided the morphological ultrasonographic signs into four grades of increasing severity (from 0 to 3). CSF flow was synchronized with respiration alone in 37 ultrasound scans, with 89% associated with normal or grade 1 findings. It was synchronized with heart beat alone in 15 cases, with 87% associated with grade 2 and grade 3 findings. It was synchronized with both respiration and heart beat in 24 cases.

Nevertheless, the Doppler spectrum changed with the evolving disease process in most infants, and even within one examination. Thus, any given CSF flow pattern does not correlate to a precise prognosis.

We studied CSF flow by pulsed Doppler in only five patients (Fig. 3.4). Peak velocities ranged from –10 to +11 cm/s. Two patients had CSF flows synchronized with heart beat and evolved toward posthemorrhagic hydrocephalus. Three patients had CSF flows independent of heart beat and had a favorable outcome (grade II hemorrhage).

In conclusion, quantitative assessment of CSF flow does not provide any main diagnostic or prognostic argument. At the contrary, detection of colored CSF flows may be very important for the early diagnosis of IVH. This investigation should be routinely performed in a high-risk premature infant without hemorrhage morphologically detected.

3.1.3
Periventricular Ischemic-Hemorrhagic Infarction

Periventricular hemorrhagic infarction is a characteristic parenchymal lesion that involves 15-25% of patients with IVH (22.5% in our series).

Where there is overt damage, morphological diagnosis is easy: a large, strongly echogenic area, rounded or fan-shaped, dorsal and lateral to the external angle of the lateral ventricle, associated with a large ipsilateral IVH. Initially described as the extension of intraventricular blood into the cerebral white matter, it is now considered to represent hemorrhagic necrosis of periventricular white matter resulting from obstruction of the veins draining the white matter (GOULD 1987; GUZZETTA 1986; TAKASHIMA 1986). Indeed, the great majority of parenchymal lesions (approximately 80%) are observed in association with large germinal matrix–IVH; when bilateral and asymmetric, it invariably occurs on the same side as the larger amount of blood, and it often develops and progresses after the occurrence of intraventricular bleeding. These data demonstrate a direct relationship between germinal matrix–IVH and periventricular hemorrhagic necrosis (GOULD 1987; VOLPE 1995).

The sequence of events might be: large subependymal or/and IVH, compression of medullary veins with impaired venous return in the veins draining white matter, followed by necrotic hemorrhagic damage in this periventricular region.

In normal infants, color Doppler provides a constant visualization of terminal veins in the subependymal region. TAYLOR (1995) has reported that displacement and/or occlusion of subependymal veins could be demonstrated by color Doppler. Our experience is similar:

- When periventricular hemorrhagic infarct had occurred, flow was not dedectable in the ispilateral terminal vein in all investigated infants (Fig. 3.5)
- In one patient, the first ultrasonographic examination was performed on day 4, and showed only a large germinal matrix hemorrhage, but flow was not visible in the ipsilateral subependymal vein. The subsequent occurrence of an ischemohemorrhagic infarction was suspected and confirmed on day 6.
- By contrast, in all cases with germinal matrix or IVH where the terminal veins were still patent (Figs. 3.6–3.8.), we did not observe subsequent development of a parenchymal infarct.

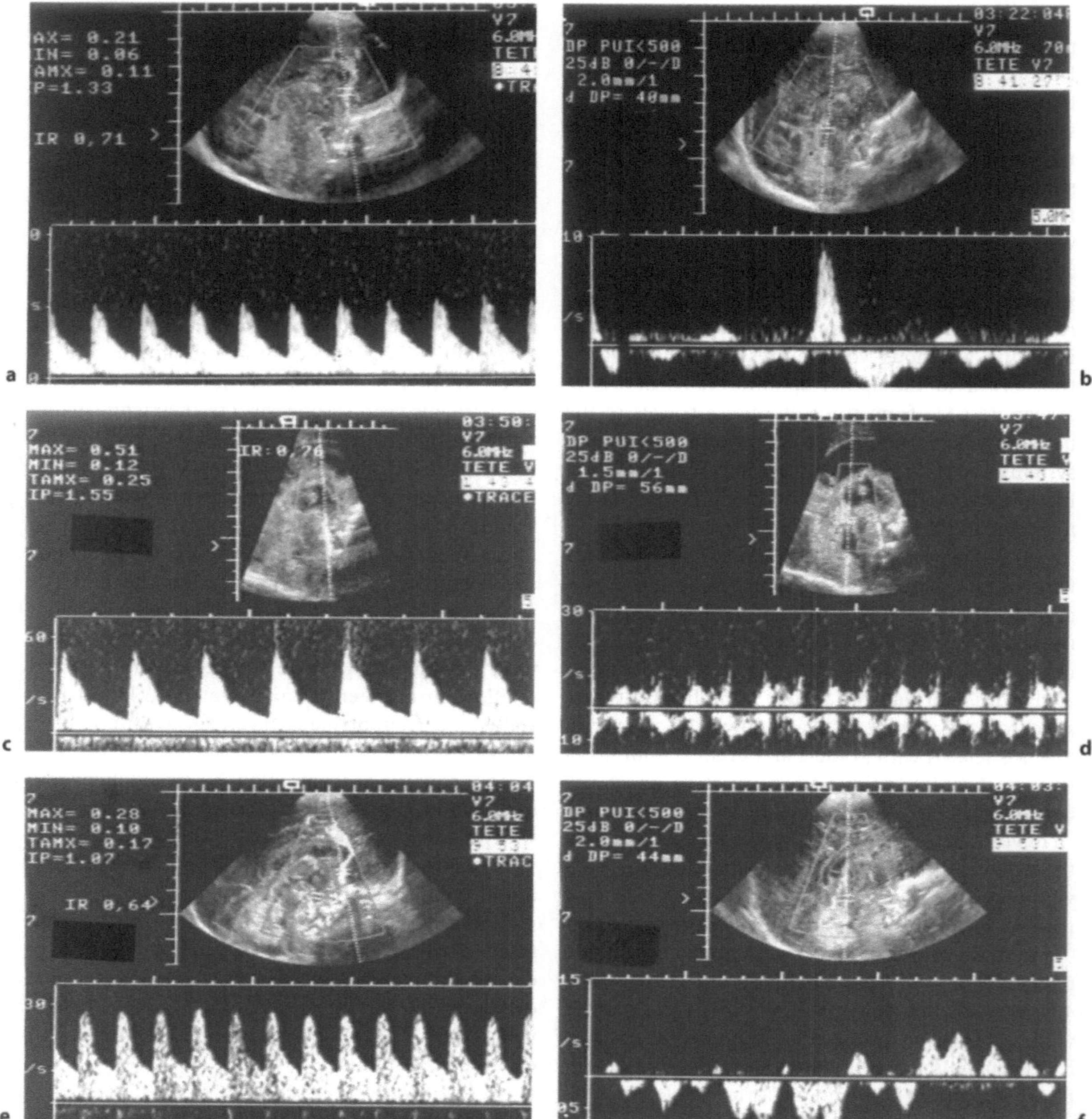

Fig. 3.4a–f. Pulsed Doppler recording of CSF flow. **a,b** Cindy. Day 4: grade II IVH, mechanical ventilation. **a** Anterior cerebral artery recording. **b** CSF flow appears synchronized with ventilation. Favorable outcome with transient dilatation and triceps hypertonia at 12 months of age. **c,d** Memphis. Grade III IVH. At day 15, moderate communicating tetraventricular dilatation without hemodynamic signs of intracranial hypertension (**c**). CSF flow exhibits a steady curve (**d**), synchronized with the heart rate, with high velocities (from –10 to +11 cm/s). After an episode of increased intracranial pressure requiring two subtractive lumbar punctures, the ventricular dilatation stabilized, followed by progressive resolution without shunting. **e,f** Cyril. Grade II IVH on day 3. Spontaneous ventilation with positive expiratory pressure. CSF flow (**f**) appears synchronized with both respiratory and heart rate (**e**): anterior cerebral artery recording. Favorable outcome

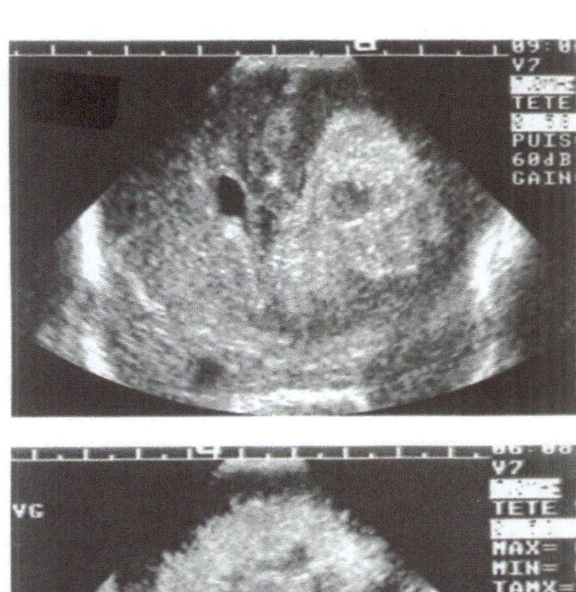

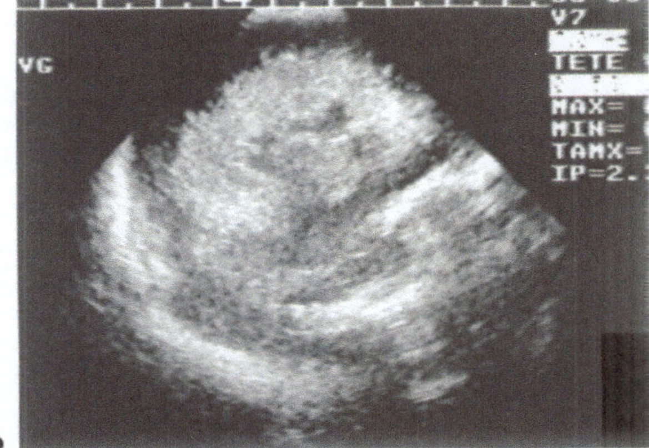

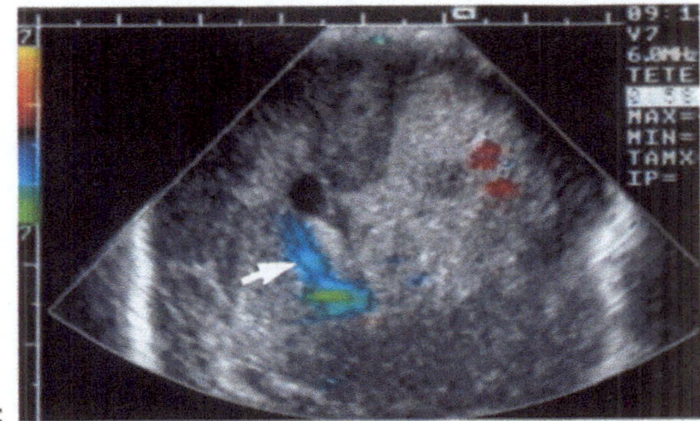

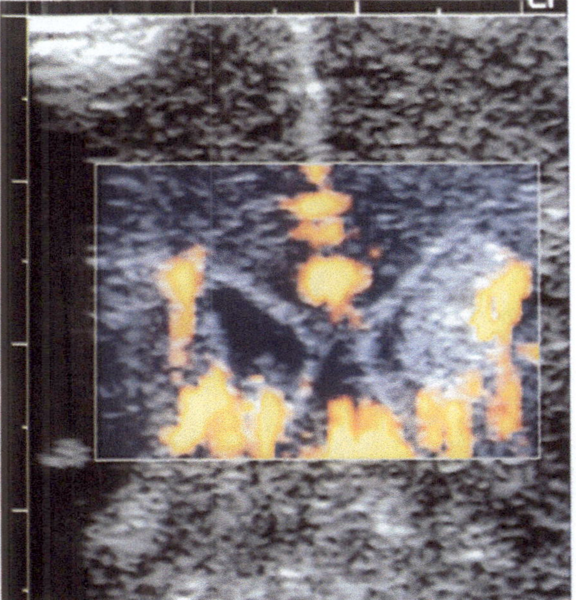

Fig. 3.5a–c. A 26 weeks' gestation preterm infant. Intubation 1 min after birth; initial clinical improvement but abrupt visceral distress on day 5 with severe hypoxia, consumption coagulopathy, and anemia. Ultrasound shows a left large IVH associated with periventricular white matter ischemic–hemorrhagic infarct (**a**), extending into the whole of the left hemisphere (**b**). **c** On color Doppler, the right terminal vein is easily visualized (*arrow*), while no flow can be detected in the left subependymal vein. The patient died on day 9

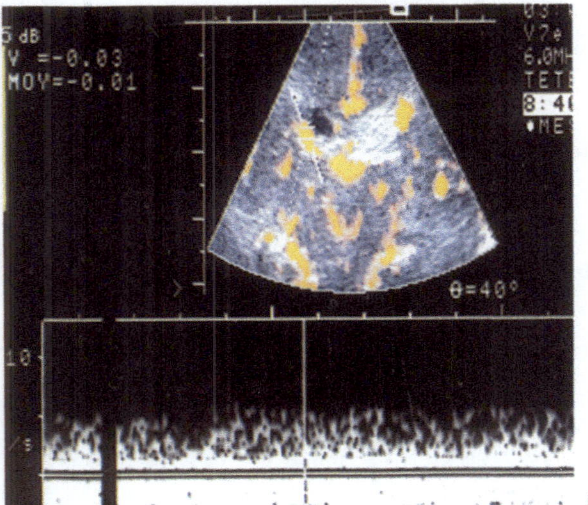

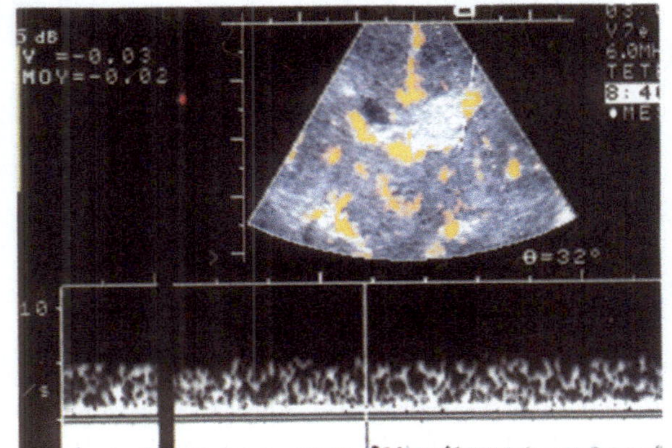

Fig. 3.6a–c. Left IVH. **a** Subependymal veins are both patent. **b,c** Flow velocities are symmetrical: 3 cm/s on both right (**b**) and left side (**c**)

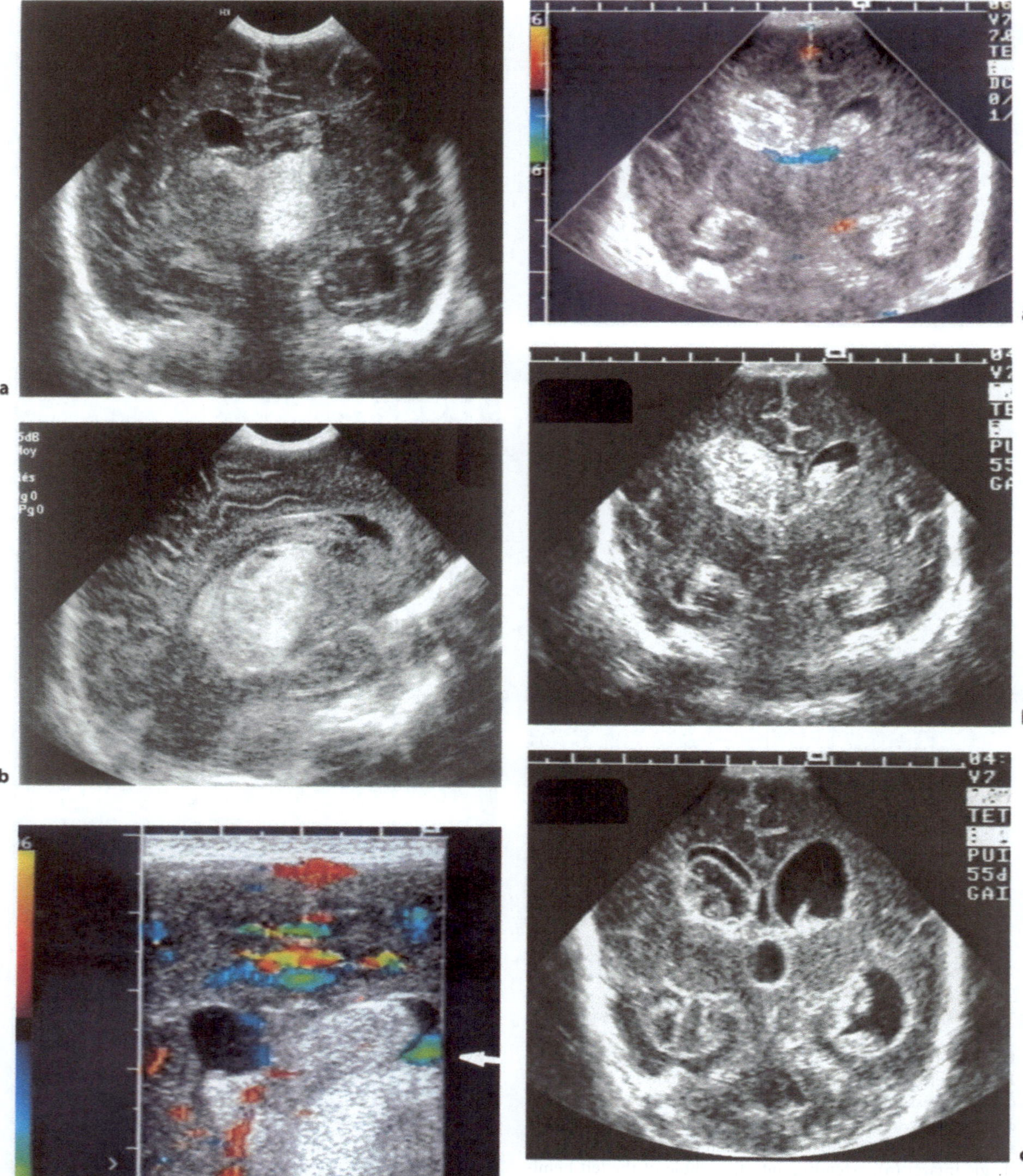

Fig. 3.7a–c. Near-term acute fetal distress. Seizures 5 h after birth. At day 1, left intraventricular and massive ganglio-thalamic ischemic–hemorrhagic lesion (**a** coronal plane, **b** parasagittal plane). **c.** Color Doppler imaging shows persistent patency of the left terminal vein (*arrow*) despite its compression by the subjacent echodense hyperechoic lesion. The ultrasonographic follow-up confirms the absence of injury to the periventricular white matter

Fig. 3.8a–c. A 30 weeks' gestation of twins: intrauterine growth retardation, maternofetal sepsis. On day 1, normal brain ultrasonography. Mechanical ventilation, exogenous surfactant therapy, instability of mean arterial blood pressure, patent ductus arteriosus resistant to indomethacin. On day 7, anemia and ultrasound follow-up showing right large IVH (**a**) with echodense hyperechoic adjacent parenchyma. (**b**) Color Doppler imaging demonstrates patency of terminal veins. (**c**) On day 20, tetraventricular dilatation, with characteristic ultrasonographic evolution of the intraluminal clot but absence of periventricular infarction

Thus, this ultrasonographic sign appears of great interest in determining the prognosis, since grade IV IVH correlates with a high mortality rate and/or severe neuromotor sequelae.

In clinical practice, when an early ultrasound examination shows a large subependymal or IVH, we routinely investigate the terminal veins by color Doppler imaging and alert the pediatricians if their flow cannot be depicted.

For other parenchymal lesions that may be associated with IVH (periventricular leukomalacia, basal ganglia and/or thalamic ischemic injury), color Doppler gives the same results, doubts, and inadequacies as for clinical conditions without hemorrhage (Chap. 5).

3.2
Pulsed Doppler Imaging

Although the pathogenesis of IVH is clearly multifactorial, among intravascular factors, disturbances of cerebral blood flow (CBF) appear to play an important role. This explains the potential value of assessing cerebral hemodynamics in the preterm infant.

3.2.1
Loss of CBF autoregulation

In the young infant as in the adult, an autoregulatory mechanism allows the maintenance of a constant CBF over a broad range of arterial pressure. Nevertheless, when arterial blood pressure becomes abnormally low or abnormally high, this mechanism may be insufficient, and the CBF evolves in parallel to systemic changes as a pressure-passive system.

Experimental animal studies (Lou 1979) have demonstrated that, in the near-term sheep fetus, cerebral autoregulation is impaired after only 20 min exposure to hypoxia, and does not recover until 7 h after restoration of normoxia. When mean arterial blood pressure is less than 30 mmHg, CBF decreases close to 0; when mean arterial blood pressure increases to 60 mmHg or more, CBF may reach six times normal values.

In the human newborn with asphyxia or varying degrees of respiratory distress syndrome, Lou (1979) has demonstrated a strong correlation between CBF (measured using the 133Xe clearance method) and arterial blood pressure, showing lack of autoregulation

and pressure-passive CBF. This may explain the direct transmission of systemic fluctuations to the cerebral circulation, the correlation between increases in CBF and in mean arterial blood pressure (MILLIGAN 1980), and the reduction in cerebral blood volume associated with bradycardia (LIVERA 1991).

Nevertheless, preterm infants undergoing intensive care may be able to maintain normal autoregulation (PRYDS 1990; ROSENKRANTZ 1988; TYSZCZUK 1998).

Several authors have used pulsed Doppler to determine whether mechanisms of autoregulation are maintained or altered in a preterm infant. AHMANN (1983) has assessed the flow–pressure relationship in the anterior cerebral artery, in conditions where pCO_2, pH, and pO_2 remain stable. If the mean anterior cerebral arterial flow velocity increases or decreases concurrently with a respective increase or decrease in mean arterial pressure, there is a pressure-passive state; whereas if the mean anterior cerebral arterial flow velocity remains unchanged despite changes in mean arterial blood pressure, or if the change in velocity is opposite to the change in pressure, autoregulation is respected.

According to JORCH (1987), loss of autoregulation may be recognized when a positive correlation between mean internal carotid arterial velocity and mean arterial blood pressure is demonstrated. The nonautoregulating group was characterized by a birth weight less than 1500 g, gestational age less than 31 weeks, and mean carotid blood velocity less than 20 cm/s; this threshold is commonly reached in this group of patients.

Pulsed Doppler seems able to detect a loss of cerebral autoregulation.

3.2.2
Fluctuating CBF

Physiological cyclical variations in CBF velocity are known in the healthy newborn (ANTHONY 1991). The cycles occur 1.5-5 times per minute and are mainly observed during the first days of life.

These are different from the beat-to-beat variability described by PERLMAN and VOLPE (1983). Using *Doppler technique*, these authors have studied CBF velocity in 50 ventilated preterm infants (weighing less than 1500 g at birth) from the first hours of life. Two groups differed:
- 27 Neonates exhibited a stable pattern, with equal peaks and troughs in systolic and diastolic flow velocity; 7 of them subsequently developed an IVH.

– 23 Neonates showed a fluctuating pattern, with marked continuous alterations in both systolic and diastolic flow velocities, varying from beat to beat; an IVH occurred in 21 of them; the CBF velocity tracings reflected similar patterns of systemic arterial blood pressure.

The authors concluded that a fluctuating pattern of CBF velocity in infants with respiratory distress syndrome indicated a high risk of IVH. This correlation has been confirmed by several groups.

These fluctuations are mainly observed when the infant is breathing out of synchrony with the ventilator, and disappear immediately after muscle paralysis (induced by curarization). They seem to be related to the mechanics of respiration in the ventilated infant. As a parallel, eliminating fluctuating CBF velocity in preterm infants with respiratory distress syndrome markedly reduces the incidence and severity of IVH (PERLMAN 1985). These data may be explained by the influence of intrathoracic and intra-abdominal pressures on the venous return, the cardiac output, and systemic arterial pressures during the respiratory cycle (COWAN 1987; HILLMAN 1987; MULLAART 1994; PERLMAN 1988). Variability of CBF velocities is significantly greater when the infant is breathing out of synchronization with the ventilator (RENNIE 1987) and lower when it is under curarization (KUBAN 1988; PERLMAN 1985).

Other conditions may correlate to the occurrence of fluctuations in CBF velocities: upper airway obstruction, pneumothorax, maneuvers of routine care, hypercarbia, patent ductus arteriosus, high concentrations of inspired oxygen, seizures, rapid volume expansion, and all causes of fluctuation in systemic blood pressure (VOLPE 1995).

All these data may explain the effect of some therapeutic agents (ROLAND 1997): phenobarbital, which reduces the number and amplitude of the peaks of mean arterial pressure, and postnatal indomethacin, which reduces the wide fluctuations resulting from patent ductus arteriosus. They also explain the inadequate efficacy of surfactant treatment on the prevalence of IVH, since it does not affect the fluctuations associated with rapid changes in lung mechanics.

In a report on a previous personal experience (VEYRAC 1987), we described the same correlations between fluctuating Doppler values and IVH and between elimination of fluctuations and reduction of the incidence of hemorrhage. A characteristic fluctuating pattern was observed in 15 premature infants, in the first 12 h of life. In 8 patients, muscular paralysis was not performed and severe IVH occurred in all of them, associated in 2 cases with ischemo-hemorrhagic parenchymal damage. The other 7 patients received pancuronium bromide (0.1 mm/kg administered intravenously); only 1 developed an IVH (after severe pneumothorax); another 1 died because of his lung disease without brain hemorrhage; while 5 had normal brain ultrasonography and a normal long-term outcome (Fig. 3.9).

In the years since that report, improvements in ventilation techniques, the common use of sedation, and the constant search for good synchronization of the infant's breathing with the ventilator have allowed

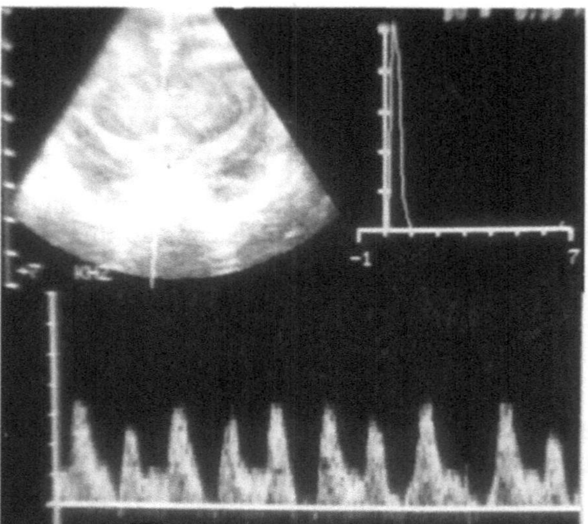

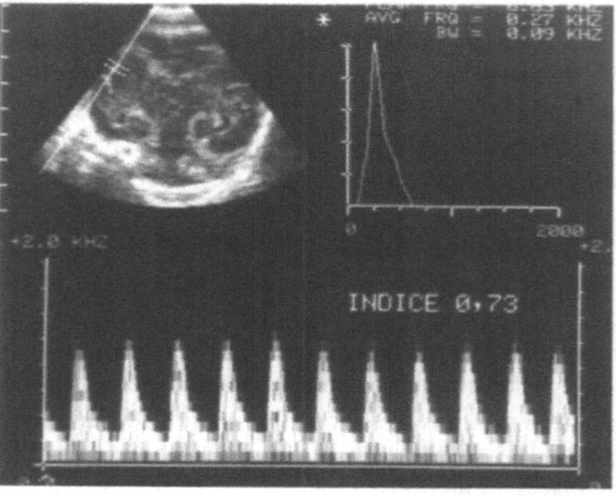

Fig. 3.9a,b. Ventilated preterm infant. Normal morphological ultrasound examination but fluctuating Doppler pattern: great variability of systolic peaks and diastolic troughs from beat to beat (**a**); concurrently, the infant is breathing out of synchronization with the ventilator. (**b**) Two minutes after muscle paralysis, the Doppler curve has become stable; resistive index (RI) is normal

the characteristic fluctuating pattern to disappear in our institution.

3.2.3
Increase in CBF

Experimental animal studies have demonstrated increased CBF. Some authors (GODDARD-FINEGOLD 1984) have reported that in the beagle puppy CBF increases by 31–42% over steady state values after 5 min hemorrhagic hypotension, and increases by 39–88% over control values after blood reinfusion. Three of the nine puppies had macroscopic IVH at autopsy. Hypertension induces a marked increase in rostral germinal matrix flow, as strikingly shown by autoradiography (PASTERNAK 1985).

In five ventilated preterm infants, MILLIGAN (1980) showed that transfusion or exchange of blood products produced a significant increase in mean arterial blood pressure and in CBF (measured by plethysmography), followed by IVH in four of them. These combined increases imply a failure of autoregulation.

Several factors may be responsible for such an elevation in CBF (VOLPE 1995):
- Rapid volume expansion, involving not only blood products but also hyperosmolar solutions
- A few noxious stimulations, such as tracheal suctioning (PERLMAN 1983)
- Some neurological disorders, such as seizures (BORCH 1998; PERLMAN 1983)
- Occurrence of pneumothorax, which correlates with a marked increase in flow velocities, especially during diastole, and in mean arterial blood pressure (especially diastolic pressure), with return to normal levels over the course of hours after resolution of the pneumothorax (HILL 1982)
- Decreased blood glucose (PRYDS 1990)
- Anemia, since CBF increases by 12% per 1 mmol/l decrease in hemoglobin levels (PRYDS 1989)
- Hypercapnia, which is a strong factor for a rise in CBF (COOKE 1980; PRYDS 1989)

This causal factor of intraventricular bleeding may explain the effect of postnatal indomethacin, which reduces baseline CBF mediated by inhibition of prostaglandin synthesis (MENT 1983; ROLAND 1997).

Doppler imaging may demonstrate the CBF increase by showing increased flow velocities, commonly accompanied by a decreased resistive index (Fig. 3.10) or pulsatility index (BADA 1979; BLANKENBERG 1997; PERLMAN 1983, VAN BEL 1987).

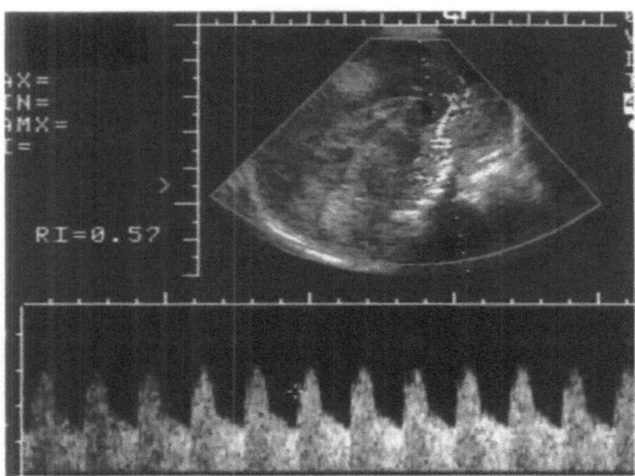

Fig. 3.10. A 30 weeks' gestation preterm infant: clinical chorioamnionitis, respiratory distress syndrome, mechanical ventilation. On day 2, grade II IVH and periventricular echodensities. Pulsed Doppler showed increased flow velocities PSV = 58 cm/s, EDV = 26 cm/s, TAV = 40 cm/s]; decrease in RI (0.57). This demonstrates an increase in CBF. Follow-up confirms periventricular leukomalacia accompanying IVH

Some authors (BLANKENBERG 1997) have reported not only increased peak systolic velocities but also greater coronal cross-sectional area of the lenticulostriate arteries in neonates with IVH than in neonates without (Fig. 3.11); however, the latter point is debatable since color/power Doppler assessment of the normal cross-section of intracerebral arteries is highly subjective.

Finally, demonstration of high cerebral flow velocities does not necessarily mean subsequent occurrence of intraventricular bleeding. As an example, JORCH (1993) investigated 16 nonasphyxiated very immature infants, intubated after birth, and reported a transitory increase in both PSV and EDV (from 29 to 35 and from 1 to 10 cm/s) during the first 5 min after birth, which occurred together with an increase in heart rate. In this series, only 3 neonates exhibited intracranial hemorrhage.

3.2.4
Decrease in CBF

The 133Xe clearance method has shown (FRIIS-HANSEN 1985) significantly lower values of CBF in the ventilated preterm infant than in "well" premature, "well" and postasphyxic mature infants, normal children, and normal adults (Table 3.1).

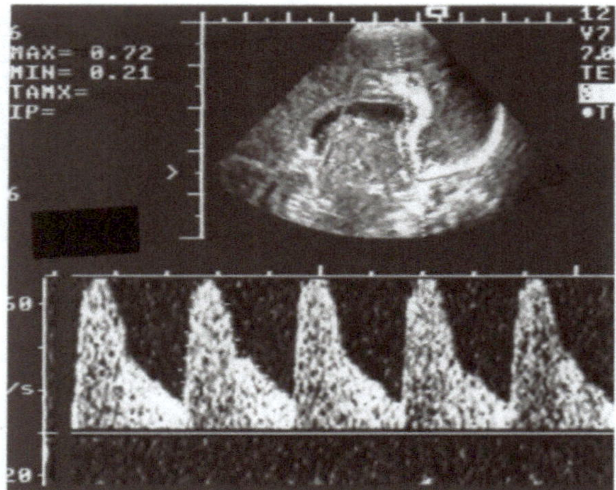

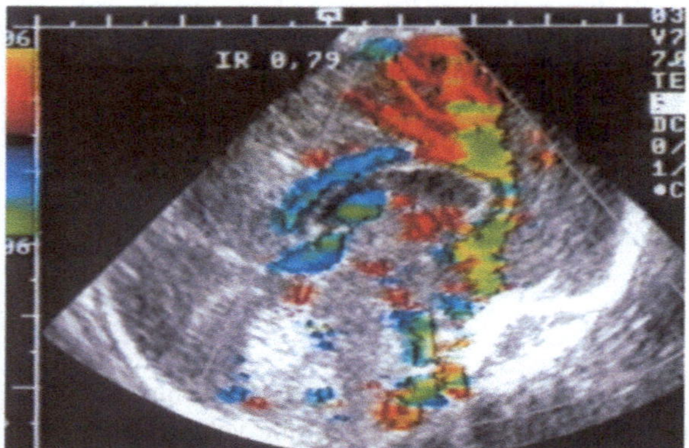

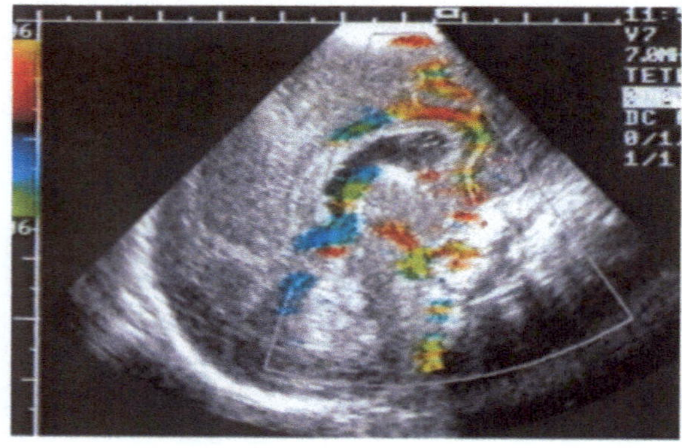

Fig. 3.11a–c. A 27 weeks' gestation preterm infant: hyaline membrane disease, transitory improvement followed by secondary clinical deterioration, grade IV ventricular hemorrhage on day 2. On pulsed Doppler (**a**), anterior cerebral artery velocities are intensely increased: PSV=72 cm/s, EDV=21 cm/s, TAV=44 cm/s, RI=0.70. On color Doppler imaging (**b**), this augmentation is evident in comparison with a normal infant of the same gestational age and birth weight, investigated with the same settings (**c**)

Table 3.1. Cerebral blood flow in "well" and stressed" premature and mature newborn infants, in postasphyxic mature infants, and in "normal" children and adults. (From FRIIS-HANSEN 1985)

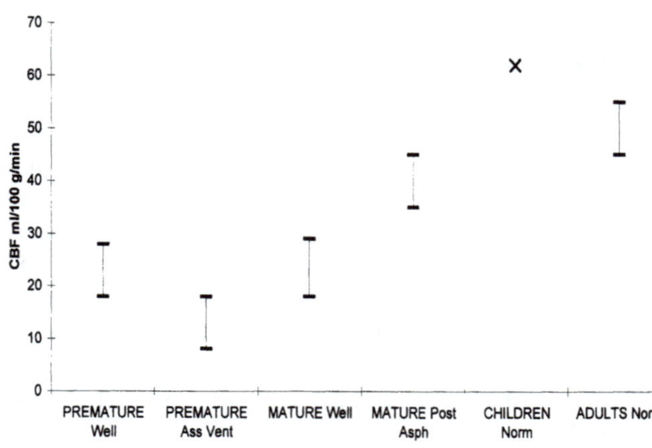

Similar results have been reported by other groups (BAENZIGER 1994). Near-infrared spectroscopic CBF measures in the neonate during the first 24 h of life also demonstrate that CBF is significantly lower in infants with germinal matrix–IVH than in those without (median 7 ml/100 g per minute versus 12.2 ml/100 g per minute), and that the most severe hemorrhagic damage correlates to the lowest CBF (MEEK 1999).

LOU (1979) determined CBF in 19 newborns a few hours after birth. Six of the ten patients with CBF of 20 mg/100 g per minute or less had developed cerebral atrophy, and four of them died with massive intracranial hemorrhage.

When intraventricular bleeding has occurred, it is also associated with decreased CBF, which a few authors (BADA 1982; BATTON 1987; FARSTAD 1994) report to be related to increased intracranial pressure.

A drop in CBF may be one of the factors that explain the strong correlation between IVH and patent ductus arteriosus (EVANS 1996; MULLAART 1997; SEPPANEN 1995). This emphasizes the value of echocardiography for measuring the aortopulmonary pressure gradient across the ductus arteriosus and identifying infants at high risk of hemorrhage (PHILLIPOS 1996; SEPPANEN 1995).

The beneficial effect of postnatal indomethacin relates to several combined mechanisms; among these are that closure of the patent ductus reduces the associated diastolic "steal" phenomenon (ROLAND 1997).

Doppler US may allow recognition of reduced CBF. In 34 newborns with intracranial hemorrhage (IVH in 26) DEEG (1987) noted a significant decrease in all flow velocities, that predominates on diastolic flow velocities, and a resultant increase in the pulsatility index.

MULLAART (1997) has shown that (1) respiratory distress, with or without hemorrhage, correlates with low flow velocities and high resistive index, (2) IVH correlates with a high cerebral pulse width (defined by PSV minus EDV), (3) the increased pulse width precedes the onset of hemorrhage, and (4) these CBF alterations can be partly attributed to ductal shunting and are improved by mechanical ventilation.

In our personal experience, Doppler detection of markedly reduced CBF velocities is rather uncommon in preterm infants with ventricular hemorrhage (5 cases from 58 patients with IVH who were studied before 3 days of life). Nevertheless, it correlates with severe damage (1 grade III and 4 grade IV hemorrhage) and very poor outcome (5 deaths) (Fig. 3.12).

3.2.5
Venous Factors

Several factors contribute to increasing cerebral venous pressure (VOLPE 1995):
- Asphyxia may induce hypoxic–ischemic cardiac failure
- Respiratory disturbances such as positive-pressure ventilation with relatively high peak inflation pressure, tracheal suctioning, pneumothorax, and any fluctuation related to ventilation being out of synchrony
- Deformations of the particularly compliant premature skull related to prolonged labor, mode of delivery, etc.

PERLMAN (1987) has well demonstrated that fluctuations in mean arterial blood pressure are associated with fluctuations in venous pressure, comparable in magnitude but variable in direction. This induces pronounced and abrupt alterations in perfusion pressure. They are related to intrathoracic pressure changes and are eliminated by muscular paralysis.

Doppler assessment of venous hemodynamics has never provided significant criteria of risk of hemorrhage. The only critical finding is the demonstration of occluded terminal veins to explain the development of ischemo-hemorrhagic infarction adjacent to IVH.

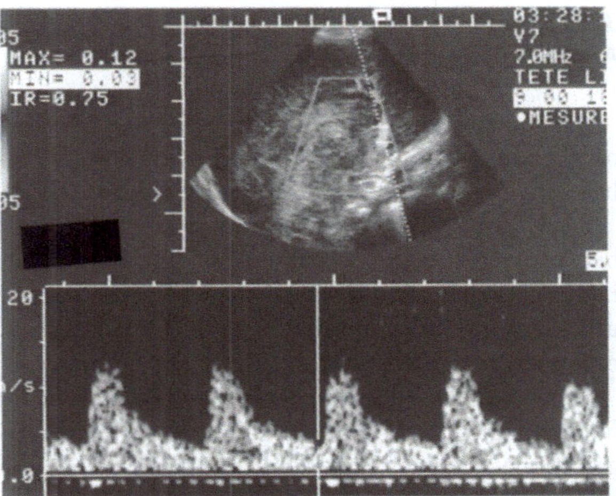

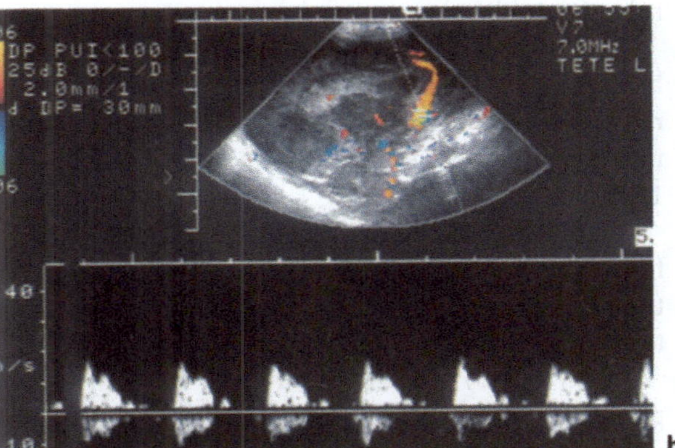

Fig. 3.12. a A 26 weeks' gestation infant: hyaline membrane disease, high frequency jet ventilation, grade IV IVH at day 1. Pulsed Doppler imaging showed extremely low flow velocities: PSV=12 cm/s, EDV=3 cm/s, TAV=6 cm/s, RI=0.75. The infant died on day 4. b A 25 weeks' gestation infant: hyaline membrane disease, high frequency jet ventilation, systemic hemodynamic instability, multivisceral distress, grade IV IVH at day 1. Pulsed Doppler imaging showed extremely low blood flow. PSV=17 cm/s, EDV=0 cm/s, TAV=5 cm/s, RI=1. The infant died on day 8

3.2.6
Other Factors

Besides the factors described above, other physiopathogenic events play an important role: coagulation disturbances, anatomic characteristics of germinal matrix vessels, metabolic factors, etc. None of these factors respond to Doppler ultrasonography, whether for diagnosis or prognosis

3.2.7
Antenatal Period

Thirty percent of hemorrhages have already occurred at 6 h of life, 55% at 24 h, and 90% at 72 h of life (VAN DE BOR 1986).

A close correlation has been demonstrated between postnatal development of IVH and increased values of some metabolites measured in the umbilical cord or amniotic fluid, which are markers of fetal hypoxia–ischemia.

In a parallel manner, the incidence and severity of hemorrhagic damage correlates strongly with low gestational age, prolonged labor, and also clinical and histological chorioamnionitis (indicating a direct role of cytokines).

Finally, in recent years, antenatal steroid therapy has been associated with a lower mortality rate, lower respiratory and blood pressure support requirements, and less severe IVH (GARLAND 1995; MOISE 1995).

Thus, it would be important to identify a group of fetuses at risk of developing IVH, in order to improve the conditions of their delivery and the acute postnatal management.

MARI (1996) studied the middle cerebral artery pulsatility index in 43 fetuses between 25 and 33.6 weeks' gestation. IVH was present in 6 of 22 newborns with a normal pulsatility index, but in none of 21 newborns with lowered pulsatility index. The mean birth weight was lower in the second group, while other criteria (gestational age, antenatal steroid treatment, antenatal exposure to magnesium, Apgar score, respiratory distress syndrome, necrotizing enterocolitis, cesarian section, sepsis in the infant) did not significantly differ between the groups.

Since fetal brain sparing effect is associated with a lower risk of neonatal IVH than is preterm labor, the identification by fetal Doppler of such hemodynamical conditions might lead to new effective strategies of perinatal care.

3.2.8
Posthemorrhagic Ventricular Dilatation

Posthemorrhagic ventriculomegaly occurs in approximately 36% of preterm infants with IVH, but spontaneous arrest or resolution is observed in 65% of these cases (VOLPE 1995). The diagnosis of ventricular dilatation is based on the morphological analysis of ventricles by ultrasound; pulsed Doppler helps in detecting increased intracranial pressure that may accompany the ventricular enlargement, by demonstrating an increase in the resistive index of the cerebral arteries. Further details are given in Chap. 4.

3.2.9
Conclusion: Role of Pulsed Doppler in the Preterm Infant with IVH

With a knowledge and understanding of the multiple different physiopathogenic mechanisms that result in the development of IVH in the preterm infant, pulsed Doppler may provide criterias indicating the risk of hemorrhage (predictive role) and the severity of brain damage (prognostic role). A Pulsed Doppler examination of the neonatal brain should search for:

- Fluctuations of the Doppler curve, leading to correction of unsynchronized ventilation, either by muscle paralysis or by other means
- Low blood flow velocities, which suggest the possibility of subsequent occurrence of hypoxic-ischemic injury or germinal matrix–IVH during the reperfusion phase
- High blood flow velocities, often associated with an increase in mean arterial blood pressure, suggesting direct rupture of germinal matrix vessels
- Lack of cerebral autoregulation, detectable in the form of intense changes in blood flow velocities concurrent with changes in mean arterial blood pressure
- Increased resistive index, which may be associated with a raise in intracranial pressure, but also with a patent ductus arteriosus, requiring echocardiography.

Unfortunately, Doppler investigation as performed in clinical practice represents the hemodynamic situation of a short period, where only abnormal results have predictive or prognostic value (SHORTLAND 1990).

References

Ahmann PA, Dykes FD, Lazzara A, Holt PJ, Giddens DP, Carrigan TA (1983) Relationship between pressure passivity and subependymal intraventricular hemorrhage as assessed by pulsed Doppler ultrasound. Pediatrics 72:665-669

Anthony MY, Evans DH, Levene MI (1991) Cyclical variations in cerebral blood flow velocity. Arch Dis Child 66:12-16

Bada HS, Hajjar W, Chua C, Sumner DS (1979) Noninvasive diagnosis of neonatal asphyxia and intraventricular hemorrhage by Doppler ultrasound. J Pediatr 95:775-779

Bada HS, Miller JE, Menke JA, Menten TG, Bashiru M, Binstadt D, Sumner DS, Khanna NN (1982) Intracranial pressure and cerebral arterial pulsatile flow measurement in neonatal intraventricular hemorrhage. J Pediatr 100:291-296

Baenziger O, Jaggi JL; Mueller AC, Morales CG, Lipp HP, Lipp AE, Duc G, Bucher HU (1994) Cerebral blood flow in preterm infants affected by sex, mechanical ventilation and intrauterine growth. Pediatr Neurol 11:319-324

Batton DG, Nardis EE (1987) The effect of intraventricular blood on cerebral blood flow in newborn dogs. Pediatr Res 21:511-515

Blankenberg FG, Loh NN, Norbash AM, Craychee JA, Spielman DM, Person BL, Berg CA, Enzmann DR (1997) Impaired cerebro-vascular autoregulation after hypoxic-ischemic injury in extremely low-birth-weight neonates: detection with power and pulse wave Doppler US. Radiology 205:563-568

Borch K, Pryds O, Holm S, Lou H, Greisen G (1998) Regional cerebral blood flow during seizures in neonates. J Pediatr 132:431-435

Bosche C, Genzel-Boroviczeny O, Hepp H, Knitza R, Versmold H, Roos R (1996) Mortality, mode of delivery, pneumothorax and intracranial hemorrhage in 859 extremely premature newborn infants between 1984-1992. Geburtshilfe Frauenheilkd 56:322-327

Claris O, Besnier S, Lapillonne A, Picaud JC, Salle BL (1996) Incidence of ischemic-hemorrhagic cerebral lesions in premature infants of gestational age less than 28 weeks: a prospective ultrasound study. Biol Neonate 70:29-34

Cooke RWI (1980) Autoregulation and intraventricular hemorrhage. Lancet 1 (8179):1197-1198

Cowan F, Thoresen M (1987) The effects of intermittent positive pressure ventilation on cerebral arterial and venous blood velocities in the newborn infant. Acta Paediatr Scand 76:239-247

Deeg KH, Rupprecht T, Segerer H (1987) Detection of reduced flow velocities in the anterior cerebral artery in premature and newborn infants and in older infants with cerebral hemorrhages using pulsed Doppler sonography. Monatsschr Kinderheilkd 135:748-757

Evans N, Kluckow M (1996) Early ductal shunting and intraventricular hemorrhage in ventilated preterm infants. Arch Dis Child Fetal Neonatal Ed 75:F183-F186

Farstad T, Odden JP, Bratlid D (1994) Effect of intraventricular hemorrhage on pulmonary function in newborn piglets. Biol Neonate 66:238-246

Friis-Hansen B (1985) Perinatal brain injury and cerebral blood flow in newborn infants. Acta Paediatr Scand 74:323-331

Garland JS, Buck R, Leviton A (1995) Effect of maternal glucocorticoid exposure on risk of severe intraventricular hemorrhage in surfactant-treated preterm infants. J Pediatr 126 .272-279

Ghazi-Birry HS, Brown WR, Moody DM, Challa VR, Block SM, Reboussin DM (1997) Human germinal matrix: venous origin of hemorrhage and vascular characteristics. Am J Neuroradiol 18:219-229

Goddard-Finegold J, Michael LH (1984) Cerebral blood flow and experimental intraventricular hemorrhage. Pediatr Res 18:7-11

Gould SJ, Howard S, Hope PL, Reynolds EOR (1987) Periventricular intraparenchymal cerebral hemorrhage in preterm infants: the role of venous infarction. J Pathol 151:197-202

Gould SJ, Howard S (1988) Glial differentiation in the germinal layer of fetal and preterm infant brain: an immunocytochemical study. Pediatr Pathol 8:25-36

Guzzetta F, Shackelford GD, Volpe S, Perlman JM, Volpe JJ (1986) Periventricular intraparenchymal echodensities in the premature newborn: critical determinant of neurologic outcome. Pediatrics 78:995-1006

Hambleton G, Wigglesworth JS (1976) Origin of intraventricular hemorrhage in the preterm infant. Arch Dis Child 51:651-659

Hill A, Perlman JM, Volpe JJ (1982) Relationship of pneumothorax to occurrence of intraventricular hemorrhage in the premature newborn. Pediatrics 69:144-149

Hillman K (1987) Intrathoracic pressure fluctuations and periventricular hemorrhage in the newborn. Aust Pediatr J 23:343-346

Jorch G, Jorch N (1987) Failure of autoregulation of cerebral blood flow in neonates studied by pulsed Doppler US of the internal carotid artery. Eur J Pediatr 146:468-472

Jorch G, Rabe H, Michel E, Engels M, Schulz V, Hentschel R, Koch HG, Hultsch E (1993) Resuscitation of the very immature infant: cerebral Doppler flow velocities in the first 20 minutes of life. Biol Neonate 64: 215-220.

Kuban KCK, Skouteli H, Cherer A, Brown E, Leviton A, Pagano M, Allred E, Sullivan KF (1988) Hemorrhage, phenobarbital and fluctuating cerebral blood flow velocity in the neonate. Pediatrics 82: 548-553

Larroche JC (1964) Hémorragies cérébrales intra ventriculaires chez le prématuré. 1ère partie: anatomie et physiopathologie. Biol Neonate 7:26-56

Livera LN, Spencer SA, Thorniley MS, Wickramasinghe Y, Rolfe P (1991) Effects of hypoxaemia and bradycardia on neonatal cerebral hemodynamics. Arch Dis Child 66:376-380

Lou HC, Lassen NA, Tweed WA, Johnson G, Jones M, Palahniuk RJ (1979) Pressure passive cerebral blood flow and breakdown of the blood-brain barrier in experimental fetal asphyxia. Acta Paediatr Scand 68:57-63

Lou HC, Lassen NA, Friis-Hansen B (1979) Impaired autoregulation of cerebral blood flow in the distressed newborn infant. J Pediatr 94:118-121

Mari G, Abuhamad AZ, Keller M, Verpairojkit B, Ment L, Copel JA (1996) Is the fetal brain-sparing effect a risk factor for the development of intraventricular hemorrhage in the preterm infant ? Ultrasound Obstet Gynecol 8:329-332

Meek JH, Tyszczuk L, Elwell CE, Wyatt JS (1999) Low cerebral blood flow is a risk factor for severe intraventricular hemorrhage. Arch Dis Child Fetal Neonatal Ed. 81:F15-F18

Ment LR, Stewart WB, Ardito TA, Madri JA (1995) Germinal matrix microvascular maturation correlates inversely with the risk period for neonatal intraventricular hemorrhage. Brain Res Dev Brain Res 84:142-149

Ment LR, Stewart WB, Duncan CC, Scott DT, Lambrecht R (1983) Beagle puppy model of intraventricular hemorrhage effect of indomethacin on cerebral blood flow. J Neurosurg 58:857-862

Milligan DWA (1980) Failure of autoregulation and intraventricular hemorrhage in preterm infants. Lancet 1 (8174):896-898

Moise AA, Wearden ME, Kosinetz CA, Gest AL, Welty SE, Hansen TN (1995) Antenatal steroids are associated with less need for blood pressure support in extremely premature infants. Pediatrics 95:845-850

Morales WJ, Koerten J (1986) Obstetric management and intraventricular hemorrhage in very-low-birth-weight infants. Obstet Gynecol 68:35-40

Mullaart RA, Hopman JC, Rotteveel JJ, Daniels O, Stoelinga GB, De Haan AF (1994) Cerebral blood flow fluctuations in neonatal respiratory distress and periventricular hemorrhage. Early Hum Dev 37:179-185

Mullaart RA, Hopman JC, Rotteveel JJ, Stoelinga GB, De Haan AF, Daniels O (1997) Cerebral blood flow velocity and pulsation in neonatal respiratory distress syndrome and periventricular hemorrhage. Pediatr Neurol 16:118-125

Nakamura Y, Okudera T, Fukuda S, Hashimoto T (1990) Germinal matrix hemorrhage of venous origin in preterm neonates. Hum Pathol 21:1059-1062

Nakamura Y, Okudera T, Hashimoto T (1991) Microvasculature in germinal matrix layer: its relationship to germinal matrix hemorrhage. Mod Pathol 4:475-480

Pape KE, Wigglesworth JS (1979) Haemorrhage, ischaemia and the perinatal brain. Clin Dev Med 69/70:11-38, 100-132

Papile LA, Burstein J, Burstein R, Koffler H (1978) The incidence and evolution of subependymal and intraventricular hemorrhage. A study of infants with birthweight less than 1500 grams. J Pediatr 92:529-534

Pasternak JF, Groothuis DR (1985) Autoregulation of cerebral blood flow in the newborn beagle puppy. Biol Neonate 48:100-109

Perlman JM, McMenamin JB, Volpe JJ (1983) Fluctuating cerebral blood flow velocity in respiratory distress syndrome. Relation to the development of intraventricular hemorrhage. N Engl J Med 309:204-209

Perlman JM, Volpe JJ (1983) Suctioning of the preterm infant: effects on cerebral blood flow velocity, intracranial pressure and arterial blood pressure. Pediatrics 72:329-334

Perlman JM, Volpe JJ (1983) Seizures in the preterm infant: effects on cerebral blood flow velocity, intracranial pressure and arterial blood pressure. J Pediatr 102:288-293

Perlman JM, Goodman S, Kreusser KL, Volpe JJ (1985) Reduction in intraventricular hemorrhage by elimination of fluctuating cerebral blood flow velocity in preterm infants with respiratory distress syndrome. N Engl J Med 312:1253-1257

Perlman JM, Volpe JJ (1987) Are venous circulatory abnormalities important in the pathogenesis of hemorrhagic and/or ischemic cerebral injury? Pediatrics 80:705-711

Perlman JM, Thach B (1988) Respiratory origin of fluctuations in arterial blood pressure in premature infants with respiratory distress syndrome. Pediatrics 81:399-403

Phillipos EZ, Robertson MA, Byrne PJ (1996) Serial assessment of ductus arteriosus hemodynamics in hyaline membrane disease. Pediatrics 98:1149-1153

Pryds O, Greisen G (1989) Effect of PaCO2 and haemoglobin concentration on day to day variation of CBF in preterm neonates. Acta Paediatr Scand 360 (Suppl):33-36

Pryds O, Greisen G, Lou HC, Friis-Hansen B (1989) Heterogeneity of cerebral vasoreactivity in preterm infants supported by mechanical ventilation. J Pediatr 115:638-645

Pryds O, Christensen NJ, Friis-Hansen B (1990) Increased cerebral blood flow and plasma epinephrine in hypoglycemic preterm neonates. Pediatrics 85:172-176

Rennie JM, South M, Morley CJ (1987) Cerebral blood flow velocity variability in infants receiving assisted ventilation. Arch Dis Child 62:1247-1251

Roland EH, Hill A (1997) Intraventricular hemorrhage and posthemorrhagic hydrocephalus. Clin Perinatol 24:589-605

Rosenkrantz TS, Diana D, Munson J (1988) Regulation of cerebral blood flow velocity in nonasphyxiated, very low birth weight infants with hyaline membrane disease. J Perinatol 8:303-308

Seppanen MP, Kaapa PO, Kero PO (1995) Hemodynamic prediction of complications in neonatal respiratory distress syndrome. J Pediatr 127:780-785

Sheth RD (1998) Trends in incidence and severity of intraventricular hemorrhage. J Child Neurol 13:261-264

Shortland DB, Levene M, Archer N, Shaw D, Evans D (1990) Cerebral blood flow velocity recordings and the prediction of intracranial haemorrhage and ischaemia. J Perinat Med 18:411-417

Sotrel A, Lorenzo AV (1989) Ultrastructure of blood vessels in the ganglionic eminence of premature rabbits with spontaneous germinal matrix hemorrhage. J Neuropathol Exp Neurol 48:462-482

Takashima S, Mito T, Anto Y (1986) Pathogenesis of periventricular white matter hemorrhage in preterm infants. Brain Dev 8:25-30

Tatsuno M, Uchida K, Okuyama K, Kawauchi A (1992) Color Doppler flow imaging of CSF flow in an infant with intraventricular hemorrhage. Brain Dev 14:110-113

Taylor GA (1995) Effect of germinal matrix hemorrhage on terminal vein position and patency. Pediatr Radiol 25:S37-S40

Trommer BL, Groothuis DR, Pasternak JF (1987) Quantitative analysis of cerebral vessels in the newborn puppy: the structure of germinal matrix vessels may predispose to hemorrhage. Pediatr Res 22:23-28

Tyszczuk L, Meek J, Elwell C, Wyatt JS (1998) Cerebral blood flow is independent of mean arterial blood pressure in preterm infants undergoing intensive care. Pediatrics 102:337-341

Van Bel F, Van de Bor M, Stijnen T, Baan J, Ruys JH (1987) Aetiological role of cerebral blood flow alterations in development and extension of peri-intraventricular hemorrhage. Dev Med Child Neurol 29:601-614

Van de Bor M, Van Bel F, Lineman R, Ruys JH (1986) Perinatal factors and periventricular intraventricular hemorrhage in preterm infants. Am J Dis Child 140:1125-1130

Veyrac C, Couture A, Baud C, Leboucq N (1987) The value of pulsed Doppler in cerebral hemorrhage of the newborn. Ann Radiol 30:463-469

Veyrac C, Couture A, Baud C (1994) Les lésions hémorragiques cérébrales. In: Couture A, Veyrac C, Baud C: Echographie cérébrale du foetus au nouveau-né: imagerie et hémodynamique. Sauramps Médical, Montpellier

Volpe JJ (1995) Neurology of the newborn, 3rd ed. Saunders, Philadelphia

Winkler P (1992a) Color-coded echographic flow imaging and spectral analysis of CSF in meningitis and hemorrhage. Part I: Clinical evidence. Pediatr Radiol 22:24-30

Winkler P (1992b) Color-coded echographic flow imaging and spectral analysis of CSF in infants. Part II: CSF-dynamics. Pediatr Radiol 22:31-42

Winkler P, Helmke K (1992c) Color-coded echographic flow imaging and spectral analysis of CSF. Part III: In vitro study of low flow velocity detection related to decreasing particle concentration (hematocrit) and tube lumen. Pediatr Radiol 22:43-47

Winkler P (1994) CSF dynamics in infants evaluated with color Doppler US and spectral analysis: respiratory versus arterial synchronization. Radiology 192:423-430

4 Hemodynamics and Hydrocephalus

ALAIN P. COUTURE

CONTENTS

Multiple scientific works and an improved analysis of CSF physiology, make it possible to propose a modern definition of hydrocephalus that takes into

A. COUTURE, MD
Department of Pediatric Radiology, Hôpital Arnaud de Villeneuve, 371 Av. Doyen Gaston Giraud, 34295 Montpellier Cédex 5, France

account our knowledge of pathogenetic mechanisms. Hydrocephalus is a progressive ventricular distension induced by a disturbance in CSF circulation/resorption or CSF production, associated with an increased intracranial pressure.

CSF production begins at the end of the 2nd month of gestation (OSAKA 1980); it is mainly secreted by choroid plexus, but there are other sites of production, particularly the ependymal floor of the ventricles and the intracranial and spinal subarachnoid spaces. In a normal state (LORENZO 1970), there is a pressure gradient between production and absorption sites. CSF circulation occurs between the lateral and third ventricles through the foramen of Monro; the CSF then pours out from the ventricular system through the foramina of Luschka and Magendie to course within the subarachnoid spaces. CSF absorption, normally equal to its production, is performed by cerebral capillaries (GREITZ 1997) and arachnoid villi or pacchionian granulations along the sagittal sinus. In infants, CSF production is 0.1 ml/min (that is 200 ml/day) and its hydrostatic pressure ranges between 5 and 15 mmHg.

In pathological situations, any increase in CSF production, any decrease in CSF resorption, or any trouble in the CSF circulation will raise the intracranial pressure. The intraventricular bulk increases and hydrocephalus occurs.

● CSF overproduction is a rarely discussed situation. This mechanism has been suggested to exist in the presence of a choroid plexus papilloma (REKATE 1986).

● Decreased CSF resorption may be observed, but its pathogenesis has not been clearly demonstrated. For example, we know that, when the sagittal sinus is thrombosed, the ventricular enlargement is due to cerebral atrophy rather than to decreased resorption of CSF. In the same way, subarachnoid effusion and external hydrocephalus are probably secondary to transient involvement of arachnoid villi, but the intimal mechanism remains unknown.

● In fact, most cases of hydrocephalus are related to CSF pathway obstruction.

Although these physiopathological definitions correspond to real observations, they seem too restrictive; the intraventricular compartment, on which the conventional definition of hydrocephalus is based, must be integrated within a wider intracranial context, as described by RAIMONDI (1994) and MORI (1995). These authors consider that hydrocephalus can be defined as "an abnormal increase in intracranial CSF volume independent of hydrostatic or barometric pressure." They believe that subarachnoid channels are the first CSF compartment to dilate in response to a hydrocephalic process, reducing CSF pressure and establishing a new balance. When this balance is broken, the increase in CSF pressure is transmitted to the ventricular system, which dilates (extraparenchymal hydrocephalus) and obliterates the subarachnoid spaces by compressing the brain against the dura mater. Thus, these authors suggest that hydrocephalus is an abnormal enlargement of intracranial fluid volume, independent of its location: intraparenchymal (cerebral edema) and/or extraparenchymal (subarachnoid, cisternal, or ventricular). This definition gives first place to the increase in parenchymal fluid volume (either primitive cerebral edema, or transependymal CSF resorption resulting from intraventricular hydrocephalus), which presents the same potential risk of parenchymal destruction and, consequently, of psychomotor retardation.

Whatever its mechanism, the discussion of a case of hydrocephalus passes through three indistinct steps:

- The positive diagnosis, with its clinical insufficiencies and uncertainties, explaining why ultrasound is best suited to make the diagnosis.

- The etiological diagnosis: the more important because there is no uniform hemodynamic pattern; the hemodynamic disturbances can be explosive in case of tumor, but slowly progressive in postinfectious or developmental hydrocephalus.

- The follow-up, with the investigation of vascular damage and the monitoring of the effect of treatment (lumbar or ventricular puncture, external drainage, fibrinolytic treatment, ventriculoperitoneal shunt): that it to emphasize the main role of Doppler imaging in this area.

4.1
Positive Diagnosis

4.1.1
Insufficiencies of Clinical Data

The clinical findings are well known: enlargement of the cranial sutures, bulging of the anterior fontanel, an excessive increase in head circumference. These signs can occur early, for example in tumoral hydrocephalus, but more often they are late, as in posthemorrhagic dilatation (DI ROCCO 1979; KIRKPATRICK 1989).

In a report of nine verified cases of posthemorrhagic hydrocephalus, LAROCHE (1972) notes a premortem increase of head circumference in only four cases. Among 22 hydrocephalic neonates evaluated on CT, 15 had no suggestive clinical findings (BURNSTEIN 1979). Finally, KOROBKIN (1975) and VOLPE (1977) observe that ventriculomegaly can precede the increase in head circumference by days or even weeks. Otherwise, symptoms are sometimes misleading, and BROMBERGER (1988) points out the occurrence of repetitive apneas at the onset of posthemorrhagic hydrocephalus.

In fact, clinical diagnosis of hydrocephalus is unreliable in newborns with a mean age of 30 days (CHAPLIN 1980). This is evidently too late, since ultrasound detection is possible in a high-risk neonate (premature, bacterial infection) as in brain abnormalities (myelomeningocele), and should be done in the first days of life.

4.1.2
Diagnosis Is Based on Neonatal Ultrasound Evaluation

● Morphological criteria are essential since the diagnosis of hydrocephalus is based on increasing ventricular volume during successive ultrasonographic examinations. We know that ventricular enlargement does not progress in a uniform manner. At the onset of the disease, dilatation first involves the occipital horns and ventricular atrium, because of local anatomic conditions (POLAND 1985; RUMACK 1982; SILVERBOARD 1980): for a long time the distending process spares basal ganglia gray matter, which explains the initially moderate dilatation of the frontal horns; by contrast, the intense edematous lesions of the white matter running along the occipital horns and atrium explain why they enlarge early (Fig. 4.1).

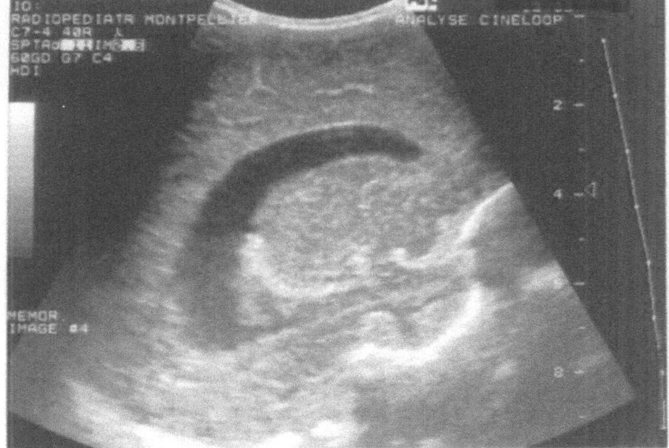

a

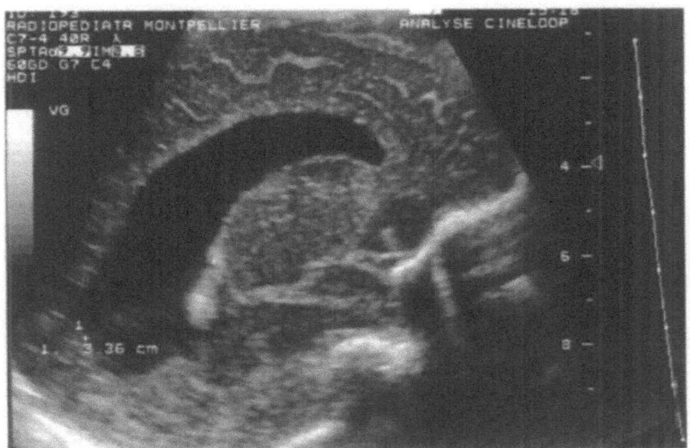

b

Fig. 4.1a,b. Myelomeningocele in a 10-day-old newborn. Predominant enlargement of the left atrium and occipital horn compared with the frontal horn (a): this is a valuable ground for diagnosing hydrocephalus. Gradual increase of the distension of the occipital horns (b) suggests progressive ventriculomegaly

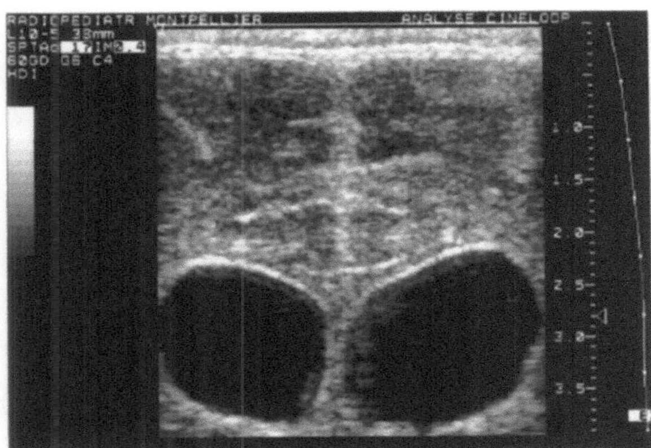

Fig. 4.2. Posthemorrhagic hydrocephalus in a 1-month-old infant. The rounded configuration of the frontal horns demonstrates the intense evolution of the hydrocephalus

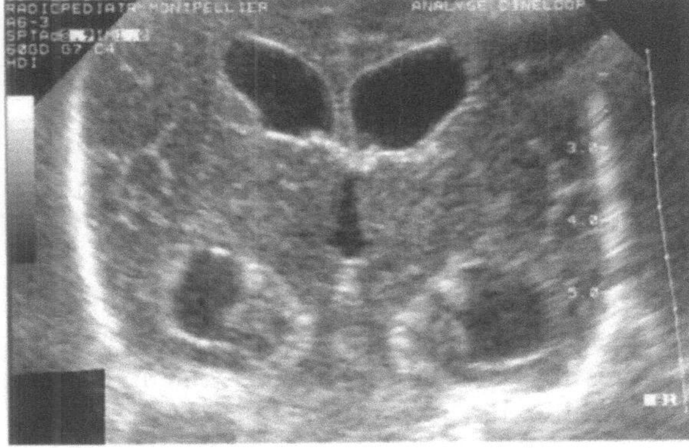

Fig. 4.3. During progressive ventriculomegaly, the temporal horns are usually less enlarged than the occipital horns and ventricular bodies

As the ventriculomegaly increases, the ventricles appear rounded, the frontal horns acquire a clubbing deformity (Fig. 4.2), and the temporal horns are simultaneously enlarged (Fig. 4.3). Finally, when dilatation is massive, the occipital horns are no longer distinguishable from the ventricular bodies (Fig. 4.4); septum lucidum fenestrations are frequent, and probably of an ischemic nature.

Dilatation of the third ventricle is first detected on a sagittal medial plane. Because the resistance of the basal ganglia prevents transverse expansion of the third ventricle, its anteroposterior enlargement is evident, with huge anterior and posterior recessus, before its transverse diameter increases (Fig. 4.5).

In the same way, the sylvian aqueduct, adjacent to the dense brain stem, has moderate possibilities of expansion; its lumen is distinct only in cases of progressive hydrocephalus.

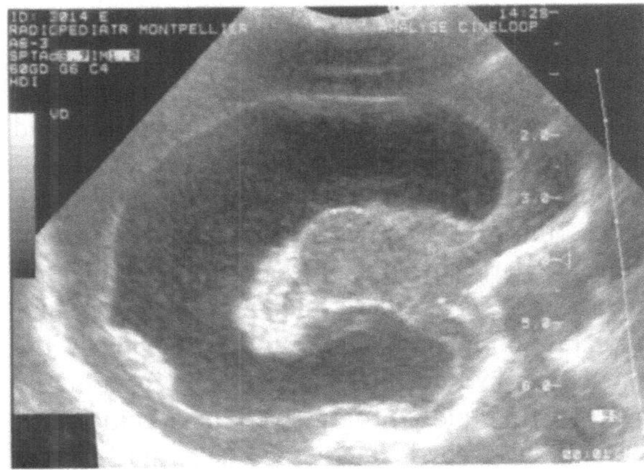

Fig. 4.4. A 1-month-old infant. Communicating tetraventricular hydrocephalus resulting from neonatal intraventricular hemorrhage. Severe dilatation involving the whole lateral ventricle except for the less enlarged temporal horns

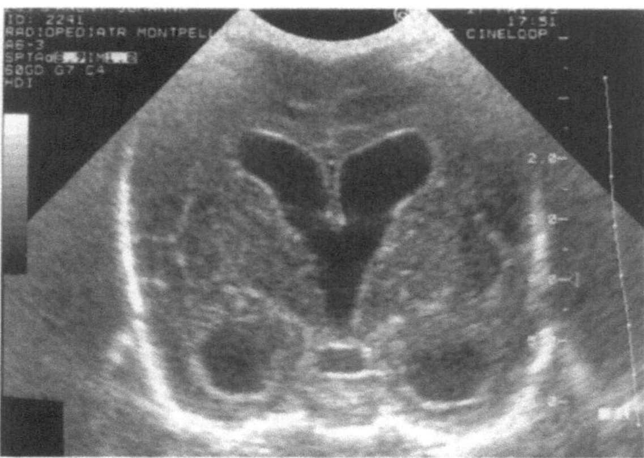

Fig. 4.5. Intraventricular hemorrhage in a premature newborn. Progressive ventriculomegaly. In a frontal plane, dilatation of the third ventricle with an enlarged foramen of Monro is evident

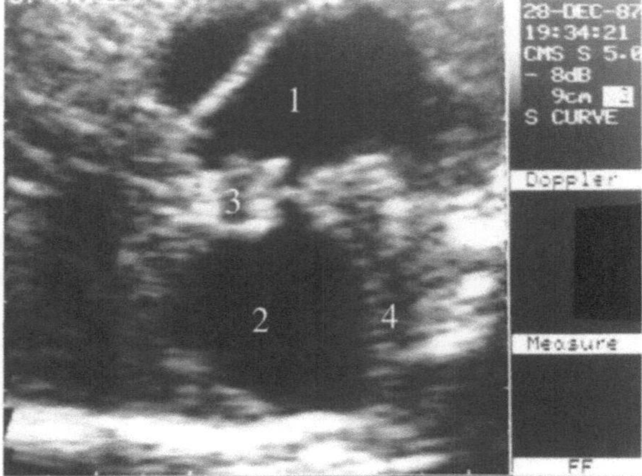

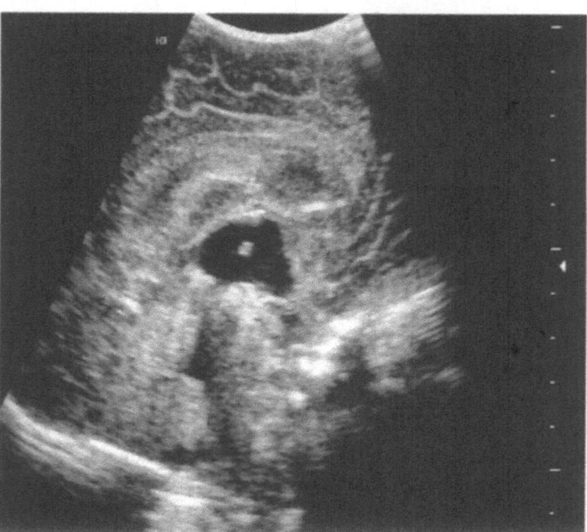

Fig. 4.6. a. Massive intraventricular hemorrhage in a premature newborn. Rounded dilated fourth ventricle, characteristic of the obstruction of foramina of Lushka and Magendie. Notice the third (*1*) and fourth (*2*) ventricular distension, good visualization of the sylvian aqueduct (*3*), and compression of the brain stem (*4*). This is the typical pattern of noncommunicating hydrocephalus. **b** Neonatal meningitis. Triangular-shaped fourth ventricle, well-visualized cisterna magna. This is the typical pattern of a communicating hydrocephalus

A triangular anechoic cavity, with an anterior floor, is the shape of a normal fourth ventricle. Its dilatation, which appears later than that of other ventricles, is usually a sign of noncommunicating hydrocephalus; it takes on a rounded configuration, compressing the brain stem, and widening backward within the less resistant cerebellar vermis (Fig. 4.6). When the hydrocephalus is communicating, the fourth ventricle and the cisterna magna are well visible, moderately enlarged, and normally shaped.

● Although morphological criteria are important in the definition of hydrocephalus, it is necessary to keep in mind that ventricular dilatation is a dynamic process: its diagnosis is also based on ventricular volume increase as seen in successive ultrasound examinations. Moreover, some objective ultrasonographic features allow to point out the rapidity with which the hydrocephalus is evolving: hyperechogenic paraventricular areas (Fig. 4.7) / ependymal lesions (Fig. 4.8), and increased vascular resistance on hemodynamic studies. Obviously, the intensity of hydrocephalus depends on its etiology: it is usually rapidly progressive after a tumor or a massive intraventricular hemorrhage, but evolves quite slowly in the case of myelomeningocele; finally, stabilization or even regression of the ventriculomegaly is often observed after a moderate ventricular hemorrhage.

4.2
Etiogical Diagnosis

Progress in antenatal diagnosis (by ultrasound and MRI) has led to profound changes in the incidences of certain etiologies: in our hospital, Dandy-Walker malformation, holoprosencephaly (Cayea 1984; Filly 1984) and developmental hydrocephalus have become less frequent. (Fig. 4.9).

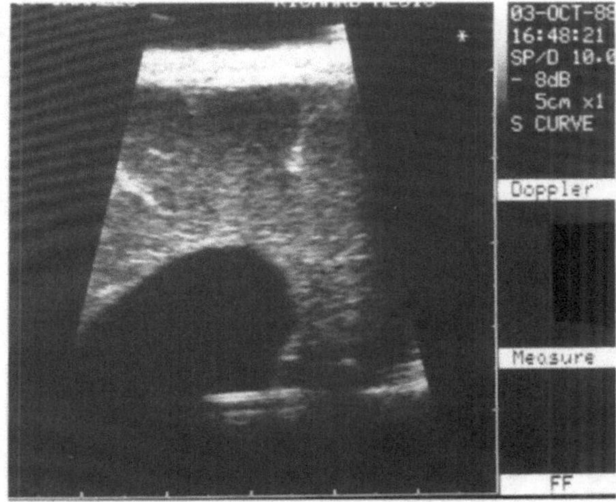

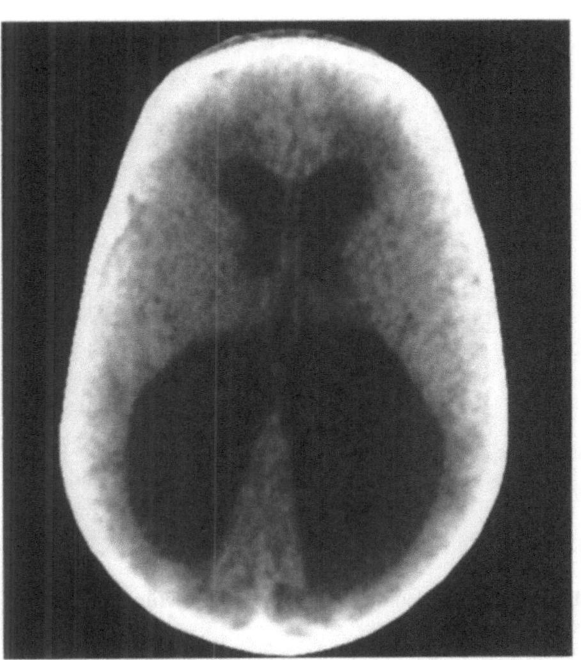

Fig. 4.7a,b. Neonatal Listeria meningitis. At 2 months of age, the patient had symptomatic intracranial hypertension. Communicating hydrocephalus on ultrasound. Notice the radial hyperechogenic images at the lateral angle of the ventricle (a). This appearance will disappear after shunting. **b** Periventricular edema is confirmed by CT

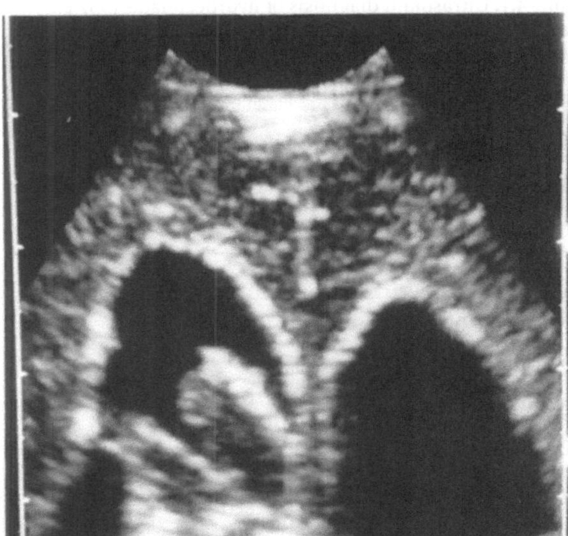

Fig. 4.8. A 12-day-old neonate with intracranial hypertension. Progressive posthemorrhagic hydrocephalus. Notice the dotted hyperechoic ventricular wall

Acquired, especially posthemorrhagic, hydrocephalus is now the most common etiological form; thus, among 307 cases of hydrocephalus diagnosed by ultrasound, intraventricular hemorrhage was the cause in more than 40% (Table 4.1).

In the hemodynamic assessment of ventriculomegaly, it is important to take care of the etiology, because the rate of progression, and consequently the severity of hemodynamic disturbances, vary according to the cause.

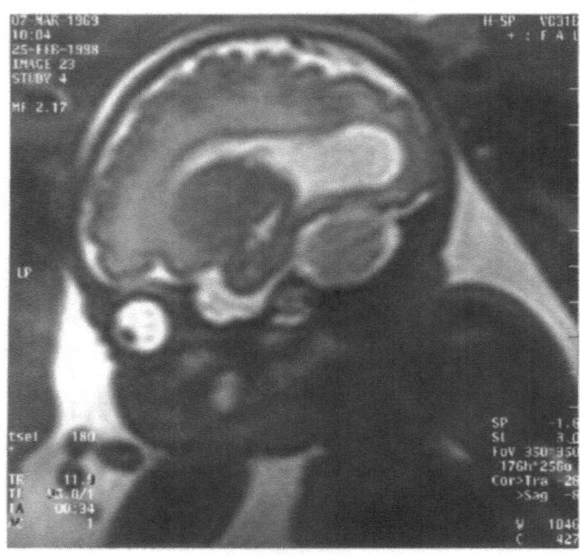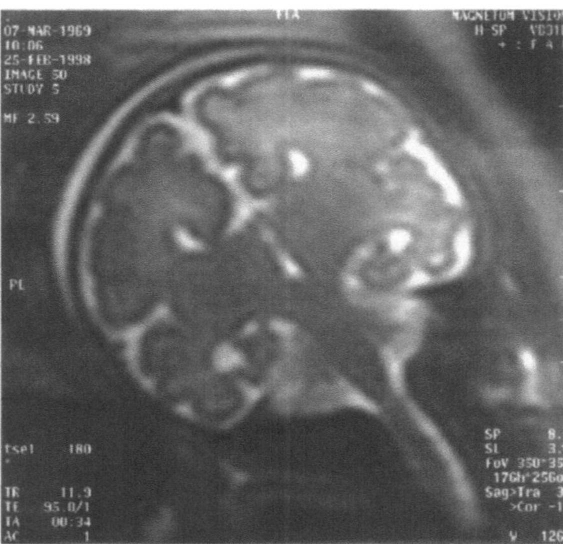

Fig. 4.9 a,b. Ventriculomegaly in a 33-week fetus. Prenatal MRI shows ventricular dilatation (a) and agenesis of the corpus callosum (b)

Table 4.1. Ultrasound diagnosis of hydrocephalus (307 cases)

Intraventricular hemorrhage	139
Infectious disease	40
– Bacterial meningitis	24
– Toxoplasmosis	10
– Cytomegalovirus	6
Brain tumor	28
Brain abnormality	100
– Myelomeningocele	62
– Aqueduct stenosis	12
– Dandy-Walker syndrome	11
– Holoprosencephaly	8
– Vein of Galen aneurysm	7

4.2.1
Ultrasound Pattern of Posthemorrhagic Hydrocephalus

Often there is a massive intraventricular bleeding, filling full the ventricular lumen. Ventriculomegaly appears immediately, probably due to bloody distension of the ventricles (BOWERMAN 1984). The hydrocephalus always occurs quickly (Fig. 4.10), and is usually due to arachnoid villous obstruction (HILL 1984); intraventricular obstruction is less frequent. In a personal study of 48 cases of neonatal post-hemorrhagic hydrocephalus, 27 were communicating and 21 noncommunicating.

In less progressive situations, neuropathological studies (BLUMHAGEN 1985; NAIDICH 1976) show that obstruction is usually due to infratentorial obliterative arachnoiditis, less frequently to clots or necrotic tissue.

4.2.2
Acute Hydrocephalus as a Frequent Complication of Bacterial Meningitis

BERMAN (1966), in a postmortem study, notes that 50% of neonates and infants with bacterial meningitis have hydrocephalus. He confirms extraventricular location as the most frequent site of obstruction: subarachnoid spaces were involved in 8 of 14 patients with hydrocephalus, while the sylvian aqueduct was obstructed in 4 and the fourth ventricle in only 2. We have observed the same: in our 10 cases of postmeningitic hydrocephalus, dilatation is communicating in 8 infants.

Finally, ventriculitis, a severe complication of bacterial meningitis (REEDER 1983) induces ventricular obstruction, while arachnoiditis leads to a communicating dilatation (HAN 1985; ROSENBERG 1983).

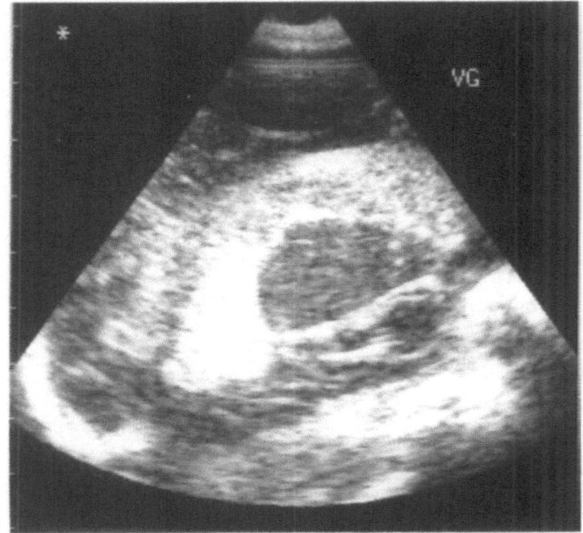

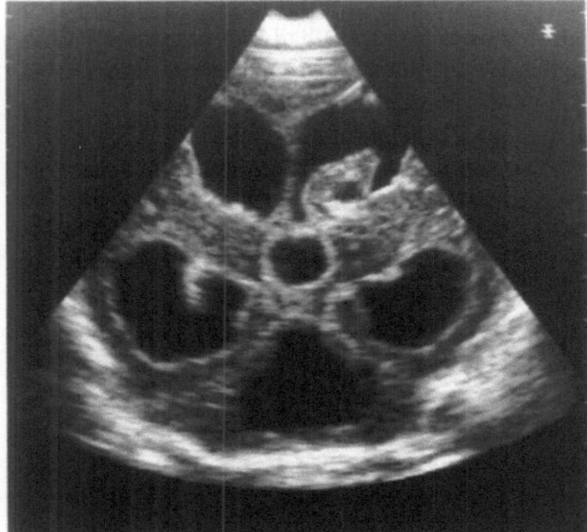

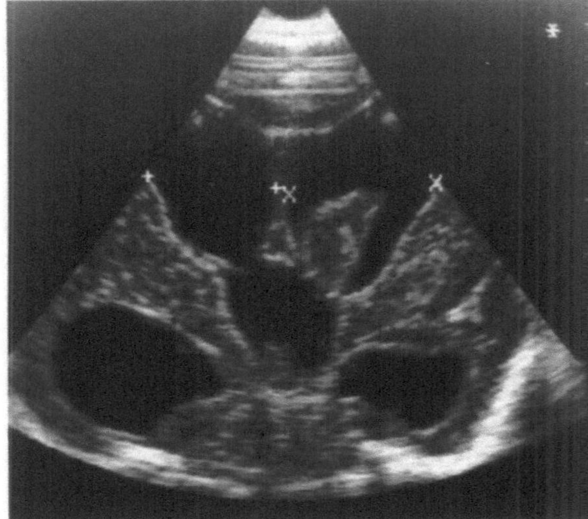

Fig. 4.10a–c. Premature newborn at 34 weeks' gestation. Hyaline membrane disease. Status epilepticus. Ultrasonography at 2 days of age (**a**) showed massive intraventricular hemorrhage, filling enlarged ventricles. Hydrocephalus will be rapidly progressive. At 13 days (**b, c**), clinical intracranial hypertension and severe hydrocephalus on ultrasonography

4.2.3
Hydrocephalus and Brain Tumor

The clinical symptoms of brain tumor in a newborn (macrocrania, intracranial hypertension) are not specific, and ultrasound plays the main role in the detection of such a tumor. Hydrocephalus is a common feature. In our experience (VEYRAC 1988), out of 36 patients with congenital brain tumor (age range from birth to 1 year old), hydrocephalus was apparent in 28 (Table 4.2).

Hydrocephalus caused by brain tumor is a noncommunicating dilatation whose extent depends on the location of the tumor. A supratentorial location, predominant in neonates and infants, was found in 24 cases; in 19 there was biventricular dilatation. Displacement of third ventricle points to a medial cr

Table 4.2. Hydrocephalus and brain tumor

Supratentorial tumors	
– Intraventricular	6
Hydrocephalus	6
– Hemispheric	11
Hydrocephalus	10
– Medial line	7
Hydrocephalus	3
Intratentorial Tumors	
– Medulloblastoma	3
Hydrocephalus	3
– Ependymoma	3
Hydrocephalus	2
– Astroglial tumor	4
Hydrocephalus	2
– Indeterminate tumor	2
Hydrocephalus	2

hemispheric tumor location. Among 12 patients with infratentorial tumors, 9 had hydrocephalus. Sylvian aqueduct or/and fourth ventricle compression and lamination induce early, often explosive, subtentorial hydrocephalus (Fig. 4.11).

Hydrocephalus in cases of choroid plexus papilloma is worth discussing. This tumor can be diagnosed on the basis of a specific ultrasound pattern: it is intraventricular, hyperechogenic, and lobulated, with alterations of the cerebral hemodynamics (Fig. 4.12). The pathogenesis of the dilatation remains under debate (REKATE 1986); considered for a long time to represent CSF overproduction by the tumor itself (EISENBERG 1971; TURCOTTE 1980), the hydrocephalus results in fact from the complex interaction of multiple mechanisms: ventricular lumen obstruction by the mass, intraventricular hemorrhagic lesion that reduces CSF absorption (GUTHKELCH 1972), increased CSF pulsation pressure within the ventricles (DI ROCCO 1979), and, lastly, CSF overproduction.

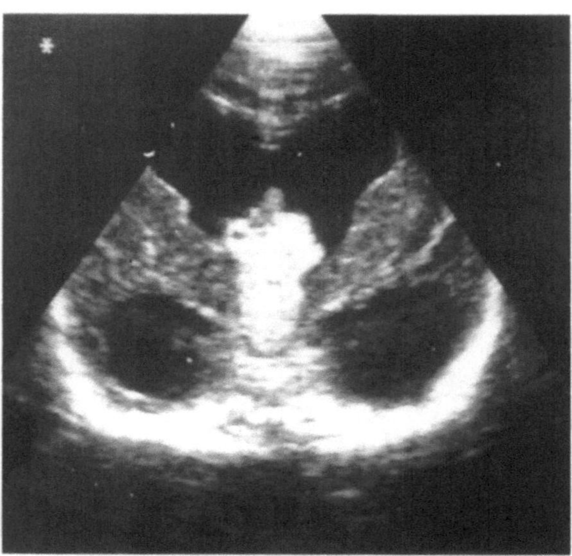

Fig. 4.12. Choroid plexus papilloma in a 3-month-old infant. Hyperechogenic tumor fills the third ventricle, causing biventricular hydrocephalus

4.2.4
Developmental Hydrocephalus

– Myelomeningocele is the most common malformation involved.
  Ventricular dilatation is a constant finding, usually biventricular, infrequently triventricular, in neonates (Fig. 4.13). It is rather a colpocephaly, the high incidence of which in fetuses is now known.

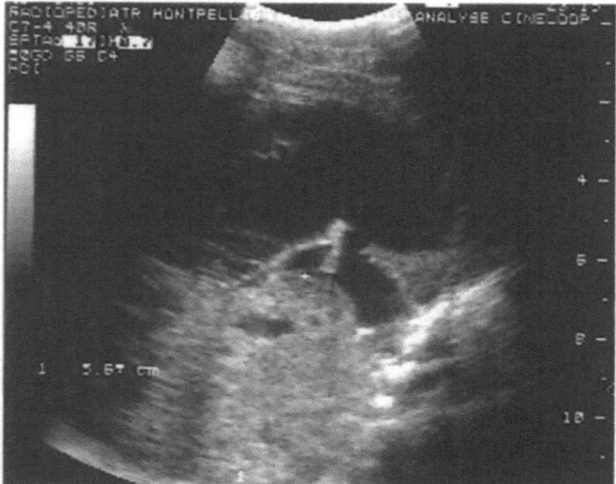

Fig. 4.11. A 9-month-old infant with acute intracranial hypertension. A large brain stem tumor is displacing the third ventricle, resulting in severe triventricular dilatation

Myelomeningocele is always associated with Arnold-Chiari malformation, and the mechanism of hydrocephalus is still debated: a communicating dilatation leading to the posterior fossa anomaly, an obstruction of CSF circulation induced by the Arnold-Chiari abnormality, and an associated sylvian aqueduct stenosis are the main suggested hypotheses. After closure of cutaneous lesion, hydrocephalus always becomes worse; clinical symptoms of intracranial hypertension appear 1–3 weeks later.

– Dandy Walker syndrome is characterized by agenesis or hypoplasia of the cerebellar vermis with fourth ventricle cystic dilatation (Fig. 4.14). Hydrocephalus is common, most often developing after birth (HIRSH 1984). Two mechanisms should be considered: changes in CSF circulation or post-delivery hemorrhage within a dilated fourth ventricle.

– Aneurysm of the vein of Galen is a rare cause of hydrocephalus (Fig. 4.15). Ventricular dilatation is explained either by compression of the sylvian aqueduct close to the large aneurysmal pouch, or by raised venous pressure, particularly within the superior sagittal sinus, which prevents normal CSF absorption. The diagnosis is suspected on clinical findings (intracranial murmur, sometimes cardiac failure) and confirmed by ultrasonography, by detection of an anechoic vascular retrothalamic mass on the medial line. This is a

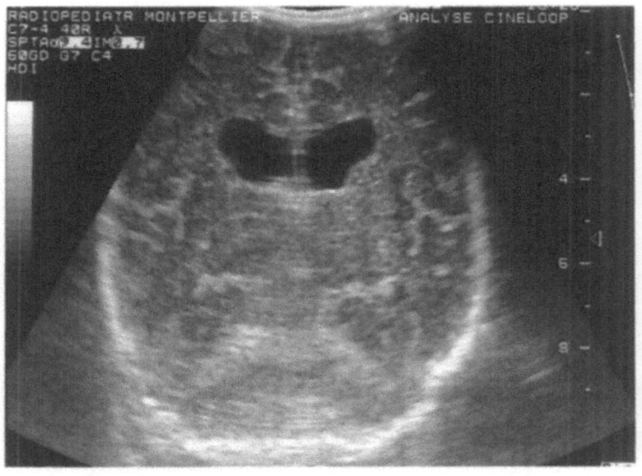

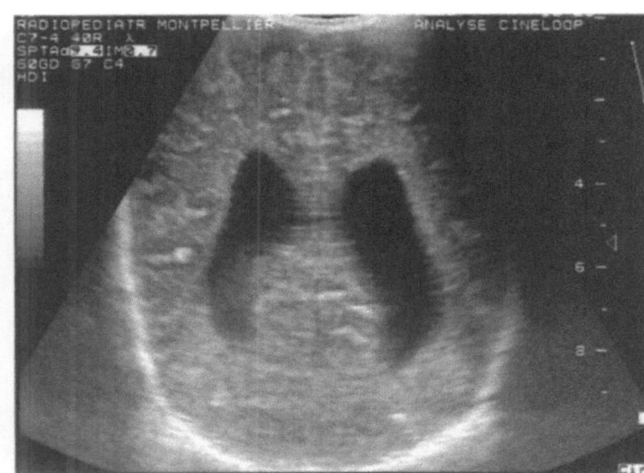

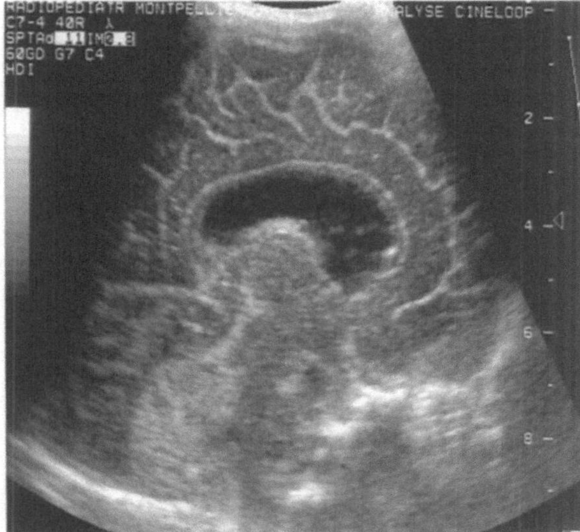

Fig. 4.13a–c. In myelomeningocele, neonatal ventriculomegaly is not severe. In this 20-day-old baby ultrasonography (a, b) was performed the day before shunting (drainage was instituted because of hemodynamic alteration and an RI of 0.92). Notice the quadrangular shape of the lateral ventricles, the ectopic fourth ventricle and cerebellar vermis, and the disappearance of the cisterna magna (c)

pathognomonic appearance (COUTURE 1981; CUBBERLEY 1982).

- Holoprosencephaly is sometimes associated with stenosis of the sylvian aqueduct. Diagnosis in utero is easy in the presence of facial malformation, single ventricle, and fusion of the thalami (CAYEA 1984; FILLY 1984).
- Stenosis of the aqueduct of Sylvius is a classical etiology of hydrocephalus. Many pathogenetic hypotheses have been suggested to explain congenital obstruction of the sylvian aqueduct.

Stenosis with gliosis is known to be a consequence of an inflammatory process, but experimental models of viral hydrocephalus never develop periaqueductal gliosis.

Stenosis without gliosis, but with a narrowed or forking aqueduct could be a developmental abnormality.

Experimentally and in humans, it has been proved that communicating hydrocephalus can provoke an aqueduct obstruction.

Lastly, sex-linked hydrocephalus of Bickers-Adams syndrome, usually considered as the model of genetic sylvian aqueduct malformation, does not constantly include aqueductal stenosis.

Thus, apart from cases where an inflammatory process is evident (toxoplasmosis, meningitis, hemorrhage), the stenotic mechanism remains in most cases obscure.

As we can see, the etiology of the hydrocephalus, which is mainly evaluated by ultrasound, is of considerable importance to guide the hemodynamic analysis. On the one hand, there is hydrocephalus that is rapidly progressive and explosive (tumoral, hemorrhagic hydrocephalus), where hemodynamic disturbances will be intense, appear early, and will require precise and repeated examination; at the opposite

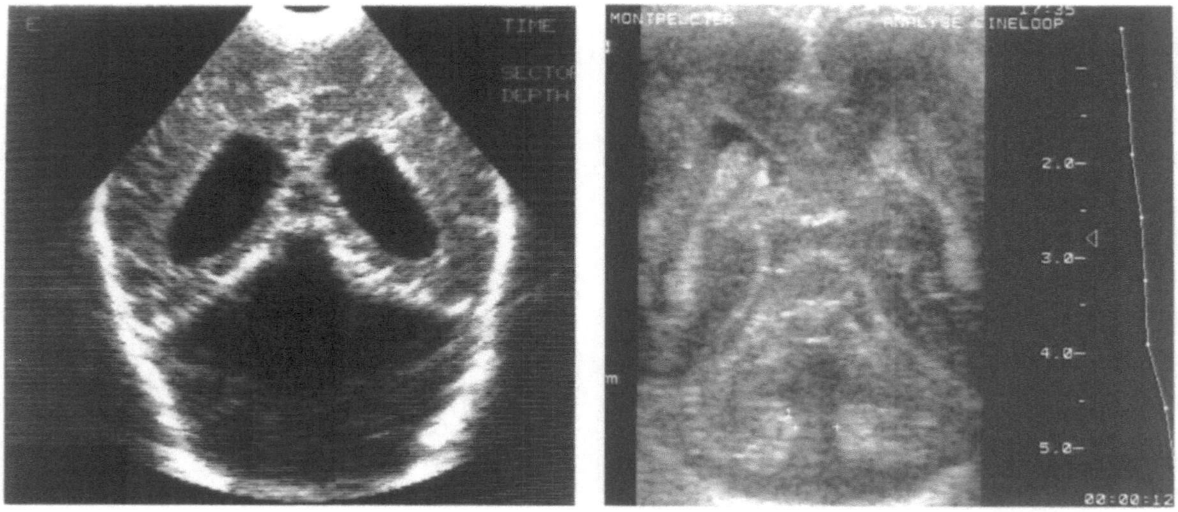

Fig. 4.14. a Dandy-Walker malformation with vermian agenesis in a 2-day-old newborn. This diagnosis is now made in the fetus (b). c Postmortem ultrasonography in a 25-week fetus: posterior fossa cyst with fourth ventricle communication. On suboccipital scan, normal-sized cerebellar hemispheres and inferior vermian agenesis

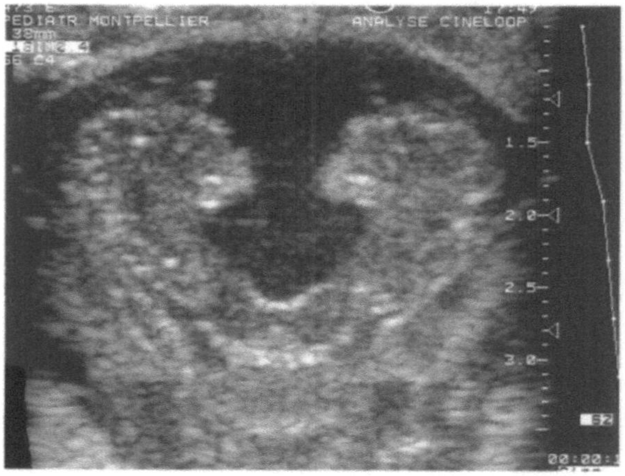

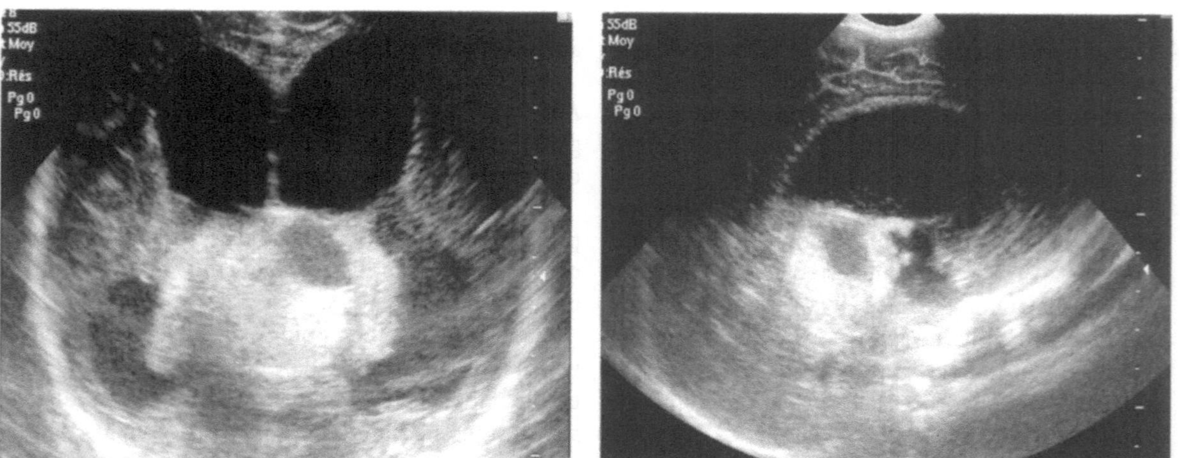

Fig. 4.15a,b. Vein of Galen aneurysm diagnosed antenatally (color Doppler and MRI). Embolization at 2 months, followed by progressive onset of triventricular dilatation with normal hemodynamics. Notice the large volume of partially thrombosed aneurysmal pouch (a) stretching the aqueduct of Sylvius (b)

extreme, postmeningitic and developmental hydrocephalus will evolve slowly with later hemodynamic signs of vascular damage.

4.3
Hemodynamic Monitoring of Hydrocephalus

During progressive ventricular dilatation, the sequence of events occurring in the cerebral parenchyma is well established. In experimental hydrocephalus, white matter edema constitutes the earliest lesion (RUBIN 1976), appearing within periventricular tissue a few hours after a ventricular obstruction; 48 h later, edema involves the subcortical white matter. The evolution is characterized by white matter destruction with a loss of glial cells, mainly astrocytes, which are the most susceptible and undergo selective swelling before disappearing. After 2 weeks, macrophagic cells gather around white matter. If the ventricular obstruction is removed, these lesions are reversible. Ultimately, oligodendroglial cell damage is observed, with axonal lengthening and unravelling of the myelin sheath (HARRIS 1994).

The observations in hydrocephalic children are similar to experimental results (RAIMONDI 1994; MORI 1995). Ventricular enlargement compresses the surrounding tissues, particularly the white matter; the most common changes in the hydrocephalic brain are atrophy, pallor and swelling, vacuolation, chromatolysis of nerve cells, hypertrophy of astrocytes, demyelinization with axonal degeneration, and loss of synapses.

In these successive stages, increased intraventricular pressure and CSF reflux into white matter play an evident role. Nevertheless, it is essential to understand that there also occurs a compression of the hemispheric vascular bed, resulting in decreased brain perfusion (RAIMONDI 1994): these disturbances probably play a main role in the genesis of neuropathological lesions and the occurrence of neurological disorders. The modalities of onset and the evolution of hemodynamic alterations should be appreciated, because their clinical consequences are important for the precision and objectivity of therapeutic management (repeated lumbar puncture, ventriculoperitoneal shunt), and for the prediction of the short- and long-term prognosis.

4.3.1
Morphological Changes in Brain Cerebral Vessels in Hydrocephalus (DE 1950; GREITZ 1968, 1969; HASSLER 1964; WOSNIAK 1975)

The vascular consequences of hydrocephalus have been well known since the experimental studies of HASSLER (1964) and WOZNIAK (1975).

DE (1950) and HASSLER (1964) were the first to analyze vascular changes during hydrocephalus induced by injecting adhesive agents into the subarachnoid spaces or the ventricular system. They observed a loss of capillaries around the dilated ventricles and concluded that induced ischemia is responsible for the parenchymal lesions. However, these studies are open to criticism: the hydrocephalus was experimentally induced, and there were too many variations between protocols: lack of uniformity in species (mongrel dogs and cats) and in techniques (kaolin and surgery).

WOZNIAK (1975) put in place a reliable experimentation, independent of artefacts occurring in induced hydrocephalus, based on the study of 20 mice with congenital hydrocephalus. He observed vascular changes depending on the duration and the severity of hydrocephalic process, and described three stages:
- Stage I (7th–14th days). This stage corresponds to moderate ventricular dilatation. The microangiogram demonstrates that there are already changes in the direction and caliber of cerebral vessels: the anterior cerebral artery is under tension, its diameter is diminished, and the number of its branches is decreased. There are architectural irregularities of vessels that supply white matter. The normal palisading pattern of cortical vessels is preserved.
- Stage II (14th–18th days). The microangiogram shows much more diffuse vascular lesions: the diameter of the anterior and middle cerebral arteries is decreased, and lenticulostriate arteries are displaced, stretched and narrowed. Backward deviation of the posterior cerebral artery is intense, and a diminished number of its branches is noticed. When the ventricles are severely dilated, there is a decrease in cortical vascularization, with distorsion of the palisading pattern. The vascularization of the brain stem and cerebellum remains preserved. The electron micrograph confirms an increase in extracellular space to 40-50% in the hydrocephalic brain, from approximately 15% in normal brain.
- Stage III (beyond the 18th day). The edema, previously restricted to white matter, now extends into the gray matter of the occipital lobe. A spontane-

ous ventriculostomy develops within the occipital lobes, connecting the ventricles with the patent subarachnoid spaces. The microangiogram demonstrates a sharp decrease in the number of branches of the posterior cerebral artery. In the brain cortex, primary and secondary vessels are markedly displaced, and there is a significant loss of the cortical capillary network. The number of tertiary vessels is reduced, the palisade configuration is disrupted. The brain stem vessels seem to be preserved.

An external drainage performed in stage 2 shows that a reduction in intraventricular pressure is associated with a return to normal of the caliber, form, and course of the cerebral vasculature.

From these observations, the authors PEREZ (1964), WOZNIAK (1975), and DA SILVA (1995) postulate a sequence of events leading to irreversible brain damage.

The first vascular change is the decrease in the diameter of vessels. Its pathophysiological mechanism is easy to understand: the progressive increase in ventricular volume, and the transependymal CSF perfusion which increases the extracellular space (SATO 1986), compress, displace, and distort the cerebral vessels. This first occurs within the white matter (Fig. 4.16), and probably results in diminished cerebral blood flow. Ultimately, there is a decrease in the number of secondary and tertiary vessels within the white and gray matter. Edema and periventricular tissue atrophy result not only from the extracellular volume increase, but also from ischemia following the compression of capillaries. That is to say, a succes-

sive sequence of events leading to irreversible brain damage may be described: ventricular volume increase, transependymal CSF flow, parenchymal vascular compression, edema, ischemia, and tissue destruction.

For the authors (WOZNIAK 1975), irreversibility of brain damage is obvious when porencephalic cysts form within the white matter during the end of stage 2. The conclusions of these experimental studies are basic:

- Increasing intracranial pressure and its consequences (ventricular dilatation, CSF transependymal perfusion) leads to a decrease in cerebral blood flow. Conversely, a decrease in intracranial pressure, achieved by ventricular drainage, is followed by an increase in the diameter of the cerebral vessels.
- It is important to perform decompression early, when the process is still reversible.
- In murine congenital hydrocephalus, the prognosis may be predicted by microangiographic studies: the presence of tertiary vessels indicates a good prognosis, whereas avascular areas will certainly result in psychomotor retardation.

In conclusion, in experimental and certainly in human hydrocephalus, there is a threshold that must not be exceeded on pain of irreversible brain damage (GOITEN 1983; SATO 1986). RAIMONDI (1994) proposes the following sequence of events: (1) increase in intraventricular CSF with a rise in hydrostatic pressure; (2) transependymal fluid flow resulting in compression of cerebral vessels; (3) ischemia and an increase in extracellular fluid, inducing communication between intraventricular and extracellular fluid; (4) cell lesions and tissue destruction.

Thus the vascular factors play a major role in the genesis of brain damage; the hemodynamic analysis of human hydrocephalus using pulsed and color Doppler ultrasonography certainly constitutes an interesting and original approach to guide the patient's management.

4.3.2
Role of Doppler Imaging in the Monitoring of Hydrocephalus

Pulsed Doppler imaging (guided by color Doppler) used to assess changes in cerebral perfusion at the onset and during the course of hydrocephalus is now a routine investigation with an essential role: first, pulsed Doppler has proven its worth in preventing

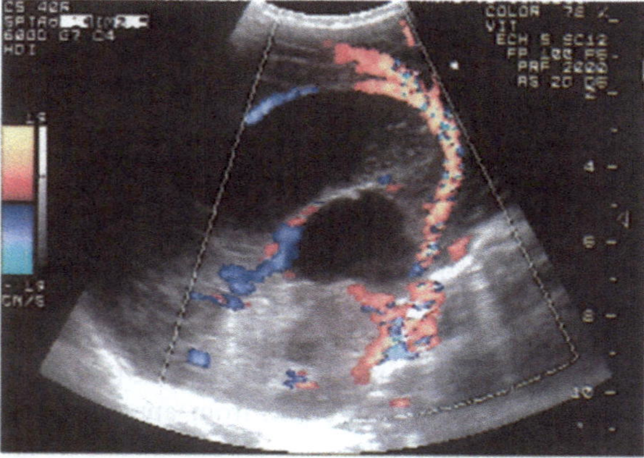

Fig. 4.16. Triventricular hydrocephalus in a 29-week premature newborn. Notice how the dilated frontal horns displace and compress the pericallosal and anterior cerebral arteries

posthemorrhagic hydrocephalus (PERLMAN 1985; VEYRAC 1987); second, it seems to be the method of choice for monitoring ventricular drainage.

Our experience is based on 91 cases of hydrocephalus (48 posthemorrhagic, 31 postmyelomeningocele, 12 postmeningitic dilatation) studied by transfontanellar Doppler.

For each case of ventriculomegaly, one or several measurements of the resistive index (RI) are done: the anterior cerebral artery is analyzed in all infants, the middle cerebral artery in some patients, and in rare cases the posterior cerebral artery, carotid arteries, and basilar artery (studies of venous flow do not bring any useful information).

In all cases where there are cerebral perfusion disturbances an increase in RI is observed, due to decreased end-diastolic velocity or even retrograde diastolic flow (Fig. 4.17) and decreased mean velocity.

Reduced end-diastolic velocity was observed in 32 cases of posthemorrhagic hydrocephalus, 20 cases of myelomeningocele and 10 cases of postmeningitic dilatation. The 16 patients with posthemorrhagic hydrocephalus without any Doppler alteration (or with a transient one) all showed a stable, stabilized, or regressive course. Finally, 11 newborns with myelomeningocele did not exhibit any change in RI: in 8 cases, this may have been due to the absence of hemodynamic monitoring during the days preceding the ventricular drainage; in the other 3 cases, Doppler measurements remained normal over several months (4–9 months), and ventriculoperitoneal shunting did not need to be performed.

4.3.2.1
Acute Hydrocephalus

Maeva was a 27-week neonate, prematurely born after chorionitis. At birth, she suffered apparent death syndrome and presented severe septic alveolitis. On her first ultrasound examination, at 2 days of life, an intraventricular hemorrhage was detected, and the RI was normal in the anterior cerebral artery (RI=0.70). During ultrasonographic monitoring, the ventricles progressively dilated, leading to tetraventricular hydrocephalus (Fig. 4.18). On her 36th day of life, alterations in cerebral hemodynamics appeared: RI=1 (Fig. 4.19). At 1.5 months her head circumference was enlarged and the RI was greatly increased (RI=1.29) (Fig. 4.20). Ventriculoperitoneal shunting was performed the next day, and clinical improvement followed.

This case report shows the characteristic hemodynamic changes observed during the course of posthemorragic hydrocephalus (COUTURE 1996), and allow some conclusions to be drawn:

- Every progressive posthemorrhagic hydrocephalus is associated with an increase in vascular resistance: the RI was abnormal in 33 patients with morphological signs of rapidly progressive ventriculomegaly, but remained normal in 15 cases where dilation progressed slowly, stabilized, or regressed.
- The time of onset of hemodynamic disturbances depends on several factors. There is a parallel between the intensity of acute intraventricular hemorrhage, the severity of ventricular dilatation, and the early onset of diastolic velocity decrease. Moreover, vascular resistance rises earlier in cases of noncommunicating hydrocephalus.

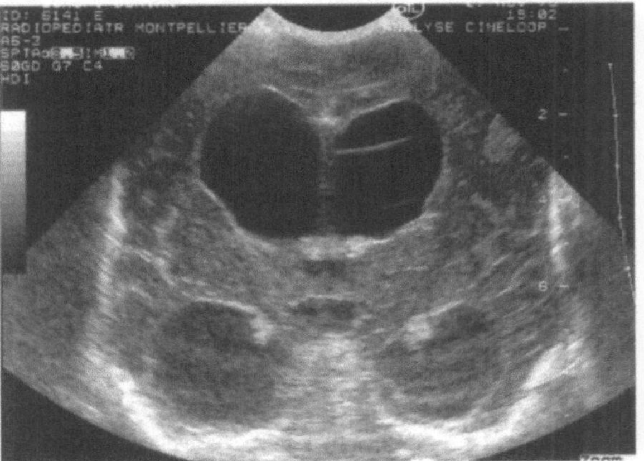
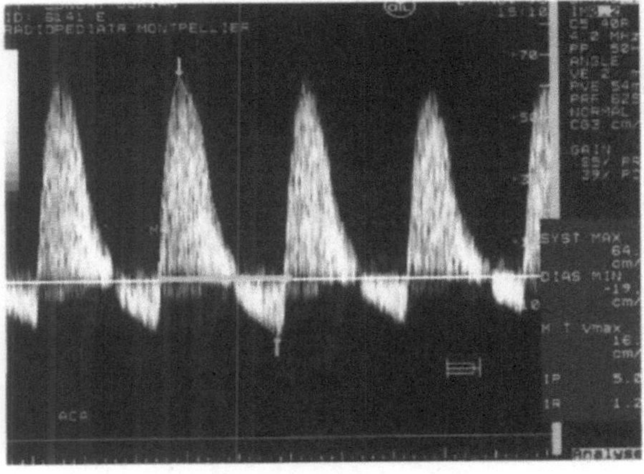

Fig. 4.17a,b. Congenital hydrocephalus with probable aqueductal stenosis. Massive triventricular dilatation (a). On day 29 (b), hemodynamic alterations: RI=1.29, PI=5. Severe decrease in mean velocities: 16.6 cm/s (normal value at this age: 36 cm/s)

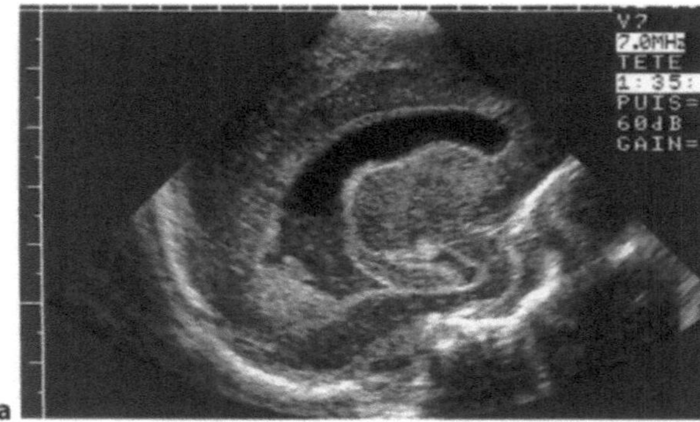
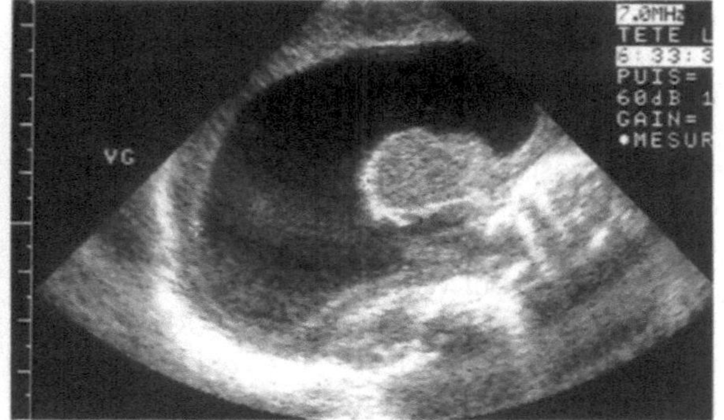

Fig. 4.18a,b. Progressive ventriculomegaly. **a** On day 2, moderate dilatation and gravity-dependent bleeding within the left ventricle. **b** At 1 month, markedly increased ventriculomegaly and slight rise in RI (RI=0.82)

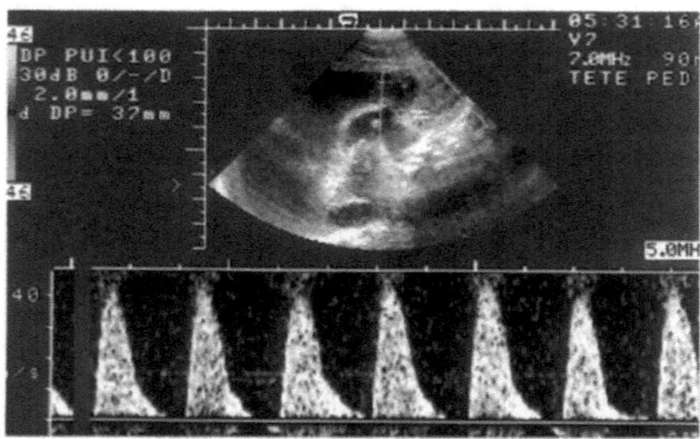
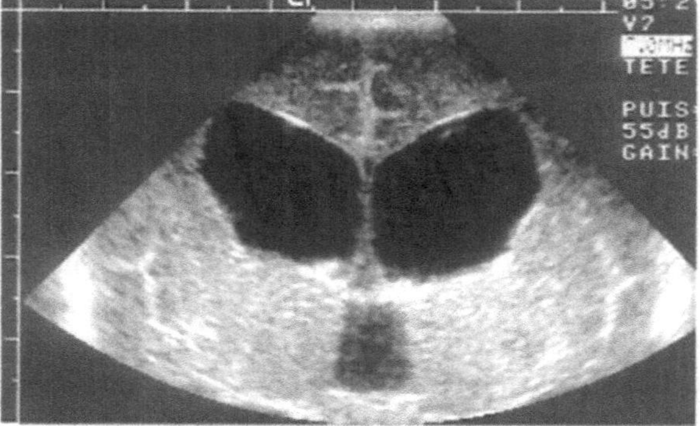

Fig. 4.19a,b. A few days later, marked hemodynamic alterations with disappearance of diastolic flow and RI=1 (**a**). **b** Severe triventricular hydrocephalus

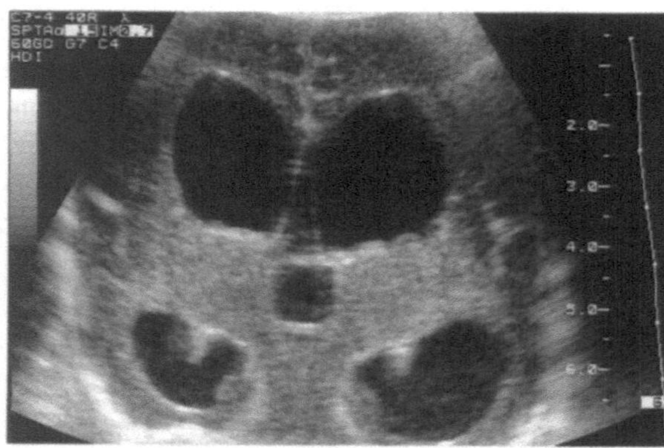
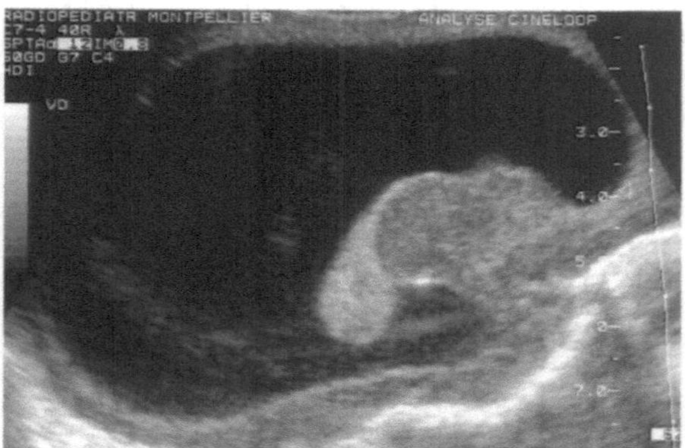
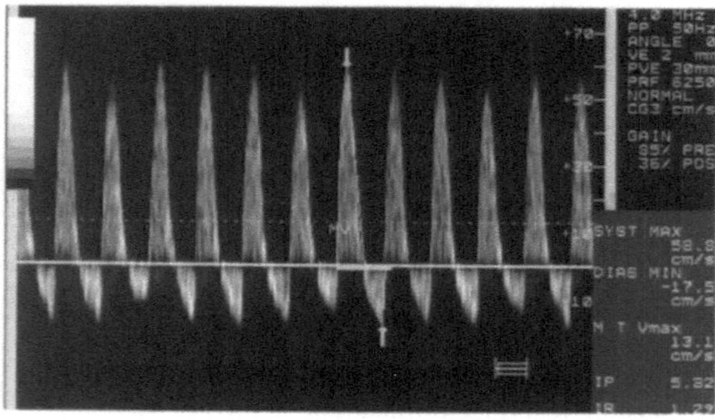

Fig. 4.20a–c. At 1.5 months, there is excessive head circumference growth and major tetraventricular hydrocephalus (**a,b**). Diastolic reverse flow and RI=1.29 (**c**) confirm intracranial hypertension

– In almost all cases, the hemodynamic alterations are severe and a good indicator of rapid progression. The RI is constantly raised (most often above 1) as a result of retrograde diastolic flow and increased downstream resistance. These alterations are often greater in the posterior cerebral artery. This is probably because dilatation is maximal in the ventricular atria and occipital horns; sometimes there is even complete disappearance of the posteromedial part of both hemispheres; this may be partially related to transtentorial herniation of the dilated temporal horns compressing the posterior cerebral artery. Pulsed Doppler analysis of this artery appears to be a reliable early indication of vascular compromise and of potential risk of ischemia (Fig. 4.21).

Whatever the mechanism of hydrocephalus and its progression rate, perfusion disturbances appear quickly in the first month of life (between 8 and 60 days), and usually when ventricular enlargement is the most intense and clinical findings the most severe.

Yannick is a 1-month-old infant evaluated after suffering neonatal streptococcal meningitis. Ultrasound detects a communicating tetraventricular dilatation, slightly asymmetric. Doppler study is normal, and RI is 0.61. Yannick is followed every week. Three weeks later, while ventricular enlargement increases gradually, obvious hemodynamic changes appear, with a striking rise in RI and a retrograde diastolic flow within branches of the anterior cerebral artery (Fig. 4.22).

Hydrocephalus is a frequent complication of bacterial meningitis in the neonate (LORBER 1966). Usually there is an extraventricular obstruction, causing progressive ventriculomegaly and necessitating subsequent ventriculoperitoneal shunting. In cases of ventriculitis, ventricular dilatation tends rather to be noncommunicating. Of our 12 patients, 10 had a rapid evolution as assessed by the early onset of hemodynamic alterations. In 2 cases, Doppler evaluation remained normal, and ventricular drainage was not required.

Jean-Baptiste was born with a lumbosacral myelomeningocele. On the first day of life, ultrasound showed a moderate triventricular dilatation and a Chiari malformation. The RI, measured within anterior cerebral artery, was normal (0.63) (Fig. 4.23). The neural plate was closed on the 2nd day of life. Ultrasound follow-up was performed on days 5, 6, 7, and showed stability of the ventricular enlargement and normality of the Doppler findings (RI was 0.70, 0.69, and 0.69 respectively). On the 8th day, the anterior fontanelle was bulging, ventricular dilatation moderately increased, but perfusion disturbances appeared marked: RI was obviously irregularly raised in all cerebral vessels, as a result of variable diastolic velocities, measuring between 0.76 and 1.18. The infant

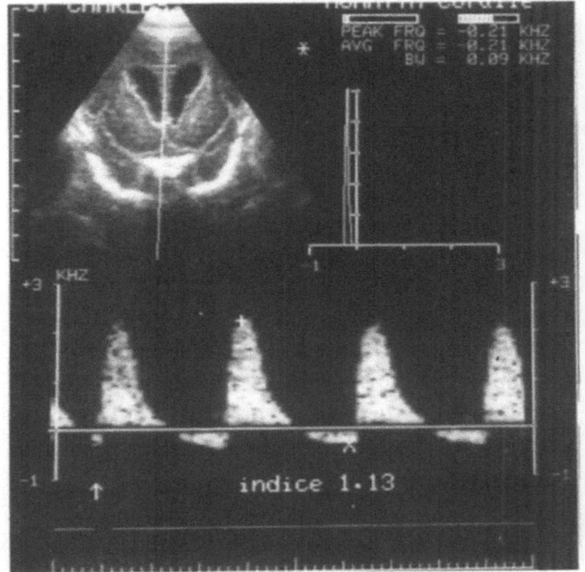
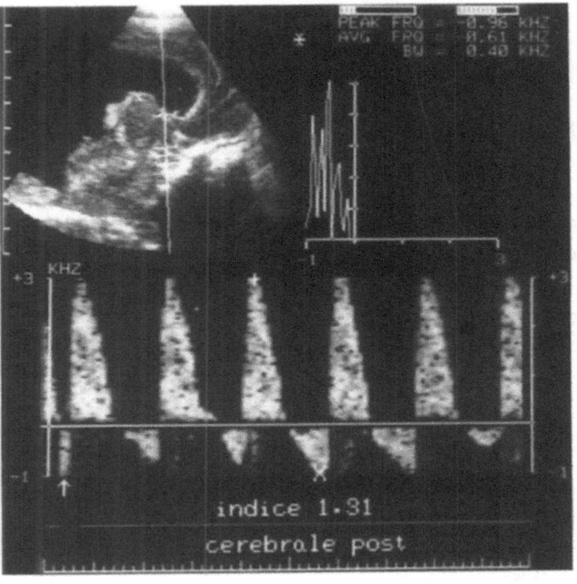

Fig. 4.21a,b. A 28 weeks' premature newborn. On day 10, massive clotted intraventricular hemorrhage. At 1 month of age, there is tetraventricular communicating hydrocephalus, RI=1.13 within the anterior cerebral artery (**a**) and 1.31 within the basilar artery (**b**)

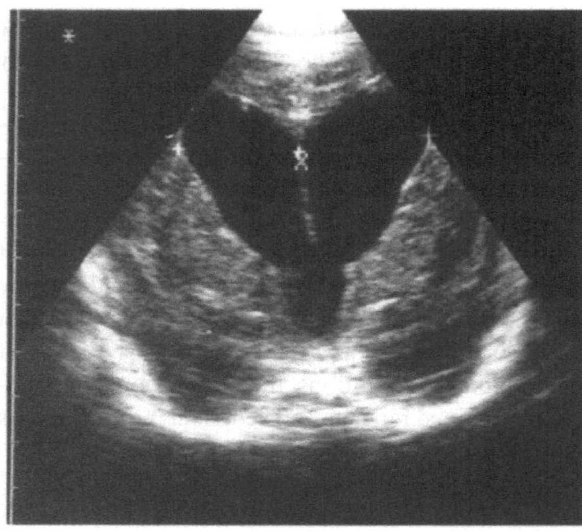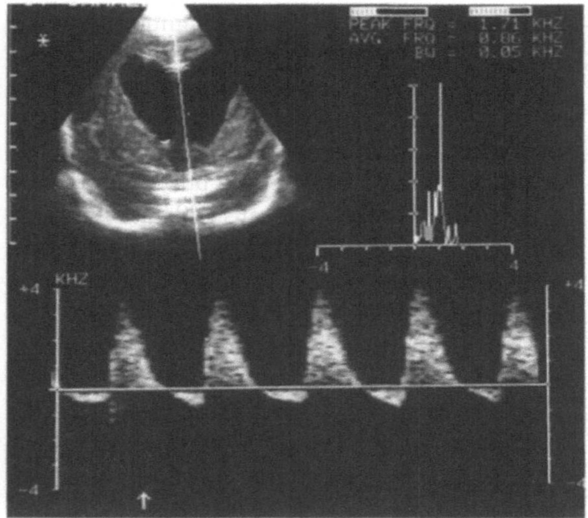

Fig. 4.22a,b. Marked lateral ventricular dilatation (**a**). Increased RI in the anterior cerebral artery: 1.10 (**b**)

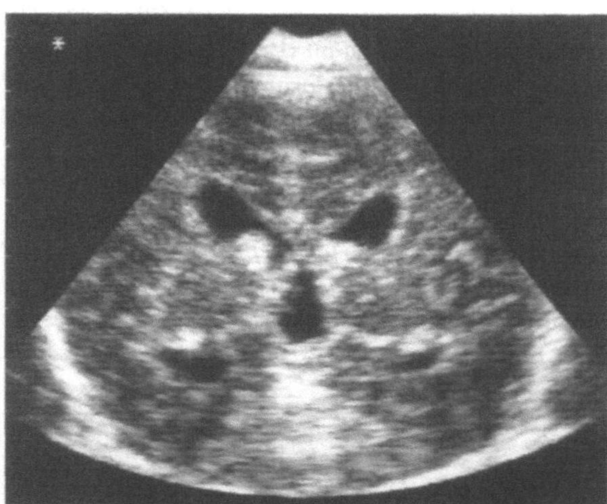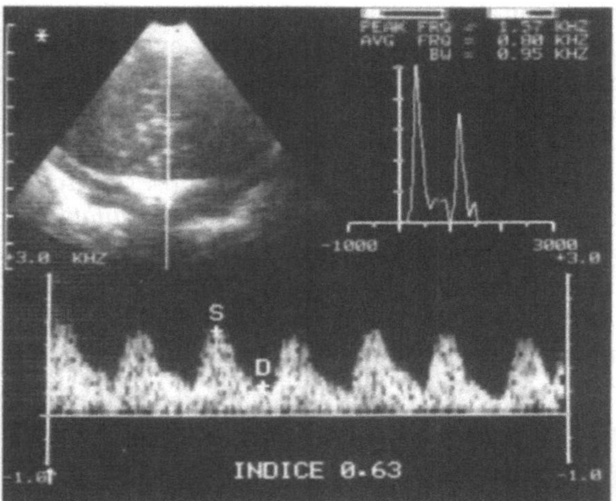

Fig. 4.23a,b Moderate triventricular dilatation (**a**). Normal RI in anterior cerebral artery (**b**)

died at 14 days of life, with unchanged hemodynamic alterations (Fig. 4.24).

This observation shows the following points to be of prime importance:

- Hemodynamic alterations are common in neonates with myelomeningocele. They were obvious in 20 patients studied before ventriculoperitoneal shunting; RI ranged from 0.80 to 1.25; in 8 newborns, diastolic velocities were irregular throughout the examination.

- These disturbances have particular characteristics:

  • At birth, except in one case (Fig. 4.25), there was no alteration of cerebral blood flow in 12 neonates analyzed on the first day of life, whereas ventricles were already enlarged in all patients. That is easily explained since it was a low-pressure hydrocephalus.

  • After surgical repair, the vascular resistance increased generally in the 15 first days (between the 6th and 21st days in the 20 patients who had Doppler monitoring). In parallel to this, a moderate accentuation of ventricular enlargement occurred. The increased RI correlated well with the raised intraventricular pressure.

These personal data are in agreement with the literature. Since the first description by Hill and Volpe (1982), many publications have confirmed the interest value of an hemodynamic assessment in hydrocephalus. Four questions have been resolved:

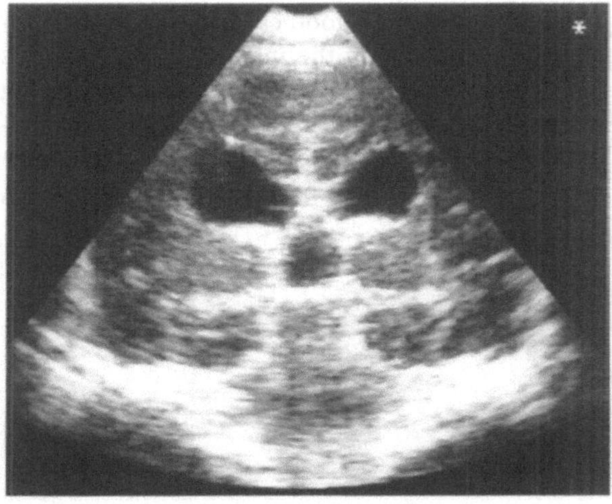

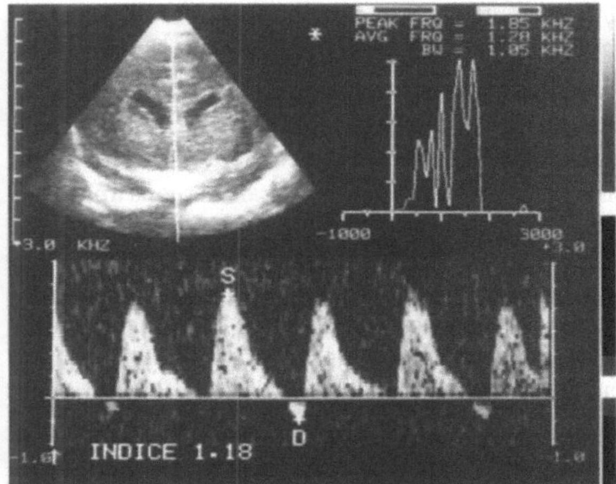

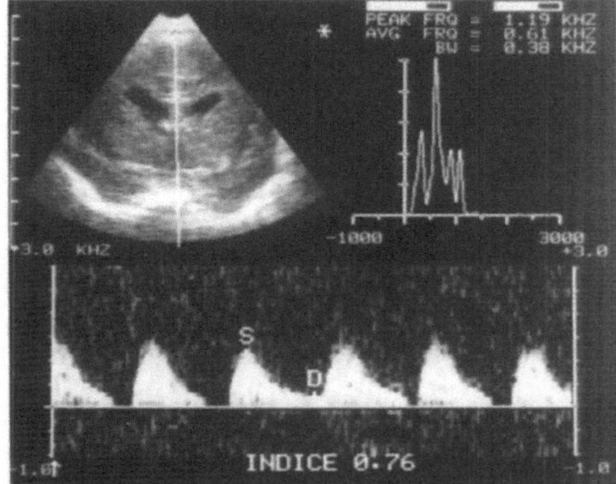

Fig. 4.24a–c. Moderate increase in ventricular enlargement (a). Severe hemodynamic disturbance (b) and fluctuating pattern of Doppler spectrum (c), probably resulting from loss of cerebral autoregulation

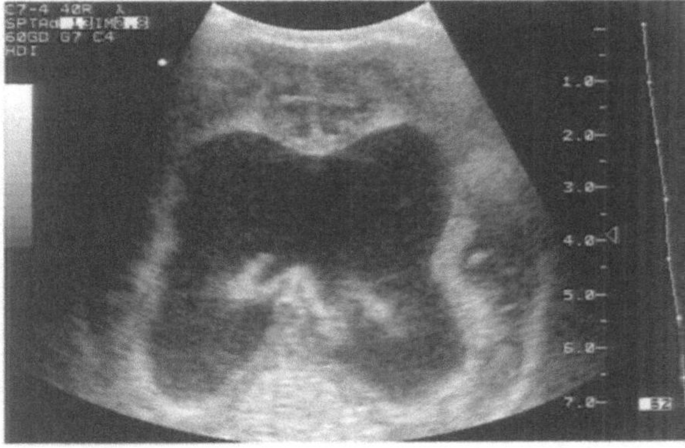

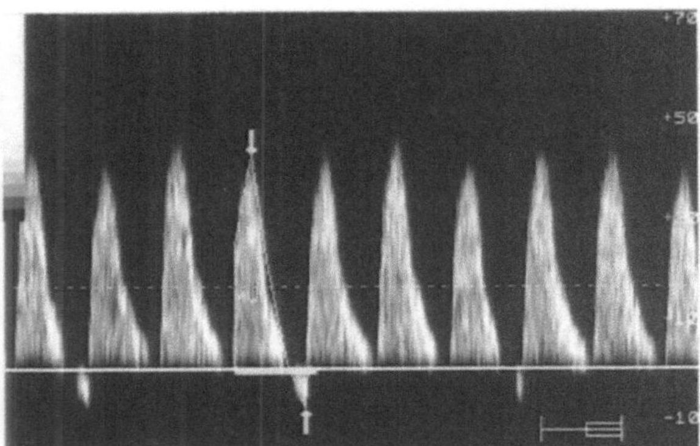

Fig. 4.25a,b. Neonatal myelomeningocele (at T12). Marked hydrocephalus with complete necrosis of the interventricular septum (a). On day 1, severe increase in RI: 1.18 (b). This case was unusual because in neonates, myelomeningocele presents a normal pressure hydrocephalus (before closure of the neural plaque) with normal hemodynamic findings

Which access?

While transfontanellar access is the best way for insonation of the anterior cerebral artery in neonates (ALVISI 1985; ANDERSON 1991; CHADDUK 1989; DEEG 1988; HILL 1982; HUANG 1991; LUI 1990; TAYLOR 1996; VAN BEL 1988), the transosseous approach (CHADDUK 1991; FISCHER 1989; GOH 1991; IACOPINO 1995; MINNS 1991; NORELLE 1989; POPLE 1992; QUINN 1989; SANKER 1991) constitutes the only access after closure of the anterior fontanelle and favors spectral analysis of the middle cerebral artery. These differences in which vessels are assessed have no practical consequences, since hemodynamic disturbances in hydrocephalic patients involve all the cerebral arteries homogeneously. In nine cases of hydrocephalus, LUI (1990) demonstrated the same Doppler alterations in all three vessels studied (anterior and middle cerebral arteries and circle of Willis). Our results, with transfontanellar ultrasonography, were the same in the anterior, middle, and posterior cerebral arteries, the basilar artery, and the lenticulostriate arteries.

Which measurements?

Two indices are most commonly employed in the literature: the Pourcelot resistive index (RI) and the Gosling pulsatility index (PI). They differ numerically, and each component can be differently affected by changes in distal resistance and cerebrovascular compliance. For this reason it is important to clarify which index has been used, and which component has contributed significantly to observed changes in the waveform (GOH 1995). Both indices are ratios designed to minimize the error in estimating arterial velocities as a result of the varying angle of insonation. This is especially important in hydrocephalus (FINN 1990) as cerebral vessels may be distorted by dilated frontal horns: calculation of true velocities is doubtful. In fact, this problem is eliminated by using color Doppler imaging (Fig. 4.26).

What results?

In a hydrocephalic brain, all authors have observed a real increase in downstream vascular resistance, particularly during progressive ventriculomegaly. In a study of nine posthemorrhagic hydrocephalic premature babies, LUI (1990) demonstrated an increased RI, with an absent or even retrograde diastolic flow in six cases. Similarly, CHADDUK (1989) reported a mean index value of 0.84 in 46 neonates with symptomatic progressive ventricular dilatation. HORIKAWA (1991), and NISHIMAKI (1991), detecting similar RI values, suggested that an index of more

than 0.80 represents a good criterion for ventriculoperitoneal drainage in the infant. Finally, NORELLE (1989), analyzing 24 infants, noticed that the Gosling index (PI) is equal to 1.06 in cases of stable ventriculomegaly, whereas it is much higher (1.72) when ventricular dilatation is progressive. That is to say,

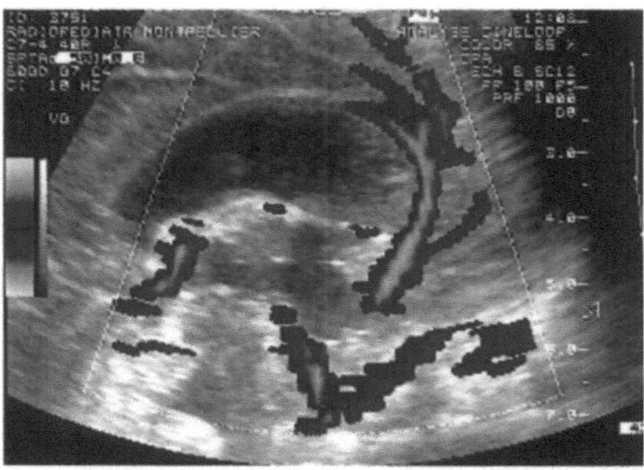

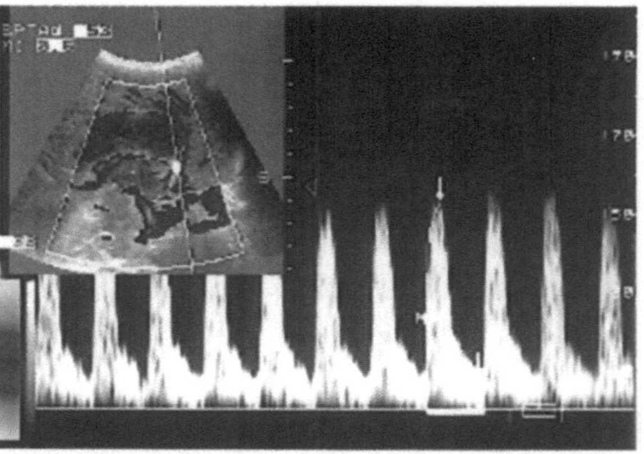

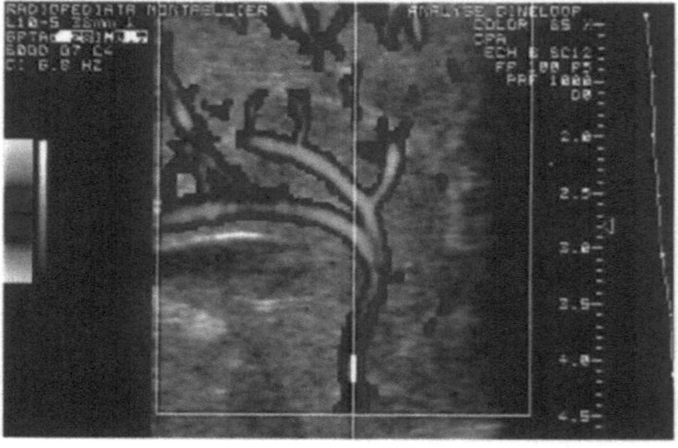

Fig. 4.26a–c. Color Doppler precisely shows changes in the direction of the anterior cerebral artery during acute hydrocephalus (**a**). Velocity values are easily obtained after correction for the insonation angle: here 32 degrees (**b**). By contrast, in a normal newborn, the anterior cerebral artery has the same axis as the ultrasound beam (**c**)

significant abnormalities of RI and PI are observed during progressive hydrocephalus.

However, ANDERSON (1991) and GRANT (1987) are in contradiction with these results, and are of the opinion that the PI does not significantly contribute to the diagnosis and the decision regarding treatment.

GRANT (1987) reported an increased PI in only 31% of infants requiring a subsequent shunting. GRANT did not detect any hemodynamic changes in 19 babies with progressive hydrocephalus.

These literature data are disturbing, but it may be that the Doppler studies were performed during periods of stable intracranial pressure.

All authors agree that the decrease in diastolic velocity is responsible for the increased indices. In our experience, the analysis of velocities, guided by color Doppler, shows unchanged systolic velocities, whereas diastolic velocities are constantly altered during progressive ventricular dilatation.

ALVISI (1985) proposes another explanation for the modifications of the spectral analysis curve: he detects a significant difference in RI between 10 neonates with progressive hydrocephalus (0.76) and 50 normal newborns (0.67); surprisingly, the rise in RI is secondary to an increase in the systolic component, whereas the diastolic value remains the same in hydrocephalic and normal brains. This author believes there is decreased cerebrovascular compliance, due to an increase in perivascular pressure, produced by cerebral edema. We know that increased perivascular pressure (AUER 1983) leads to a reduction in transmural pressure, usually balanced by increased systolic velocity.

The observation of ALVISI probably corresponds to a different hemodynamic situation: in his experience, the cerebrovascular system is able to counteract the fall in transmural pressure by increasing systolic velocity, in order to maintain a normal cerebral blood flow. This could be the first stage of hemodynamic alteration. In fact, as confirmed by the literature as a whole, when the cerebrovascular system can no longer maintain a normal cerebral blood flow, vascular resistance rises, and the diastolic component significantly decreases (DEEG 1988; GOH 1992, 1995; HUANG 1991).

How are we to explain the increased vascular resistance during hydrocephalus?

In 1982, HILL and VOLPE, using continuous Doppler in ten hydrocephalic newborns, provide a first explanation. Without ruling out the role of intracranial pressure, which is increased simultaneously with the

vascular resistance in eight cases, they propose a mechanical theory: the abnormal diastolic flow could be the result of compression and distorsion of cerebral vessels by the enlarged ventricles. They give three arguments:
- Two infants had an increased RI, while intracranial pressure was normal, measured by fontanometry
- The 4 infants with the most severe ventriculomegaly also had the highest index
- During normal-pressure hydrocephalus in adults, decreased flow is noted within the anterior cerebral artery, normalizing after drainage (GREITZ 1969; RUBIN 1976).

SALIBA (1985), studying eight hydrocephalic babies, argued the same pathogenetic hypothesis by detailing the hemodynamic assessment of two cases of developmental unilateral dilatations: he detected an increased RI in the middle cerebral artery on the side of the dilatation, whereas the contralateral spectral analysis curve remained normal. Finally, he noted that the more severe dilatation, of more rapid onset, was associated with a higher RI. He concluded that the hemodynamic alterations seem to be the result of stretching and compression of vessels by ventricular enlargement more than the result of a rise in intracranial pressure.

Among nine hydrocephalic neonates, LUI (1990) noted an absent or even retrograde diastolic flow in the four cases where ventricular dilatation was most marked. However, in two cases of moderate ventriculomegaly, RI was equal to 1.

In agreement with most of the authors, our experience speaks against a mechanical pathogenesis (VEYRAC 1987), and we think rather that intracranial pressure plays the main role in the occurrence of hemodynamic disturbances. This is based on multiple arguments:
- The hemodynamic evolution of a myelomeningocele shows a close relationship between intracranial pressure and cerebral blood flow changes. At birth, myelomeningocele presents with a low-pressure dilatation. Doppler studies performed on the first day of life, before closure of the neural plate, always demonstrate normal Doppler indices (RI=0.60–0.70), although all these babies have a ventricular dilatation. After closure of the neural plate, which results in a rise in intracranial pressure, RI increases after 1 or 2 weeks' evolution.

Otherwise, the progression rate of ventricular enlargement is rather slow during myelomeningocele and all patients present a moderate triventricular dilatation at the time of ventriculoperitoneal drainage. This morphological and hemodynamic behavior, which is peculiar to the neonatal myelomeningocele, demonstrates that cerebral circulation and its disturbances follow the increase in intracranial pressure. The role of ventriculomegaly in the genesis of vascular alterations seems moderate, or even absent.

- During the neonatal management of hydrocephalus, the hemodynamic evolution accounts for central role of intracranial pressure. After a lumbar or ventricular puncture is performed in progressive hydrocephalus, vascular resistance immediately decreases, even if only transiently. We know that this procedure has few consequences for ventricular volume and we may reasonably think the improvement in blood flow velocities is related to a decrease in intracranial pressure (DRAYTON 1986; GOH 1991; MINNS 1991). The same observations are made after ventriculoperitoneal shunting: diastolic velocities return to normal values, within the first hours following the drainage, while ventricular volume is not significantly changed. These data demonstrate a close correlation between cerebral blood velocities and intracranial pressure (CHADDUCK 1991; FISCHER 1989; HORIKAWA 1991; IACOPINO 1995; NADVI 1994).
- During stable or slowly progressive major dilatation, cerebral hemodynamics often remain normal (DEEG 1988; HUANG 1991; NORELLE 1989). There is probably a precarious balance between intraventricular pressure and cerebral blood flow that explains the absence of vascular alteration. In these circumstances, the ventricular enlargement does not appear to be an important factor.
- In cases of asymmetrical hydrocephalus, we have never observed any asymmetry in vascular resistance; indices are either normal or disturbed, but are equivalent on both sides (Fig. 4.27).
- Finally, although it is evident that an increase in ventricular distension and in intracranial pressure induces combined harmful consequences on cerebral vessels, it is also evident that the effect of ventricular volume on the hemodynamics is frequently moderate or absent. There are cases of moderate ventriculomegaly with markedly disturbed RI, and others where Doppler indices are completely normal despite massive ventriculomegaly (Fig. 4.28).

Since intracranial pressure has not been directly measured in our experience, our conclusions are not proven, but all these observations argue in favor of the role of intracranial pressure in hemodynamic disturbances. Moreover, our experience is corroborated by data from the literature. SEIBERT (1989) measured intracranial pressure in four dogs with a fiberoptic monitor with simultaneous Doppler recordings and found a direct correlation between intracranial pressure, cerebral perfusion pressure, and RI. In the hydrocephalic infant, measurements of transfontanellar pressure by fontanometry (HORIKAWA 1991; HANLO 1995) and measurements of intracranial pressure by lumbar tap or intracranial reservoir puncture (GOH 1991; CHADDUK 1991) demonstrate a clear relationship between intracranial pressure and hemodynamic pattern.

Vascular alterations reflect an acute, highly progressive disease, whatever its etiology. Most often, they accompany large ventriculomegaly and a marked rise in intracranial pressure. Their development reveals progression of the hydrocephalus and should suggest a danger of ischemic damage resulting from vascular distorsion and increased blood flow resistance. Obviously hemodynamic follow-up is important for deciding the best management: alteration of cerebral blood flow during acute hydrocephalus is an emergency requiring rapid decompression if irreversible ischemic damage is to be avoided (Fig. 4.29).

To conclude this overview of an acute progressive hydrocephalus, the diagnostic strategy appears straightforward: the detection of a zero or negative diastolic velocity indicates a rapid drainage.

4.3.2.2
Slowly Progressive, Stable, Stabilized, or Regressive Hydrocephalus

Anthony was a 32 weeks' premature baby, delivered after unexplained membrane rupture and development of Streptococcus B chorionitis. It was a breech presentation and bradycardia was noticed during labor. Neonatal respiratory distress (grade II hyaline membrane disease) required 6 days' ventilation. On day 8, ultrasound revealed posthemorrhagic triventricular dilatation (Fig. 4.30). Doppler study showed a minimal increase in vascular resistance (RI=0.80 in the anterior cerebral artery). A series of lumbar punctures was begun, with weekly ultrasound monitoring. Progressive triventricular dilatation developed on day 22, then stabilized and regressed; during this period, RI remained normal in every cerebral artery studied (Fig. 4.31). The last examination, at 2 months of age, shows biventricular enlargement and a normal RI (0.70 in the anterior cerebral artery) (Fig. 4.32). The infant showed good psychomotor development at 6 months, and the ventricular enlargement remained unchanged.

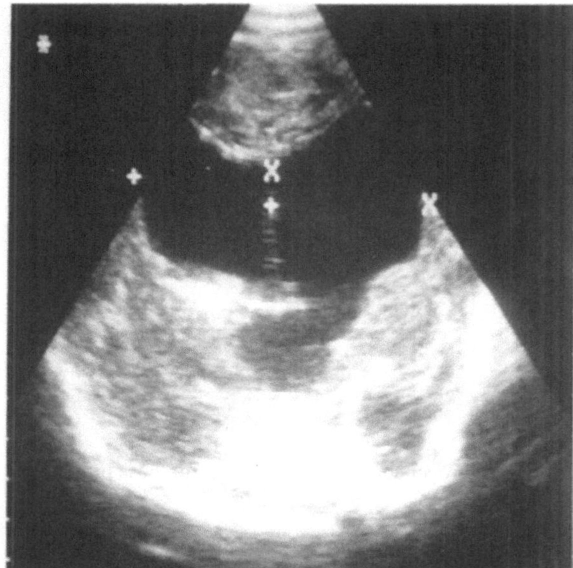

Fig. 4.27a–c. A 3-month-old infant with myelomeningocele. A ventriculoperitoneal shunt has been in place since the neonatal period (a). There is progressive triventricular dilatation with asymmetric lateral ventricles. Vascular resistances remain symmetric: RI=0.66 on the right (b) and 0.64 on a temporal branch of the left middle cerebral artery (c)

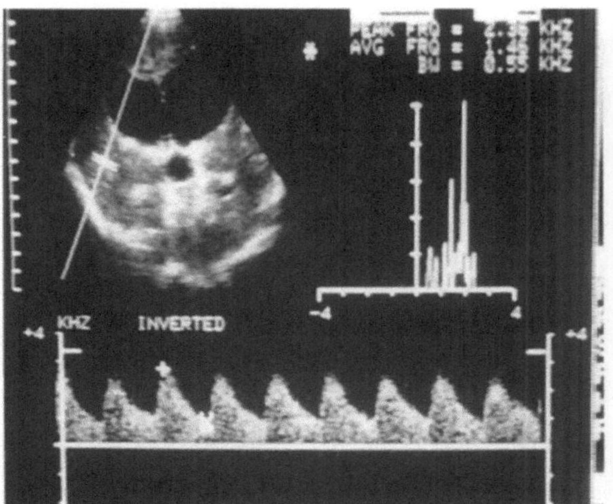

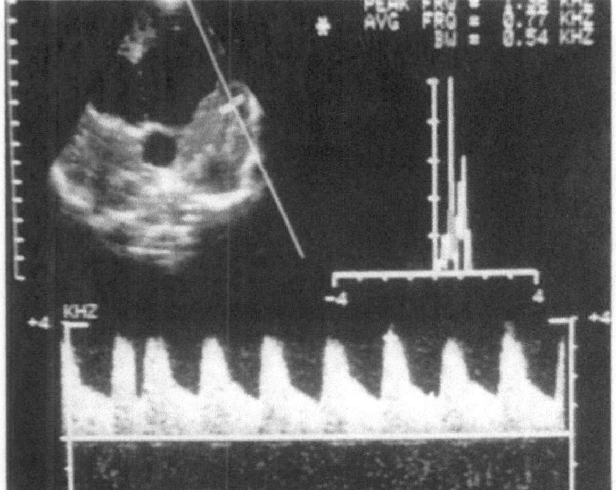

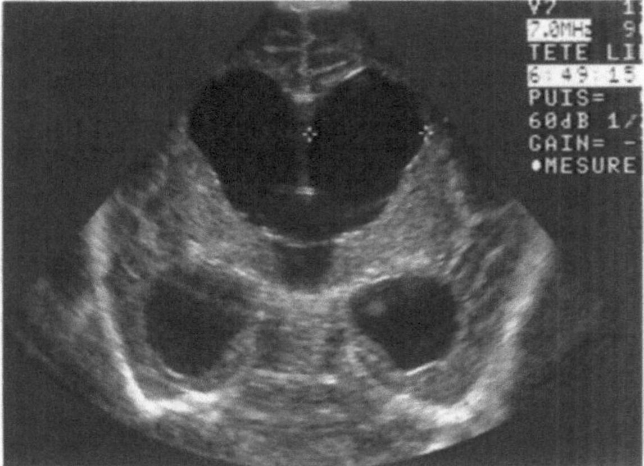

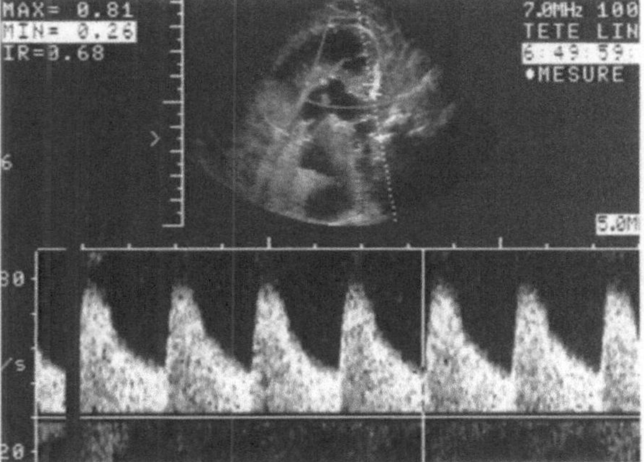

Fig. 4.28a,b. Progressive posthemorrhagic hydrocephalus. At 2 months, large ventriculomegaly (a) with normal RI=0.68 (b). However, clinical signs of intracranial hypertension required ventriculoperitoneal shunting at the age of 4 months

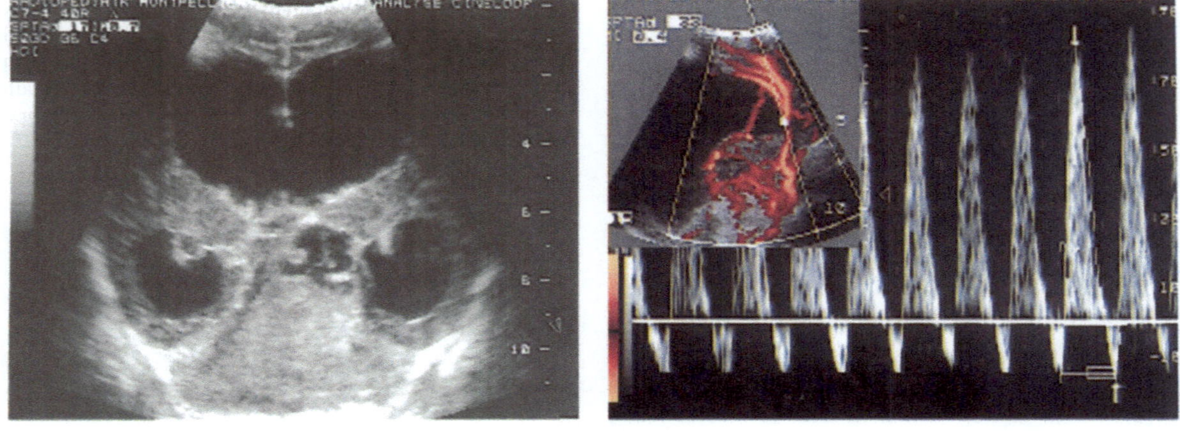

Fig. 4.29a,b. A 9-month-old infant with acute intracranial hypertension. A heterogeneous large brain stem tumor is present (**a**). Reverse diastolic flow with RI=1.22 confirms the clinical findings (**b**)

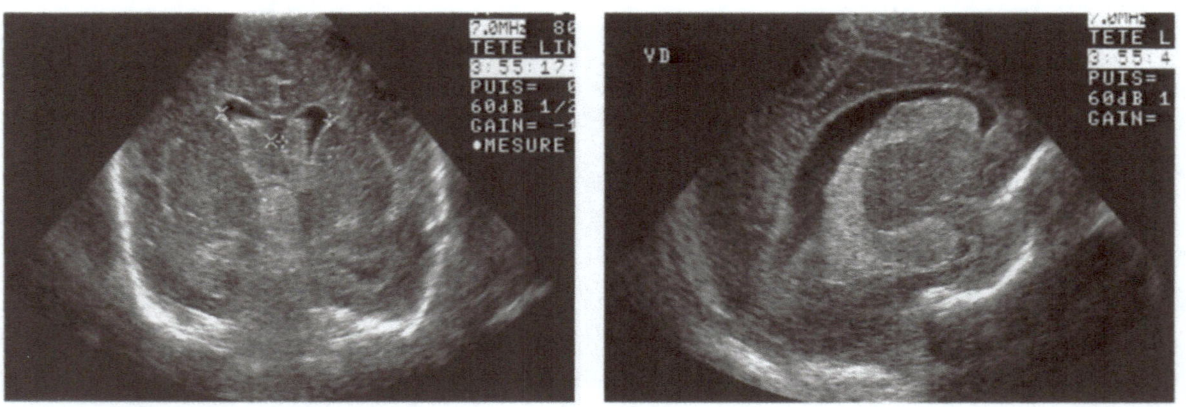

Fig. 4.30a,b. Severe lateral (**a**) and third ventricular (**b**) clotting, resulting in early ventricular dilatation

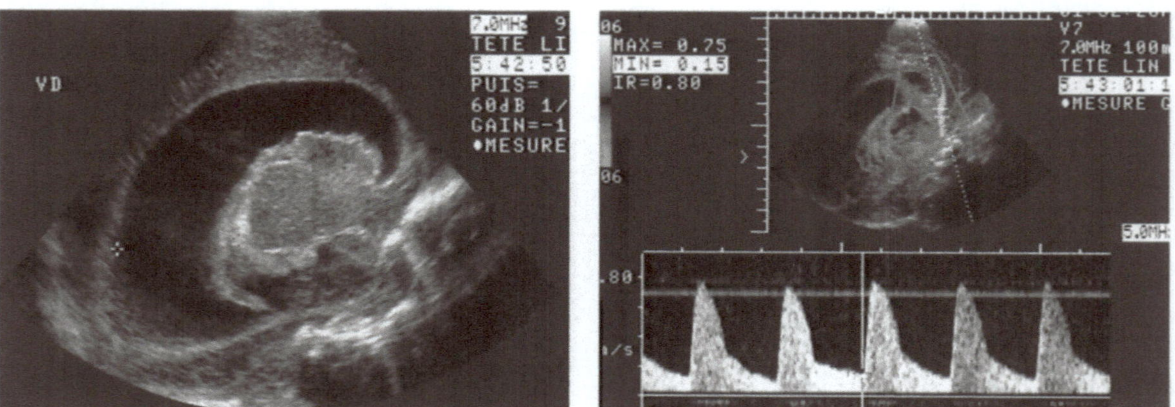

Fig. 4.31a,b. The ventricular dilatation has increased (**a**). RI=0.80 (**b**)

This case shows that vascular resistance is normal when ventriculomegaly is poorly progressive, stable, or regressive.

In these circumstances, the pathological process and the compensatory mechanisms (transependymal CSF resorption, cranial vault expansion, cerebral atrophy, decreased CSF production (the occurrence of which reality is under debate) (LORENZO 1970; SAHAR 1969) are in balance. Such a balance usually occurs when ventricular obstruction is incomplete: in addition to the mechanisms described above, other unaltered sites of absorption operate and compensate the abnormal situation. This is rather observed in communicating hydrocephalus (as in Anthony's case). In obstructive hydrocephalus, this phenomenon is infrequent.

In poorly progressive hydrocephalus, sometimes with successive periods of stabilization, the treatment decision is difficult, but pulsed Doppler analysis does not help. Despite compression of the cerebral vessels, some mechanisms of circulatory adaptation allow apparently normal vascular resistance.

In neonatal hydrocephalus, it seems that a threshold value exists, below which no abnormality is found, and which depends on multiple factors: the etiology of the ventriculomegaly, the degree of ventricular enlargement, whether the hydrocephalus is communicating or noncommunicating, and the progression rate.

There are other difficulties:

- We have seen some cases of ventriculomegaly where sudden rises in inracranial pressure rapidly spontaneously resolve, and are followed by a favorable course (Fig. 4.33).
- We have also known some rare cases in which the clinical situation indicates ventriculoperitoneal shunting while the hemodynamic assessment remains normal (Fig. 4.34).

These pitfalls and difficulties of interpretation lead to a few questions:

- Should treatment be proposed when hemodynamic alteration is alone and transient and unaccompanied by other change. In our experience, five newborns (2 with myelomeningocele and 3 with posthemorrhagic dilatations) developed asymptomatic episodes of absent (2 cases) or negative (3 cases) diastolic flow that quickly resolved. The two patients with myelomeningocele do not require any discussion, but the three with posthemorragic dilatations are interesting: the initial ventricular hemorrhage was severe in one patient and moderate in two; all three babies had a communicating dilatation; hydrocephalus was progressive during the first month of life, then unchanged in three cases and regressive in two; hemodynamic disturbances which certainly correspond to infraclinical intracranial pressure rises occurred twice during the progressive phase of the dilatation and once during the stabilization phase; and finally, two patients were treated with serial lumbar punctures.

In these three cases of posthemorrhagic hydrocephalus, there were no absolute indications of severity: the moderate volume of ventricular hemorrhage explains the slow progression of the dila-

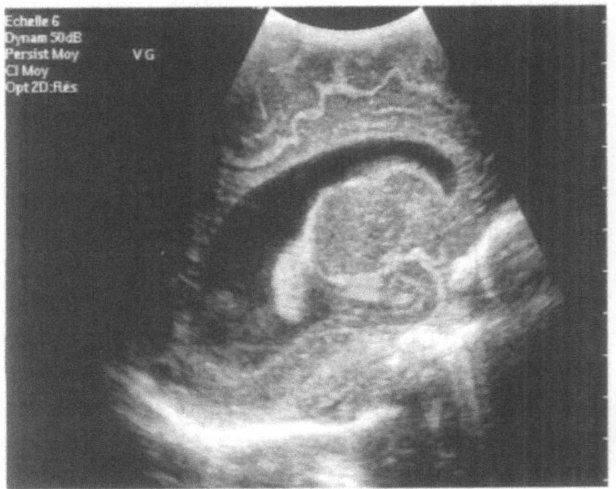

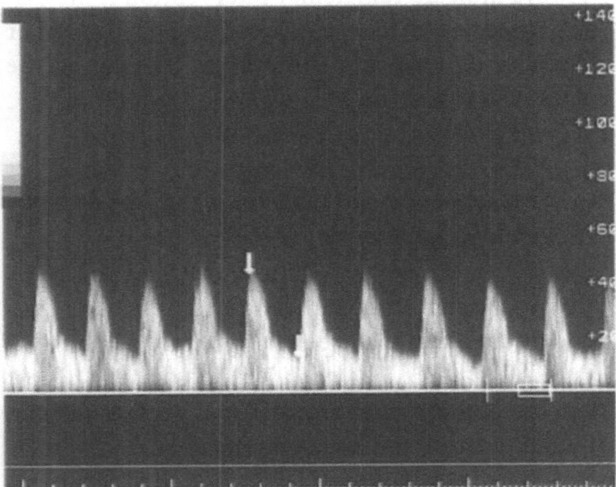

Fig. 4.32a,b. The ventricular enlargement is more moderate (a) and RI is normal=0.71 (b)

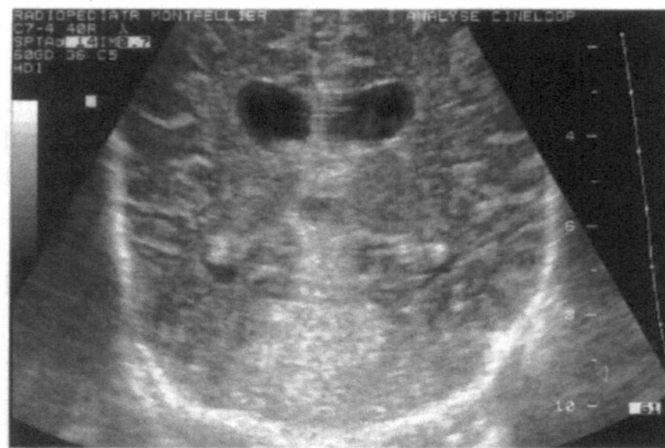

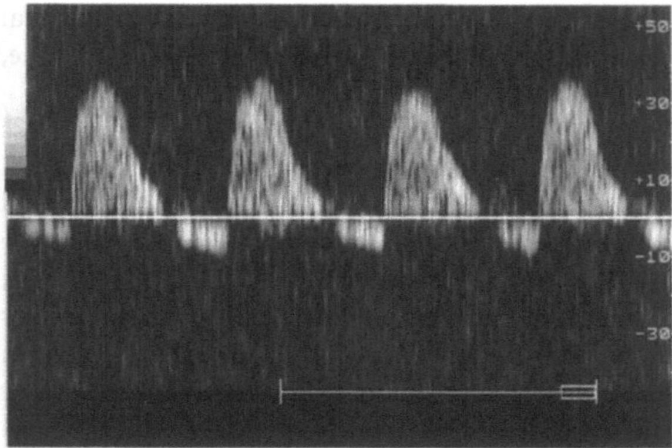

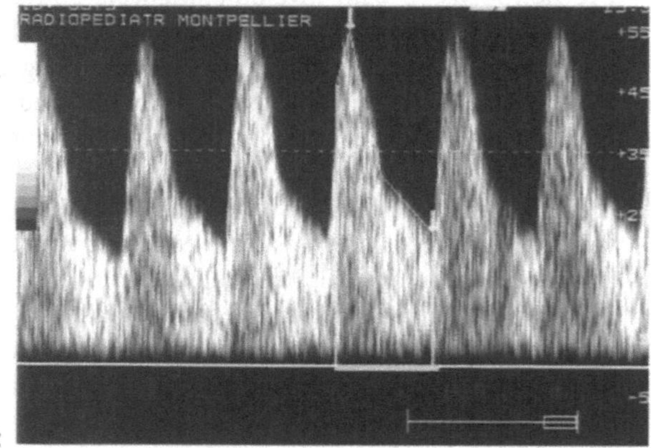

Fig. 4.33,a–c. Neonatal myelomeningocele with normal hemodynamic assessment. On day 3, the neural plate is closed. During follow-up, triventricular dilatation occurs with normal Doppler findings (RI ranges from 0.70 to 0.76). At 1 month of age, while ventricular enlargement is moderate (**a**), recording of the anterior cerebral artery shows retrograde diastolic flow (RI=1.10) (**b**), despite absence of obvious intracranial hypertension. The alterations disappear quickly; at 4 months, RI is normal (0.60) (**c**)

tation; hydrocephalus requiring ventriculoperitoneal drainage is rarely communicating in character; the favorable ultrasonographic course (4-months follow-up in the 3 cases) suggests that the peak of intracranial hypertension was, in fact, a nonpejorative harmless epiphenomenon. This demonstrates that the detection of abnormal hemodynamics in a hydrocephalic brain does not always indicate ventricular intervention if the disturbance remains unaccompanied by other changes and quickly disappears, so long as the patient is closely monitored.

How are normal Doppler studies during progressive hydrocephalus to be explained?

Normal Doppler studies during progressive hydrocephalus are a real fact frequently reported in the literature (GOH 1995; HANLO 1995; TAYLOR 1996). Most often, the authors offer the explanation that normal arterial velocities are usually associated with slowly progressive ventriculomegaly. In fact, the interpretation of quantitative results is difficult because there is a wide range of reference values in the normal prema-

ture infant of less than 35 weeks' gestational age (HORGAN 1989).

On the other hand, near-normal or mildly elevated RI values in hydrocephalus may be due to partial compensation by the neonatal skull: the bone and dura mater can accommodate the additional intracranial volume, inducing an accelerated rate of head growth but only a modest increase in intracranial pressure. Reports of pressure–volume (compliance) studies suggest that the capacity to compensate an intracranial volume increase is greater in hydrocephalic infants than in healthy infants with a similar head size (SHAPIRO 1985).

In these difficult situations, the recent study of TAYLOR (1996) is very valuable. This author proposes sensitizing the hemodynamic assessment by applying fontanellar compression. The aim is to determine whether the hemodynamic response to fontanellar compression during Doppler ultrasonography can be used to indirectly assess the intracranial pressure and, thus, help define whether there is a need for shunt placement. He investigated 14 newborns (11 with posthemorrhagic and 3 with idiopathic hydrocephalus) of gestational ages ranging from 24 to 40 weeks. All babies received acetazolamide, furo-

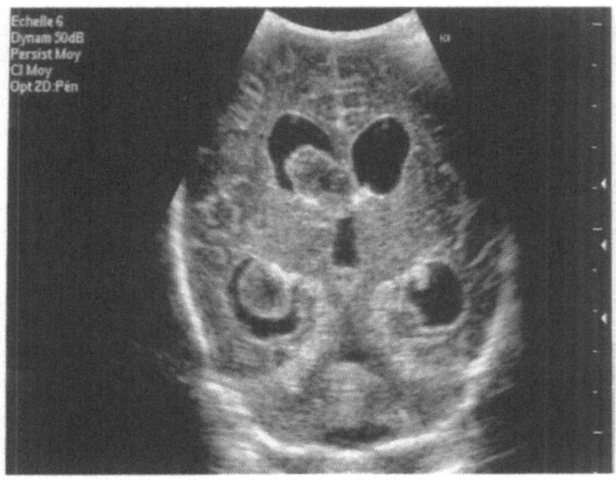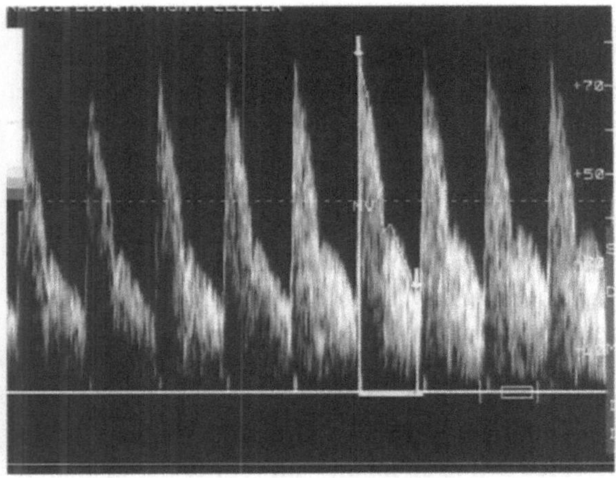

Fig. 4.34a,b. Intraventricular hemorrhage treated by serial lumbar puncture (a). There is progressive communicating hydrocephalus, which then stabilizes. At 3 months, RI is normal (0.63) (b). Two days later, clinical findings indicate intracranial hypertension and a ventriculoperitoneal shunt is required

semide, and serial lumbar punctures. RI was not considered to determining the need for ventricular drainage. Criteria for ventricular catheter placement were signs of failed medical management, rapid increase in head circumference, full fontanelle, and neurological signs such as apnea. The Doppler study was performed on the anterior cerebral artery, by transfontanellar access, with spectral analysis before and during fontanellar compression.

The results of this study are extremely interesting:

- Three measures were obtained: baseline RI, RI during fontanellar compression, and percentage change in RI, or ΔRI, defined as:

$$\frac{Fontanellar\ compression\ RI - baseline\ RI}{baseline\ RI}$$

ΔRI is obviously the best predictor of intracranial hypertension.

- The results are statistically significant: all infants who required ventricular drainage had a maximum preoperative ΔRI of 45% (mean: 75% ± 10%; range: 47%–132%), compared with 18% ± 5% (range: 3%–29%) in infants who did not require surgical intervention. Moreover, baseline RI varied considerably and correlated poorly with intracranial pressure measures.
- Although therapeutic intervention (lumbar puncture, ventriculoperitoneal shunt, or ventricular drainage) reduced intracranial hypertension, it also resulted in a mean decrease in ΔRI, from 44% ± 6% before drainage to 21% ± 2% after drainage, while baseline RI remained unchanged

(0.72 ± 1). Finally, marked changes in hemodynamic response were observed in ten neonates after removal of CSF, despite minimal differences in ventricular volume.

To confirm this trend of development, TAYLOR presents an argument based on conflicting reports of the literature. Several authors have demonstrated an increased RI in hydrocephalic infants and a subsequent drop after ventricular drainage (SEIBERT 1989; COUTURE 1994); however, other investigations found no difference in the RI values before and after treatment (TAYLOR 1994), and poor correlation between RI and intracranial hypertension (GOH 1992); finally, some authors note a large overlap between pre- and postpuncture RI measures (GOH 1991).

This shows the importance of studying the hemodynamic consequences of fontanellar compression in the hydrocephalic brain compared with the results in normal babies. In healthy infants, the hemodynamic response to fontanellar compression is minimal. TAYLOR (1992), in a study of 23 normal infants, found a ΔRI of only 7% during the procedure. The volume-pressure relationship can be described with a compliance curve with a long, flat initial portion in which a small intracranial pressure increase occurs with increasing intracranial volume, and a steep portion in which small increments in volume result in progressively larger elevations in intracranial pressure. As we know that the volume of the brain (CSF, blood, and other intracranial components) is constant, it is plausible that, initially, a change in intracranial volume is offset with volume shifts in other components such that the intracranial pressure remains unchanged. When the capacity for volume shift is exceeded, however, a further increase in volume results in elevation of the intracranial pressure. During graded fontanellar compression in normal infants, a moderate increase in RI and a slight reduction in mean velocity are observed. This effect is much greater in infants with decreased cerebral compliance (especially hydrocephalic newborns) since their intracranial volume is already increased and the pressure–volume relationship already altered.

In conclusion, TAYLOR (1996) considers that an increased ΔRI in an infant with ventricular dilatation suggests the presence of intracranial hypertension and is an important argument for placing a ventriculoperitoneal shunt. Fontanellar compression seems to sensitize the hemodynamic assessment when baseline results are normal or borderline, as shown in the following example:

Florian was a 28 weeks' gestation premature baby. On day 4, acute anemia was noted (hemoglobin: 7 g/l) and a clotted intraventricular hemorrhage detected, with lateral ventricular enlargement. A series of lumbar punctures was decided on, with ultrasonographic morphological and hemodynamic follow-up, for 3 months (25 examinations). The ventricular dilatation increased during the first month of life, then stabilized (Fig. 4.35).

The hemodynamic course was as follows:
- *In the anterior cerebral artery, the baseline RI was measured 16 times before ventriculoperitoneal shunting and 3 times after shunt placement. Its*

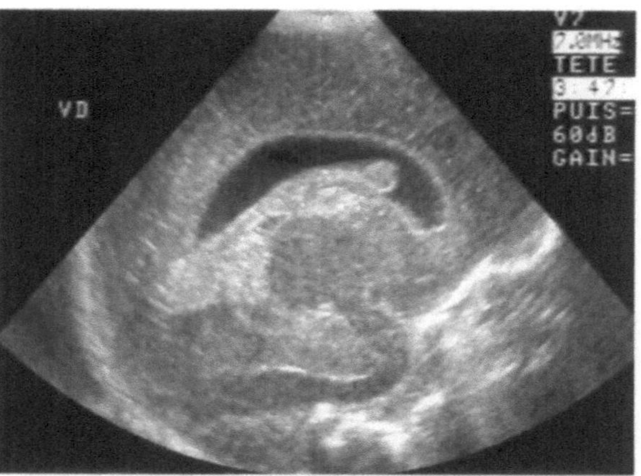

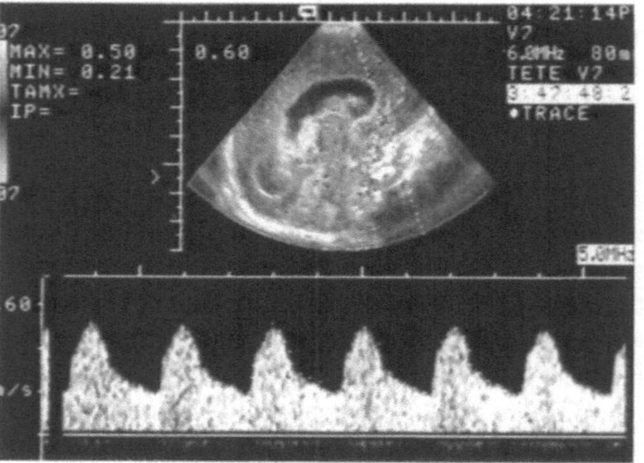

Fig. **4.35a,b.** Day 10. Large right intraventricular clot (**a**). Normal hemodynamic findings: RI=0.60, mean velocity=33 cm/s (**b**)

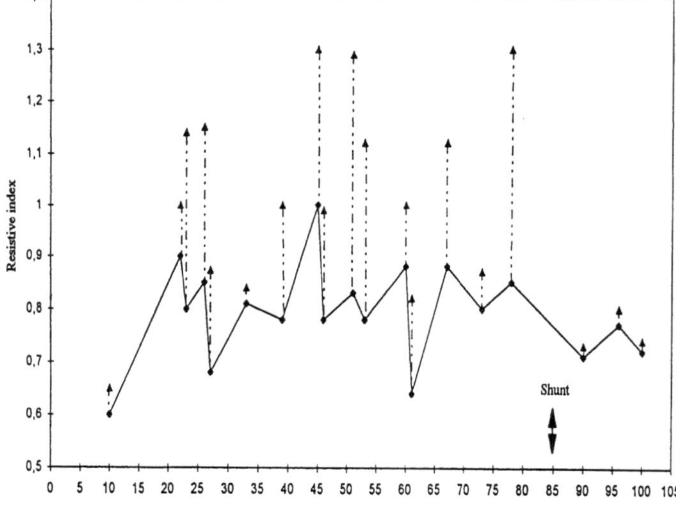

Graph **4.1.** Resistive index in anterior cerebral artery before (●) and after (▲) fontanellar compression

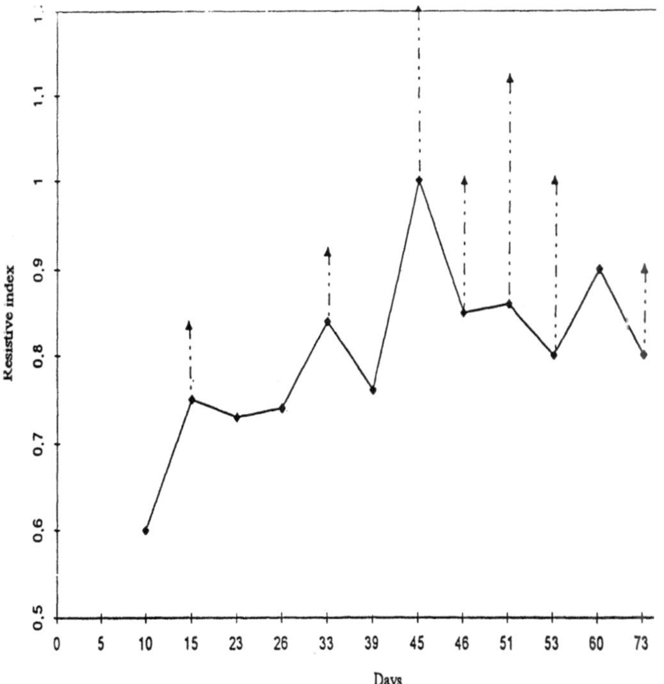

Graph 4.2. Resistive index in anterior cerebral artery before (●) and after (▲) fontanellar compression

mean value was 0.80 (range: 0.60–0.80, 9 times and 0.80–1, 7 times) (Graph 4.1). Parallel to this, RI was measured 12 times in the basilar artery; its mean value was 0.78 (range: 0.60–0.80, 7 times and 0.80–1, 5 times) (Graph 4.2; Fig. 4.36).

- *Hemodynamic response to fontanellar compression was studied 16 times in the anterior cerebral artery and 7 times in the basilar artery. Under compression, the diastolic component became zero or negative 11 times in the anterior cerebral artery and 4 times in the basilar artery. ΔRI was more than 27% 11 times in the anterior cerebral artery (Graph 4.3) and 3 times in the basilar artery. Mean velocities dropped significantly as measured 9 times in the anterior cerebral artery, mean values going from 25.5 cm/s to 16.8 cm/s during compression.*

- *RI and mean velocities values correlated closely with removal of CSF (Graph 4.4): cerebral hemodynamics improved significantly when measurements were performed immediately or a few hours after the lumbar tap. However, when velocities were measured later (after 40 h or more), the benefit of CSF removal had disappeared. Lumbar tap did not change ΔRI.*

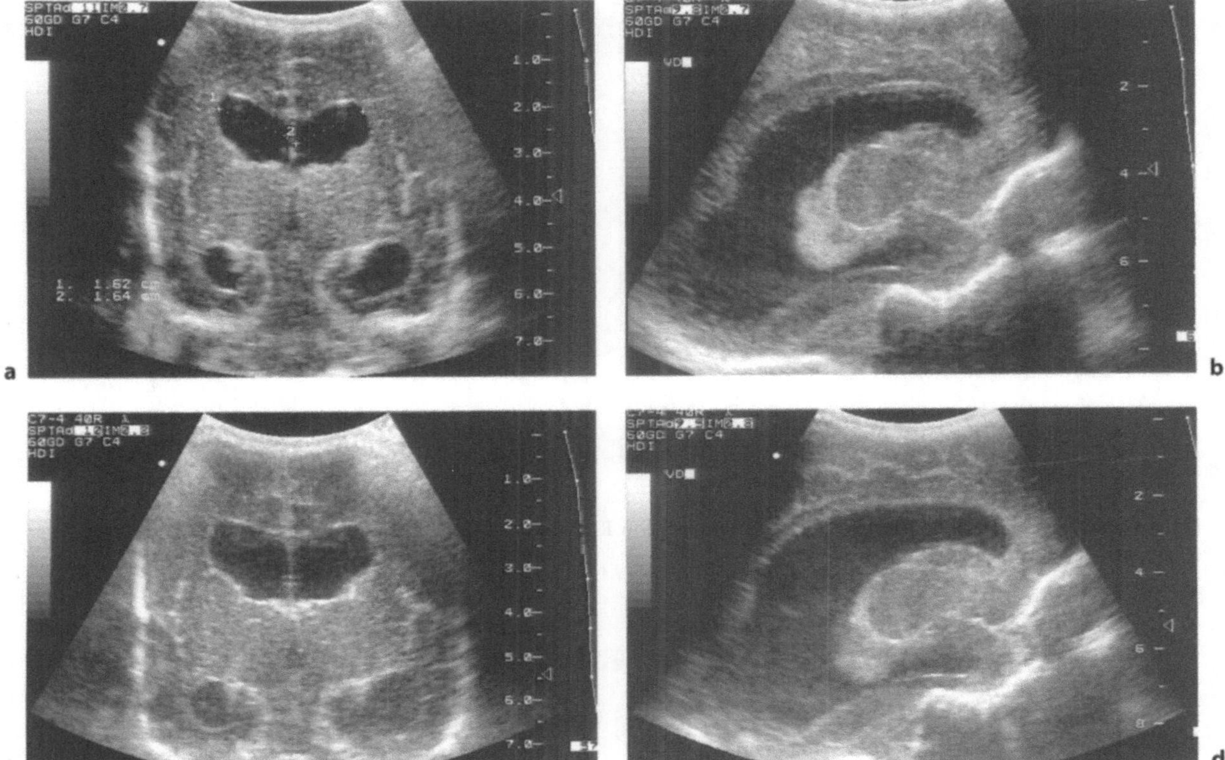

Fig. 4.36 a–d. Day 40: Ventricular dilatation is no more evolving (**a,b**). Day 60: ventriculomegaly (**c,d**)

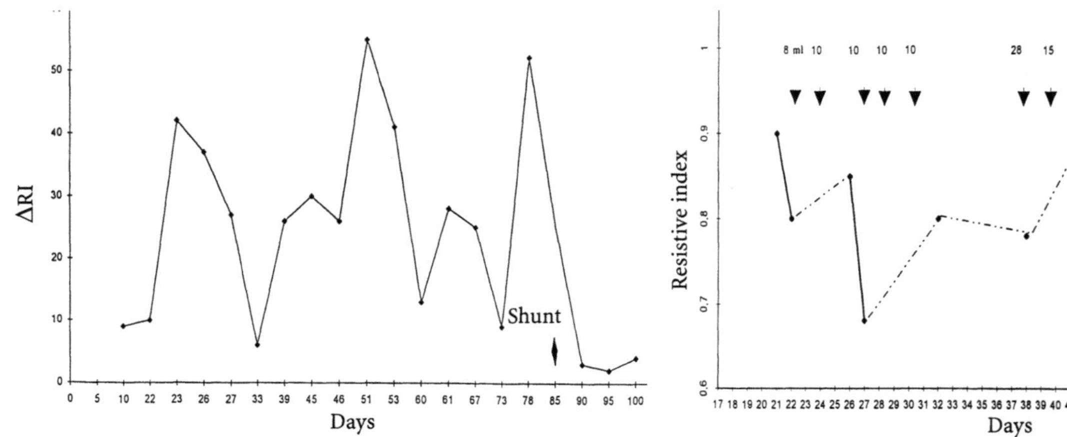

Graph 4.3. Evolution of RI differential (ΔRI) in anterior cerebral artery

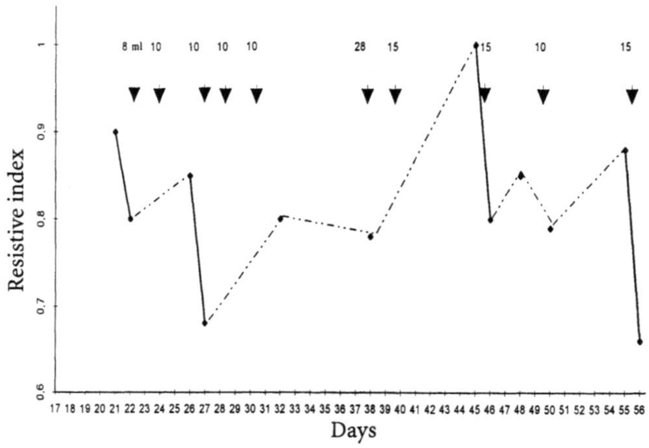

Graph 4.4. Evolution of RI in anterior cerebral artery; repeated lumbar punctures

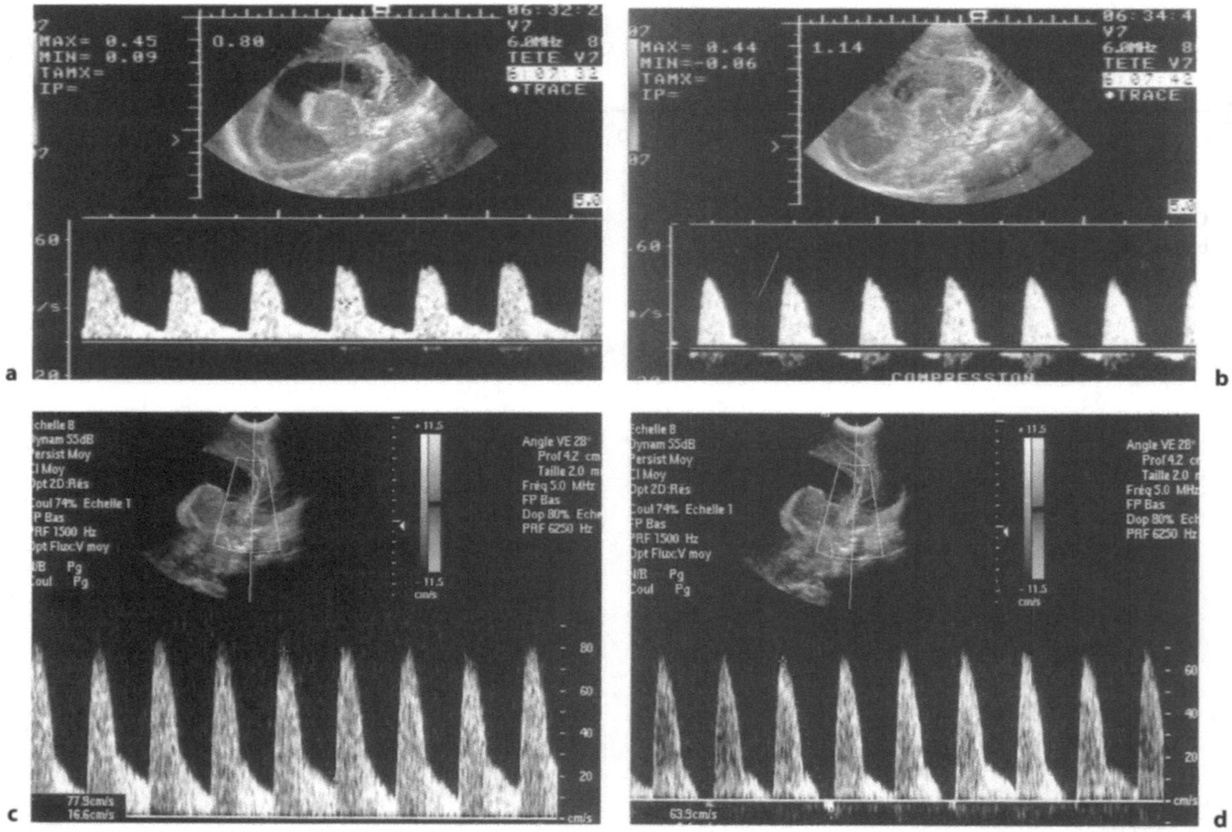

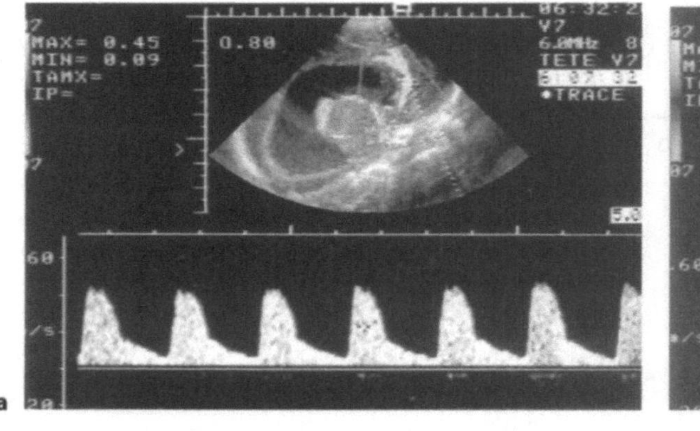

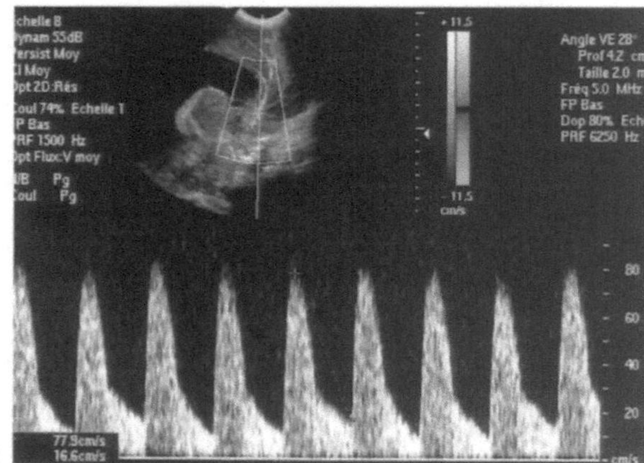

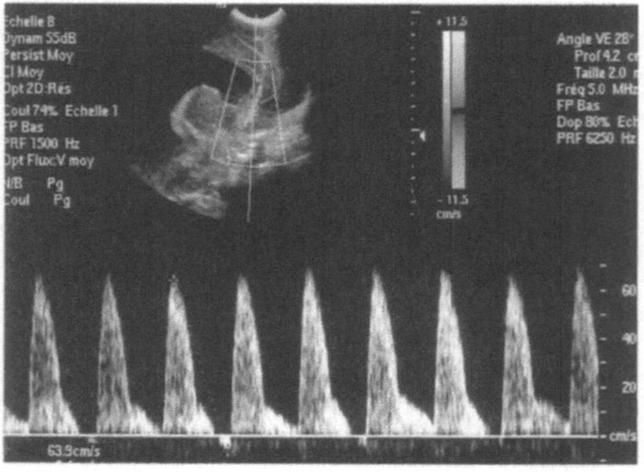

Fig. 4.37a–d. Day 23. Baseline RI=0.80 (a). After compression RI=1.14 (b), ΔRI is 42%. Day 53: baseline RI is 0.79 (c). After compression, RI=1.10 (d), ΔRI is 40%

- *At 3 months of life, ventriculoperitoneal shunting was decided on, faced with a new infraclinical episode of hemodynamic disturbance: baseline RI was 0.85, going to 1.30 during fontanellar compression, and ΔRI was 52% (Graph 4.3). After shunting, Doppler indices improved dramatically, with ΔRI ranging from 2% to 4% (Fig. 4.37).*

Florian represents a typical case where the decision regarding surgery is very difficult since there is no rationale for the decision: intracranial hypertension was clinically latent, ventriculomegaly stabilized at 1 month of age, and baseline Doppler indices not significantly altered. Three points merit discussion:

- In this premature infant, baseline RI (ranging from 0.60 to 0.90) was insufficient to evaluate the severity of intracranial hypertension; marked hemodynamic alteration (diastolic velocity: 0, RI=1) was noted in only one examination, quickly resolving after lumbar tap.
- RI measures should be interpreted according to the timing of CSF withdrawal: in our experience, RI always drops immediately after lumbar puncture. This favorable effect is transient and usually disappears within 48 h. During Florian's monitoring, several RI measurements were performed early after lumbar tap, and the severity of hemodynamic alterations may have been underestimated (Graph 4.4).
- In reality, the Doppler results after fontanellar compression seem to be the most appropriate measure by which to appreciate cerebral compliance alterations and to quantify the degree of intracranial hypertension (Graph 4.1). ΔRI, which seems a reliable and accurate measure, was more than or equal to 25% at 11 measurements (out of 16). These results do not reach the values put forward by TAYLOR (≥ 45%), but they are significantly greater than those in normal newborns. In a personal study of 23 neonates, aged from birth to 4 months and with normal compliance, the mean ΔRI was 7% (range: 1%-19%). Finally, in contrast to baseline RI, ΔRI remained unchanged after CSF removal.

Thus, like TAYLOR, we think that an increased ΔRI detected during the course of a ventricular dilatation suggests intracranial hypertension. It seems to be the best criterion by which to distinguish infants who require ventriculoperitoneal shunting from those who do not.

Finally, both TAYLOR (1996) and our personal observations show that fontanellar compression and ΔRI measurement are valuable in the detection of intracranial hypertension when serial punctures to remove CSF are performed; in such cases, changes in baseline RI and intrathecal pressure are obviously underestimated.

Compression of the anterior fontanelle requires accurate technique:
- The pressure delivered to the fontanelle should be brief (no more than 5 s), enough to obtain a Doppler spectrum; if this condition is observed, the procedure is well tolerated even by a premature baby with neurological distress.
- The compression should not be repeated, because there is a diminished response after repeated compressions, due to partial accommodation of the increased intracranial volume.
- A firm pressure is required, delivered by a trained operator, using the same transducer, because a partial or incomplete fontanellar depression results in underestimation of intracranial pressure. To avoid these drawbacks, TAYLOR (1994) proposed using an ophthalmodynamometer, applying a reproducible scanning pressure. However, two persons are required for this method. By contrast, a single operator is sufficient for fontanellar compression. If the technique is correctly carried out, the hemodynamic findings are reliable: although the exact amount of pressure applied is unknown, the amount by which the volume transiently increases appears much greater than what is necessary.

In conclusion, the assessment and follow-up of hydrocephalus obviously require a careful sequential analysis of its hemodynamic sequelae. Several facts are now certain:
- Increased vascular resistance reflects acute progressive hydrocephalus; the risk of ischemic damage resulting from decreased cerebral blood flow is evident: shunting is needed. Neurosurgeons now have an additional argument to their decision making.
- This alarm sign is absent during moderately progressive, stable, or regressive ventricular dilatation. There certainly exists a phenomenon of accommodation and a threshold of vascular compression below which Doppler studies remain normal. This is why the hemodynamic response to fontanellar compression seems a valuable form of assessment.

4.3.2.3
Prognosis and Hemodynamics

Hemodynamic studies have obvious prognostic potentialities:

- The poor long-term neurological development of hydrocephalic infants with shunts in place is known. Persisting inferior limb spasticity is the result of axonal compression by the enlarged ventricles, but ischemic insult, especially in the territory of the anterior cerebral artery, certainly contributes to the brain damage; the main lesion occurs within the periventricular arterioles and capillaries. In the future, detailed neurodevelopmental assessment of infants with shunts placed according to hemodynamic criteria will be necessary. It is extremely difficult to determine the outcome of shunted infants (FLETCHER 1997; FERNELL 1990; GUZZETTA 1995; HANLO 1997; KIRKINEN 1996; LEVITSKY 1995; LUMENTA 1995; SMITH 1982), but the severity and duration of hemodynamic alterations play an obvious role in the brain integrity.

- This consideration is important when reading the report of HANLO (1997). Nineteen hydrocephalic newborns were followed for at least 27 months, with assessment of intracranial pressure (by fontanometry), degree of myelination and ventricular dilatation (by MRI), and neurodevelopmental testing. His conclusions are:
  • Increased intracranial pressure (and its duration) is closely related to developmental outcome, through the process of myelination.
  • The delay in myelination can be partially or totally reversible, depending on the timing of ventricular drainage.
  • Finally, CSF volume is of minor importance in regard to neurological development.

These results show the chief role of intracranial hypertension and its duration in neurodevelopmental alterations. As cerebral Doppler measurements (velocity, RI, fontanellar compression RI, ΔRI) indirectly reflect intracranial pressure, we conceive their value in determining the best moment for intervention in order to improve the short- and long-term outcome is obvious.

4.3.2.4
Fetus and hemodynamics

Hemodynamic assessment of a ventriculomegalic fetus should help the physician in the difficult decision about management. To detect fetal ventriculomegaly is easy; much more difficult is confirming the diagnosis of hydrocephalus. The whole problem is to define early criteria of progressiveness and of brain damage, especially since the benefit of antenatal ventricular shunting has never been proved (MANNING 1986).

In the neonate, it has been demonstrated that stable ventriculomegaly is not associated with hemodynamic disturbances and that vascular alterations are observed during acute hydrocephalus. It is probably the same in the fetus.

In fact, the few hemodynamic studies of fetal hydrocephalus give conflicting results. For example, MAI (1995) detects a positive diastolic frequency

within the anterior cerebral artery and an increased PI in only 4 of 23 hydrocephalic fetuses. By contrast, VOIGT (1995), studying 143 cases of fetal hydrocephalus, considered that detection of increased vascular resistance should be an indication for premature delivery, in order to perform ventricular shunting in the best conditions.

The prognosis of fetal hydrocephalus is rather poor (CHERVENAK 1983; KIRKINEN 1996; LEVITSKY 1995; NYBERG 1987; OI 1990; PRETORIUS 1985; ROSSEAU 1992), but it is necessary to identify which fetuses require hemodynamic investigation: those with stable or progressive dilatation, normal biparietal diameter for gestational age, absence of CNS malformation, absence of detectable morphological abnormality, and normal karyotype.

In these selected cases, a protocol of sequential Doppler studies is necessary, as in the newborn, to detect the occurrence of intracranial hypertension, since a single sample signifies nothing at all (Fig. 4.38).

4.4
Treatment of Hydrocephalus and Hemodynamic Monitoring

Gaelle was born at 34 weeks' gestation by cesarian delivery because of acute fetal distress with meconium-stained amniotic fluid; she also presented intrauterine growth retardation (birth weight: 1820 g). At birth, neonatal asphyxia required immediate tracheal tube placement. For the first hours, her neurological state remained worrying, with severe hypotonia. On day 2, the first ultrasound examination revealed a massive IVH, with moderate tetraventricular dilatation; RI was 0.62 in the anterior cerebral artery. Ultrasonography was repeated twice a week during the first month of life (Graph 4.5).

Rapid clotting of ventricular blood was associated with a progressive noncommunicating dilatation with a huge rounded fourth ventricle. Until day 10, Doppler indices remained normal (RI=0.72). On day 16, RI increased to 1 in the anterior cerebral artery. Because of the continuous progression of the ventricular enlargement, and the severe hemodynamic alterations (RI=1.10 on day 20), a ventricular puncture was performed on day 20, with 10 ml CSF removed, followed by immediate improvement of the cerebral hemodynamics (RI=0.74). This effect was transient; 10 days later, RI reached 1, and on day 36 it was 1.10. After a repeat removal of CSF (10 ml), RI returned to 0.72. On

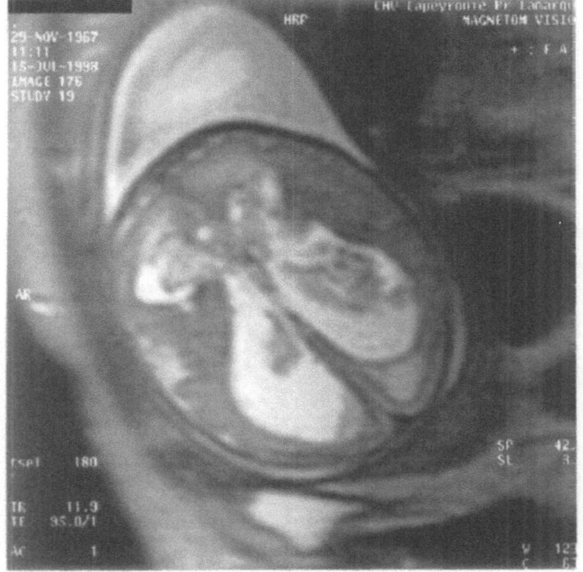

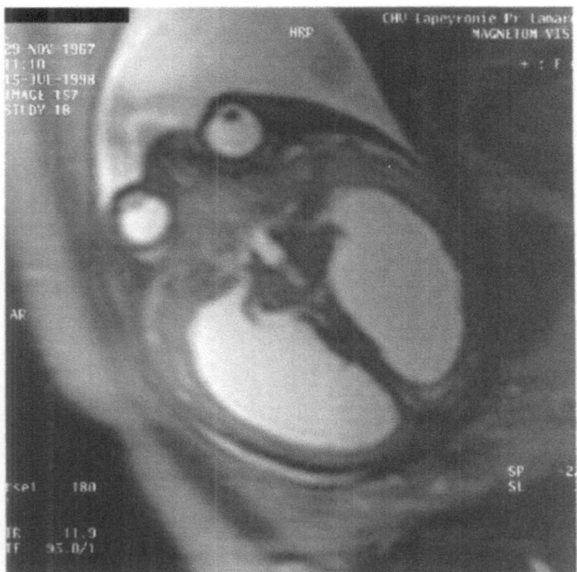

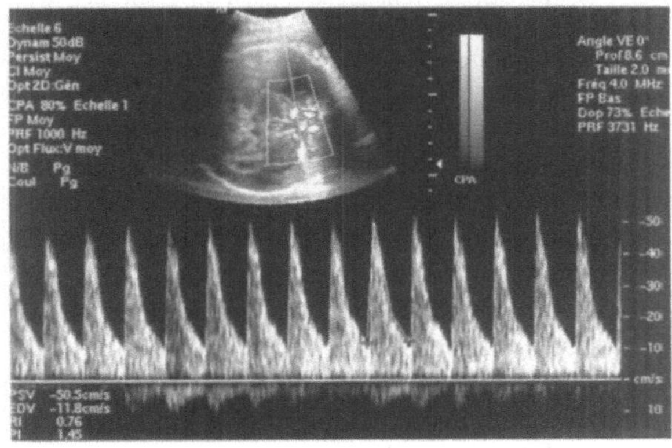

Fig. 4.38a–c. A 30-week fetus. Triventricular dilatation with probable intraventricular bleeding detected by ultrasound. At 34 weeks, MRI shows the severity of IVH and hydrocephalus (a, b). Surprisingly, velocities and RI (0.70) are normal within the middle cerebral artery (c)

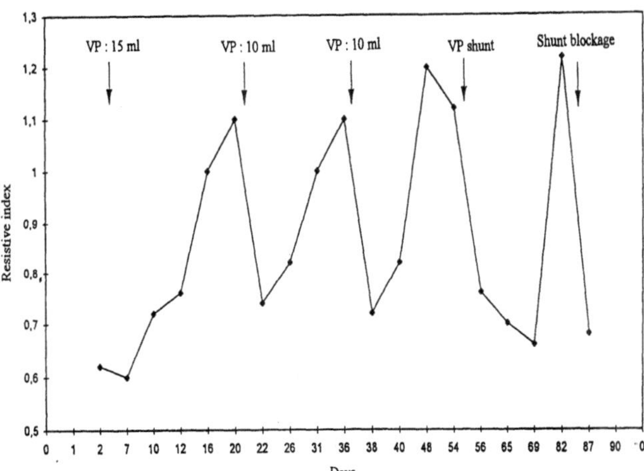

Graph 4.5. Hemodynamic evolution in the anterior cerebral artery VP Ventricular puncture, VP shunt ventriculoperitoneal shunt

day 40, the dilatation was severe but its progression seemed reduced, and ventricular clots had disappeared. Eight days later, an acute rise of intracranial pressure was observed (obvious macrocrania, full fontanelle, poor feeding). Ultrasound and Doppler results agree: accentuation of hydrocephalus, high RI (1.20), fluctuating Doppler spectrum, and bradycardias revealing brain stem postcompression insult (Fig. 4.39).

Ventriculoperitoneal shunting was performed on day 55. Postdrainage follow-up showed that diastolic velocity had improved, while ventricular volume was almost unchanged; the ventricular shunt was found within the left frontal horn. A new acute intracranial hypertension syndrome occurred at 2.5 months, with altered Doppler indices (RI=1.22) (Fig. 4.40) and exclusion of the right ventricle. CT confirmed transependymal CSF resorption.

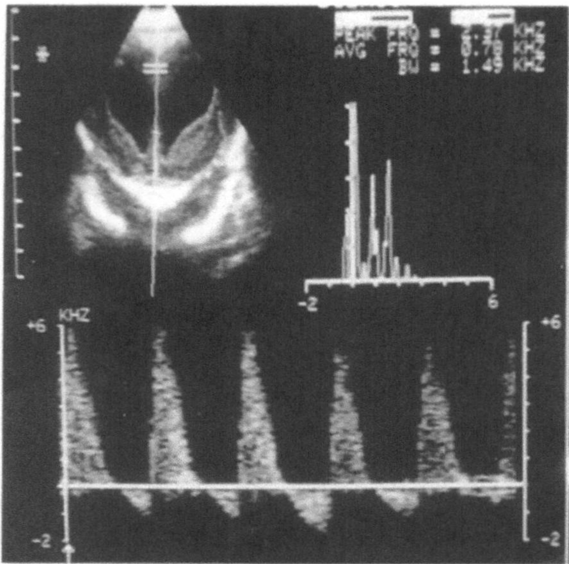

Fig. 4.39. Increased vascular resistance with reverse diastolic flow and fluctuating systolic–diastolic velocities (especially diastolic velocities)

Fig. 4.40. Increase in ventricular dilatation associated with increased vascular resistance: there is obvious malfunction of the ventriculoperitoneal shunt

A second shunt was placed within the excluded ventricle. Hemodynamic normalization was immediate, followed by gradual decrease of the ventricular enlargement. At 4 months of age, ultrasound follow-up of the residual dilatation gives a normal hemodynamic assessment.

This case history effectively summarizes the influence of modern Doppler imaging on the monitoring of hydrocephalus and its therapeutic management.

The decision to place a shunt in tumoral, infectious, or developmental hydrocephalus is usually easy to take; drainage of a posthemorrhagic dilatation, on the other hand, is most often controversial. The technical difficulties of shunting in a premature infant and the frequency of mechanical or infectious complications are arguments to be taken into account. This explains the development of other therapeutic possibilities undertaken to stabilize or decrease the ventriculomegaly in these fragile newborns: serial lumbar or ventricular taps, or the use of diuretic or osmotic agents, anticoagulant therapy, or drugs that decrease CSF production (SHERMAN 1986).

For this reason, the case of Gaelle well demonstrates the difficulties that are encountered in the management of posthemorrhagic dilatations, and the usefulness of ultrasound imaging, particularly Doppler studies:

– Progressive ventriculomegaly and hemodynamic disturbances require urgent treatment

– Use of lumbar and ventricular tap has a favorable but transient effect on cerebral hemodynamics
– Efficiency of a ventriculoperitoneal shunt is proven by immediate normalization of the cerebral hemodynamics and a subsequent slower reduction in ventricular volume
– Postshunt complications, especially blockage, can be detected by ultrasonographic and hemodynamic long-term follow-up.

In conclusion, after hydrocephalus is diagnosed, ultrasound evaluation and follow-up provides the main further information that may determine on which to base management and the best treatment: repeated lumbar or ventricular punctures, ventricular reservoir placement, ventriculoperitoneal shunting, or shunt revision if mechanical complications occur.

4.4.1
Differential Diagnosis: Role of Hemodynamics

Ventriculomegaly mean different things: of course, it may be caused by progressive obstructive hydrocephalus, but it may also result from cerebral atrophy, postischemic loss of white matter, a large IVH, transient disturbance of CSF dynamics, or a stabilized ventricular dilatation. Prognosis and treatment differ for these etiologies, since ventriculoperitoneal drainage is obviously not indicated in patients with atrophic ventriculomegaly. The value of Doppler investigations is well demonstrated by HUANG (1991). He studied 14 ventriculomegalic infants, aged from 7 days to 8 months (9 postmeningitic cases, 3 posthemorrhagic cases, 2 congenital cases), all shunted and followed up for 1 year. The patients were divided into two groups: group I (9 infants) with an obvious decrease in ventricular volume, and group II (5 infants) with no apparent change in ventricular size. The results were:

- Before shunt, RI in group I was significantly higher than in group II, although the ventriculomegaly of group I was smaller than that of group II; there was no significant difference in intracranial pressure between the two groups.
- Changes in systolic and diastolic velocities and RI 3 days before and 1 month after shunt placement were shown: in group I, diastolic velocity increased and RI significantly decreased, whereas Doppler variables remained unchanged in group II.
- At 1 year neurological follow-up, significant differences were observed between the two groups: in group I neurological development was normal in four cases, mildly abnormal in four other cases, and one infant died; in group II, severe retardation with microcephaly was noted in four patients out of five.

HUANG's conclusions (1991) are interesting, and the main points should be emphasized:
- "Clinical findings rarely make much contribution: in atrophic ventriculomegaly, clinical symptoms are often occult; intracranial pressure may be normal or mildly increased during progressive hydrocephalus; finally, in ventricular enlargement of mixed etiology, it is difficult to form a conclusion on the basis of clinical and morphological criteria alone." In the opinion of FLODMARK (1981), when ventricular dilatation occurs in an infant without evident symptoms of progressive hydrocephalus, it should be considered as atrophic ventriculomegaly unless ultrasonography demonstrates persisting accentuation of ventricular size or loss of brain parenchyma. In the history of a case of spontaneously stabilized or slowly increasing hydrocephalus, some suggestive features may be noticed: moderate macrocrania or slight signs of intracranial hypertension. Thus, clinical findings are often insufficient as a basis for deciding on a therapeutic strategy.
- "Ventricular size is not a reliable enough indicator to predict resolution of the dilatation after ventriculoperitoneal shunt." This assertion may appear excessive, since the lateral ventricles are frequently different in shape in hydrocephalus and atrophy:

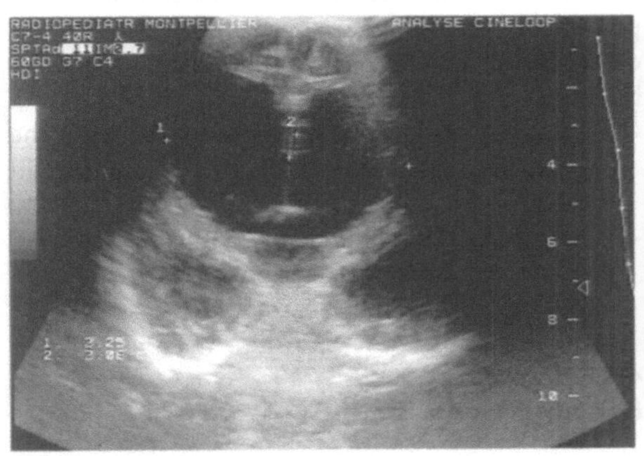

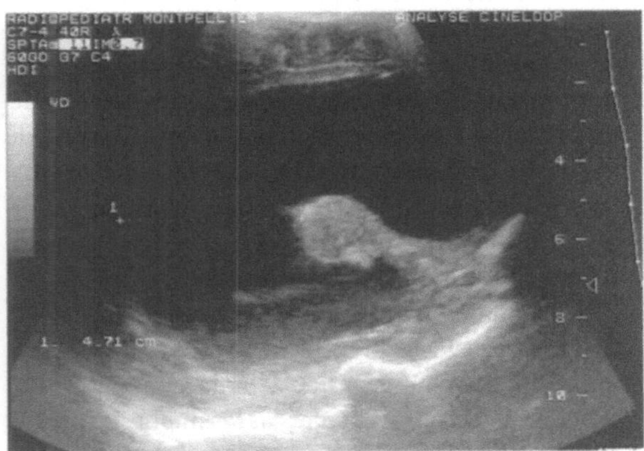

Fig. 4.41a–c. A 4-month-old infant with massive ventriculomegaly (a). Doppler imaging is normal, RI is 0.59. Is drainage required? In fact, this dilatation is the result of cerebral atrophy and does not require any shunt. Its atrophic nature is suggested by two characteristics: the predominant enlargement of the frontal horns (b) and of the interhemispheric fissure (c)

in the latter, the predominant dilatation is of the frontal horns, whereas in the former the occipital horns are more enlarged.

The second finding is just useful: atrophic ventriculomegaly is not progressive and may regress over sequential examinations; however, some cases of true hydrocephalus may present a regressive course.

The third criterion appears later, but demonstrates cerebral atrophy directly: the decrease in brain volume is shown in closer detail by high frequency probes as a subarachnoid expansion of CSF within the interhemispheric fissure. This ultrasonographic sign is never observed during hydrocephalus unless there is associated ischemic damage. Nevertheless, hydrocephalus may present minimal or moderate dilatation, and cerebral atrophy may show intense dilatation. Thus, ventricular size is not a reliable criterion by which to differentiate hydrocephalus from atrophic ventriculomegaly.

This gives great value to hemodynamic investigations, as demonstrated by HUANG (1991). This author believes that distorsion, compression, and stretching of the anterior cerebral artery depends not only on the degree of dilatation of the frontal horns, but also on the intrinsic biochemical properties of the cerebral parenchyma: RI may be a good measurement of both. A unelevated normal RI with ventriculomegaly means that the anterior cerebral artery is not stretched, and the elastic nature of the cerebral parenchyma is damaged; this is the case in cerebral atrophy. By contrast, the RI is increased in progressive hydrocephalus because the anterior cerebral artery is stretched. After shunting, RI significantly decreases in hydrocephalus with preserved parenchymal elasticity, whereas no significant changes in RI are found in atrophic ventricular enlargement. Thus, sequential cerebrovascular assessment is useful for differentiating hydrocephalus from atrophic dilatation and for deciding on shunting procedures.

4.4.2
Repeated Removal of CSF

Attempts to prevent hydrocephalus by serial CSF removal (using lumbar or ventricular tap) are controversial, since recent large studies provide contradictory results. The first report by PAPILE (1980) suggests that serial lumbar punctures are effective:

among 12 treated premature babies, 6 showed a decrease in ventricular size, 5 had a stabilization of the dilatation, and only 1 infant required a ventriculoperitoneal shunt. On the other hand, MANTOVANI (1982) reports failure of the procedure in 19 neonates and concludes that CSF removal is inefficacious. In fact, these authors study too small a number of patients and their inclusion criteria are disparate.

The process by which serial CSF removal arrests the progression of hydrocephalus is unknown. GOLDSTEIN (1976) attributes the beneficial effect to the lowering of CSF pressure and facilitation of CSF absorption due to decreasing protein content of the CSF. The recent study of KREUSSER (1985) is more interesting, because she analyzes some criteria of selection. Her study included 16 newborns with posthemorrhagic progressive dilatation without intracranial hypertension. The effectiveness of daily lumbar tap was followed by measuring lateral ventricular size and intracranial pressure (obtained at the anterior fontanelle); Doppler ultrasonography was not performed. In 12 patients, ventricular volume and intracranial pressure decreased after each lumbar tap; in these infants, progression of hydrocephalus stopped, as shown by regression or stabilization of the ventricular dilatation. In four infants, the failure of treatment with daily CSF removal resulted in definitive ventriculoperitoneal shunt placement. According to this author, two features determine a transient or definitive efficiency of lumbar punctures:

- First, there must be communication between the ventricular system and the lumbar subarachnoid space.
- Second, a critical volume of CSF must be removed in order to obtain a reduction in ventricular volume.

4.4.2.1
Hemodynamic Assessment

Our personal experience is based on the management of 28 hydrocephalic babies (25 posthemorrhagic, 2 postmeningitic, and 1 with myelomeningocele). The number of lumbar taps performed ranged from 5 to 20, with a mean of 8 ml CSF removed (range 2–30 ml) at each puncture. In 6 cases, the detection of a noncommunicating dilatation resulted in ventricular punctures. In the 17 most recent cases, the effectiveness of the treatment was followed by Doppler ultrasonography. The effect of CSF removal appeared rather disappointing: in five cases, the ventricular enlargement decreased sharply; in four more cases, a moderate improvement was observed, but the dilatation continued to evolve in 19 infants, resulting in subsequent shunt placement.

On the other hand, in all cases Doppler variables showed a reduction in downstream vascular resistance, whatever the clinical outcome.

Mathieu was a 34-weeks' gestation premature infant presenting with a maternofetal Streptococcus infection, with normal CSF at lumbar tap. On day 14, routine ultrasonography showed tetraventricular communicating dilatation with predominant enlargement of the ventricular atria and occipital horns. Doppler imaging showed the RI to be slightly raised (0.83). The presence of a left germinal matrix hemorrhage suggested posthemorrhagic hydrocephalus. Treatment by serial lumbar punctures was begun. After 5 punctures, at each of which 5 ml CSF was removed, ultrasound follow-up was performed (day 20). The result was impressive: the ventriculomegaly was markedly reduced and the Doppler indices were normal (Fig. 4.42). The treatment was carried on for 9 days,

and the total amount of CSF removed was 70 ml. At 10 months, the infant was reviewed and noted to have excellent neurological development and a moderate remaining dilatation.

This example summarizes the objective selection criteria required in order to obtain a clear favorable effect of lumbar punctures. This newborn presented with mild IVH and slowly progressing dilatation without any clinical or hemodynamic symptom of intracranial hypertension; finally, he had a communicating dilatation, as shown by the postpuncture regression.

This is in agreement with the work of KREUSSER (1985), confirming the absence of value of hemodynamic investigation as normal as expected in these clinical circumstances with these imaging findings.

Maxime was the first baby of a twin gestation; he was born at 28 weeks, after an uneventful delivery, and showed diffuse hypotonia. The first ultrasound examination, performed on day 3, showed a left germinal matrix hemorrhage and a right intraventricu-

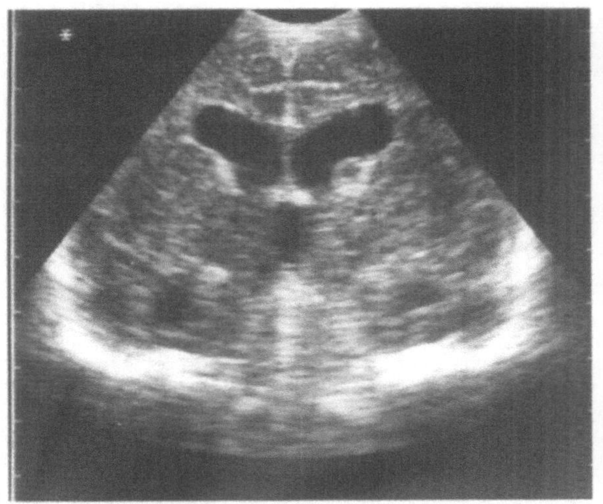

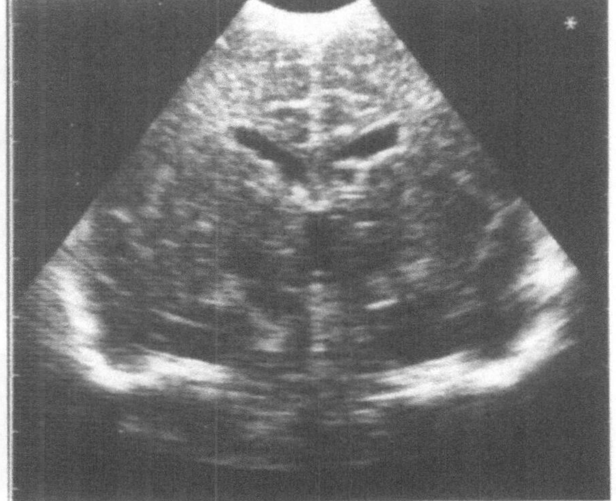

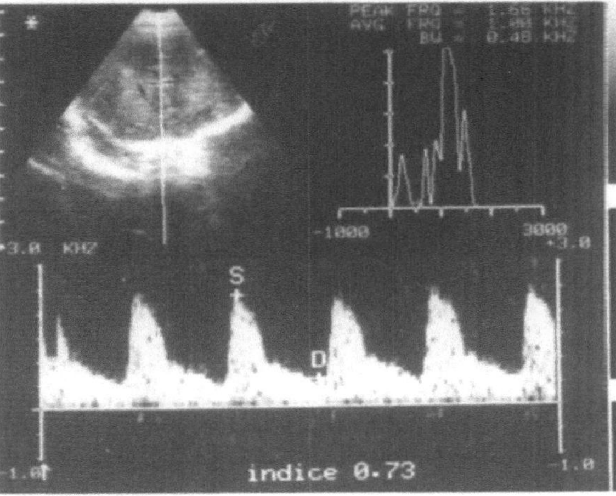

Fig. 4.42. a Day 14. Lateral and third ventricular dilatation. After a program of serial lumbar punctures is begun, lateral ventricular volume starts to decrease (b, day 20), with normal RI (c)

lar hemorrhage. Communicating triventricular dilatation quickly occurred, and a daily program of subtractive lumbar punctures was decided on at day 25.

Fifteen lumbar taps were performed, removing 5 ml CSF at each procedure. With this treatment, the clinical and sonographic course was characterized by:
- *A slightly excessive growth in head circumference without a sudden rise in intracranial pressure.*
- *A gradual, moderate increase in ventricular dilatation. Parallel to this, hemodynamic alterations were detected, with obviously increased vascular resistance, showing subclinical intracranial hypertension. Despite this, the punctures appeared to be efficacious, since each tap was followed by an improvement in vascular resistance, even though transient (Fig. 4.43).*

At 1.5 months, lumbar tap became unproductive and the treatment was stopped; head circumference growth and hemodynamic results progressively returned to normal, and the ventricular enlargement stabilized. The infant was reviewed at 18 months and macrocrania was noted; his psychomotor performance was evaluated at 15 months.

This case report is interesting because it asks the question of the real effect of the lumbar punctures since the ventricles enlarged moderately but gradually during the subtractive treatment, and this dilatation stabilized quite a long time after CSF removal ceased.

This supports the hypothesis of spontaneous regression of the hydrocephalus in our case (DYKES 1989). In the literature (ALLAN 1984), spontaneous arrest of the hydrocephalic process with partial or

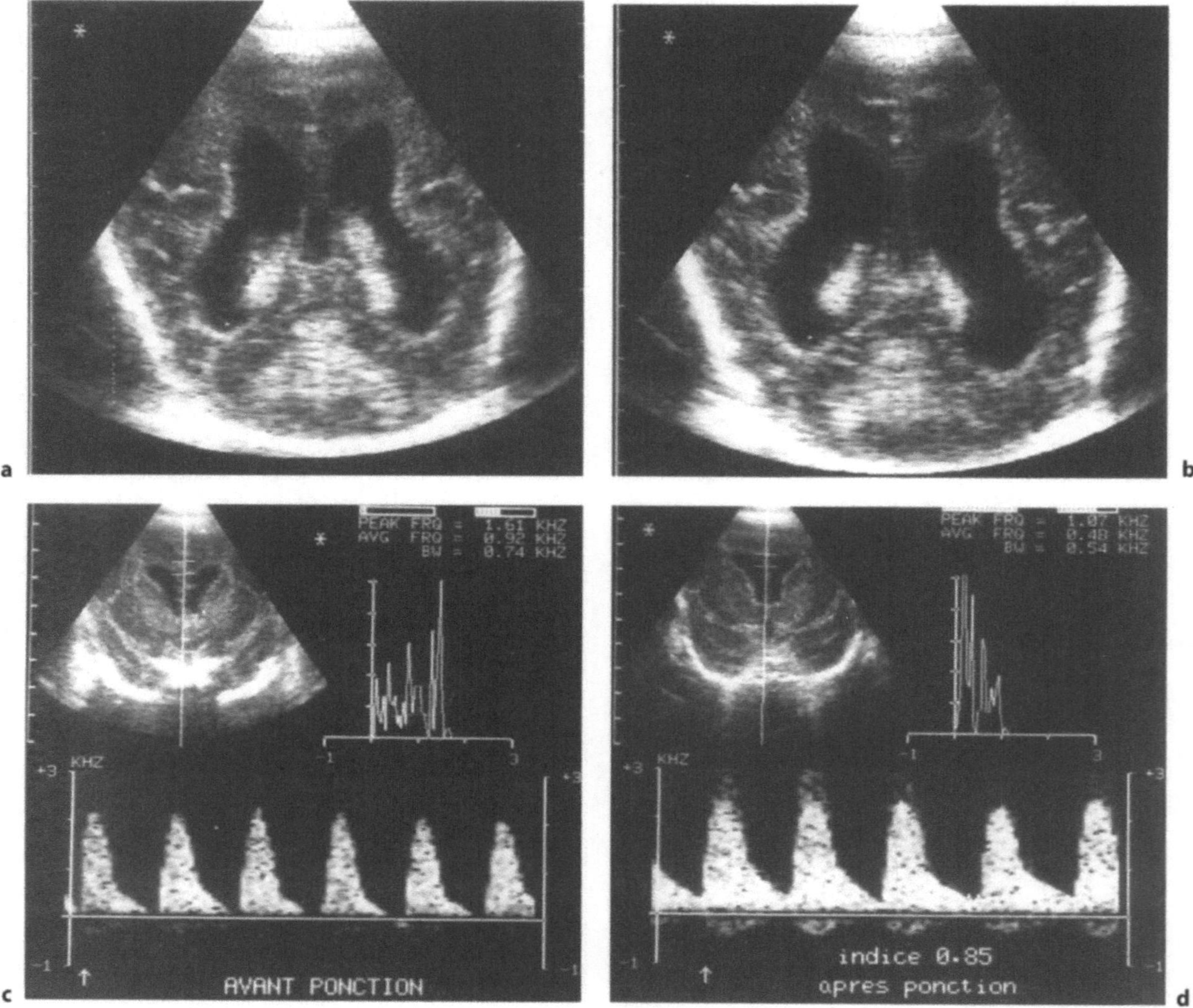

Fig. 4.43a–d. Day 25. Symmetric lateral ventricular dilatation (**a**). A program of daily lumbar punctures is begun, without result, since ventricular dilatation is moderately increased by day 33 (**b**). Parallel to this and simultaneously (day 32), hemodynamic alterations occur (**c**), which decrease (**d**) or disappear after withdrawal of CSF

complete resolution of ventriculomegaly has been described in approximately 40% of cases of posthemorrhagic hydrocephalus. This is why it is extremely difficult to assess the effectiveness of lumbar punctures: such a treatment seems always uneasy to indicate in this kind of gradually evolving ventricular dilatation.

In this infant, it is also interesting to note that, although the ventricular volume remained unchanged after the lumbar punctures, the cerebral vascularization was improved: immediately after CSF withdrawal, vascular resistance decreased and even returned to normal. This benefit is transient and lasts usually 12–24 h, sometimes 48 h.

During hydrocephalus managed by serial lumbar punctures, hemodynamic assessment allows several conclusions:

- First, it confirms communication between the ventricular system and the lumbar subarachnoid spaces when vascular resistance decreases after lumbar CSF removal. In our series of 17 patients, all Doppler studies performed after the puncture demonstrated an obvious improvement in cerebral hemodynamics, in respect of both RI and velocities (especially diastolic velocities). Results published by others are the same (DRAYTON 1986; GOH 1991; MINNS 1991).
- Second, even if they have no effect on ventricular volume, lumbar punctures appear justified when hemodynamic alteration is detected. We know that vascular resistance analyzed by pulsed Doppler is a reliable reflection of intracranial pressure. Thus, when CSF removal reduces vascular resistance, it improves intracranial pressure, reducing vascular damage. Nevertheless, the vascular data during the hemodynamic assessment of a patient with progressive hydrocephalus should be interpreted with care: if Doppler imaging is performed immediately after CSF puncture, it may lead to a false sense of security (Graph 4.4). For patient management, it is better to rely on results obtained after a delay after puncture.

4.4.2.2
Failure of Lumbar or Ventricular Puncture

Failure of treatment by CSF removal was obvious in 19 patients (17 posthemorrhagic, 1 postmeningitic, and 1 with myelomeningocele). In all these cases, progressive ventriculomegaly required definitive ventriculoperitoneal shunting, despite serial lumbar punctures. All the cases of posthemorrhagic hydrocephalus followed massive intraventricular bleeding

and the ineffectiveness of CSF withdrawal is not surprising. Nevertheless, some comments about this procedure are necessary:

- The treatment may have failed because too small an amount of CSF was removed (mean 8 ml). All authors (KREUSSER 1985; PAPILE 1980) stress the importance of removing a critical volume of CSF: KREUSSER (1985) withdraws 50–90 ml CSF per week, for a total duration of 4 weeks.
- In all these babies, sudden rises of intracranial pressure occur, with obvious clinical signs and sharp increase in vascular resistance on Doppler imaging. If the analysis is done immediately after a puncture, improvement of the hemodynamic situation is shown. On the other hand, it is unchanged when CSF removal is zero, low, or delayed. The benefit for cerebral vascularization (and for intracranial pressure), although transient, is clear.
- Since posthemorrhagic hydrocephalus cannot be shunted early because of intraventricular clotting, lumbar punctures may be an effective waiting procedure, on the condition that a strict protocol is precisely adhered to: daily punctures, with a sufficient volume of CSF withdrawn, guided by Doppler imaging, in order to determine the best time, the best frequency, and the best duration of the procedure.

Following same idea, since RI has been shown to correlate reliably with intracranial pressure, DRAYTON (1986) and GOH (1995) tried to demonstrate that this index may be a useful landmark by which to assess the simultaneous hemodynamic changes during the puncture, and the exponential relationship between intracranial volume and intracranial pressure.

DRAYTON (1986), the first, showed in a single patient with posthemorrhagic ventricular dilatation that, during CSF drainage by lumbar tap, the PI follows an exponential pattern of decline, decreasing sharply at the beginning of the drainage and rapidly reaching a plateau before the end of the drainage.

Later, GOH examined the pattern of decline in RI in 16 patients sequentially during CSF subtraction. Theoretically, this exponential curve reflects the response of blood flow velocity to volume changes, and allows an estimation of a half volume i.e., the volume of CSF withdrawn when half the observed changes in RI have occurred. In his report, GOH (1995) suggests that, after only a small volume of CSF (1.25 ml) has been drained, significant hemodynamic changes may be observed.

This study should be carried further to better identify which hydrocephalic patients will benefit from ventriculoperitoneal shunting.

4.4.3
Ventriculoperitoneal Shunt and Hemodynamic Follow-Up

Ventriculoperitoneal shunting constitutes a definitive modality the indication for which may be targeted by ultrasonography.

4.4.3.1
Hemodynamic Monitoring of Ventriculoperitoneal Shunt Efficiency

During follow-up of a shunt, morphological ultrasonography must be accompanied by Doppler imaging of the cerebral vessels. Our experience is based on the assessment of 62 patients with shunted hydrocephalus (31 posthemorrhagic, 24 with myelomeningocele, and 7 postmeningitic).

In all cases where shunt placement was decided on because of progressive hydrocephalus and hemodynamic disturbances, normalization of Doppler variables was observed in the first few hours after surgery (Fig. 4.44).

Of course, it is important to show the tip of the shunt, which ideally is located within the frontal horn. The progressive reduction in ventricular volume must also be assessed. In early-shunted infants, ventricular diameter decreases during the first week: the third ventricle returns to normal size the day after shunt placement, while the volume of the lateral ventricles gradually decreases, the occipital horns being the last dilated. This is confirmed by SMITH (1982), who found in 74% of 37 cases a great reduction in ventricular volume in the first week after surgery.

Beside these observations, hemodynamic assessment by pulsed Doppler imaging constitutes an earlier, more efficient, and more objective modality that may prove the effectiveness of a ventriculoperitoneal shunt (Fig. 4.45).

Graph 4.6 shows the results we found in 14 patients with shunted hydrocephalus (9 posthemorrhagic, 1 postmeningitic, and 4 with myelomeningocele) during the examination performed the day after surgery. These personal data confirmed other published reports.

Thus, in 46 neonates with symptomatic progressive hydrocephalus, CHADDUCK (1989) noted a mean RI value of 0.84, which decreased to 0.72 after shunting. NORELLE (1989) reported a mean PI value of 1.06 for stable ventriculomegaly, while it was 1.72 for progressive ventricular dilatation, and 1.02 after shunt placement.

All authors (DEGG 1988; FRANK 1988; GOH 1991; HANLO 1995; NISHIMAKI 1991; RIFKINSON-MANN 1994; VAN BEL 1988) observe that normalization of RI after shunting is the result of a significant increase in diastolic velocity compared with systolic velocity, suggesting a decrease in cerebrovascular resistance. The association with increased mean velocity supports the idea that cerebral blood flow increases.

The experience of IACOPINO (1995) is worth recalling. This author assessed cerebral blood flow changes during ventricular shunting by means of intraoperative monitoring in three hydrocephalic children (aged 2 months, 14 months, and 8 years, respectively), under standardized conditions (general anesthesia, continuous Doppler recording of the middle cerebral

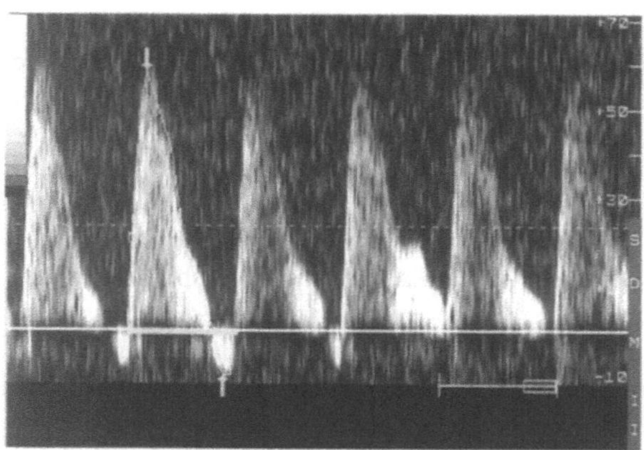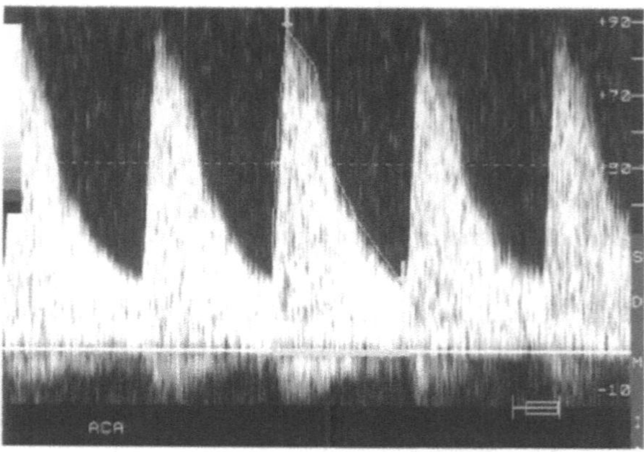

Fig. 4.44. a Neonatal myelomeningocele. Severe hemodynamic disturbance, RI=1.16. A few hours after shunt placement, normalization of the Doppler curve (**b**) confirms the efficacy of shunting

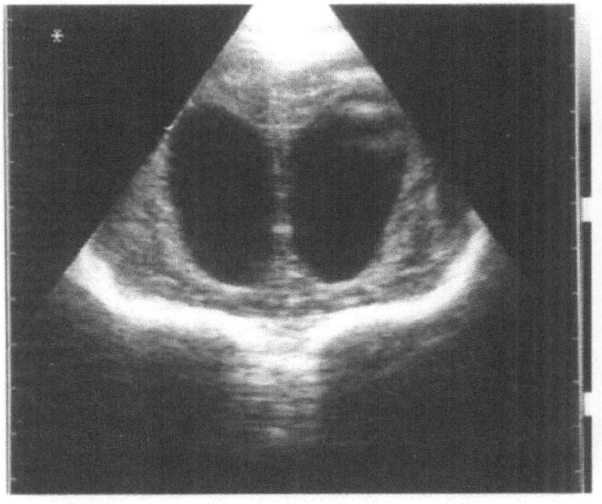

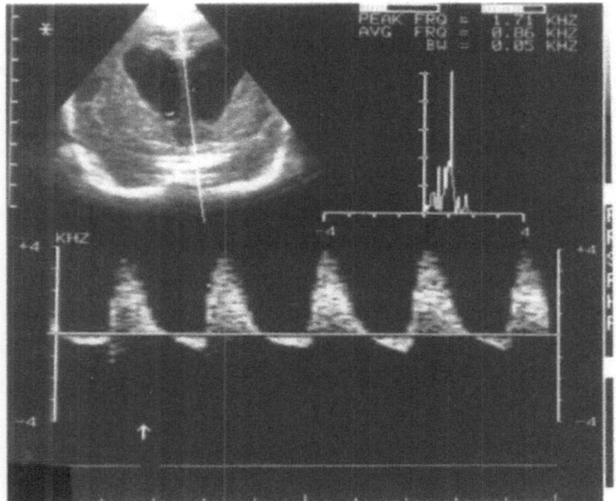

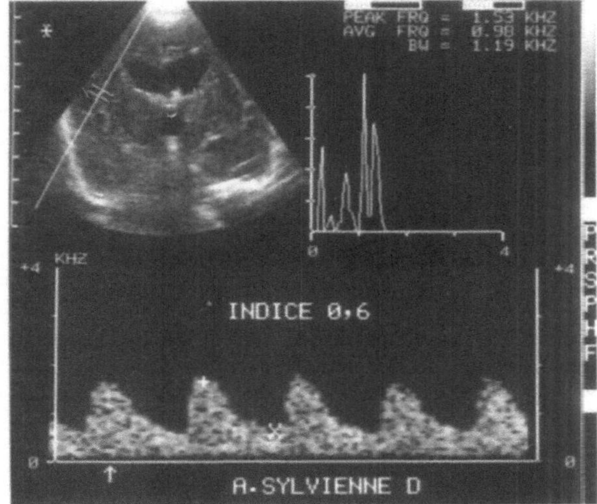

Fig. 4.45. a Postmeningitic hydrocephalus. Severe increase in vascular resistance with reverse diastolic flow (b), prompting immediate shunting. On day 1 and day 7, Doppler indices are normal, despite the still enlarged frontal horns (c)

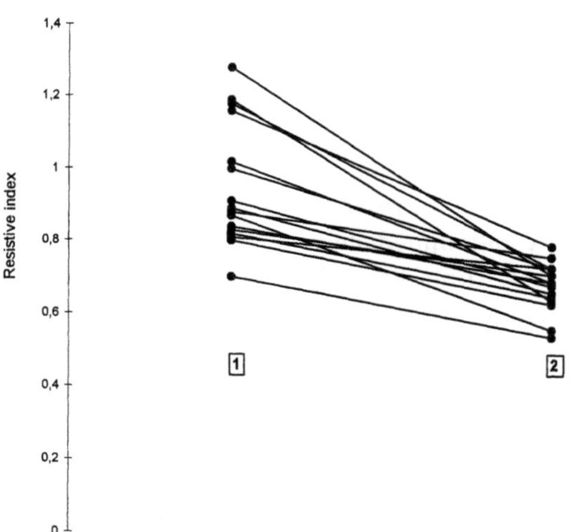

Graph 4.6. Resistive index before (1left) and after (2right) ventriculoperitoneal shunting

artery). In all the patients, in the first minutes that followed shunting, a clear and sudden increase in mean velocity by more than 30% was detected, as well as a significant decrease in RI. These results supply additional evidence of the close relationship between hydrocephalus, intracranial pressure, and cerebrovascular alterations.

4.4.3.2
Hemodynamics During Complications of Ventriculoperitoneal Shunt

All authors emphasize the frequency and variable pattern of shunt complications, 80% of which are due to obstruction and dysfunction. Shunt complications are a major problem of pediatric neurosurgery. SEKHAR (1982) detailed the multiple causes of 200 shunt revisions in 119 infants and reported possible blockage by abnormal proliferation of choroid plexus or ependymal cells. This was confirmed by HAKIM (1969), who found choroidal cells in 80% of 15 examined catheters, and by HOCKLEY (1982), who detected choroidal material in 10 of 16 obstructed catheters studied by electron microscopy. The presence of choroidal material is partially explained when the ventricular catheter is located behind the foramen of Monro, where the choroid plexus is prominent. A ventriculoperitoneal shunt works better when it is placed within the frontal horns, which are free of the choroid plexus (VIRES 1980).

SEKHAR (1982) observed that leptomeningeal, glial, or connective tissue, and neural tissue (subependymal astrocytes, neurons, and white matter) may also be obstructive material. Brain tissue is probably introduced into the catheter during shunt placement. Finally, cotton fibers, hair, or talc powder may induce inflammatory granulomas around the tip of the catheter.

In the diagnosis of shunt malfunction, the ultrasound examination (together with the skull X-ray and abdominal plain film) plays an important role.

Ectopic or aberrant location of the ventricular tip is easily shown by ultrasound. HARWOOD-NASH (1982) notes that shunts placed in the temporal horn or third ventricle, or incarcerated in brain parenchyma, most often suffer dysfunction. It is also possible for a shunt to migrate as the head grows, even if it was previously correctly situated. Finally, the presence of septa within a dilated ventricle can result in shunt malfunction.

Diagnosing shunt blockage is not always easy:
- First, because clinical findings vary and are often occult. In a personal study of 32 patients with myelomeningocele who we followed during their first year of life, the clinical pattern was latent in 20 out of 40 shunt obstructions.
- Second, because ventricular dilatation may occur and increase slowly.
- Third, because the value of hemodynamic investigation seems actually to be moderate. We did not notice any change in eight patients with shunt blockage (6 with myelomeningocele and 2 with posthemorrhagic dilatation). However, we found increased vascular resistance in three patients with acute obstruction, suggesting that hemodynamic alteration reflects only an acute ventricular complication (Figs. 4.46, 4.47).

As a matter of fact, our experience, so far disappointing, may well improve if we may judge by the more optimistic literature.

POPLE (1992) reports, in 11 infants with suspected shunt malfunction requiring surgical revi-

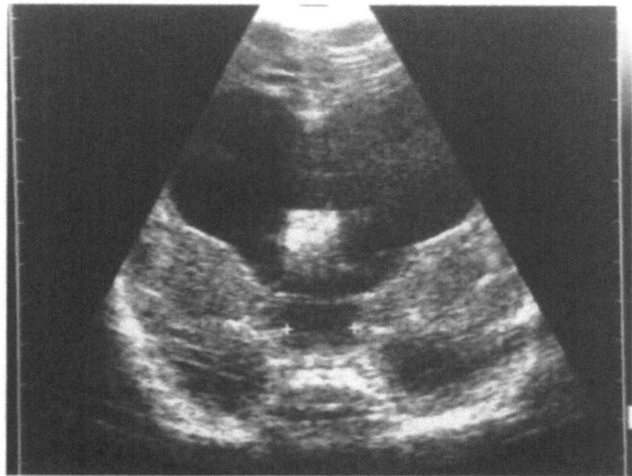

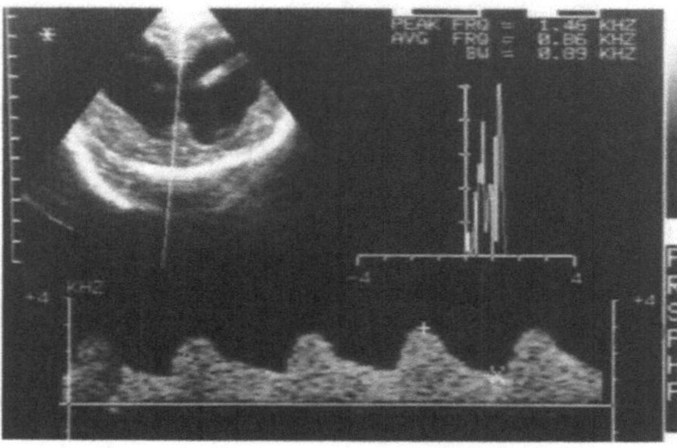

Fig. 4.46a,b. Shunted posthemorrhagic hydrocephalus. Shunt functioned well for 3 months. Progressive ventriculomegaly without any change in cerebral hemodynamics. Two days before shunt revision, ultrasonography showed evident ventriculomegaly (**a**), despite normal vascular resistance (**b**)

sion, a significant increase in RI in nine cases, but he does not specify whether the blockage is acute or slowly evolving. In slowly progressive blockage, fontanellar compression will probably sensitize the investigation.

The experience of HUANG (1991) is interesting too. In two patients with recurrent ventriculomegaly due to distal shunt obstruction, he applied repeated manual pumping of the reservoir for 3 min, and measured RI before and immediately after the pumping test. In both cases, RI markedly decreased, indicating shunt malfunction. This result was similar to that described by MEYER (1984), who showed by xenon 133 inhalation that cerebral blood flow in frontal and temporal gray matter increased after CSF pressure was reduced by lumbar puncture, in patients with normal-pressure hydrocephalus. This test seems a valuable tool to sensitize the detection of dysfunction, particularly when the clinical pattern and morphological characteristics of the ventriculomegaly are not significant.

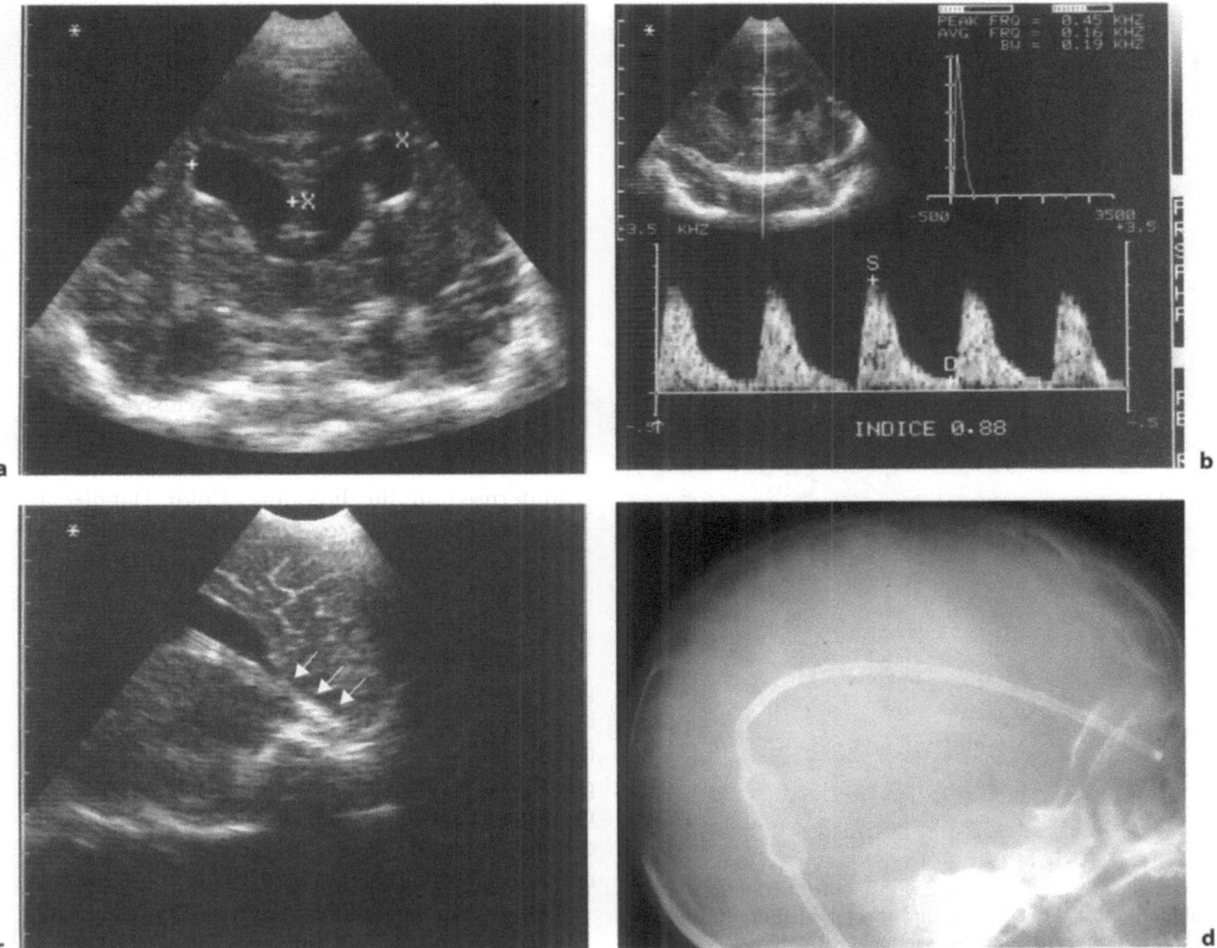

Fig. 4.47a–d. In this 3-month-old shunted infant with myelomeningocele, clinical findings of intracranial hypertension (vomiting, bulging fontanelle) suggested acute shunt blockage, confirmed by the presence of ventricular dilatation (a) and raised RI (b). Shunt exclusion was diagnosed, since the ventricular tip (c) was shown within the frontal parenchyma (arrow). Confirmation by lateral skull X-ray (d)

Finally, we should pay attention to the recent experience of Sgouros (1996), who tries to assess the patency of ventriculoperitoneal shunts by Doppler imaging. In 17 infants, aged 3 months to 12 years, 20 investigations were performed. In 13 cases, CSF flow was identified through the shunt tube; flow velocities between 5 and 7 cm/s were measured. No CSF flow was visualized in 7 patients, 3 of whom were being examined before revision for a blocked shunt. In 1 case, a colored signal was noted at the outlet of the peritoneal end of the shunt. The reservoir was insonated, first distal to the valve, then in the lumen of the tube in the anterior chest wall, and over the outlet of the peritoneal tube.

The conclusions to be drawn from this experience seem surprising for several reasons:

– CSF is ultrasonically invisible because of the complete absence of any reflective particles (Widder 1986), and it is difficult to understand how it can produce a colored Doppler signal. As an explanation, the author proposes, in the 13 cases where a flow was identified, the presence of microbubbles generated at points of turbulence, and of choroid plexus debris small enough to pass through the valve.
– It is surprising too, to detect a colored flow at the peritoneal end of the shunt. Despite a previous X-ray examination, localization of the free end of the tube in peritoneal cavity is not always easy.
– It is technically difficult to identify a flow and obtain a Doppler spectrum in a lumen with a cross-sectional diameter of only 1 mm. We tried to record several Doppler curves within the chest

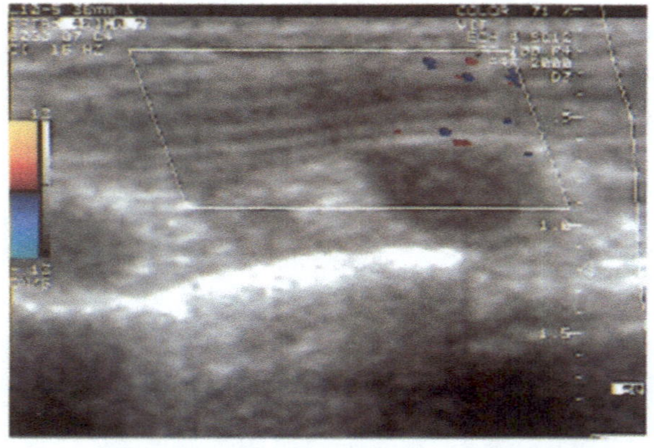

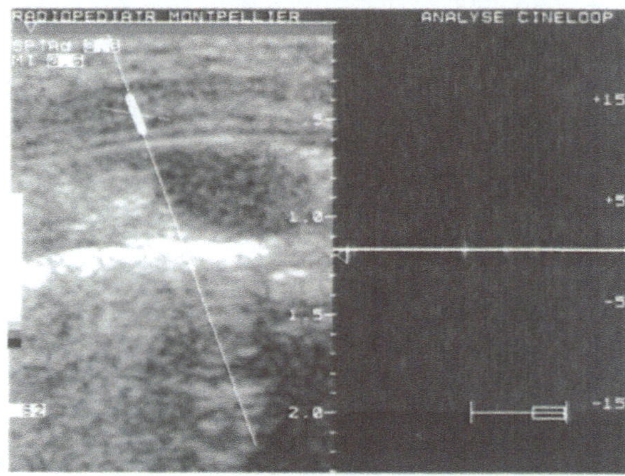

Fig. 4.48a,b. A 3-year-old child with a well-functioning ventriculoperitoneal shunt. Ultrasound was targeted on the anterior chest wall tube, whose cross-sectional diameter is 1.5 mm (a). No spectral analysis was obtained, despite a long wait (b)

wall tube, before and after pumping the reservoir, but never detected any Doppler signal (Fig. 4.48).
- Finally, a positive result indicates a functioning shunt, but a negative one does not automatically indicate a blocked shunt. The clinical application of this investigation is limited at this time.

4.5
Conclusion

Several pieces of evidence suggest that cerebral arterial velocities are a reliable reflection of intracranial pressure. Nervertheless, some questions and difficulties still remain:
- The interpretation of RI values is open to criticism, because there is a wide range of reference values in the normal neonate, and especially in the premature baby. To avoid misinterpretation, sequential determination of multiple indices in the same infant is recommended.
- Doppler study and direct measurement of intracranial pressure provide only brief samples of intracranial velocities and pressure, and normal and abnormal variations of these two values are poorly known. Perhaps, as HANLO (1995) suggests, cerebral velocities and intracranial pressure should be simultaneously recorded over several hours in order to appreciate the occurrence and duration of hemodynamic alterations during rises in intracranial hypertension.
- To favor RI and PI measures as exclusive diagnostic criteria is a mistake. We should be interested in the arterial velocities themselves, always underused in the literature. Color Doppler, by determining the insonation angle of the vessel, allows reliable measurements of systolic, diastolic, and mean velocities.

Despite these limitations, the neurosurgeons are progressively acquiring the habit of employing hemodynamic investigations before deciding on therapeutic management: lumbar or ventricular punctures, or ventriculoperitoneal shunt, etc. This requires a precise detailed protocol for morphological and Doppler analysis in the hydrocephalic neonate:
- In the newborn and the infant, the best ultrasonographic approach is by transfontanellar access. Transcranial ultrasonography is used in the older child, after one has learned to detect the middle cerebral artery, which is easier with color Doppler.
- Proper follow-up requires three or four Doppler examinations a week and must be continued for 3 months, especially when the ventricular enlargement appears to be stabilized or slowly evolving.
- Hemodynamic results may present different patterns:
  • Detection of hemodynamic alterations in progressive hydrocephalus should prompt urgent ventricular drainage.
  • In cases of slowly progressive or stabilized dilatation, the hemodynamic assessment (velocities and indices) is usually normal; a sensitization test by fontanellar compression should then be performed, with measurement of pre and postcompression RI and of ΔRI; if cerebral compliance is disturbed, shunting is required.
- Hemodynamic investigation gives the best measure of the effectiveness of the treatment and should be routinely done after lumbar tap, ventricular tap, or ventriculoperitoneal shunting.

– Finally, hemodynamic follow-up of shunt placement is necessary. If shunt blockage is suspected, the Doppler examination should be sensitized by fontanellar compression and reservoir pumping.

References

Alan H, Volpe JJ (1982). Decrease in pulsatile flow in the anterior cerebral arteries in infantile hydrocephalus. Pediatrics 69:4-7

Allan WC, Dransfield DA, Tito AH (1984) Ventricular dilatation following periventricular-intraventricular hemorrhage. Outcome at age 1 year. Pediatrics 73:158-162

Alvisi C, Cerisoli M, Giulioni M, Monari P, Salvioli G, Sandri F, Lippi C, Bovicelli L, Pilu G (1985) Evaluation of cerebral blood flow changes by transfontanel Doppler ultrasound in infantile hydrocephalus. Child's Nerv Syst 1:244-247

Anderson JC, Mawk JR (1991) Intracranial arterial duplex Doppler waveform analysis in infants. Child's Nerv Syst 4:144-148

Auer LM, Samaya I (1983) Intracranial pressure oscillations (B-waves) caused by oscillations in cerebrovascular volume. Acta Neurochir 68:93-100

Berman PH, Banker BQ (1966) Neonatal meningitis: a clinical and pathological study of 29 cases. Pediatrics 38:215-226

Blumhagen JD, Mack LA (1985) Abnormalities of the neonatal cerebral ventricles. Radiol Clin North Am 23:13-27

Bowerman RA, Donn SM, Silver TM, Jaffe MH (1984) Natural history of neonatal periventricular/intraventricular hemorrhage and its complications: sonographic observations. Am J Neuroradiol 5:527-538

Bromberger P, James H, Saunders B, Schneider H (1988) Sudden infant apnea and insidious hydrocephalus. Child's Nerv Syst 4:241-243

Burnstein J, Papile LA, Burnstein R (1979) Intraventricular hemorrhage and hydrocephalus in premature newborns: a prospective study with CT. Am J Roentgenol 132:631-635

Cayea PD, Balcar L, Alberti O, Jones T (1984) Prenatal diagnosis of semilobar holoprosencephaly. Am J Roentgenol 142:401-402

Chadduck WM, Seibert (1989) Intracranial duplex Doppler: practical uses in pediatric neurology and neurosurgery. J Child Neurol 4:77-86

Chadduck WM, Crabtree HM, Blankenship JB, Adametz JR (1991) Transcranial Doppler ultrasonography for the evaluation of shunt malfunction in pediatric patients. Child's Nerv Syst 7:27-30

Chaplin ER, Goldstein GW, Myerberg D, Hunt J, Tooley W (1980) Post-hemorrhagic hydrocephalus in the preterm infants. Pediatrics 65:901-909

Chervenak FA, Berkowitz RL, Romero L (1983) The diagnosis of fetal hydrocephalus. Am J Obstet Gynecol 147:703-716

Couture A, Ferran JL, Senac JP, Castan E, Bonnet H (1981) Image ultrasonore d'un anévrysme de la Veine de Galien. Arch Fr Pediatr 38:55-57

Couture A, Veyrac C, Baud C (1994) Echographie cérébrale, du foetus au nouveau-né. Sauramps Médical, Montpellier, pp 409-467

Couture A, Veyrac C, Baud C, Ferran JL (1996) Le Doppler cérébral en pédiatrie. JEMU 17:21-29

Cubberley DA, Jaff RB, Nixon GW (1982) Sonographic demonstration of Galenic arteriovenous malformations in the neonate. Am J Neuroradiol 3:435-439

Da Silva M, Michowicz S, Drake J, Chumas P (1995) Reduced local cerebral blood flow in periventricular white matter in experimental neonatal hydrocephalus restoration with CSF shunting. J Cereb Blood Flow Metab 15:1057-1065

De S (1950) A study of the changes in the brain in experimental hydrocephalus. J Pathol Bacteriol 62:197-207

Deeg KH, Paul J, Rupprecht T, Harms D, Mang C (1988) Pulsed Doppler sonographic determination of absolute flow velocities in the anterior cerebral artery in infants with hydrocephalus in comparison with a healthy patient sample. Monatsschr Kinderheilkd 136:85-94

Di Rocco C, Ditrapani G, Pettorossi WE (1979) On the pathology of experimental hydrocephalus induced by artificial increase in endoventricular CSF pulse pressure. Child's Brain 5:81-95

Di Rocco C, Caldarelli M, Ceddia A (1989) "Occult" hydrocephalus in children. Child's Nerv Syst 5:71-75

Drayton MR, Skidmore R (1986) Doppler ultrasound in the neonate. Ultrasound Med Biol 12:761-772

Dykes FD, Dunbar B, Lazarra A, Ahmann PA (1989) Posthemorrhagic hydrocephalus in high-risk preterm infants: natural history management and long term outcome. J Pediatr 114:611-618

Eisenberg HM, McComb JG, Lorenzo AV (1971) Cerebrospinal fluid overproduction and hydrocephalus associated with choroid plexus papilloma. J Neurosurg 35:427-430

Fernell E, Hagberg G, Hagberg B (1990) Infantile hydrocephalus: the impact of enhanced preterm survival. Acta Paediatr Scand 79:1080-1086

Filly R, Chinn DH, Callen PW (1984) Alobar holoprosencephaly: ultrasonography prenatal diagnosis. Radiology 151:455-459

Finn JP, Quinn MW, Hall-Craggs MA, Kendall BE (1990) Impact of vessel distorsion on transcranial Doppler velocity measurements: correlation with magnetic resonance imaging. J Neurosurg 73:572-575

Fischer AQ, Livingstone JN (1989) Transcranial Doppler and real time cranial sonography in neonatal hydrocephalus. J Child Neurol 4:64-69

Fletcher J, Landry S, Bohan T, Davidson K, Brookshire B, Lachar D, Kramer L, Francis D (1997) Effects of intraventricular hemorrhage and hydrocephalus on the long term neurobehavioral development of preterm very low birth weight infants. Dev Med Child Neurol 39:596-606

Flodmark O, Scotti G, Harwood-Nash DC (1981) Clinical significance of ventriculomegaly in children who suffered perinatal asphyxia with or without intracranial hemorrhage: an 18 months follow-up study. J Comput Assist Tomogr 5:663-673

Frank VB, Margot VDB, Jan B, Theo B, Jan HR (1988) Blood flow velocity pattern of the anterior cerebral arteries: before and after drainage of the posthemorrhagic hydrocephalus in the newborn. J Ultrasound Med 7:553-559

Fusch C, Ozdoba C, Kuhn P, Durig P, Remonda L, Muller C, Kaiser G, Schroth G, Moessinger A (1977) Perinatal ultrasonography and magnetic resonance imaging findings in congenital hydrocephalus associated with fetal intraventricular hemorrhage. Am J Obstet Gynecol 177:512-518

Goh D, Minns RA, Pye SD, Steers AJ (1991) Cerebral blood flow velocity changes after ventricular taps and ventriculoperitoneal shunting. Child's Nerv Syst 1:452-457

Goh D, Minns R, Pye S (1991) Transcranial Doppler (TCD) ultrasound as a noninvasive means of monitoring cerebrohemodynamic change in hydrocephalus. Eur J Pediatr Surg 1(Suppl 1):14-17

Goh D, Minns RA, Hendry GM, Thambyayah M, Steers AJ (1992) Cerebrovascular resistive index assessed by duplex Doppler sonography and its relationship to intracranial pressure in infantile hydrocephalus. Pediatr Radiol 22:246-250

Goh D, Minns RA, Pye SD, Steers AJ (1992) Cerebral blood flow velocity and intermittent intracranial pressure elevation during sleep in hydrocephalic children. Dev Med Child Neurol 34:676-689

Goh D, Minns RA (1995) Intracranial pressure and cerebral arterial flow velocity indices in childhood hydrocephalus: current review. Child's Nerv Syst 11:392-396

Goiten KJ, Amit V, Mussafi H (1983) Intracranial pressure in central nervous system infections and cerebral ischemia in infancy. Arch Dis Child 58:184-186

Goldstein GW, Chaplin ER, Maitland J, Norman D (1976) Transient hydrocephalus in premature infants: treatment by lumbar punctures. Lancet 1(7958):512-514

Grant EG, White EM, Schellinger D, Choyke PL, Sarcone AL (1987) Cranial duplex sonography of the infant. Radiology 163:177-185

Greitz TV, Cronqvist S (1968) Angiographic evaluation of cerebral circulation time and regional cerebral blood flow. A comparative study. Scand J Clin Lab Invest Suppl 102:11-A

Greitz TV (1969) Cerebral blood flow in occult hydrocephalus studied with angiography and the 133 xenon clearance method. Acta Radiol Diagn 8:376-384

Greitz D, Greitz T, Hindmarsh T (1997) A new view on the CSF-circulation with the potential for pharmacological treatment of childhood hydrocephalus. Acta Paediatr 86:125-132

Guthkelch AN, Critchley M (1972) High pressure hydrocephalus. Scientific Foundations of Neurology. Davis, Philadelphia, pp 296-301

Guzzetta F, Mercuri E, Spano M (1995) Mechanisms and evolution of the brain damage in neonatal post-hemorrhagic hydrocephalus. Child's Nerv Syst 11:293-296

Hakim S (1969) Observations on the physiopathology of the CSF pulse and prevention of ventricular catheter obstruction in valve shunts. Dev Med Child Neurol (Suppl 20):42-48

Han BK, Babcock DS, McAdams L (1985) Bacterial meningitis in infants: sonographic findings. Radiology 154:645-650

Hanlo P, Gooskew R, Nijhuis T, Faber J, Peters R, Van Huffelden AC, Tulleken C (1995) Value of transcranial Doppler indices in predicting raised ICP in infantile hydrocephalus. A study with review of the literature. Child's Nerv Syst 11:595-603

Hanlo PW, Peters RJ, Gooskens RH, Heethaar RM, Keunen RW, Van Huffelden AC, Tulleken CA, Willemse J (1995) Monitoring intracranial dynamics by transcranial Doppler. A new Doppler index: transsystolic time. Ultrasound Med Biol 21:613-621

Hanlo AN, Gosskens RJ, Van Schooneveld M, Tulleken CA, Van Der Knaap MS, Faber JA, Willemse J (1997) The effect of intracranial pressure on myelination and the relationship with neurodevelopment in infantile hydrocephalus. Dev Med Child Neurol 39:286-291

Harris NG, Jones HC, Patel S (1994) Ventricle shunting in young H-Tx rats with inherited congenital hydrocephalus: a quantitative histological study of cortical gray matter. Child's Nerv Syst 10:293-301

Harwood-Nash DC (1982) Radiology of shunt complications in childhood hydrocephalus. Monogr Neural Sci 8:26-33

Hassler O (1964) Angioarchitecture in hydrocephalus. An autopsy and experimental study with the aid of microangiography. Acta Neuropathol 4:65-74

Hill A, Volpe JJ (1982) Decrease in pulsatile flow in the anterior cerebral artery in infantile hydrocephalus. Pediatrics 69:4-7

Hill A, Shackelford GD, Volpe JJ (1984) A potential mechanism of pathogenesis for early posthemorrhagic hydrocephalus in the premature newborn. Pediatrics 73:19-21

Hirsh JF, Kahn AP, Renier D, Sainte-Rose C, Hoppe-Hirsh E (1984) The Dandy Walker malformation. A review of 40 cases. J Neurosurg 61:515-522

Hockley AD (1982) Histological response to ventricular catheters. Monogr Neurol Sci 8:63-65

Horgan JG, Rumack CM, Hay T, Manco-Johnson ML, Merenstein GB, Esola C (1989) Absolute intracranial blood flow velocities evaluated by duplex Doppler sonography in asymptomatic preterm and term neonates. Am J Roentgenol 152:1059-1064

Horikawa M (1991) Usefulness of Doppler method for evaluating intracranial hemodynamics in infantile hydrocephalus. No To Hattatsu 23:200-206

Huang CC, Chio CC (1991) Duplex color ultrasound study of infantile progressive ventriculomegaly. Child's Nerv Syst 7:251-256

Iacopino DG, Zaccone C, Molina D, Todaro C, Tomasello F, Cardia E (1995) Intraoperative monitoring of cerebral blood flow during ventricular shunting in hydrocephalic pediatric patients. Child's Nerv Syst 11:483-486

Kirkinen P, Serlo W, Jouppila P, Rynanen M, Martikainen A (1996) Long term outcome of fetal hydrocephalus. J Child Neurol 11:189-192

Kirkpatrick M, Engelman H, Minns RA (1989) Signs and symptoms of progressive hydrocephalus. Arch Dis Child 64:124-128

Kokkonen J, Serlo W, Saukkonen AL, Juolasmaa (1994) Long term prognosis for children with shunted hydrocephalus. Child's Nerv Syst 10:384-387

Korobkin R (1975) The relationship between head circumference and the development of communicating hydrocephalus in infants following intraventricular hemorrhage. Pediatrics 56:74-77

Kreusser KL; Tarby TJ, Kovnar E, Taylor DA, Hill A, Volpe J (1985) Serial lumbar punctures for at least temporary amelioration of neonatal posthemorrhagic hydrocephalus. Pediatrics 75:719-724

Larroche JC (1972) Posthemorrhagic hydrocephalus in infancy: anatomical study. Biol Neonate 20:287-299

Levistsky DB, Mack LA, Nyberg DA, Shurtleff DB, Shields LA, Nghiem HV, Cyr DR (1995) Fetal aqueductal stenosis diagnosed sonographically: how grave is the prognosis. Am J Roentgenol 164:725-730

Lorber J, Pickering D (1966) Incidence and treatment of postmeningitic hydrocephalus in the newborn. Arch Dis Child 41:44-50

Lorenzo AV, Page LK, Watters GV (1970) Relationship between cerebrospinal fluid formation, absorption and pressure in human hydrocephalus. Brain 93:679-692

Lui K, Hellman J, Sprigg A, Daneman A (1990) Cerebral blood flow velocity patterns in post-hemorrhagic ventricular dilatation. Child's Nerv Syst 6:250-253

Lumenta CB, Skotarczak U (1995) Long term follow-up in 233 patients with congenital hydrocephalus. Child's Nerv Syst 11:173-175

Mai R, Rempen A, Kristen P (1995) Color flow mapping of the middle cerebral artery in 23 hydrocephalic fetuses. Arch Gynecol Obstet 256:155-158

Manning FA, Harrison MR, Rodeck C (1986) Catheter shunts for fetal hydronephrosis and hydrocephalus. Report of the international fetal surgery registry. N Engl J Med 315:336-340

Mantovani JF, Pasternak JF, Mathew OP, Allan WC, Mills MT, Casper J, Volpe JJ (1980) Failure of daily lumbar punctures to prevent the development of hydrocephalus following intraventricular hemorrhage. J Pediatr 97:278-281

Meyer JS, Tachibana H, Hardenberg JP, Dowell RE, Kitagawa Y, Mortel K (1984) Normal pressure hydrocephalus influences on cerebral hemodynamic and cerebrospinal fluid pressure – clinical autoregulations. Surg Neurol 21:195-203

Minns RA, Goh D, Pye S, Steers AJ (1991) A volume–blood flow velocity response (VFR) relationship derived from CSF compartment challenge as an index of progression of infantile hydrocephalus. In: Matsumoto S, Tamali N (eds) Hydrocephalus: pathogenesis and treatment. Springer, Tokyo Berlin Heidelberg, pp 270-278

Mori K (1995) Current concept of hydrocephalus: evolution of new classifications. Child's Nerv Syst 11:523-532

Nadvi SS, Du Trevou MD, Van Dellen JR, Gouws E (1994) The use of transcranial Doppler ultrasonography as a method of assessing intracranial pressure in hydrocephalic children. Br J Neurosurg 8:573-577

Naidich TP, Epstein F, Lin JP (1976) Evaluation of pediatric hydrocephalus by computed tomography. Radiology 119:337-345

Nishimaki S, Kawamaki T, Akamatsu H, Iwasaki Y (1991) Cerebral blood flow velocities in the anterior cerebral arteries and basilar artery. Investigation in hydrocephalus (part 2). No To Hattatsu 23:560-566

Norelle A, Fischer AQ, Flannery AM (1989) Transcranial Doppler: a noninvasive method to monitor hydrocephalus. J Child Neurol 4:87-90

Nyberg DA, Mack LA, Hirsch J, Pagon RO, Shepard TH (1987) Fetal hydrocephalus: sonographic detection and clinical significance of associated anomalies. Radiology 163:187-190

Oi S, Matsumoto S, Katayama K, Mochizuki M (1990) Pathophysiology and postnatal outcome of fetal hydrocephalus. Child's Nerv Syst 6:338-345

Osaka K, Handa H, Matsumoto S, Yasuda M (1980) Development of the cerebrospinal fluid pathway in the normal and abnormal human embryo. Child's Brain 6:26-38

Papile LA, Burstein J, Burstein R, Koffler H, Koops BJ, Johnson JD (1980) Post-hemorrhagic hydrocephalus in low birth weight infants: treatment by serial lumbar punctures. J Pediatr 12:445-448

Perez CA, Hodges FJ, Margolis AR (1964) Microangiography in experimental cerebral edema in rats. Radiology 82:529-535

Perlman JH, Goodman S, Kreusser KL, Volpe JJ (1985) Reduction in intraventricular hemorrhage by elimination of fluctuating cerebral blood flow velocity in preterm infants with respiratory distress syndrome. N Engl J Med 312:1353-1357

Poland RI, Slovis TL, Shankaran S (1985) Normal values of ventricular size as determined by real time sonographic techniques. Pediatr Radiol 15:12-14

Pople IK (1992) Doppler flow velocities in children with controlled hydrocephalus: reference values for the diagnosis of blocked cerebrospinal fluid shunts. Child's Nerv Syst 8:124-125

Pretorius DH, Davis K, Manco-Johnson ML, Manchester D, Meier P, Clewell WH (1985) Clinical course of fetal hydrocephalus: 40 cases. Am J Roentgenol 144:827-831

Quinn MW (1989) Intracranial arterial duplex Doppler waveform analysis in infants. Child's Nerv Syst 5:54-58

Raimondi AJ (1994) A unifying theory for the definition and classification of hydrocephalus. Child's Nerv Syst 10:3-12

Reeder JD, Sanders RC (1983) Ventriculitis in the neonate: recognition by sonography. Am J Neuroradiol 4:37-41

Rekate HL, Erwood S, Brodkey JA, Chizeck HJ, Spear T, Ko W, Montague F (1986) Etiology of ventriculomegaly in choroid plexus papilloma. Pediatr Neurosci 72:186-201

Rifkinson-Mann S, Leslie D, Goraj B, Kasoff S (1994) Transcranial Doppler ultrasonography in the evaluation of shunt function in the patient with hydrocephalus and spina bifida. Eur J Pediatr Surg 4 (Suppl 1):46

Rosenberg HK, Levine RS, Stoltz K, Smith DR (1983) Bacterial meningitis in infants: sonographic features. Am J Neuroradiol 4:822-825

Rosseau GL, Mc Cullough DC, Joseph AL (1992) Current prognosis in fetal ventriculomegaly. J Neurosurg 77:551-555

Rubin RC, Hoschwald G, Liwnicz B (1976) Hydrocephalus I: histological and ultrastructural changes in the preshunted cortical mantle. Surg Neurol 5:109-114

Rumack CM, Johnson ML (1982) Real time ultrasound evaluation of the neonatal brain. J Clin Ultrasound 10:179-202

Sahar A, Hochwald GM, Ransohoff J (1969) Alternative pathway for cerebrospinal fluid absorption in animals with experimental obstructive hydrocephalus. Exp Neurol 25:200-207

Saliba E, Santini JJ, Arbeille Ph, Chergui A, Gold F, Pourcelot L, Laugier J (1985) Mesure non invasive du flux sanguin cérébral chez le nourrisson hydrocéphale. Arch Fr Pediatr 42:97-102

Sanker P, Richard KE, Weigl HC, Klug N, Leyen K (1991) Transcranial Doppler sonography and intracranial pressure monitoring in children and juveniles with acute brain injuries or hydrocephalus. Child's Nerv Syst 7:391-393

Sato H (1986) Experimental congenital hydrocephalus. Pathogenetic processes in differentiating brain. Neurol Med Chir (Tokyo) 26:11-18

Seibert JJ, McCowan TC, Chadduck WM, Adametz JR, Glasier CM (1989) Duplex pulsed Doppler US versus intracranial pressure in the neonate: clinical and experimental studies. Radiology 171:155-159

Sekhar LN, Moosy J, Guthkelch N (1982) Malfunctioning ventriculoperitoneal shunts. J Neurosurg 56:411-416

Sgouros S, John P, Walsha, Hockley AD (1996) The value of colour Doppler imaging in assessing flow through ventriculoperitoneal shunts. Child's Nerv Syst 12:454-459

Shapiro K, Fried A, Marmarou A (1985) Biomechanical and hydrodynamic characterization of the hydrocephalic infant. J Neurosurg 63:69-75

Sherman JL, Citrin CM, Gangarosa RE, Bowen BJ (1986) The MR appearance of CSF flow in patients with ventriculomegaly. Am J Neuroradiol 7:1025-1031

Silverboard G, Horder MH, Ahmann PA (1980) Reliability of ultrasound in diagnosis of intracerebral hemorrhage and post-hemorrhagic hydrocephalus: comparison with CT. Pediatrics 66:507-512

Smith JR, Haber K, Reynolds AF, Weinstein PR (1982) Ultrasonic evaluation of post-ventricular shunt dynamics in infants and young children. Radiology 145:133-138

Smith J, Bannister C, Stellman-Ward C (1995) Long term outcome of 53 children with post-haemorrhagic hydrocephalus. Eur J Pediatr Surg 5 (Suppl 1):48

Taylor GA (1992) Effect of scanning pressure on intracranial hemodynamics during transfontanellar duplex Doppler examinations. Radiology 185:763-766

Taylor GA, Phillips MD, Ichord RN, Carson BS, Gates JA, James CS (1994) Doppler evaluation of intracranial compliance in infants. Radiology 191:787-791

Taylor G, Madsen J (1996) Neonatal hydrocephalus: hemodynamic response to fontanelle compression correlation with intracranial pressure and need for shunt placement. Radiology 201:685-689

Turcotte JF, Copty M, Bedard F (1980) Lateral ventricle choroid plexus papilloma and communicating hydrocephalus. Surg Neurol 13:276-279

Van Bel F, Van De Bor M, Baan HJ, Stijnen T, Ruys JH (1988) Blood flow velocity pattern of the anterior cerebral arteries before and after drainage of post-hemorrhagic hydrocephalus in the newborn. J Ultrasound Med 7:553-559

Veyrac C, Couture A, Baud C, Leboucq N (1987) Value of pulsed Doppler in cerebral hemorrhage of the newborn. Ann Radiol 30:463-469

Veyrac C (1988) Imagerie des tumeurs cérébrales du nouveau-né et du foetus. In: Couture A, Veyrac C, Baud C. Les malformations congénitales: diagnostic anténatal et devenir. Sauramps Medical, Montpellier, pp 240-247

Voigt H, Deeg K, Rupprecht T (1995) Cerebral Doppler ultrasound in fetal hydrocephalus. Z Geburtshilfe Perinatol 199:23-29

Volpe J, Pasternak JF, Allan CW (1977) Ventricular dilatation preceding rapid head growth following neonatal intracranial hemorrhage. Am J Dis Child 131:1212-1215

Vries JK (1980) Endoscopy as an adjunct to shunting for hydrocephalus. Surg Neurol 13:1212-1215

Widder DJ, Davies KR, Taveras JM (1986) Assessment of ventricular shunt patency by sonography: a new noninvasive test. Am J Neuroradiol 7:439-442

Wozniak M, McLone D, Raimondi AJ (1975) Micro and macrovascular changes as the direct cause of parenchymal destruction in congenital murine hydrocephalus. J Neurosurg 43:535-554

5 Anoxic-Ischemic Cerebral Damage

Alain P. Couture

CONTENTS

A. COUTURE
Department of Pediatric Radiology, Hôpital Arnaud de Villeneuve, 371 Av. Doyen Gaston Giraud, 34295 Montpellier Cédex 5, France

Clinical and experimental studies have shown that hemodynamic and gas exchange disorders occurring within the fetoplacental unit and neonatal brain may induce severe CNS damage, which frequently results in long-term neuropsychomotor sequelae (BROWN 1974; FINER 1983; SHANKARAN 1991; VANNUCCI 1997).

Hypoxic–ischemic encephalopathy involves several specialists of neonatal management:

- The obstetrician and prenatal sonographer (and now fetal MRI specialist) who gradually discover intrauterine brain lesions of circulatory origin (Fig. 5.1), and their scars mimicking developmental lesions (Fig. 5.2): porencephaly, multicystic encephalomalacia, hydranencephaly.
- The pediatrician in the intensive care unit, who knows that reducing the ischemic risk and improving the outcome require prevention of intrauterine ischemia, preservation of adequate ventilation perfusion and metabolism, and control of seizures.
- The pediatric radiologist, who is faced every day with the diagnosis and prognostic evaluation of ischemic brain damage.

The morphological approach to anoxic–ischemic lesions is known to be difficult because of the complexity and multiplicity of the lesions, the frequently associated neuropathological lesions (cortical necrosis, parasagittal infarction, porencephaly, periventricular and subcortical leukomalacia, arterial infarction, multicystic encephalomalacia, hydranencephaly), and because some lesions (status marmoratus) are described macroscopically rather than on imaging. In reality, improvement of the diagnosis requires the use of MRI and high-frequency ultrasound transducers (7.5 or 10 MHz). Ultrasonogra-

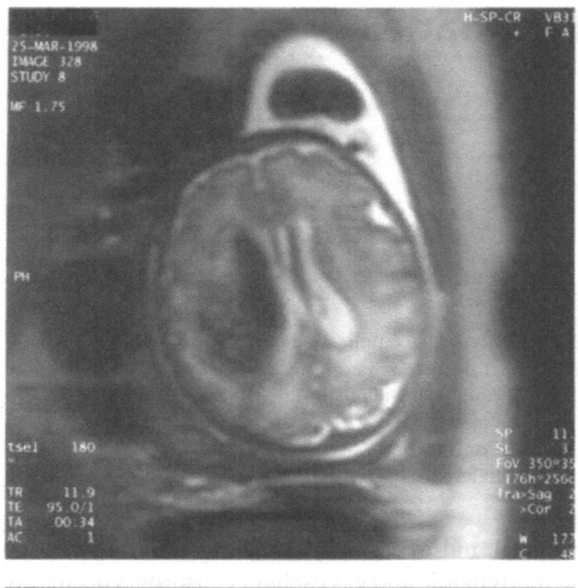

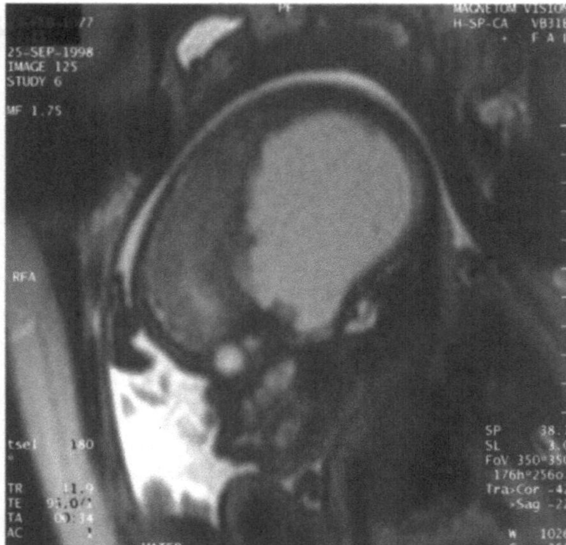

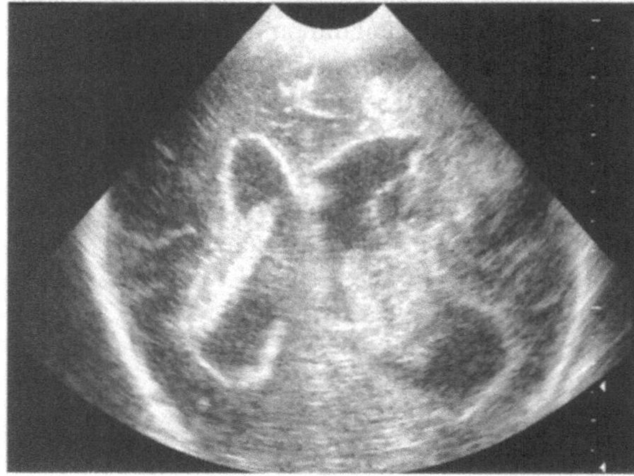

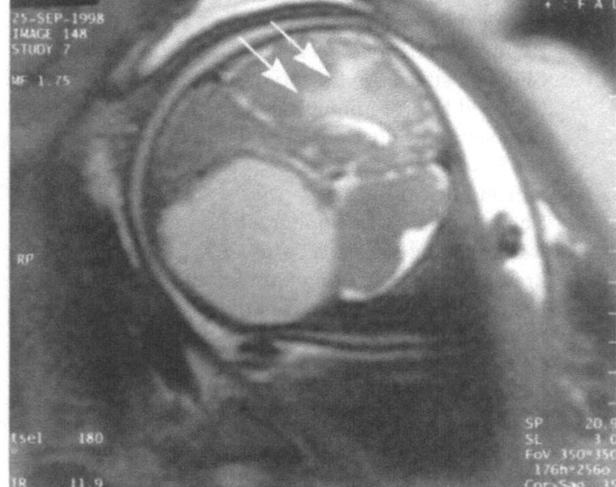

Fig. 5.1a,b. 31 weeks of gestation. Fetal ultrasonography detected a left periventricular hyperechoic area. MRI showed intraventricular hemorrhage and hemorrhagic infarct in the territory of the middle cerebral artery (**a**). The pregnancy was interrupted. Ischemic damage was confirmed by post-mortem ultrasonography (**b**)

Fig. 5.2a,b. Thirty-eight weeks' gestation. Ultrasound detection of left hemispheric cavity. Irregular and thickened edges, persistent perilesional ring of parenchyma, hyperintense signal (arrows) within contralateral centrum semiovale on T2-weighted MRI suggest an ischemic porencephalic cyst, confirmed at autopsy

phy, which remains of little interest to several authors (BABCOCK 1995; BARKOVICH 1997; SIEGEL 1984), nowadays, is a remarkable imaging modality for the evaluation of ischemic brain injury. Nevertheless, morphological description is no longer sufficient, being a passive investigation, unable to assess the progressiveness of the disease and suggest an early prognostic evaluation.

- It is essential to understand that the anoxic-ischemic process is related to changes in cerebral blood flow (CBF). This is why a hemodynamic study (pulsed, color, power Doppler) is required: it is an active investigation that can be orientated toward an early diagnosis and prognosis. Thus the pediatric radiologist should use Doppler ultrasonography together with gray scale ultrasonography in order to evaluate the severity of brain injury.

- Although ultrasonography and pre- and postnatal MRI constitute the main pillars of the diagnosis, the hemodynamic data add to this the assessment of an anoxic-ischemic encephalopathy: determination of arterial velocities, appreciation of the spectral analysis curve, color Doppler study of ischemic tissue, and understanding of brain ischemia physiopathology.

5.1
Pathogenesis

Cerebral blood flow changes play a main role in the development of neurological and neuropathological abnormalities resulting from perinatal asphyxia.

5.1.1
Experimental Data

The sequential events of perinatal asphyxia have been described in experimental models (ASHWAL 1980, 1984; BERHMAN 1970; CAVAZUTTI 1982; DUFFY 1982; GOLPERUD 1989; PURVES 1969; ROSENBERG 1985; ROSENBERG 1986; TWEED 1986; VANNUCCI 1993). Initially there is a preferential distribution of cardiac output to the brain, associated with an increase in arterial pressure and CBF; in parallel to this, cerebral autoregulation disappears. If asphyxia persists, systemic hypotension arises, with, as a consequence, a decrease in CBF.

5.1.1.1
Redistribution of Fetal Circulation

Immediately after the onset of asphyxia in fetal primate or lamb, there is a redistribution of cardiac output to the brain and coronary vessels (ASHWAL 1980; BALL 1994; BERHMAN 1970; RUDOLPH 1984).

5.1.1.2
Increase in Cerebral Blood Flow

This protective mechanism is initial in experimental models, and CBF increases by 50–500% (ASHWAL 1984; CAVAZUTTI 1982; COHN 1974; DUFFY 1982; JOHNSON 1979; PURVES 1969; ROSENBERG 1988). The increase is related to vasodilatation secondary to hypercapnia or/and hypoxemia. Indeed, arterial PCO_2 is known as one of the most powerful stimuli of CBF (BATTON 1983).

The response to hypercapnia and hypoxia varies widely among brain regions, depending on their metabolic demand, and gradually decreases in the brain stem, cerebellum, cortical gray matter, and white matter (CAVAZUTTI 1982; DUFFY 1982; JOHNSON 1979; GOPLERUD 1989; LEFFLER 1989; McPHEE 1985; MUJSCE 1989; ROSENBERG 1990; SZYMONOWICZ 1990). Thus there is poor adaptation of white matter to hypoxia (YOUNG 1982), especially in premature newborn (VOLPE 1997).

5.1.1.3
Loss of Cerebral Autoregulation

CBF is regulated by a remarkable mechanism which maintains a constant blood flow in the brain over a broad range of perfusion pressure. This constancy of CBF, called autoregulation, is due to arteriolar vasoconstriction with increased perfusion pressure and vasodilatation with decreased perfusion pressure.

Experimental studies have established (HERNANDEZ 1980; PAPILE 1985) that in preterm animal models, the autoregulatory mechanism is efficient only in a narrow range of arterial blood pressure. In the preterm lamb (PAPILE 1985), CBF remains unchanged for carotid mean arterial pressure ranging from 45 to 80 mmHg; above and below these values, CBF changes linearly with systemic arterial pressure, as a pressure-passive relationship.

Cerebral autoregulation is constantly impaired during perinatal asphyxia. Using the radioactive microsphere technique and producing asphyxia (pH 6.8–7.0) in term fetal sheep by partial occlusion of umbilical vessels, LOU (1979) demonstrated that CBF passively follows systemic arterial pressure changes: when mean arterial pressure rises to 60–70 mmHg, CBF increases up to six times normal, whereas when arterial pressure is lowered to 30 mmHg, CBF declines to close to zero in cortical areas.

In fetal animals, cerebral autoregulation appears to be extremely sensitive to asphyxia and its hallmarks, which are hypoxemia and hypercapnia.

Finally, in experimental conditions, the autoregulatory protective mechanisms depend on the arterial blood pressure level and follow regional variations. ARNOLD (1991) demonstrated in fetal lamb that the upper limits of arterial pressure that are associated with efficient autoregulation are the same in all brain regions, in contrast to the lower limits, which may fall very low in brain stem and basal ganglia.

5.1.1.4
Systemic Hypotension and Decrease in CBF

The rapidity and severity of systemic hypotension and the drop in CBF depend on the duration and severity of asphyxial insult.

The decrease in cardiac output, probably resulting from myocardial impairment, leads to systemic hypotension. The consequences for the brain may be devastating because loss of autoregulation leaves CBF at the mercy of systemic deficiency.

REIVICH (1972) demonstrated a severe decrease in CBF, particularly in the parasagittal areas of the cerebral hemispheres, in fetal monkeys subjected to severe and prolonged asphyxia. Similarly, white matter of newborn dogs has been shown to be particularly sensitive to a decrease in CBF (YOUNG 1982).

5.1.1.5
Postasphyxial Reperfusion

Several authors (CHIAMULERA 1993; FELLMAN 1997; HAMMERMAN 1998; LINNIK 1993; VANNUCCI 1997) have studied the hemodynamic events which follow asphyxial insult in animal models. ROSENBERG (1990) has described, in newborn lamb, initial cerebral hyperemia, followed after 30–60 min by hypoperfusion associated with an excess of vasoconstrictor molecules (KARLSSON 1994; PALMER 1995) and/or the presence of free radicals.

This secondary hypoperfusion is probably multifactorial, and the mechanisms implicated are endothelial impairment due to inflammatory injury, edema (PETITO 1982; PLUTA 1994), influx of granulocytes in microvessels (DEL ZOPPO 1991; ZHANG 1994), and intravascular clotting (THOMAS 1993).

Experimental studies have demonstrated the serious effect of delayed postasphyxial hypoperfusion, especially as loss of cerebral autoregulation and a reduction in oxygen consumption are associated with it.

Taken together, experimental models show the precise hemodynamic changes which follow asphyxia:
- *First*, compensatory adaptive response with redistribution of circulation to brain and a rise in CBF
- *Second*, a cascade of events leading to a fall in CBF and ischemic insult
- *Third*, worsening of lesions reinforced by CBF reduction

5.1.2
Pathogenesis in the Human Newborn

Cerebral autoregulation disturbances have been well demonstrated in the asphyxial newborn (BLANKENBERG 1997; PANERAI 1995). LOU (1979), using the xenon clearance technique in 19 asphyxial neonates, reported a linear relationship between CBF and mean arterial pressure. This pressure-passive relationship suggests inoperative autoregulation, similar to what is obtained in experimental models.

Thus, cerebral vascular autoregulation does exist in the human newborn, and represents a vulnerable, fragile, and labile process, especially in the premature

infant (MULLIGAN 1980). Moderate hypoxia is sufficient to impair autoregulation for more than 7 h (LOU 1979). Hypercapnia and hypoxia induced by perinatal asphyxia are mainly responsible for these alterations. An increase in CBF of 8.6% per 1 mmHg increase in arterial PCO_2 has been shown (LEAHI 1980).

In the same way, COOKE (1979) reports a direct relationship between CBF and arterial PCO_2 in 13 preterm neonates with respiratory distress.

The clinical implications of these data may be imagined: a drop in cardiac output necessarily results in reduced CBF, with subsequent irreversible brain damage (leukomalacia in preterm infants, parasagittal injury in full-term newborns).

Most authors think with LOU (1979) that 20 ml/100 mg per minute constitutes the critical threshold value of CBF that correlates with irreversible ischemic brain damage.

Finally, in contrast to the experimental animal models, a pronounced sustained cerebral hyperemia is observed after perinatal asphyxia, propably due to vasoplegia (PRYDS 1990), and appearing from 6 to 130 h after the insult (ARCHER 1986; RAMAKAERS 1990).

5.1.3
Practical Consequences

The practical consequences are obvious: a fetus or preterm or full-term newborn presenting severe asphyxia requires analysis of CBF. Several techniques have been proposed for obtaining this information. Some utilize inert gas (N_2O) or radioactive xenon (xenon-133), administered either by intravenous or intra-arterial injection or by inhalation; but this for investigation is criticized for being invasive and exposing the patient to radiation. Other techniques allow the study of changes in intracranial volume after brief occlusion of the jugular veins (plethysmography), but present multiple causes of error with underestimation of CBF. These difficulties point up the usefulness of Doppler ultrasonography, which provides serial information about cerebrovascular resistance and flow velocities, especially in perinatal asphyxia (COUTURE 1987, 1994, 1996; LIVES 1998).

5.2
Hypoxic–Ischemic Encephalopathy

Hypoxic–ischemic encephalopathy is defined as a deficit in oxygen supply to neural tissue. Two major mechanisms are distinguished, hypoxemia and ischemia, which occur in different circumstances.

Hypoxia is caused by intrauterine asphyxia, respiratory distress, recurrent apneic spells, or severe right-to-left shunts secondary to heart disease or persistent fetal circulation. Ischemia is the result of cardiac failure, secondary to intrauterine asphyxia, recurrent apneic spells, large patent ductus arteriosus, severe congenital heart disease, or vascular collapse.

This distinction also relates to the neuropathological consequences (Diagram 5.1): hypoxia is responsible for neuronal necrosis or status marmoratus of the basal ganglia or thalami, while ischemia induces either periventricular leukomalacia in the premature infant, parasagittal injury in the full-term newborn, or cerebral focal necrosis (porencephaly, multicystic encephalomalacia, hydranencephaly).

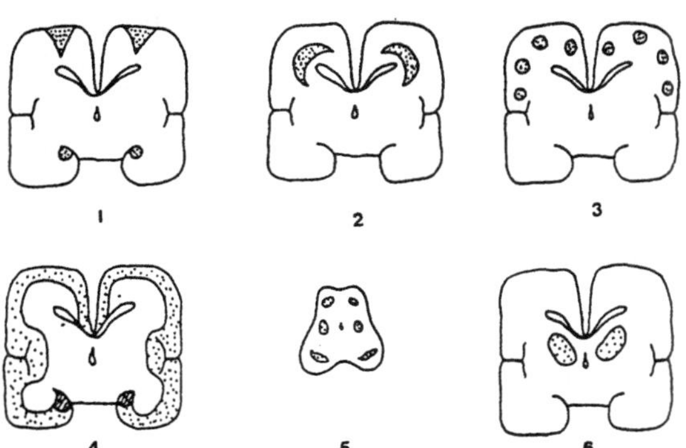

Diagram 5.1. Hypoxic–ischemic encephalopathy. Neuropathological patterns (LEVENE 1987)
  1 Parasagittal cerebral injury
  2 Periventricular leukomalacia
  3 Subcortical leukomalacia
  4 Cortical ischemia
  5 Brain stem ischemia
  6 Basal ganglia and thalamus ischemia

5.2.1
Clinical Pattern: An Essential Guide for Neonatal Neuroradiological Investigations
(RIVKIN 1997; ROLAND 1995; VOLPE 1995)

Anoxic–ischemic encephalopathy is a frequent and severe complication of perinatal asphyxia (FENICHEL 1983; GRAY 1983; LEVENE 1987; VOLPE 1976). In many cases the immediate prognosis remains dreadful (EKERT 1997; FINER 1983). The long-term sequelae are significant (DE SOUZA 1978; ISHIKAWA 1987; KORNBERG 1985; MULLIGAN 1980; ROBERTSON 1993; SCOTT 1976): motor deficits are common, mental retardation is often evident, seizures are frequent. The incidence, timing and clinical circumstances are essential to precise.

– According to different reports (BROWN 1974; ERGANDER 1983; FINER 1983; MACDONALD 1980; NELSON 1981; VANNUCCI 1997), 2.9–9‰ full-term newborns suffer asphyxia at birth, while 6‰ develop anoxic–ischemic damage (BROWN 1974; LEVENE 1987) and 1‰ suffer severe encephalopathy. These data point up the importance of neuroradiological investigations, especially by ultrasound, in an attempt to gain a better assessment of the severity of the disease in neonate.

– The timing of vascular injury is important to know (Table 5.1). VOLPE (1995) and other authors (BROWN 1974; LOW 1985, 1997) have shown the predominance of ante- and perinatal difficulties. VOLPE (1995) reported that antepartum events (maternal hypotension, often with major uterine hemorrhage) account for approximately 20% of cases. Intrapartum events (traumatic delivery, prolonged labor, acute placental or cord disturbances) occur in approximately 35% of cases. In an additional percentage (35%), intrapartum disturbances (fetal heart alterations, meconium-stained amniotic fluid) are present, often associated with antepartum difficulties (maternal diabetes, preeclampsia, intrauterine growth retardation). Finally, postnatal insults (recurrent apneic spells, cardiac failure, respiratory distress) affects approximately 10% or less of infants. These results are confirmed by BROWN (1974), who found the same incidences (antepartum 50%, intrapartum 40%, postpartum 10%) in a large series of asphyxial newborns.

Table 5.1. Anoxic–ischemic encephalopathy in full-term neonate (VOLPE 1995)

Timing of insult	Approximate % of total
Antepartum	20
Intrapartum	35
Intra +/- antepartum	35
Postnatal	10

It is clear that anoxic–ischemic encephalopathy is predominantly related to intrauterine asphyxia.

– The severity of anoxic–ischemic encephalopathy is closely related to the intensity and duration of antenatal, perinatal, or postnatal asphyxia. Several authors (FINER 1983; HILL 1989; LEVENE 1985; ROBERTSON 1985; SARNAT 1976) have proposed a classification by grades of increasing severity (Table 5.2):

Table 5.2. Classification of hypoxic–ischemic encephalopathy (From SARNAT 1976)

Grade I:	Normal consciousness
	Jitteriness
	Tone: mild disorders
	Seizures: none
	EEG: normal
Grade II:	Lethargy
	Hypotonia
	Seizures: focal or multifocal
	EEG: epileptiform activity – voltage suppression
Grade III:	Coma or deep stupor
	Severe hypotonia
	Status epilepticus
	EEG: Burst suppression pattern

● *Grade I or mild encephalopathy* is characterized by jitteriness, hyperalert state, and short periods of sleep. Sympathetic overactivity is noticed with dilated reactive pupils and tachycardia (SARNAT 1976). Muscle tone is mildly disturbed (axial hypotonia). These symptoms may disappear in 48 h.

● Lethargy, irritability, poor feeding, tone disorders, disappearance of primary reflexes, and seizures controlled by anticonvulsive therapy characterize *grade II or moderate encephalopathy*. These symptoms usually disappear at the end of the first week, but 20%–40% of these infants will develop long-term sequelae, especially if the first clinical signs persist for longer than 1 week.

● In *grade III or severe encephalopathy* deep stupor or coma is associated with major hypotonia, brain stem disturbances, generalized seizures, and increased intracranial pressure. This pattern is invariably followed by a poor outcome; status epilepticus or generalized seizures are often resistant to anticonvulsive therapy, and severe neurological features persist after 1 week: deep coma, often associated with apneic spells, brain stem dysfunctions (abnormal pupillary response and oculomotor movements) which appear in the first 3 days of life, and medullary impairment (swallowing and sucking disturbances) which develops later and is sustained. After the first week, a generalized hypotonia of limbs and a major decrease of spontaneous movements are commonly observed.

To summarize, although seizures obviously increase the risk of long-term sequelae (FINER 1983; MULLIGAN 1980; ROBERTSON 1985; SARNAT 1976), the duration of neurological anomalies is the main criterion of the severity of hypoxic–ischemic encephalopathy (ROBERTSON 1985; SARNAT 1976; SCOTT 1976). This hallmark is reliable, but a precise clinical prediction of the outcome for the infant is not always possible in the first days of life.

This underlines the importance of an early ultrasound evaluation which may provide not only diagnostic findings, but also some of prognostic value.

5.2.2
Ultrasound Evaluation: Value, Limitations, and Potentialities

Doppler ultrasound investigation (color, power, and pulsed Doppler) is of most value when it is used to complete a morphological assessment of cerebral ischemia (by ultrasound or MRI): an appreciation of the prognosis of subcortical ischemia, detection of low blood flow or velocimetric disturbances (heart rate disorders, fluctuating Doppler, spectral analysis curve alterations, disappearance or reversal of diastolic flow), the search for thrombosis in an arterial infarction, and more. An accurate morphological examination is the compulsory preliminary to a high-quality hemodynamic exploration.

5.2.2.1
Morphological Imaging

Ultrasonography has a bad reputation in the diagnosis of hypoxic–ischemic encephalopathy in the full-term newborn, (BABCOCK 1995; BARKOVICH 1997; BLANKENBERG 1996; HOPE 1988; O'SHEA 1993; RUTHERFORD 1994; SHANKARAN 1993; SIEGEL 1984; VOLPE 1995).

VOLPE (1987) noted that ultrasound cannot detect selective neuronal necrosis because cortical lesions are too restricted (Fig. 5.3) and brain stem lesions too far from the transducer; the same holds for parasagittal cerebral injury, which is too peripherally located.

SIEGEL (1984), studying 32 patients with anoxic-ischemic encephalopathy, observed that cerebral hyperechogenicity usually corresponded to a poor outcome, but there was no correlation between sonographic and neuropathological findings: five cases of cortical neuronal necrosis were observed at post-mortem examination without a sonographic correlate in any.

Finally, neonatal cerebral ischemia (BABCOCK 1995; SIEGEL 1984; SLOVIS 1984) does not seem to correspond to a specific sonographic pattern:
– The diffuse hyperechogenicity of cerebral parenchyma shadowing sulci and fissures is the main feature of anoxic–ischemic encephalopathy (Fig. 5.4) (GUPTA 1983; MARTIN 1983).

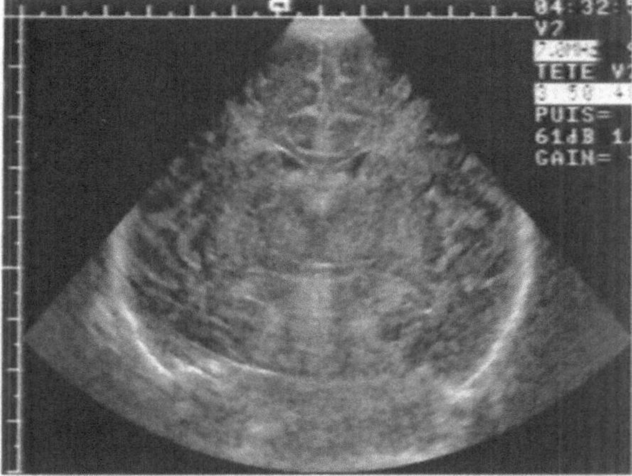

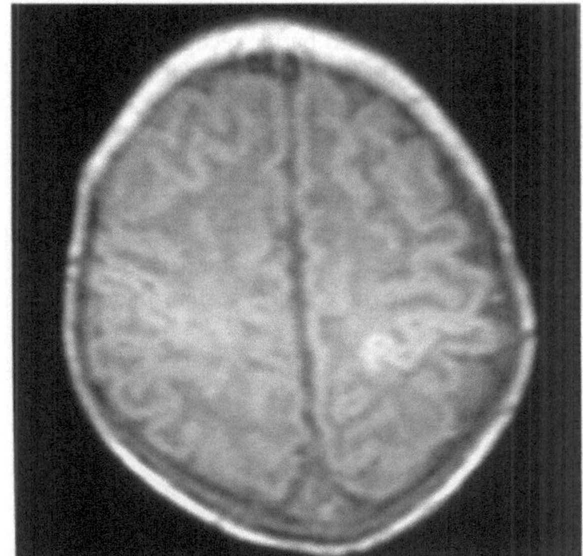

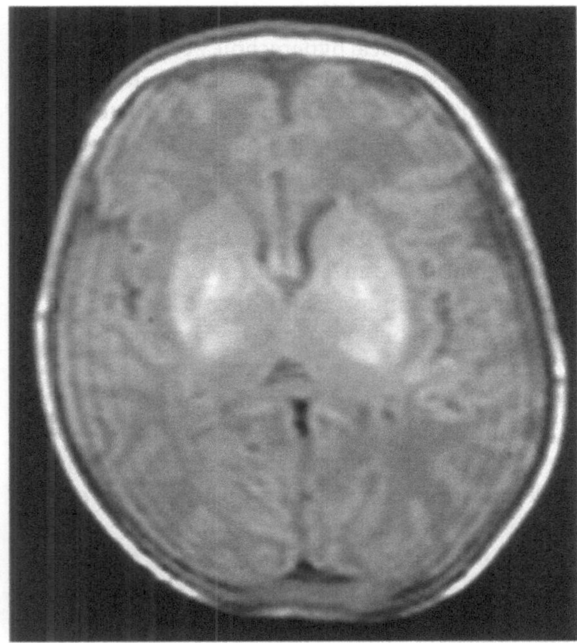

Fig. 5.3a,b,c. 9 days old newborn. Acute fetal distress secondary to cord prolapse. US (a): Ganglio thalamic and subcortical ischemia are detected. Simultaneous MRI (b) confirms these lesions (hyperintense foci on T1–weighted sequence) and reveals associated damage of cortical gray matter in left central gyrus (c). These structures which are myelinated at birth are commonly damaged in severe asphyxia, and their location (superficial and posterior) makes them difficult or impossible to detect sonographically

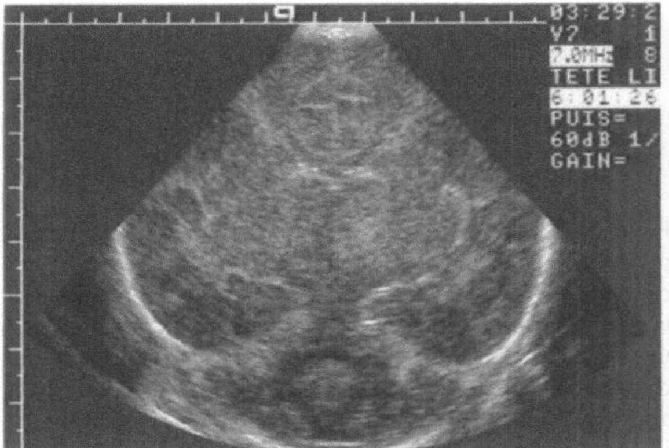

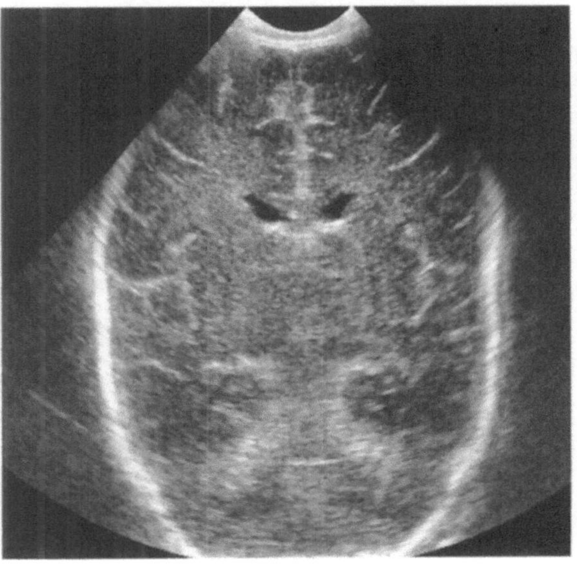

Fig. 5.4a,b. A 2-day-old neonate. Anoxic–ischemic encephalopathy with status epilepticus. Brain parenchyma was hyperechoic, sulci had disappeared, ventricles had collapsed (a). These anomalies were striking as compared with the normal neonatal pattern (b)

Nevertheless, this pattern lacks specificity and fails to recognize focal hyperechoic peripheral lesions (cortical gray matter ischemia, parasagittal injury). However, ultrasound is conclusive in the detection of injury to the basal ganglia and thalami (CABANAS 1991). Thus, appreciation of an ischemic brain requires wide experience, because changes in the echo structure may be subtle. BARR (1996) has suggested quantitative measurement of tissue echogenicity in order to improve the diagnosis.

HILL (1991) believes that the interpretation of sonographic changes in full-term newborn ischemia is often subjective, which explains the poor sensitivity of ultrasonography as reported by BABCOCK (1995). By contrast ultrasound is clearly effective in the demonstration of postischemic sequelae: cerebral atrophy, porencephalic cyst, and others.

- Early prediction of the prognosis on the basis of morphological features is a difficult challenge because simple edema, irreversible ischemia, hematoma, and even tumor have the same sonographic appearance (Fig. 5.5). Detection of collapsed lateral ventricles during perinatal asphyxia is of little diagnostic value since it is frequently observed in normal newborns (BABCOCK 1995; SIEGEL 1984). These observations are not to be discussed and explain the difficulty in interpreting the ultrasound examination to diagnose anoxic-ischemic encephalopathy.

- Our experience shows that ultrasound does not have the place it deserves in the diagnosis of cerebral ischemia; the routine use of high-frequency probes has completely changed the morphological diagnosis (COUTURE 1994). The sonographic description of focal or diffuse ischemic lesions relies nowadays on objectively reproducible features, and the main neuropathological entities (neuronal necrosis, parasagittal injury, basal ganglia ischemia, periventricular leukomalacia) are becoming better and better recognized on ultrasonography and MRI (BARKOVITCH 1995; CHRISTOPHE 1994; HUPPI 1997; MERCURI 1999; RUTHERFORD 1995, 1996).

● Selective Neuronal Necrosis

Selective neuronal necrosis probably results from oxygen deprivation in the perinatal period. The sites of predilection are the cerebral cortex, diencephalon

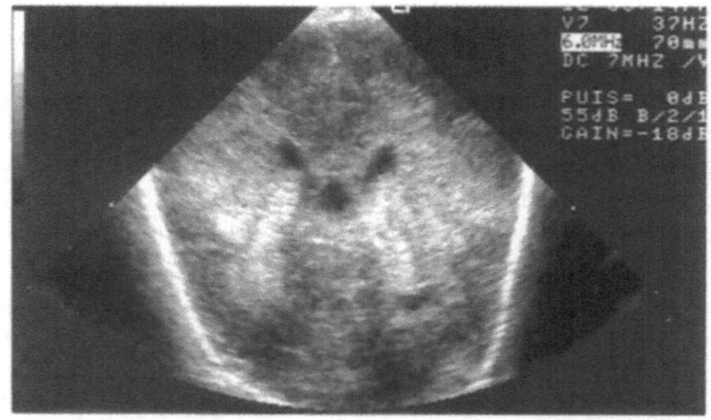

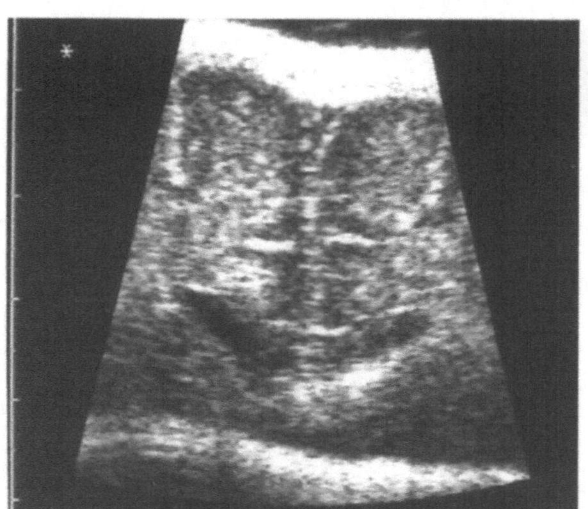

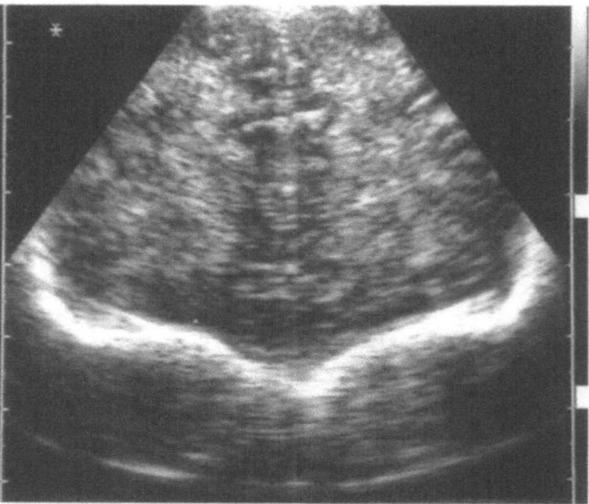

Fig. 5.5a–c. These three newborns show similar abnormal parenchymal echogenicity, but their clinical histories and courses differ, allowing a precise diagnosis. a A 29-weeks' gestation preterm baby. Severe hyaline membrane disease. First ultrasound exam suggested extensive periventricular and subcortical leukomalacia. At 1 month, periventricular cysts appeared. b A full-term newborn. Perinatal asphyxial injury. Repeated seizures. White matter was obviously hyperechoic but hemodynamics appeared normal. Subcortical densities rapidly resolved with signs of reversible edema. Psychomotor development was normal at 2 years of age. c Neonatal status epilepticus. Diffuse subcortical hyperechogenicity and hyperperfusion on pulsed Doppler: subcortical ischemic damage, as confirmed by CT. The patient died on day 6

(WILSON 1982), brain stem (ROLAND 1988; RORKE 1992), cerebellum, and spinal cord (CLANCY 1989). The neurological presentation mainly depends on the location of the lesions. Disturbances of consciousness (coma) are attributable to involvement of the cerebral hemispheres and reticular activating system in the brain stem and diencephalon. Seizures relate to hypoxic injury of the cerebral cortex. Cerebral or/and cerebellar cortical or spinal injury may explain the intense hypotonia. Finally, oculomotor disorders and sucking and swallowing impairments are probably due to brain stem cranial nerve nuclear involvement.

The long-term sequelae are striking and including mental retardation, spastic quadriparesis, and seizure disorders. The severity of these sequelae show why early detection of damage to the cerebral cortex, cerebellar cortex, basal ganglia, or brain stem is important. Although ultrasonography is effective in several circumstances (QUIOGUE 1987), it is obviously inadequate when the cerebral cortex, cerebellum, or brain stem is involved, and this is where MRI is extremely valuable (BARKOVITCH 1995; CASTILLO 1995) (Fig. 5.3).

Ultrasonography will show fronto-parietal cortex necrosis, which appears as hyperechoic gray matter close to the fissures, corresponding to cortical hyperintensity on T1-weighted MRI.
- When hypoxic injury is massive, the gray matter of the interhemispheric surface, gyri of the convexity, and basal ganglia look like an hyperechoic patchwork, often extending to the subcortical white matter (Fig. 5.6). The diagnosis is easy, the prognosis disastrous. On the convexity, the cortex appears as a discontinuous hyperechoic ribbon, contrasting with the relative hypoechogenicity of subjacent white matter (Fig. 5.7).
- High-frequency probes (10 mHz) are necessary to detect focal and superficial cortical necrosis in the frontal lobe; low-frequency probes are required to appreciate lesions of the occipital, parietal and temporal cortex (Fig. 5.8).
- Finally, ultrasound diagnosis of infratentorial cortical necrosis remains extremely difficult. In rare circumstances, ultrasonography may reveal acute infratentorial ischemia (Fig. 5.9) or porencephalic atrophy of the cerebellum or brain stem following fetal asphyxia. Of course, the gold standard is MRI (BARKOVITCH 1995).

● **Parasagittal Ischemia** (PASTERNAK 1987)
This entity refers to a lesion of the cerebral cortex and subcortical white matter with a characteristic

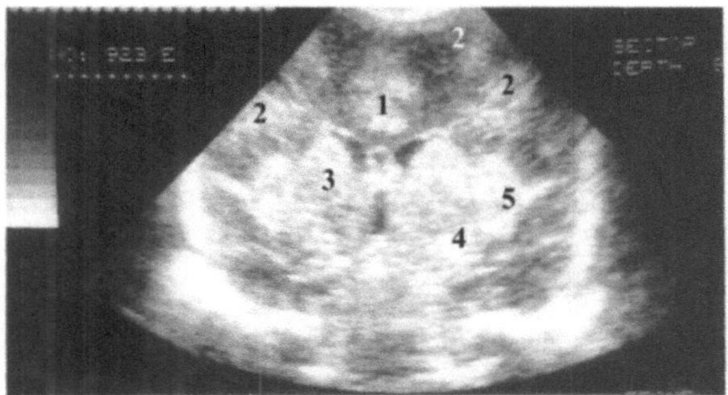

Fig. 5.6. A full-term newborn, 3 days old. Severe neurological distress. Gray matter involvement along the interhemispheric fissure (*1*) and on the brain surface (*2*) appears as wide and poorly limited hyperechoic areas. Note the severe impairment of the caudate nucleus (*3*), genu of internal capsule, lenticulate nuclei (*4*), external capsule, claustrum, extreme capsule, and insular cortex (*5*)

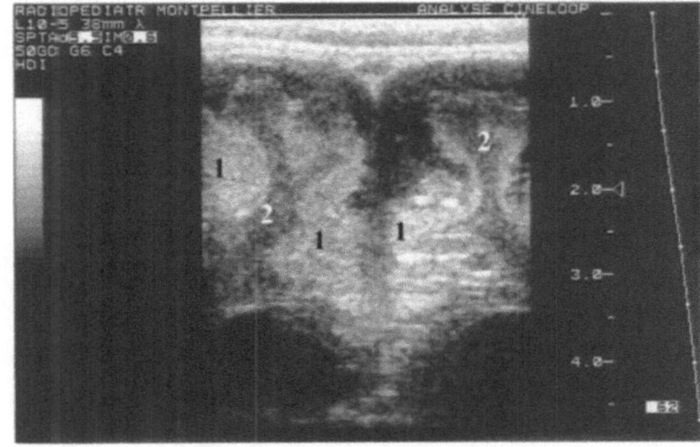

Fig. 5.7. A 5-month-old infant. Status epilepticus. Selective neuronal necrosis appears as a thick hyperechoic ribbon (*1*) surrounding normal hypoechoic subcortical white matter (*2*)

parasagittal distribution (Diagram 5.2) i.e., superior-medial aspects of the cerebral convexities. It is bilateral and affects especially the parieto-occipital areas, the most vulnerable regions. Parasagittal injury is characterized by necrosis of the cortex and the subjacent white matter, and is the principal ischemic lesion of the full-term newborn. In fact, it is rarely isolated and most often constitutes the main damage of more diffuse ischemia.

In the opinion of VOLPE (1977), parasagittal injury is extremely common during hypoxic-ischemic encephalopathy, as shown by positron emission tomography. It results from a low blood flow within the border zones between the end-fields of the anterior, middle, and posterior cerebral arteries (Diagram 5.2). Suggestive clinical findings include a particular weakness of the proximal limbs, more

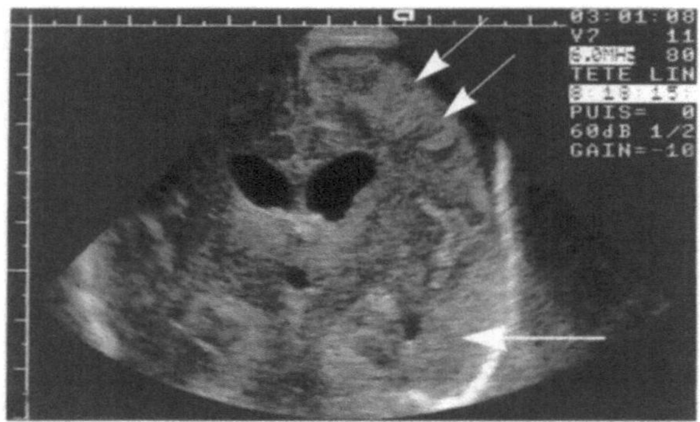

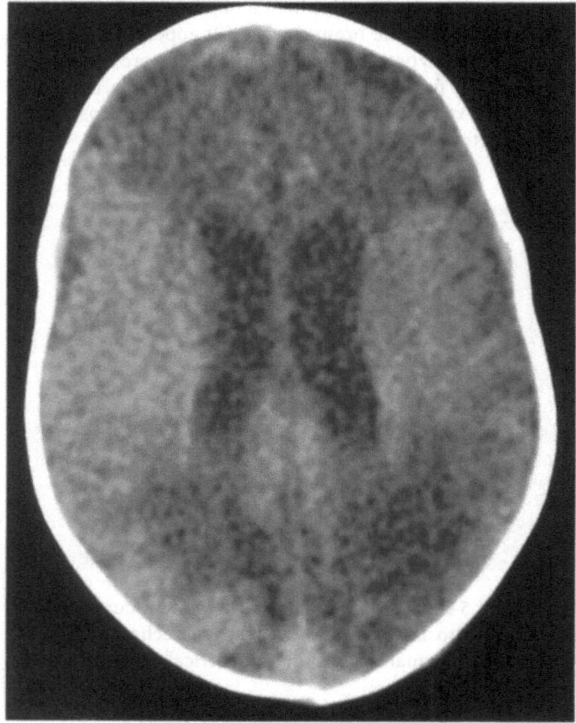

Fig. 5.8a,b. A 3-month-old infant. *Neisseria meningitidis* meningitis. Damage to frontal (*double arrow*) and temporal (*long arrow*) gray matter (**a**). Confirmation by CT (**b**)

prominent in the upper than in the lower extremities. The long-term sequelae are poorly known, but VOLPE (1995) reported that spastic quadriparesis and disorders in the development of language or visual-spatial abilities are frequent.

VOLPE (1995) emphasized the value of positron emission tomography, which demonstrates a reduction in CBF to parasagittal regions, more marked posteriorly than anteriorly.

The ultrasound appearance of this lesion is poorly described in the literature (HUANG 1987; LEVENE

1987), and the relative ineffectiveness of ultrasonography is due to several reasons:

– Access to the cortical gray matter and subcortical white matter is difficult in the supero-medial parenchyma, especially the posterior cerebrum, and transfontanellar ultrasonography cannot reach the damaged areas. This is where MRI is valuable.
– Moreover, the lesion is often obscured within a diffuse hyperechoic atmosphere of gray and white matter. In our experience, when isolated, it appears on high-frequency ultrasonography as bilateral wedge-shaped hyperechoic images within parasagittal areas (Fig. 5.10), followed by rapid onset of cerebral atrophy or cortico-subcortical cysts (Fig. 5.11).

● **Ischemic Lesions of Basal Ganglia and Thalami**
Ischemic lesions of basal ganglia and thalami affect more full-term than premature infants and seem to be very frequent (KOTAGAL 1983; PASTERNAK 1991;

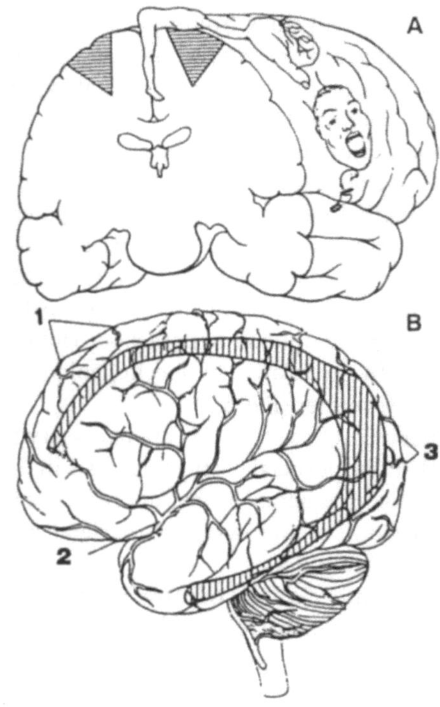

Diagram 5.2A,B. Parasagittal cerebral injury From VOLPE (1995)
Superior medial aspects of the cerebral convexity are involved (**A**) and areas of necrosis appear at the end-fields of the anterior, middle, and posterior cerebral arteries.

  1 Anterior cerebral artery
  2 Middle cerebral artery
  3 Posterior cerebral artery

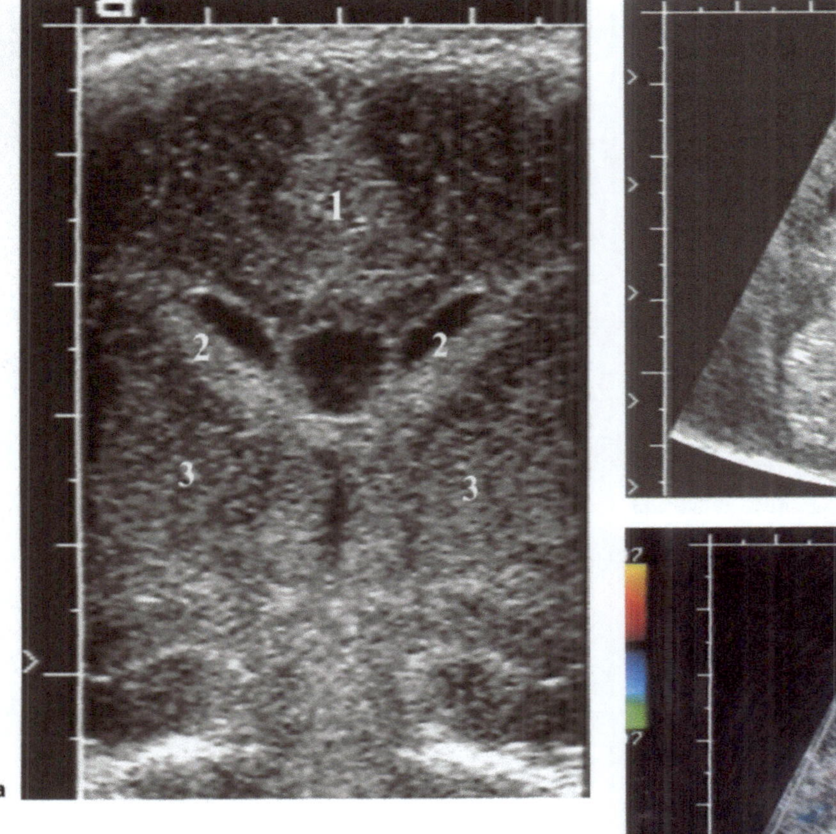

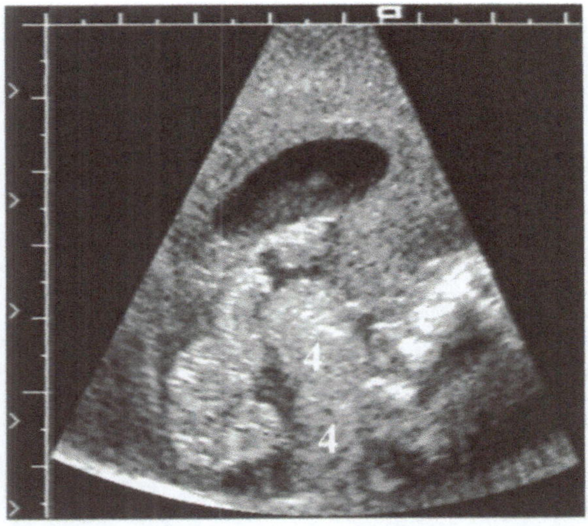

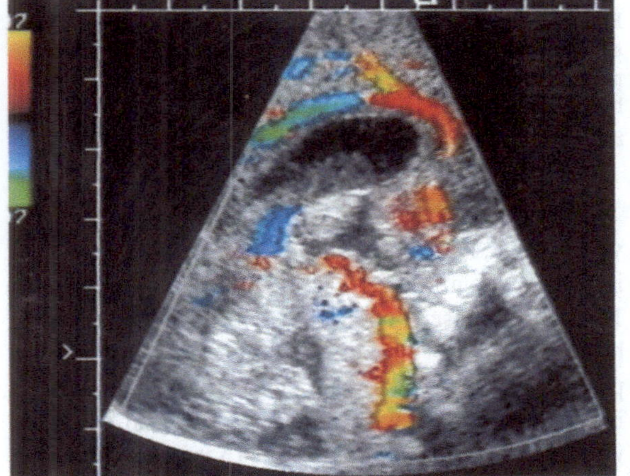

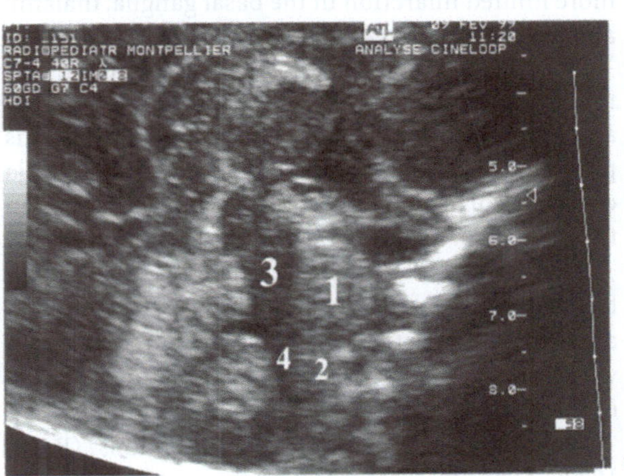

Fig. 5.9a–d. A 29-weeks' gestation preterm infant. Apparent stillbirth. EEG silence. Diffuse ischemia (a) with associated cortical necrosis (*1*), hyperechogenicity of caudate nuclei (*2*) and thalami (*3*), and enlarged hyperechoic midbrain (*4*) (b) with basilar artery compression (c). This is the sign of a major midbrain ischemia (pons and medulla) and explains the clinical pattern: absence of spontaneous ventilation and movements, absence of cough reflex. This location of ischemia is infrequent and sonographic diagnosis is easy if the normal appearance is well known (d): the ventral portion of the pons (*1*) and medulla (*2*) are hyperechoic, probably representing both decussation of the pyramidal tract and the presence of inferior olivary nuclei which produce strong interfaces. The dorsal portion of the pons (*3*) and medulla (*4*) have low echogenicity, probably corresponding to the more homogeneous structure of the longitudinal fibers with fewer interfaces

VOIT 1987). The most commonly involved nuclei are the putamen, the caudate, and the thalamus, which is impaired in 80%–90% of cases (MALAMUD 1950), while the globus pallidus is frequently but less severely involved.

Basal ganglia are particularly vulnerable to severe ischemia, as demonstrated by experimental studies after umbilical cord compression (MYERS 1975) and by follow-up on ultrasonography (CABANAS 1991; SHEN 1984), CT (KOTAGAL 1983) and MRI (BARKO-

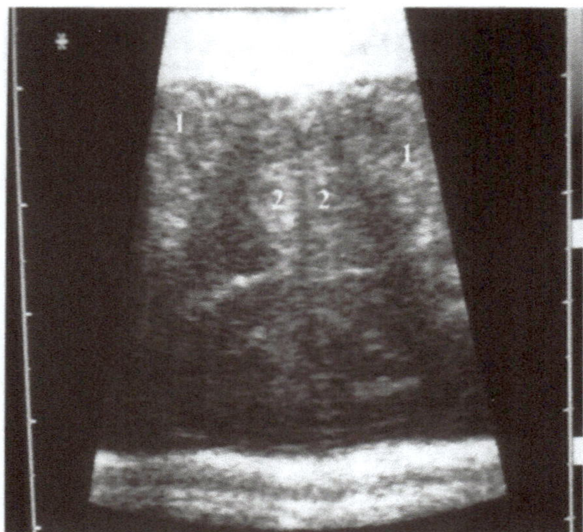

Fig. 5.10. A 5-month-old infant. Cardiorespiratory arrest and status epilepticus. Ultrasonography showed a characteristic parasagittal injury with wedge-shaped cortico-subcortical hyperechogenicity (*1*). Note the neuronal necrosis within the gray matter close to the interhemispheric fissure (*2*)

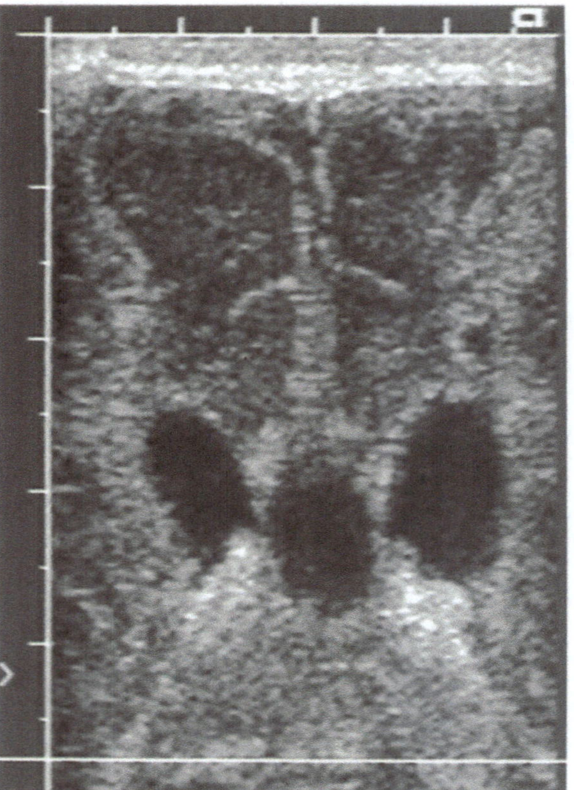

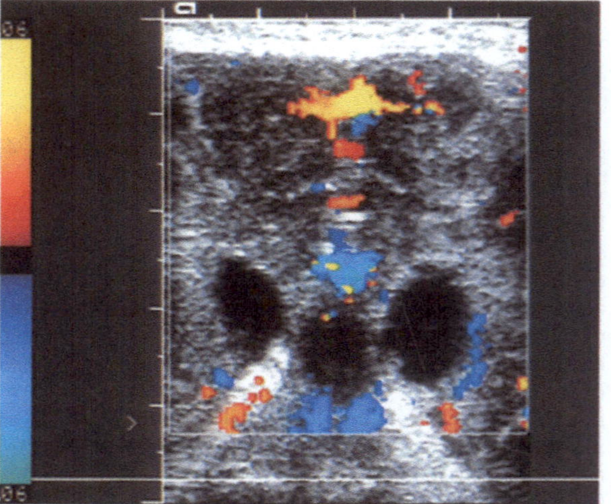

Fig. 5.11a,b. A full-term infant. Apparent stillbirth requiring 10 min cardiac resuscitation. At 1 month of age, parasagittal injury was diagnosed, appearing as posterior cortico-subcortical hyperechoic areas. Note left cystic necrosis (**a**). On color Doppler imaging, lesions were avascular (**b**). MRI confirmed the diagnosis

VITCH 1995; RUTHERFORD 1995). Experimental studies by MYERS and others (BRANN 1975; MYERS 1969, 1975) have described the distribution of ischemic lesions during anoxic–ischemic encephalopathy: prolonged partial asphyxia (1–3 h) results in diffuse infarction (cortex, white matter, and basal ganglia), while acute total asphyxia (10–15 min) produces a more limited infarction in the basal ganglia, thalami, and brain stem (ROLAND 1998).

In human neonatal pathology, basal ganglia and thalami ischemia is rarely isolated but is most often associated with cortical and subcortical damage. This probably explains why injury of the basal ganglia does not correlate with a precise clinical pattern in the neonate (VOLPE 1995).

MALAMUD (1950) reported the long-term neurological sequelae; these are mainly extrapyramidal abnormalities, particularly bilateral choreoathetosis, which appears to be related to bilateral involvement of the basal ganglia and intact pyramidal tracts.

Dyskinetic and dystonic manifestations (BRUN 1979; FOLEY 1992) seem to be a consequence of bilateral globus pallidus involvement. Finally, it has been proven that thalamic injury is critical in causing intellectual deficits, which are common in these children (KYLLERMAN 1982).

All authors (CABANAS 1991; CONNOLLY 1994; KREUSSER 1984; NAIDICH 1986; SHANKARAN 1991; SHEN 1984) have reported the great value of ultra-sonography in diagnosing ischemic lesions of the basal ganglia. SHEN (1984) describes in six severely asphyxiated newborns a special sonographic appearance termed "bright thalamus"; this is a diffuse hyperechogenicity seen all over the thalamus, with sharp regular margins, distinguishing it from the appearance of hemorrhagic necrosis which appears strongly echogenic with irregular margins.

CABANAS (1991) reported three patients with gangliothalamic hyperechogenicity, and showed cerebral atrophy specifically located in the thalamus and basal ganglia characterized by an irregular inner border of the ventricular wall which contributes to ventriculomegaly. These patients had a poor outcome.

Finally, NAIDICH (1988) detailed precisely the topography of lesions within the basal ganglia and thalami.

Our experience relies on the sonographic study and follow-up of 108 patients with gangliothalamic ischemic involvement (age range 0–4 months), isolated in 41 cases (Table 5.3) and associated with more diffuse parenchymal damage in 67 cases: corticosubcortical ischemia in 28, white matter ischemia in 26, neuronal necrosis in 11, and parasagittal injury in two. This diffuse involvement correlated with severe clinical findings, as is reported in the literature (CABANAS 1991; MALAMUD 1950; SHEN 1984).

Table 5.3. Basal ganglia and thalamic injury (108 cases)

Isolated	41 cases
Associated	67 cases
parasagittal injury	2
neuronal necrosis	11
white matter ischemia	26
cortico-subcortical ischemia	28

The thalamus was the most frequently damaged nucleus (78 cases, i.e., 73%), while putamen, pallidum, and caudate were equally involved; in 13 cases, the internal capsule appeared hyperechogenic (Table 5.4).

Table 5.4. Location of lesions within thalami and/or basal ganglia (108 patients)

Thalamus	78
Putamen	35
Pallidum	30
Caudate nucleus	38
Internal capsule	13

During asphyxia, gangliothalamic injury demonstrates a hyperechogenicity (Fig. 5.12), the meaning

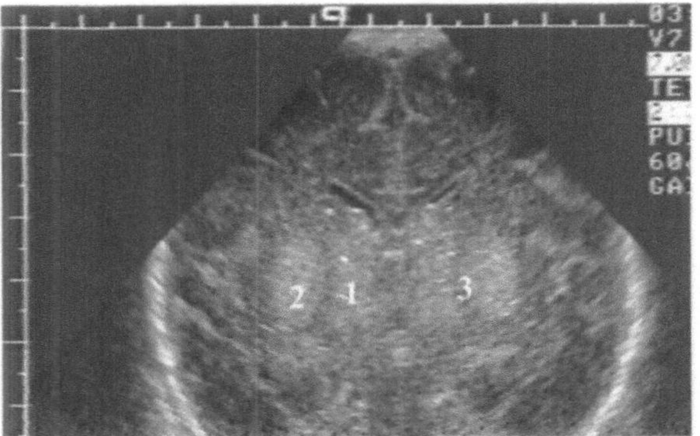
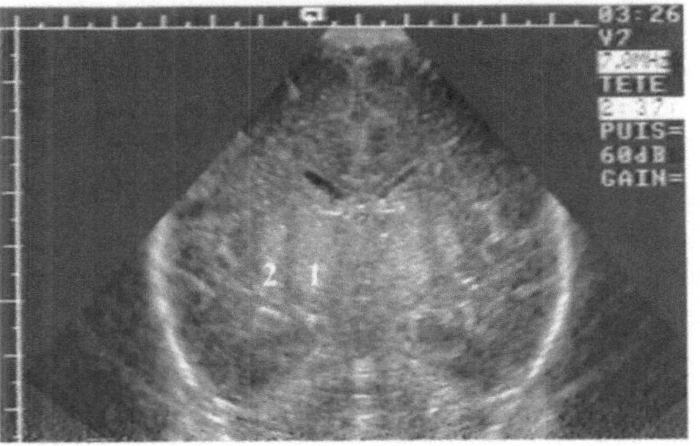

Fig. 5.12a,b. Acute fetal distress. Status epilepticus in a premature infant of 35 weeks' gestation. Well-delineated hyperechoic ischemic lesions involving the thalamus (*1*) and lenticulate nuclei (*2*). Note that the posterior limit of the internal capsule remains normal, i.e., hypoechoic (*3*)

of which is unclear: sonographic–anatomic correlations usually reveal hemorrhagic necrosis in these cases (ADAMS 1988; KREUSSER 1984).

In fact, infarction is predominant, as shown by the suggestive clinical findings, the subsequent development of atrophy (GIROUD 1995), and the poor neurological outcome (Fig. 5.13).

The sonographic appearance and location of lesions depend on the intensity of the asphyxial insult. During anoxic–ischemic encephalopathy, parenchymal and associated gangliothalamic involvement, without constant respect of pyramidal tracts (Fig. 5.6), constitute the most common possibility. The prognosis is disastrous, and ultrasound is an excellent tool to appreciate the severity and progressiveness of the damage (Fig. 5.14).

When isolated, ischemic lesions of the thalami and basal ganglia are sometimes diffuse, often focal (Fig. 5.15).

A thalamic lesion may be observed after a moderate insult, as noted by PARISI (1983), who reported a gangliothalamic injury in a newborn in whom the only relevant history was a maternal fall during the

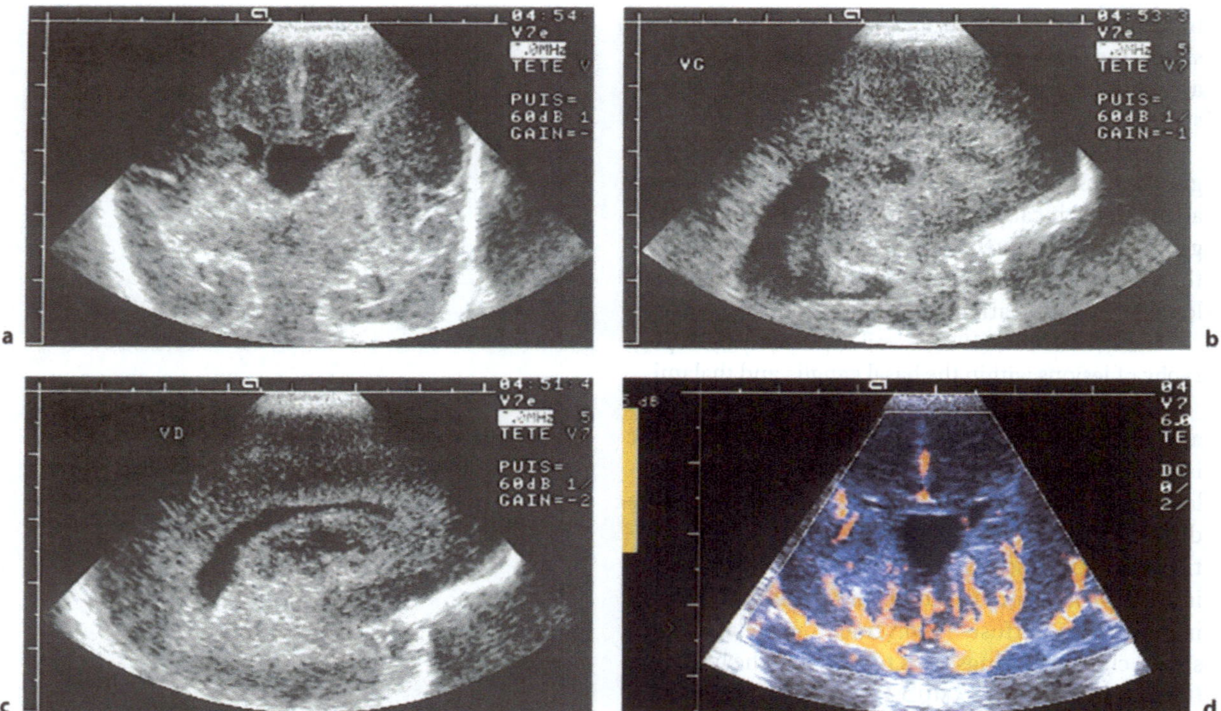

Fig. 5.13a–d. A 25-weeks' gestation preterm infant. At 15 days of life, lenticulate nuclei hyperechogenicity was detected. At 1 month, the basal ganglia were atrophic (**a–c**) and necrotic damage was obvious on the right side (**c**). On color Doppler imaging, the lenticulostriate arteries have become less well visualized on the right side

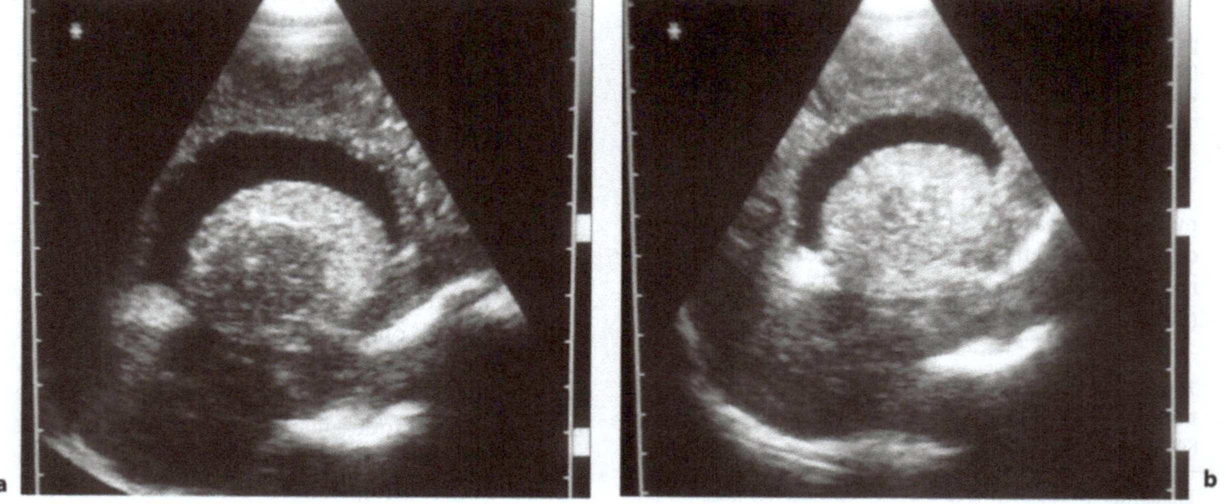

Fig. 5.14a,b. An 8-month-old infant. Cardiorespiratory arrest. Two days later, ultrasonography showed hyperechoic caudate and lenticulate nuclei (**a**). On day 3, gangliothalamic involvement was total (**b**)

last trimester of pregnancy. This is explained by the particular vulnerability of this structure when it has the highest rate of vascularization and oxygen consumption.

Finally, ultrasonography is remarkably effective in locating the damage precisely. An isolated thalamic injury does not have the same prognosis as putaminal or caudate damage.

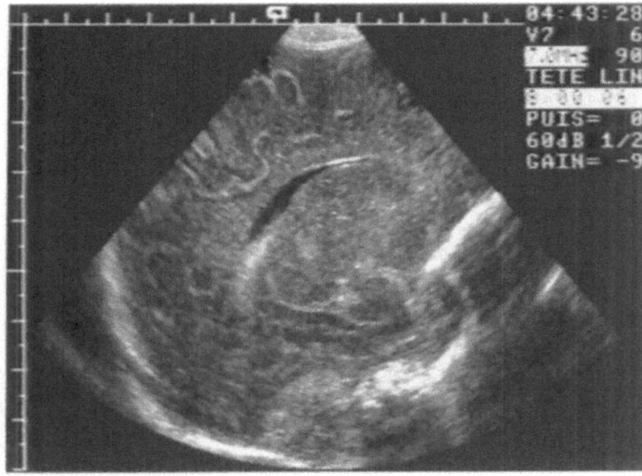
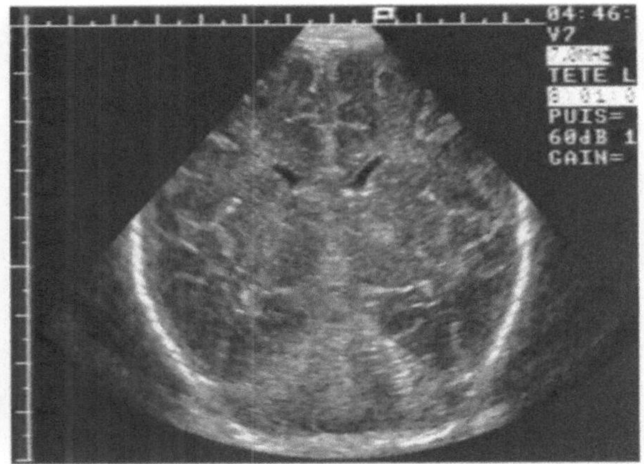

a
b

Fig. 5.15a,b. A premature baby (34 weeks' gestation). Perinatal neurological distress. A focal hyperechoic lesion is seen within the left thalamus (**a,b**)

To sum up, ultrasonography is the main investigation to perform in order to diagnose gangliothalamic anoxic–ischemic lesions, and in the ten most recent cases the sonographic results correlated perfectly with those of MRI (Fig. 5.3).

● *Cortical and Subcortical Ischemic Injury: Value of High-Frequency Probes*

Cortical and subcortical ischemic injury is the most common injury occurring after fetal or perinatal asphyxia. Its sonographic appearance is well known: hyperechoic areas contrast with normal hypoechoic parenchyma, giving a characteristic patchwork effect (COUTURE 1994). However, the transducers that are usually employed lack the sensitivity to determine the extent and exact location of the lesions. High-frequency probes (10 mHz) provide a very valuable and necessary alternative. In normal brain, on either side of the interhemispheric fissure and on the cerebral convexity, white and gray matter have a slightly different echogenicity: the subcortical area is slightly more echogenic than the cortex (Fig. 5.16). When an ischemic insult occurs, ultrasonography reveals either an increase in the cortico-subcortical differentiation (Fig. 5.17), a sign of subcortical ischemia, or else disappearance of this differentiation, a consequence of a diffuse increase in the echogenicity of both white and gray matter (Fig. 5.18). This pattern is accurate; among 29 patients with anoxic–ischemic encephalopathy studied by CT or MRI (Table 5.5), the ultrasound diagnosis was confirmed by CT in 26 cases and MRI in three cases. Thus, when ischemic damage is suspected, high-frequency probes are a necessity in the sonographic examination.

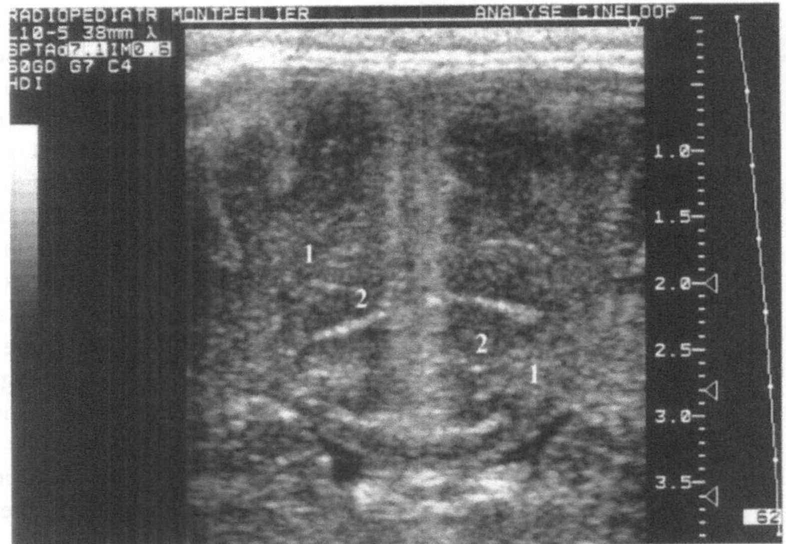

Fig. 5.16. A normal newborn. High-frequency transducer (10 mHz). White (*1*) and gray matter (*2*) have slightly different echostructures

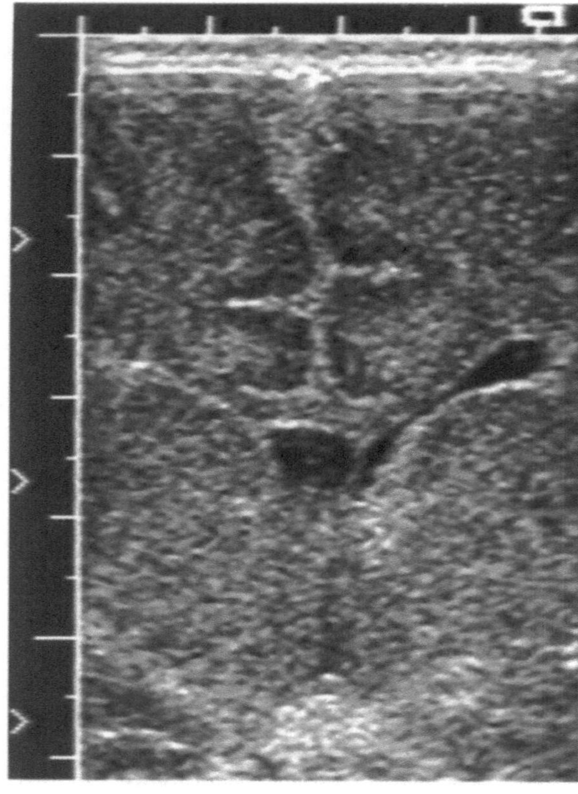

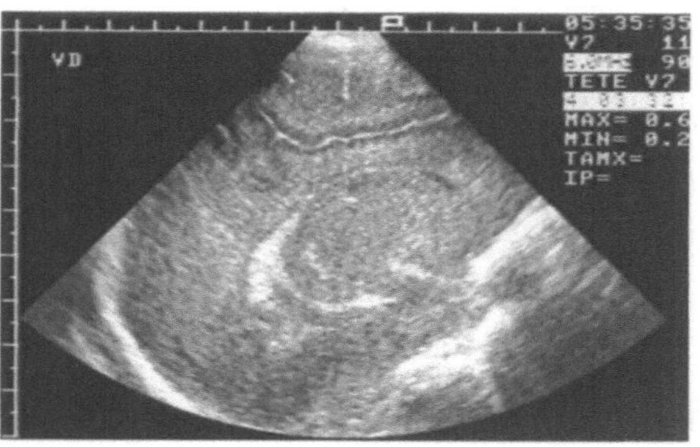

Fig. 5.17a,b. Full-term newborn: esophageal atresia and prolonged intraoperative anoxia. White matter is obviously hyperechoic, indicating subcortical ischemia. Notice that gray
matter hypoechogenicity is preserved, close to the interhemispheric fissure (**a**) and sulci (**b**). Death occurred on day 8

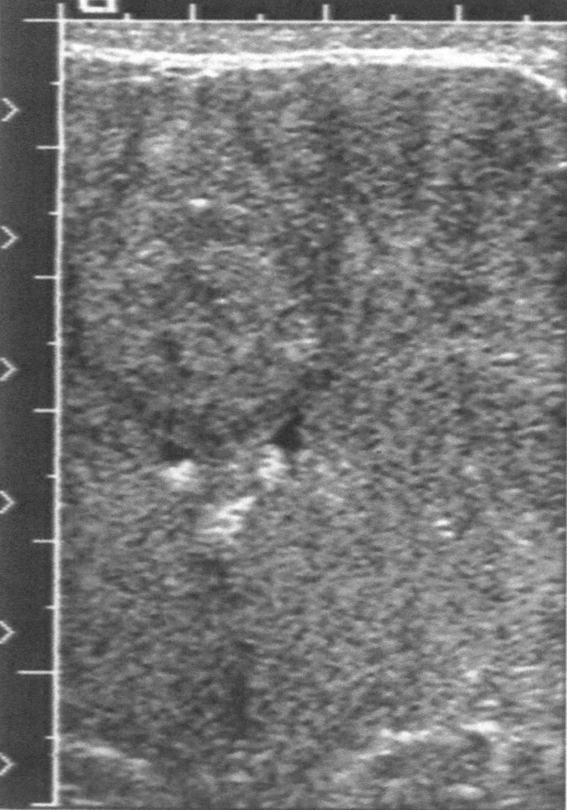

Fig. 5.18. Fetal anoxic–ischemic encephalopathy: status epilepticus. Diffuse hyperechogenicity with disappearance of cortico-subcortical differentiation, indicating diffuse ischemia.
The patient died on day 6

5.2.2.2 Hemodynamic Ultrasonography: A Compelling Necessity

Faced with a case of anoxic–ischemic encephalopathy, the question is how to evaluate the severity of
neonatal brain ischemic damage as a basis for deciding about resuscitation?

This decision is often difficult. Although the clinical assessment of perinatal insult (SARNAT 1976) and
the severity of EEG alterations (HOLMES 1982; MER-
CURI 1999; SCHER 1993) and biological disturbances
constitute the main indications of short-term outcome, they are not always decisive: the poor specificity of the Apgar score and umbilical cord pH results
(RUTH 1998) are well known and explain the difficulty of assessing the neurological status of a sedated
ventilated newborn. This only underlines the value of
ultrasonography, which allows accurate analysis of
parenchymal lesions by using high-frequency probes
coupled with the detection of hemodynamic disorders by pulsed Doppler imaging.

● **Material and Methods** (Table 5.5)

Our experience is based on the clinical and ultrasonographic evaluation of 82 patients: 78 full-term newborns (gestational age range 34–43 weeks) and 4 infants aged 1, 2, 3, and 5 months respectively. The risk factors were postmaturity (14 cases), perinatal collapse (11 cases), maternal toxemia (7 cases), and umbilical cord disease (prolapse, 7 cases). Severe asphyxia with seizures was observed in 60 patients.

Clinical analysis showed grade III encephalopathy in 61 newborns and grade II encephalopathy in 21 neonates and infants.

Asphyxia began in the fetal or perinatal period in 68 neonates (82%) and in the postnatal period in 14 patients (from day 1 to 5 months of age).

The first ultrasound investigation was performed in the intensive care unit, during the first hours of life in 41 neonates, and between day 2 and day 5 in 37 neonates. Routine ultrasound examination consisted in all cases of a morphological analysis (with high-frequency probes) and a hemodynamic study (with pulsed Doppler guided by color Doppler). Ultrasonography was repeated during the first 10 days of life, with a mean of 3 examinations per patient (range 1–5).

CT was performed in 26 cases and MRI in three cases.

Table 5.5. Anoxic–ischemic encephalopathy (82 cases)

CASE	CLINICAL FINDINGS	US (hyperechogenicity)	DOPPLER Day	RI	CT (hypoattenuation)	OUTCOME
1	39 Weeks Grade III	Cortico-subcortical	D2 D3 D4	0.24 0.33 0.36	Cortico-subcortical	Death D4
2	35 Weeks Grade II	Cortico-subcortical	D2	0.50		Death D3
3	3 Months Grade III	Subcortical Gangliothalamic	D1 D3	0.40 0.75	Subcortical	Death D4
4	34 Weeks Grade III	Cortico-subcortical Gangliothalamic	D1	0.30		Death D2
5	39 Weeks Grade III	Cortico-subcortical	D1 D3 D6	0.46 0.51 0.57	Subcortical	Death D10
6	40 Weeks Grade III	Cortico-subcortical Gangliothalamic	D2	0.30		Death D3
7	40 Weeks Grade III	Subcortical	D1 D3	0.46 0.65		Death D4
8	38 Weeks Grade III	Subcortical Gangliothalamic	D1 D3	0.40 0.60		Death D7
9	38 Weeks Grade III	Subcortical	D1 D4	0.40 0.66		18 Months psycho-motor retardation strabismus
10	40 Weeks Grade III	Subcortical Gangliothalamic	D1 D6	0.38 0.48		Death D7
11	36 Weeks Grade III	Cortico-subcortical Gangliothalamic	D1 D2 D7	0.67 0.68 0.45		Death D10
12	39 Weeks Grade III	Subcortical	D4	0.40		9 Months spasticity of inferior limbs

CASE	CLINICAL FINDINGS	US (hyperechogenicity)	DOPPLER Day	RI	CT (hypoattenuation)	OUTCOME
13	41 Weeks Grade II	Subcortical	D3 D7	0.47 0.65		6 Months hypertonia
14	39 Weeks Grade III	Subcortical Gangliothalamic	D3	0.50		Death D12
15	1 Month Grade III	Cortico-Subcortical	D1 D4	0.37 0.63		Death D10
16	39 Weeks Grade III	Cortico-subcortical Brain stem Cerebellum	D5 D6 D10	0.43 0.49 0.50	Cortico-subcortical	Death D10
17	42 Weeks Grade III	Cortico-subcortical	D1 D2 D3 D4 D5	0.36 0.26 0.35 0.53 0.52	Cortico-subcortical	Death D6
18	40 Weeks Grade III	Subcortical	D1 D6 D10	0.50 0.50 0.65	Subcortical	6 Months spastic tetraparesis strabismus
19	39 Weeks Grade III	Subcortical	D1 D3 D5	0.45 0.48 0.50	Subcortical	Death D6
20	36 Weeks Grade III	Subcortical	D1 D2 D3 D7	0.48 0.50 0.51 0.61	Subcortical	Death D8
21	42 Weeks Grade III	Subcortical	D1 D2 D5 D7	0.48 0.40 0.57 0.55	Subcortical	6 Months spastic tetraparesis comitial encephalopathy
22	42 Weeks Grade III	Subcortical	D1 D2 D5 D6	0.40 0.43 0.46 0.54	Subcortical	Death D12
23	40 Weeks Grade II	Subcortical	D3 D9	0.45 0.65		8 Months normal
24	40 Weeks Grade III	Subcortical	D2	0.50		Death D5
25	43 Weeks Grade III	Subcortical Gangliothalamic	D1 D3 D7	0.40 0.50 0.51		6 Months spasticity lower limbs dystonia upper limbs
26	40 Weeks Grade III	Subcortical	D1 D10	0.38 0.56		Death D12
27	43 Weeks Grade II	Subcortical	D1	0.42		6 Months normal
28	39 Weeks Grade II	Subcortical	D3	0.50		10 Months normal

CASE	CLINICAL FINDINGS	US (hyperechogenicity)	DOPPLER Day	RI	CT (hypoattenuation)	OUTCOME
29	38 Weeks Grade II	Subcortical	D1 D3 D7	0.43 0.43 0.40	Subcortical	Death D14
30	40 Weeks Grade III	Subcortical	D1 D7	0.47 0.67	Subcortical	8 Months normal
31	39 Weeks Grade II	Subcortical	D1 D10	0.46 0.56		7 Months normal
32	40 Weeks Grade II	Subcortical	D8 D10 D14	0.36 0.75 0.65		11 Months normal
33	40 Weeks Grade III	Cortico-subcortical Gangliothalamic	D2 D3	0.35 0.45		Death D4
34	40 Weeks Grade III	Cortico-subcortical	D1 D3 D5 D11	0.41 0.41 0.50 0.62		10 Months psychomotor retardation spastic tetraparesis
35	42 Weeks Grade III	Subcortical	D3	0.45		Death D8
36	37 Weeks Grade III	Cortico-subcortical	D2 D6	0.30 0.48	Cortico-Subcortical	Death D7
37	39 Weeks Grade II	Subcortical	D1 D5	0.47 0.50	Subcortical	12 Months normal
38	38 Weeks Grade III	Subcortical Gangliothalamic	D1 D3	0.45 0.46		Death D5
39	42 Weeks Grade III	Cortico-subcortical Gangliothalamic	D1	0.35		Death D4
40	40 Weeks Grade III	Cortico-subcortical	D1	0.45		Death D3
41	39 Weeks Grade III	Subcortical	D2	0.42		Death D8
42	36 Weeks Grade III	Cortico-subcortical	D4 D7 D15	0.54 0.78 0.90	Cortico-subcortical	Death D18
43	40 Weeks Grade III	Subcortical Gangliothalamic	D1	0.42		Death D2
44	40 Weeks Grade III	Cortico-subcortical Gangliothalamic	D2 D5	0.50 0.51		Death D5
45	40 Weeks Grade II	Subcortical	D2 D3	0.36 0.41		6 Months normal
46	40 Weeks Grade III	Subcortical Gangliothalamic	D1 D2	0.31 0.44	Cortico-subcortical Gangliothalamic	Death D17
47	40 Weeks Grade III	Subcortical Gangliothalamic	D2	0.48		Death D2

CASE	CLINICAL FINDINGS	US (hyperechogenicity)	DOPPLER Day	RI	CT (hypoattenuation)	OUTCOME
48	40 Weeks Grade II	Subcortical Gangliothalamic	D1 D4	0.31 0.50		4 Months normal
49	38 Weeks Grade III	Subcortical Gangliothalamic	D1 D2 D3 D4	0.53 0.48 0.43 0.62	MRI: Gangliothalamic Subcortical	Death D8
50	35 Weeks Grade II	Subcortical	D2	0.54		6 Months hypertonia
51	39 Weeks Grade III	Subcortical Gangliothalamic	D2 D3 D4	0.37 0.42 0.77	Subcortical Gangliothalamic	Death D18
52	34 Weeks Grade III	Cortico-subcortical Gangliothalamic	D3 D5	0.58 0.52		Death D7
53	43 Weeks Grade III	Cortico-subcortical	D3 D5	0.48 0.49		Death D6
54	38 Weeks Grade II	Subcortical	D3 D9	0.45 0.71		11 Months normal
55	42 Weeks Grade III	Cortico-subcortical	D2 D7	0.37 0.75		17 Months psychomotor retardation strabismus left hemiparesis
56	40 Weeks Grade II	Subcortical	D2 D5 D15	0.47 0.49 0.86		5 Months, normal
57	40 Weeks Grade III	Cortico-subcortical Gangliothalamic	D2 D3	0.47 0.39		Death D8
58	2 Months Grade III	Cortico-subcortical Gangliothalamic	D1	0.51	Cortico-Subcortical Gangliothalamic	Death 2 months 10 days
59	36 Weeks Grade III	Subcortical Gangliothalamic	D1 D3	0.57 0.54	Subcortical Gangliothalamic	Death D14
60	42 Weeks Grade III	Cortico-subcortical Gangliothalamic	D3	0.54		Death D6
61	40 Weeks Grade III	Subcortical Gangliothalamic	D3 D7	0.47 0.47		Death D8
62	40 Weeks Grade II	Subcortical	D3 D11 D21	0.49 0.51 0.63	MRI: Gangliothalamic	12 Months hypertonia
63	41 Weeks Grade III	Cortico-subcortical Gangliothalamic	D3 D8	0.44 0.70	Cortico-subcortical	Death D16
64	40 Weeks Grade II	Subcortical	D2 D5	0.60 0.54	Subcortical	23 Months spastic diplegia
65	40 Weeks Grade III	Subcortical Gangliothalamic	D2 D5	0.49 0.52		Death D10

CASE	CLINICAL FINDINGS	US (hyperechogenicity)	DOPPLER Day	RI	CT (hypoattenuation)	OUTCOME
66	40 Weeks Grade II	Subcortical	D1	0.42		Death D13
67	40 Weeks Grade III	Subcortical Gangliothalamic	D1 D7	0.69 0.48		Death D10
68	40 Weeks Grade II	Subcortical	D1 D3 D8	0.60 0.49 0.60		2 Months hypertonia
69	41 Weeks Grade III	Cortico-subcortical Gangliothalamic	D4 D8	0.49 0.49	Cortico-subcortical Gangliothalamic	Death D18
70	42 Weeks Grade III	Cortico-subcortical Gangliothalamic	D1 D4	0.51 0.37	MRI: cortico-subcortical Gangliothalamic	Death D10
71	35 Weeks Grade III	Cortico-subcortical	D1 D3 D6	0.70 0.52 0.79	Cortico-subcortical	Death D12
72	40 Weeks Grade II	Subcortical	D3	0.51		4 Months hypertonia
73	40 Weeks Grade II	Subcortical	D3 D7	0.50 0.82	Subcortical	1 Year normal
74	39 Weeks Grade III	Cortico-subcortical Gangliothalamic	D3	0.48		Death D2
75	39 Weeks Grade II	Cortico-subcortical Gangliothalamic	D2	0.52	Cortico-subcortical	Death D11
76	39 Weeks Grade III	Subcortical Gangliothalamic	D4	0.46		Death D6
77	38 Weeks Grade III	Cortico-subcortical Gangliothalamic	D2 D4 D6	0.63 0.47 0.69		Death D8
78	40 Weeks Grade III	Subcortical Gangliothalamic	D1 D4 D8 D10	0.72 0.53 0.47 0.67		Death D13
79	40 Weeks Grade III	Cortico-subcortical Gangliothalamic	D5	0.31		Death D7
80	37 Weeks Grade III	Cortico-subcortical Gangliothalamic	D4 D6 D8 D10	0.48 0.88 0.71 0.76		Death D12
81	37 Weeks Grade III	Cortico-subcortical Gangliothalamic	D3 D5	0.39 0.55		Death D6
82	5 Months Grade III	Cortico-subcortical Gangliothalamic	D1 D3 D5 D7 D11	0.60 0.36 0.39 0.41 0.77		Death 5 months 15 days

● *Results*

In the whole group, gray-scale ultrasonography detected hyperechoic lesions involving white matter in 49 neonates and 1 infant, and gray and white matter in 29 neonates and 3 infants; basal ganglia and thalami were also damaged in 37 children. CT confirmed the sonographic data by showing subcortical or cortico-subcortical hypoattenuated areas.

In all cases, Doppler ultrasonography of the cerebral arteries revealed a decrease in resistive index (RI) resulting from an increase in diastolic amplitude: RI was less than 0.55 (range 0.25–0.54) (Table 5.5). This alteration may be observed at birth; it was recognized in the first hours of life in 41 babies with perinatal asphyxia, and lasted from 4 to 6 days.

Velocimetry was performed in the 44 most recent cases. If the increase in peak systolic velocities was moderate, a major increase in end-diastolic and mean velocities was observed, a sign of luxury perfusion.

In our experience, anoxic–ischemic encephalopathy has a poor prognosis: death occurred in 54 neonates (between day 2 and day 14) and the 4 infants (with a delay ranging 2 to 23 months). Two examples demonstrate the interest of this US evaluation.

Jade was a full-term newborn with congenital abnormalities (cleft palate, type III esophageal atresia). Neonatal ultrasonography was normal, RI was 0.74, systolic and diastolic velocities were in the normal range. During surgery, prolonged hypoxia occurred, followed by postoperative multiorgan distress. On day 4, ultrasound showed diffuse subcortical white matter hyperechogenicity and pulsed Doppler revealed low RI and increased arterial velocities. The newborn died on day 10 (Fig. 5.19).

Tarik, a post-term newborn, required immediate neonatal ventilation because of neurological distress. Severe anemia was discovered, probably due to fetomaternal transfusion. At birth, the anterior cerebral artery Doppler imaging showed a marked increase in the diastolic component with RI=0.26 (Fig. 5.20), and extensive cortico-subcortical ischemic lesions were demonstrated. The hemodynamics remained disturbed until the infant died on day 6. On macroscopic examination, multiple ischemic and necrotic foci were found in the edematous parenchyma.

● Discussion

– *Alterations in the Doppler curve allow immediate evaluation of the prognosis.*

During perinatal asphyxia, Doppler recording of the anterior cerebral artery demonstrates an early and prolonged drop in RI by increased diastolic amplitude and increased velocities. This appearance

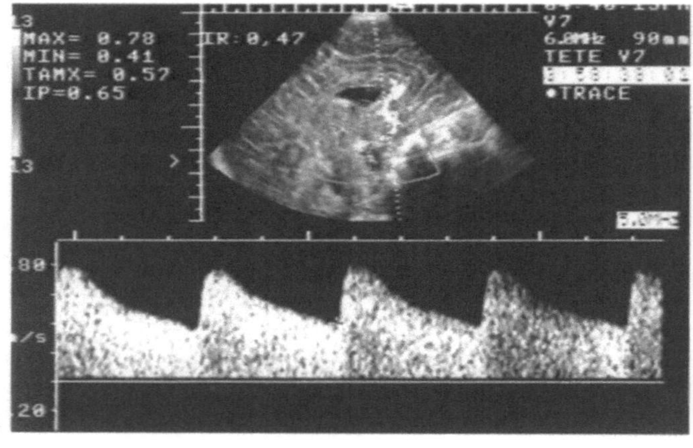
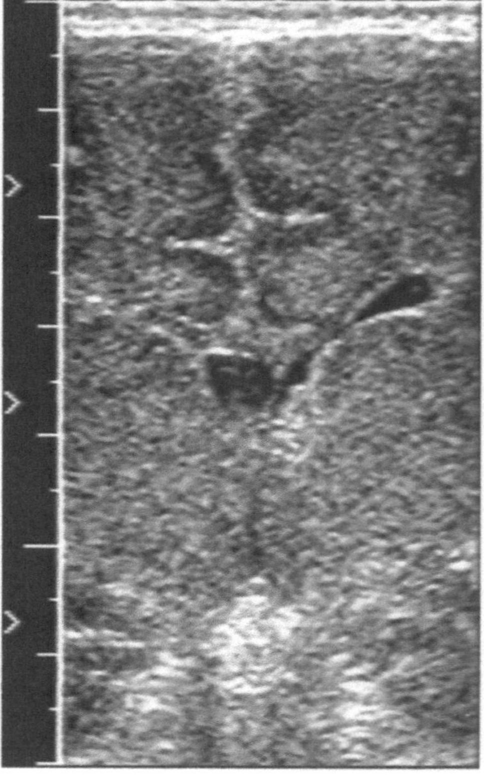

Fig. 5.19. a Doppler recording of the anterior cerebral artery. Diastolic amplitude is highly increased, RI is 0.47. Velocities are raised: peak systolic velocity: 78 cm/s; end-diastolic velocity: 41 cm/s; time average mean velocity: 57 cm/s. **b** White matter is obviously hyperechoic: subcortical ischemia with cortical integrity

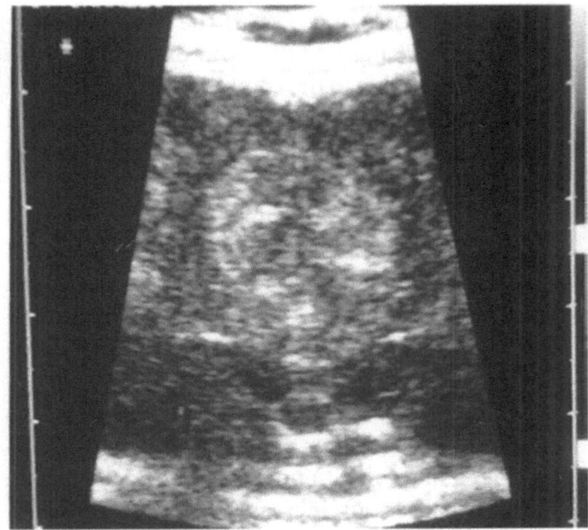
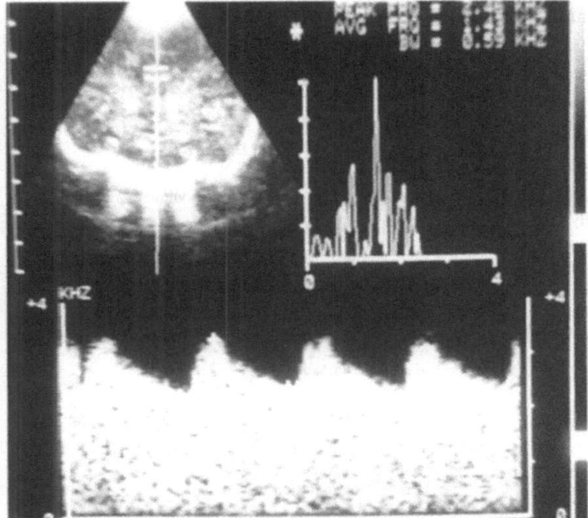

a b

Fig. 5.20. a Cortico-subcortical differentiation has disappeared, due to gray and white matter ischemia (diffuse hyperechogenicity). **b** On day 2, RI has fallen to 0.26. Two days before death, it remains low at 0.35

is also observed in the carotid artery, basilar artery, and small peripheral cortical and lenticulostriate arteries (Fig. 5.21). These neonatal disturbances reflect arterial vasodilatation, the mechanisms of which are complex and multifactorial (Table 5.6).

Fetomaternal distress leads rapidly to hypoxemia, hypercapnia, and fetal acidosis, which cause cerebral arterial vasodilatation. This safeguarding response, well known by pediatricians, may be detected in utero (ARBEILLE 1987; CHANDRAN 1993; SCHERJON 1993).

In parallel to this, bradycardia and low blood flow are frequent during fetal asphyxia. In fact, the loss of cerebral autoregulation plays the main role in the development of ischemic lesions. Vasodilatation resulting from biological alterations and low cardiac output secondary to bradycardia induces a linear variation between CBF and systemic arterial pressure. The severity of lesions arbitrated by the loss of autoregulation balances between protective vasodilatation and ischemia-inducing low blood flow.

At birth, resuscitation improves and normalizes the biological and hemodynamic parameters and reduces the disturbances that alter cerebral autoregulation. When arterial pressure has recovered, and normocapnia and normoxia are obtained, it is impor-

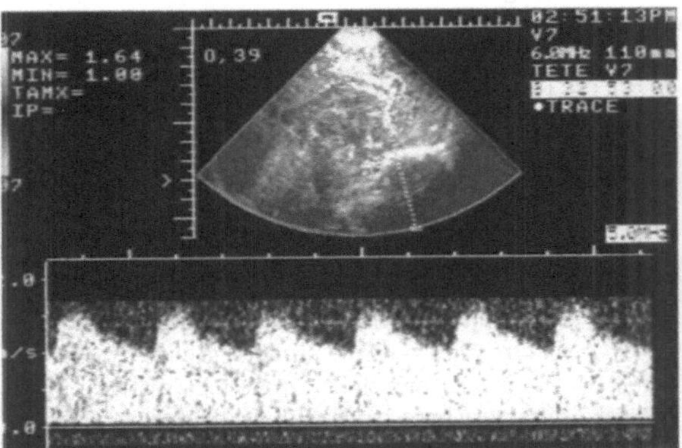
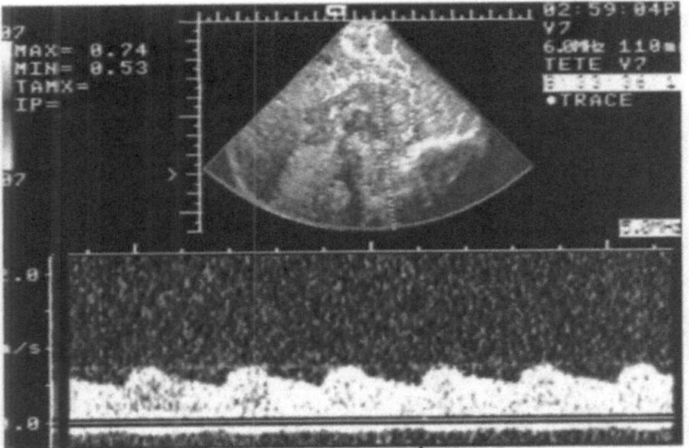

a b

Fig. 5.21a,b. A 5-month-old infant. Repeated seizures of unknown cause. First gray scale and Doppler ultrasonography are normal. On day 2, striking sonographic alterations are seen with cortico-subcortical and basal ganglia ischemic damage. There is luxury perfusion in all cerebral arteries. In the anterior cerebral artery (**a**), PSV=164 cm/s, EDV=100 cm/s, TAV=142 cm/s, and RI=0.39. In a branch of the callosomarginal artery (**b**) the same alterations are present: RI 0.28, PSV 74 cm/s; EDV 53 cm/s, TAV 60 cm/s

Table 5.6

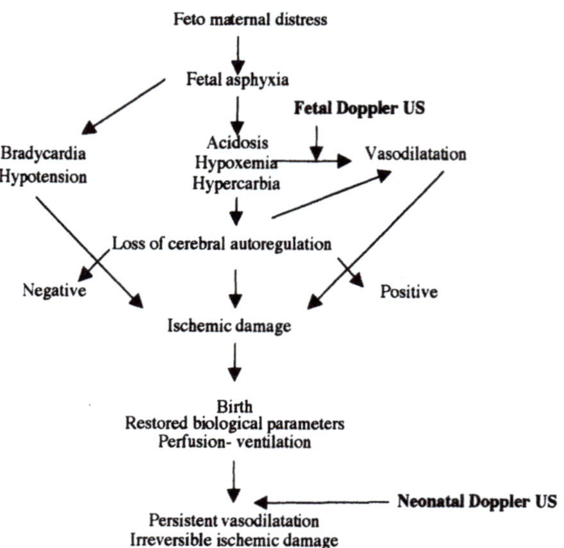

tant to evaluate the neonatal hemodynamics (LEVENE 1989). Hypoxia (Fig. 5.22) and hypercapnia are strong vasodilators and may by themselves explain a decreased RI and increased diastolic component, similar to what is observed during perinatal insult (Fig. 5.23).

Persistence of vasodilatation, as revealed by the spectral analysis curve (Fig. 5.24) during the first days of life, is probably due to acidosis and is a sign of tissue necrosis. Called luxury perfusion (LASSEN 1966; PRYDS 1990), it apparently reflects the reality of irreversible ischemic lesions (ARCHER 1986; COUTURE 1994; HELMANN 1987; LEVENE 1989; VAN BEL 1987).

In the literature, several physiopathological hypotheses have been discussed:

– In the opinion of VOLPE (1995), the onset of postischemic hyperemia is difficult to explain. He suggests it may be due to the combined effect of stored vasodilating agents and vascular wall damage, and reports that this response is never observed in experimental studies.
– Among 30 patients with anoxic–ischemic neonatal encephalopathy, LEVENE (1989) noted a low RI combined with an increased CBF in 17 cases. In his view, these alterations reflect paralysis of arteriolar vasomotricity and irreversible cerebral damage.
– Other authors (DEEG 1990; SEIBERT 1989; VAN BEL 1987) propose another explanation. DEEG (1990) ascribes a main role to postischemic edema: brain swelling causes an increase in tissue pressure, which compresses brain vessels, resulting in a protective increase in diastolic flow, as he observed in seven patients (among 25 with cerebral edema). When cerebral edema became higher than perfusion pressure (particularly in diastole), he detected an absent or even negative diastolic flow in six cases; these alterations signify a poor prognosis (three patients died, two suffered major neurodevelopmental retardation, one had mild mental retardation).

In reality, cerebral edema probably plays a secondary role, because of the great compliance of the neonatal skull; most often, increased blood flow velocities and decreased vascular resistances are observed in the follow-up of neonatal anoxic–ischemic encephalopathy. By contrast, increased vascular resistance with an absent or negative diastolic component is only exceptionally encountered in the newborn (Fig. 5.25), but it is essential to detect it when it does occur, because of its bad prognosis.

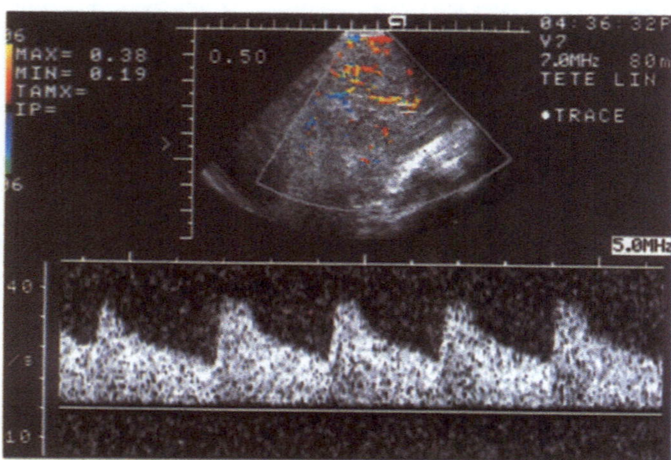

Fig. 5.22. A 34-weeks' gestation preterm infant: premature rupture of membranes; group B *Streptococcus* pneumonitis with respiratory distress. Major refractory hypoxemia with death on day 2. This situation of refractory hypoxemia is well documented after maternofetal infection with group B *Streptococcus* and *Mycoplasma pneumoniae*, and induces cerebral vasodilatation with RI=0.50. This emphasizes how important it is to know the PO_2, PCO_2 and pH before beginning any interpretation of the hemodynamic studies

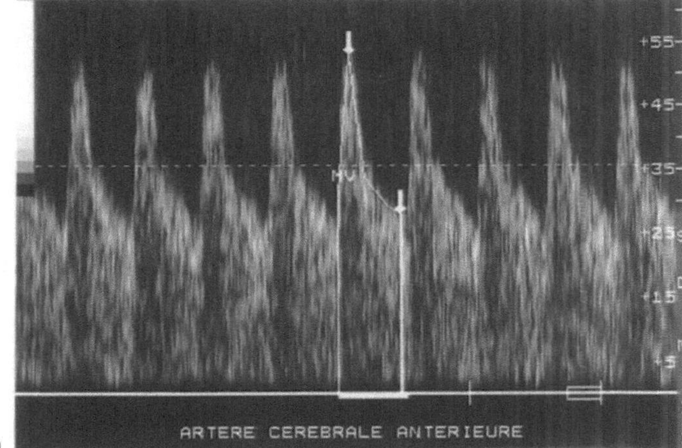

a

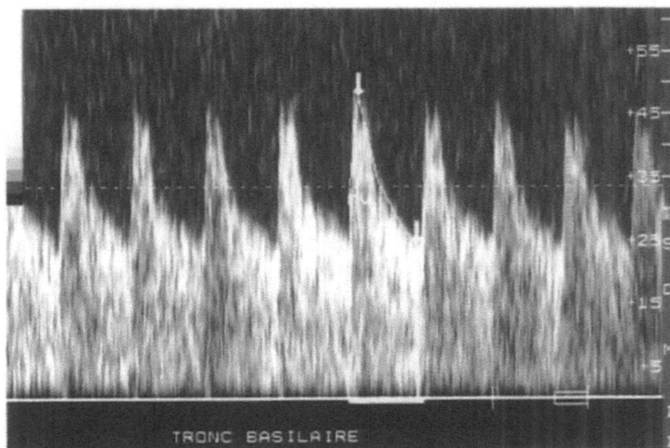

b

Fig. 5.23a,b. A full-term newborn: acute anemia and bilateral adrenal hematoma; extended thrombosis of the inferior vena cava. The final diagnosis is protein C deficiency. Neonatal evaluation shows hemodynamic alterations, with increased diastolic velocities and decreased RI [0.47 in the anterior cerebral artery (a) and 0.49 in basilar artery (b)]. These alterations lasted 48 h, and ultrasonography was normal at 8 days of life. The neonatal neurological state remained normal, as did arterial blood pressure, PO_2, and PCO_2. In summary, a case of neonatal hemodynamic alterations which mimic ischemic damage

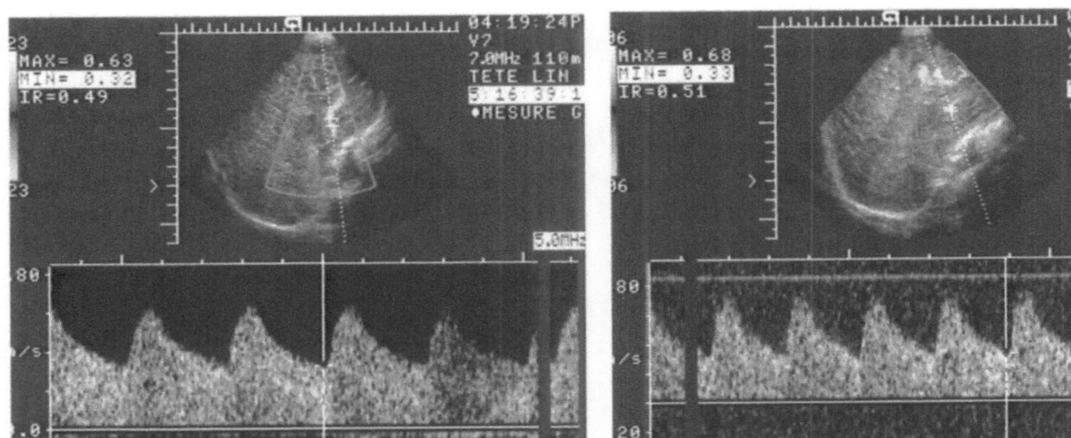

a   b

Fig. 5.24a,b. A full-term newborn: meconium aspiration, seizures, hypotonia. First ultrasound study on day 2 (**a**): white matter ischemia, high velocities, RI=0.49. Six days later (**b**), biological parameters are normal, RI= 0.51

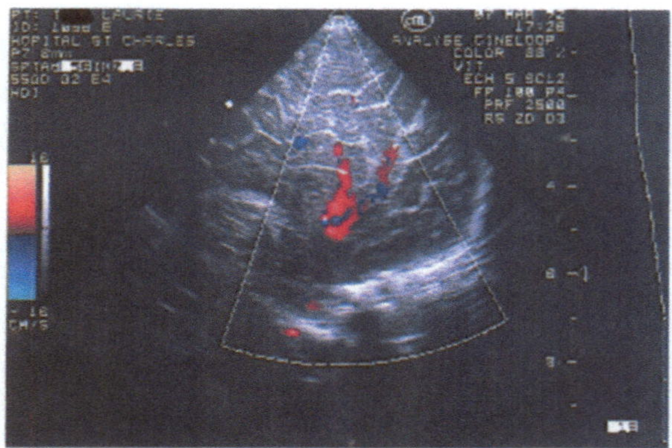

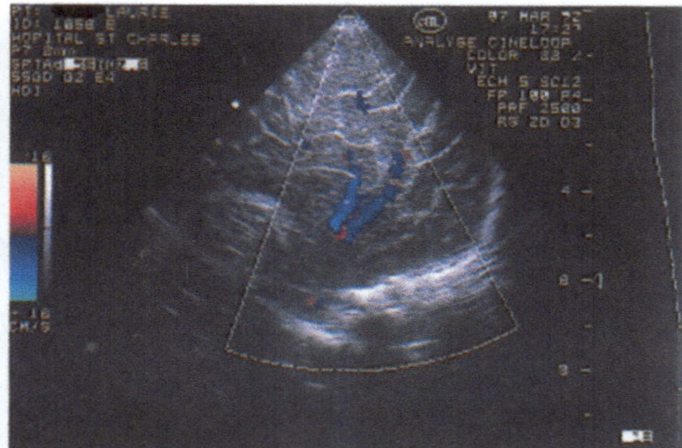

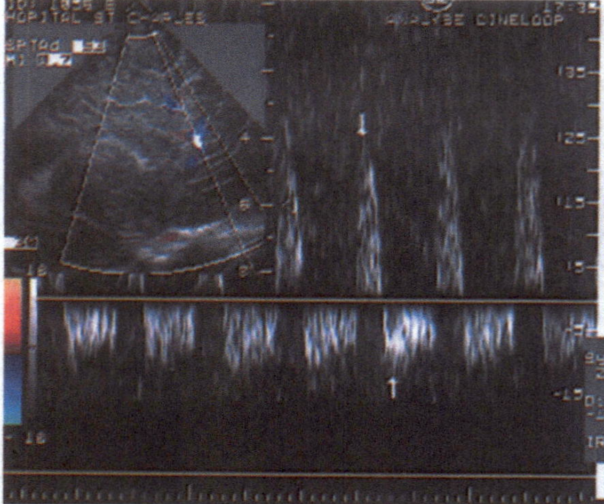

Fig. 5.25a–c. A 2-month-old infant: seizures, apneic spells, cardiac arrest. Major damage was present, with diffuse neuronal necrosis and gangliothalamic ischemia. On color Doppler, reverse diastolic flow appeared as a change in the colored signal (**a,b**); this demonstrated increased downstream resistance, and was confirmed by spectral analysis; RI=1.32 (**c**). Assessment of velocities showed low blood flow (PSV=24 cm/s). Two days later, no colored signal was detected on color Doppler imaging

- *The hemodynamic alterations in asphyxial injury nowadays represent an objective reality*

Doppler investigation plays a major role in the accurate prognostic evaluation of anoxic–ischemic neonatal injury. We know that early imaging may be misleading (GONZALES DE DIOS 1995) since sonographic morphological anomalies require 24–48 h to appear. Thus, in a suggestive clinical context, a decreased RI with increased velocities and diastolic amplitude constitutes the only ground for determining the immediate potential severity and guiding resuscitation. Among 16 patients with anoxic-ischemic encephalopathy, STARK (1994) observed a decreased RI during the first day of life, whereas imaging findings remained normal in half of the cases. The diagnostic reliability of postasphyxial hyperemia has now been demonstrated (Fig. 5.26), and several authors have emphasized the importance of Doppler analysis. ARCHER (1986) reported an early prolonged drop in vascular resistance during perinatal asphyxia, correlated with a poor prognosis: out of 12 patients with grade III postasphyxial

encephalopathy, hemodynamics were altered in nine, with poor outcome (seven deaths and two cases of severe retardation); by contrast, in three patients the hemodynamics remained normal, none of whom had an adverse outcome. Several reports have now confirmed the value of these Doppler techniques (BENNHAGEN 1998; COUTURE 1994; DEEG 1990; EKEN 1995; GONZALES DE DIOS 1995; HELMANN 1987; LEVENE 1989; LIVES 1998; PRYDS 1990; SALIBA 1996; SEIBERT 1989; STARK 1994; VAN BEL 1987).

- *Should velocimetric measures be favored over the resistive index in evaluating the prognosis?*

LEVENE (1989) was the first to confirm the value of velocimetric measurements, which improve the predictive value of neonatal hemodynamic alterations. Following 21 patients with moderate or severe anoxic–ischemic encephalopathy, he described a decreased RI associated with significantly increased mean flow velocity in 17 cases and an obvious decrease in this value in four cases. Correlations

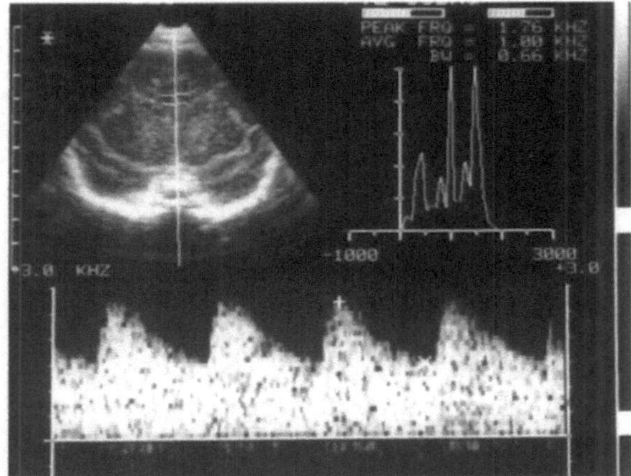

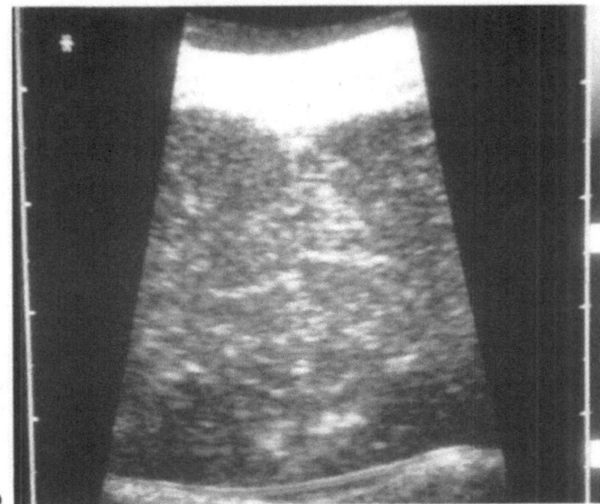

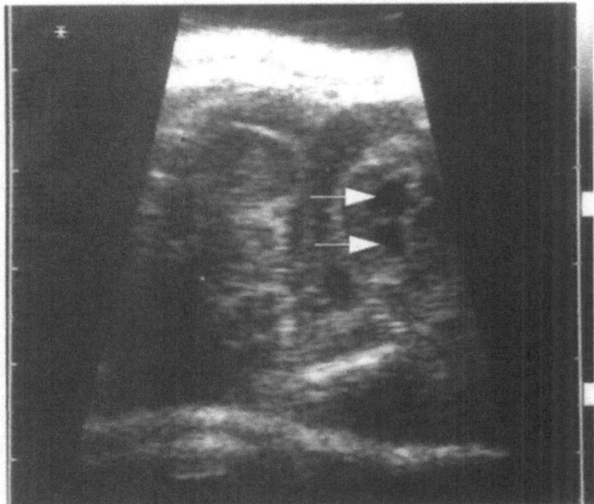

Fig. 5.26a–c. A full-term newborn, day 2. Repeated seizures. Morphological ultrasonography was normal, but the spectral analysis was worrying, with RI=0.41 (**a**). The day after, diffuse cortico-subcortical hyperechogenicity was obvious (**b**). At 2 months of life (**c**), follow-up ultrasonography demonstrated the severity of the injury: cerebral atrophy and porencephalic cysts (*arrow*) within the left frontal white matter, detected by high-frequency probes

between blood flow velocity and outcome are impressive: no infant with a velocity measurement more than three standard deviations above the mean survived without severe cerebral palsy; three of the four infants with low flow velocity (>2 SD below the mean) died. In this author's study, the positive predictive value of abnormal CBF velocity for an adverse outcome was 94%, compared with 83% for a single low RI. This was the first report to demonstrate the importance of measuring systolic, diastolic, and mean velocities during an acute asphyxial event (Fig. 5.27).

Several authors have now confirmed that high velocities provide more precise information than low RI for the prediction of neurological outcome (STARK 1994; EKEN 1995). Recently, LIVES (1998) reported, in 39 full-term newborns with perinatal asphyxia, that velocities were altered earlier than RI: out of eight neonates with severe encephalopathy, six had very high velocities (>3 SD) within the first 12 h of life, whereas only two infants had a low RI. RI was disturbed in association with high velocities at 24 h of life. Thus, in the first 12 h, measuring RI alone was insufficient.

Our personal experience confirms these data. In a complete hemodynamic assessment guided by color Doppler imaging (anterior cerebral artery, basilar artery, internal carotid artery, and sometimes cortical arteries), we measured systolic, diastolic, and mean velocities in the 44 most recent cases (42 newborns and 2 infants) among 82 patients with anoxic–ischemic encephalopathy.

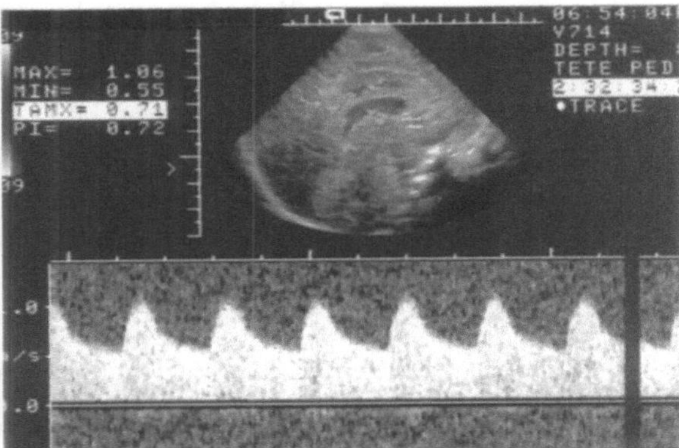

Fig. 5.27. Acute fetal distress. Apparent stillbirth, followed by immediate seizures. There was diffuse ischemic involvement of white matter and gangliothalamic nuclei. On pulsed Doppler imaging, RI=0.48 and CBF velocities were increased: PSV=106 cm/s, EDV=55 cm/s, TAV=71 cm/s. These diffuse alterations were also observed within small cortical arteries. The infant died on day 10

Compared with the normal range in full-term newborns, the first hemodynamic alterations (appearing from some hours to 5 days of life) in the 42 neonates were homogeneous:
- The median of systolic, diastolic, and time average velocities were high above normal values (40 control patients); this related to the anterior cerebral artery (42 cases), basilar artery (13 cases), and internal carotid artery (7 cases) (Table 5.7).

Table 5.7. Anoxic–ischemic encephalopathy (42 patients) Arterial velocities (cm/s)

	Normal newborn (40 cases)			Encephalopathy (42 cases)		
	PSV	EDV	TAV	PSV	EDV	TAV
Anterior cerebral artery (42 cases)	45.4	12.3	24.3	58.3	31	45
Basilar artery (13 cases)	44.7	12	24	55.3	30.5	36.6
Carotid artery (7 cases)	50	12.9	26.6	71	39	47

- This luxury perfusion was mainly the result of highly increased diastolic velocities (range 15–64 cm/s in anterior cerebral and basilar arteries), compared with normal values (Table 5.8).
- Peak systolic velocities were also increased, but to a lesser degree. In the anterior cerebral artery, they were above the normal range in 30 cases, and below it in 12 cases (range 34–94 cm/s). For the basilar artery, they were above the normal range in ten cases, and below it in five (range 34–106 cm/s) (Table 5.9).
- Mean velocities probably represent the most reliable criteria of luxury perfusion, and were constantly high above the normal range (range 26–82 cm/s in anterior cerebral and basilar arteries) (Table 5.10).
- Finally, comparing grade II and grade III encephalopathies, there were interesting differences in anterior cerebral artery recordings between the two groups: in grade II damage (12 cases), systolic,

Table 5.8. Anoxic–ischemic encephalopathy (42 patients) End-diastolic velocities (EDV) in anterior cerebral artery

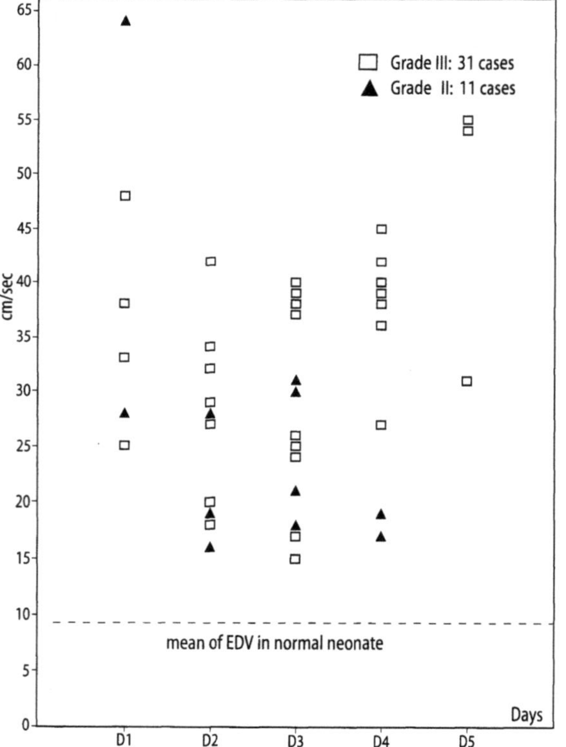

Table 5.9. Anoxic–ischemic encephalopathy (42 patients) Peak-systolic velocities (PSV) in anterior cerebral artery

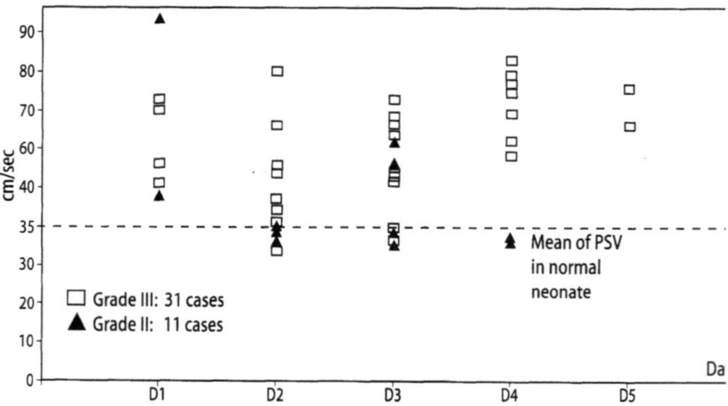

Table 5.10. Anoxic–ischemic encephalopathy (23 patients) Time-average velocities (TAV) in anterior cerebral artery

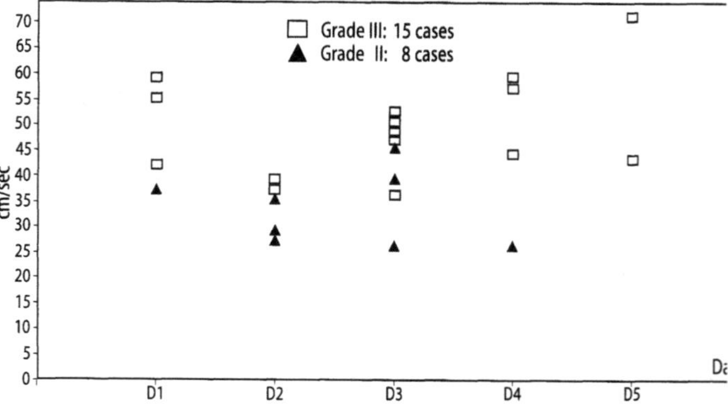

diastolic, and mean velocities were markedly below those of grade III (30 cases) (Tables 5.8, 5.9, 5.10, 5.11). These data are particularly important since RI had the same value in both groups: 0.46 in grade II, 0.45 in grade III. When hemodynamic assessment was repeated over several days, we noted that luxury perfusion lasted longer in grade III injury than in grade II. This allows some conclusions to be drawn:

● In our series, RI and velocities were simultaneously disturbed, but velocimetric alterations appeared as the most reliable guarantee of an accurate early prognostic assessment (Fig. 5.28).

Early, severe, and prolonged postischemic hyperemia indicates a disastrous, irreversible prognosis: this is the rule in grade III injury. When hyperemia is less severe and less prolonged, the prognosis is much more difficult to predict: this is usually the pattern in grade II encephalopathy.

Concerning the duration of luxury perfusion, experience remains too limited. However, its severity seems to be a good criterion for distinction between grade II and grade III injuries (Table 5.11).

Table 5.11. Anoxic-ischemic encephalopathy (42 cases) Arterial velocities (cm/s)

	GRADE II 12 cases			GRADE III 30 cases		
	PSV	EDV	TAV	PSV	EDV	TAV
Anterior cerebral artery	46	26	33.8	63	34.5	46.3

● Moreover, very early study of velocities may help in better understanding of the physiopathology of anoxic–ischemic encephalopathy, as demonstrated by this example:

Jean Baptiste was born in a great emergency: a cesarean delivery was decided on when umbilical cord

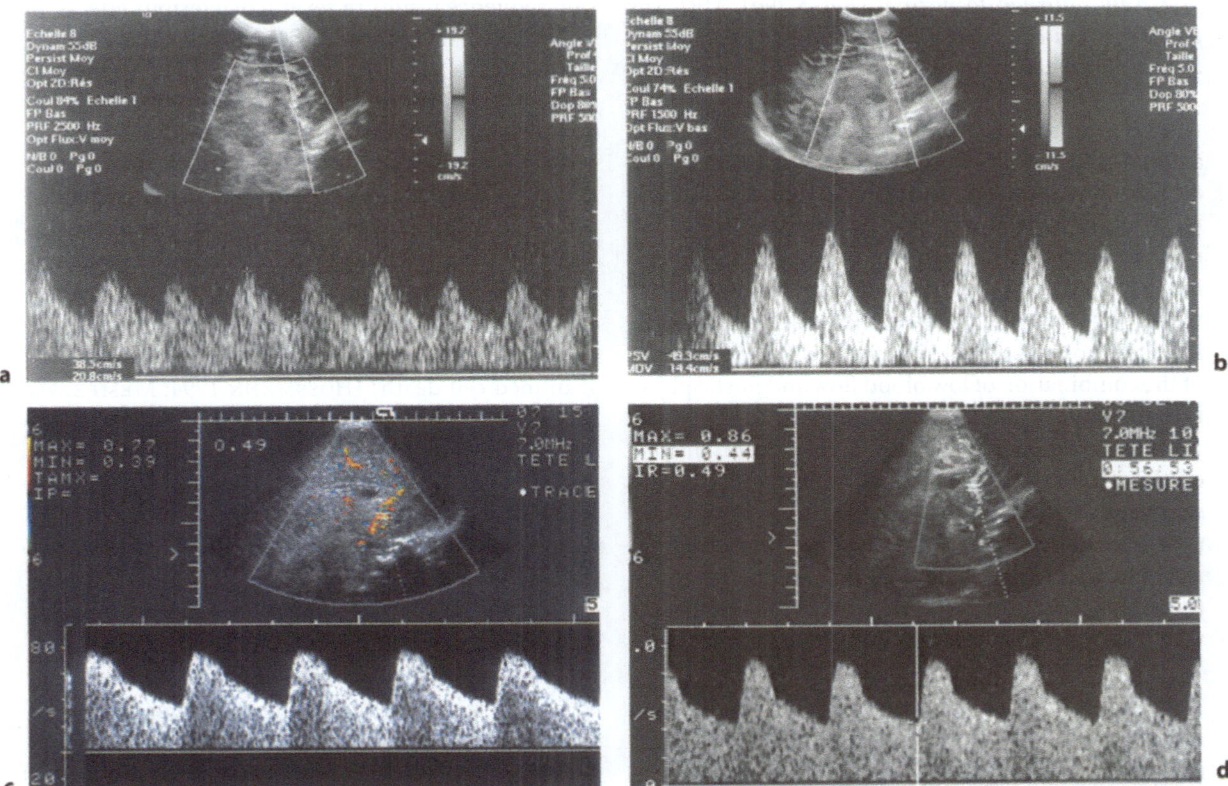

Fig. 5.28. a,b A 38-weeks' gestation newborn, apparently still born, then showing clonic seizures which rapidly resolved: grade II encephalopathy. Hyperechoic white matter. **a** On day 3: RI=0.46, PSV=38 cm/s, EDV=20 cm/s (mildly increased). **b** On day 6: normal hemodynamic data: RI=0.71. PSV=49 cm/s, EDV=14 cm/s. Normal examination at 3 months. **c,d** A post-term neonate with repeated seizures: grade III encephalopathy. The hemodynamics are completely different: **c** on day 3, RI=0.49. Velocities are highly increased: PSV=77 cm/s, EDV=39 cm/s. **d** On day 8 the findings are the same: RI=0.49, PSV=86 cm/s, EDV=44 cm/s. The infant died on day 18

prolapse with fetal bradycardia occurred. He suffered a neonatal clinical and EEG status epilepticus. Ultrasonography was performed at 3 h of life and showed moderate hyperechogenicity of white matter, but the spectral analysis curve was severely disturbed: in the anterior cerebral artery, RI was low (0.53) but all velocities had dropped (Fig. 5.29a), suggesting seriously low blood flow. This was confirmed in the basilar artery (PSV=13 cm/s, EDV=7 cm/s) and carotid artery (PSV=13 cm/s, EDV=5 cm/s).

The next day, the hemodynamic situation was completely different: a typical luxury perfusion pattern was found, with increased blood flow in the anterior cerebral, basilar, and lenticulostriate arteries (Fig. 5.29b). The morphological appearance had changed too, showing diffuse white matter hyperechogenicity and casting doubt on the integrity of the basal ganglia.

On day 3, the hemodynamic alterations were unchanged (Fig. 5.29c), and subcortical white matter and gangliothalamic ischemia was confirmed (Fig. 5.30). Finally, on day 4, the hemodynamics progressively returned to normal (Fig. 5.29d). MRI was performed on day 6, and demonstrated the ischemic lesions. The baby died on day 8.

This example shows the value of early study of the arterial velocities. Cerebral hypoperfusion, detected at H3, corresponded probably to low blood flow resulting from fetal bradycardia, and was obviously responsible for the subsequent ischemic lesions. The following luxury perfusion indicates the severity of the anoxic–ischemic insult. In his study of 39 asphyxiated newborns, Lives (1998) emphasizes the severity of the combination of low blood flow and postasphyxial hyperemia.

In the example just described, the natural history of the cerebral damage seems well shown by the sequential hemodynamic assessment: low blood flow, postischemic luxury perfusion, parenchymal ischemic lesions, death. This demonstrates that a protocolized early Doppler examination is important when ischemic insult occurs in the neonatal period.

● In the literature, contradictory information is reported about CBF alterations during anoxic-ischemic encephalopathy. Most authors confirm the frequency and severity of postischemic hyperemia. Others (Fellman 1997; Lives 1998; Van Bel 1993) note cerebral hypoperfusion during the hours following neonatal asphyxia.

Lives (1998) is of the opinion that this is most often observed during moderate asphyxial injury, but

Van Bel (1993) reports hypoperfusion during severe insult. Using near-infrared spectroscopy in five severely asphyxiated newborns during the first 12 h of life, he detected a marked decrease in cerebral blood volume. These data do not support the results of an earlier study (Van Bel 1987), in which he found increased CBF velocity. In fact, however, this seems to be only an apparent contradiction, since Doppler imaging investigates the major cerebral arteries whereas spectroscopy assesses cerebral blood volume and oxygenation within the cortex and adjacent subcortical white matter in the parietal regions of the brain. Thus, it is possible that, in the early postischemic period, hypoperfusion at a microvascular level coexists with luxury perfusion due to vasoparalysis (Fellman 1997).

Other authors (Hammerman 1988; Vannucci 1997; Volpe 1995) have studied the paradoxical bad consequences of postasphyxial reperfusion. It has now been established that increased blood flow and high oxygen levels are the major determinants of cerebral lesions and cell death. The ischemia/reperfusion sequence results in several deleterious effects on brain cells, including release of reactive oxygen metabolites and free radicals, ATP depletion, glutamate concentration, intracellular calcium accumulation, and inflammatory response with cytokines activating vascular endothelial alterations that decrease tissular flow. It is clear that hypoxic-ischemic brain damage is an evolving process which begins during the insult and extends after resuscitation. When infarction occurs, the immediate parenchyma surrounding the infarct (penumbra) consists of neurons undergoing necrosis and apoptosis (programmed cell death) (Hossmann 1994; Memezawa 1992).

Apoptosis is a major physiological process; the whole of development depends on the induction of cells toward apoptosis (for example, T-lymphocytes within the fetal thymus). The regulation of apoptosis plays a role in several pathological states, especially cerebral ischemia (Charriaut-Marlangue 1996; Edwards 1997). Apoptosis is defined by morphological characteristics which differ from those of necrosis: cell shrinkage, membrane blebbing, chromatin condensation, and DNA fragmentation (Li 1995).

It has been shown that, after arterial occlusion, apoptotic cells appear in the ischemic area, at the periphery of the infarct, while necrotic cells are predominant within the infarct. Some neurons initiate apoptosis before any sign of necrosis, indicating a maturation of neural death.

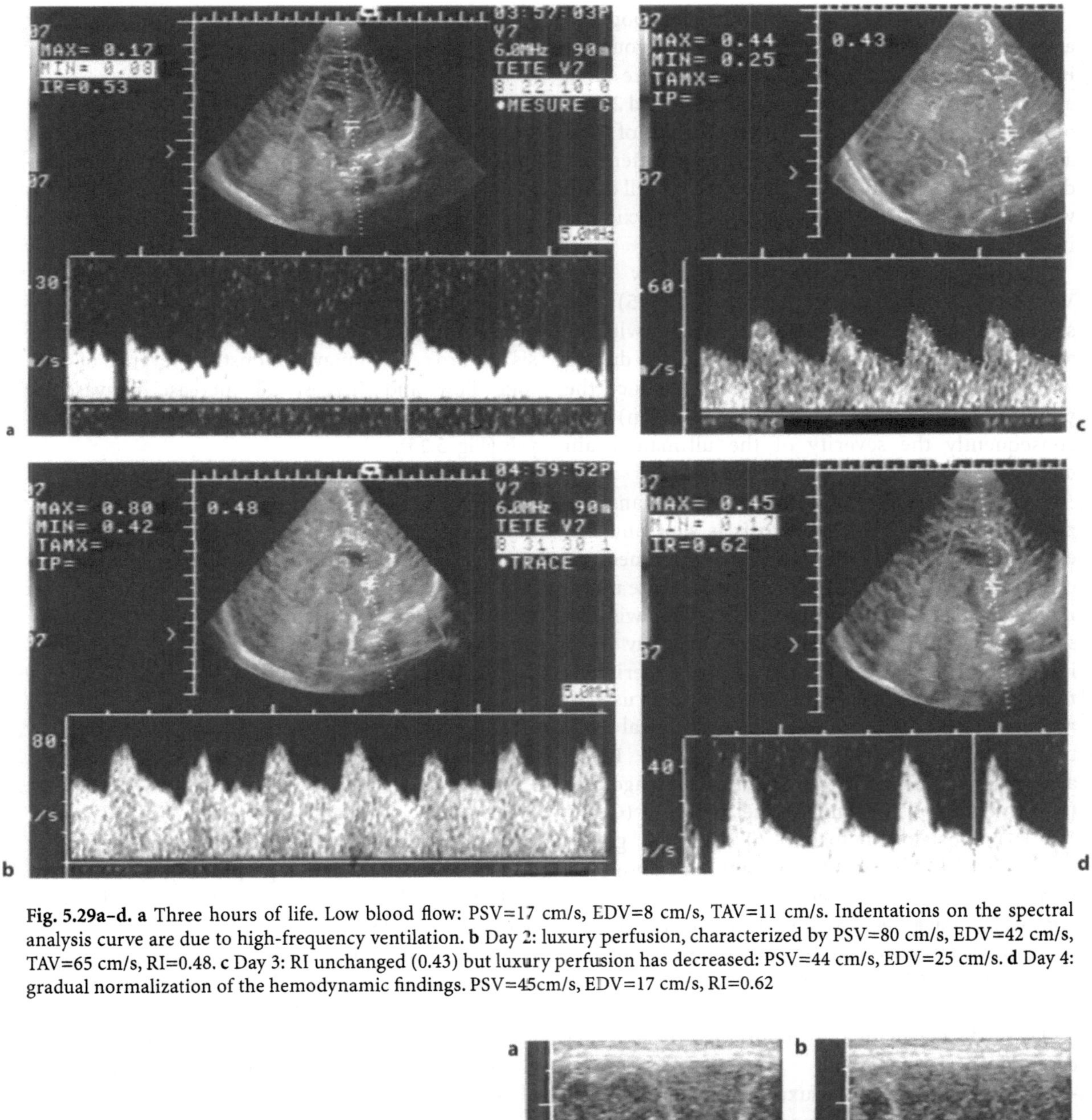

Fig. 5.29a–d. a Three hours of life. Low blood flow: PSV=17 cm/s, EDV=8 cm/s, TAV=11 cm/s. Indentations on the spectral analysis curve are due to high-frequency ventilation. **b** Day 2: luxury perfusion, characterized by PSV=80 cm/s, EDV=42 cm/s, TAV=65 cm/s, RI=0.48. **c** Day 3: RI unchanged (0.43) but luxury perfusion has decreased: PSV=44 cm/s, EDV=25 cm/s. **d** Day 4: gradual normalization of the hemodynamic findings. PSV=45cm/s, EDV=17 cm/s, RI=0.62

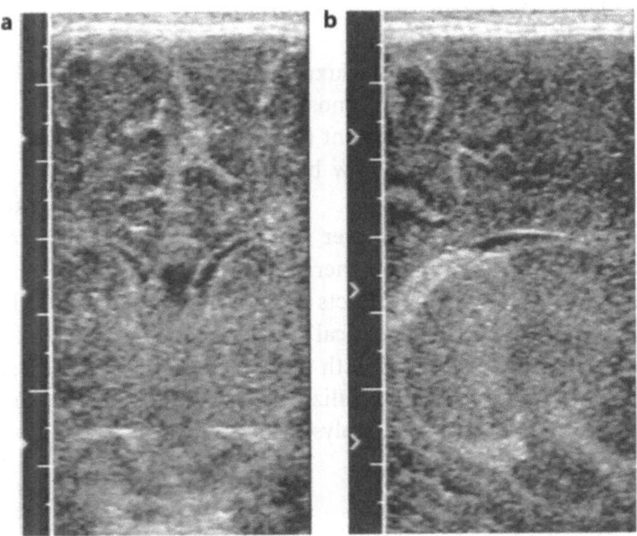

Fig. 5.30 a,b. On day 4, parenchymal damage was obvious, with hyperechogenicity of subcortical white matter (**a**), basal ganglia, and thalami (**b**)

Finally, EDWARDS (1997) has quantified apoptosis and necrosis in the cingulate gyrus of two groups of infants. In six newborns who suffered severe birth asphyxia, he found 8.3% of apoptotic cells and 20.8% of necrotic cells, compared with proportions of 6.7% and 3% respectively in six stillborn babies (after sudden intrauterine death at or close to term); cell death was apoptotic in 26% of cells after birth asphyxia and in 78% of cells in stillborn infants

Recently, several reports (HAMMERMAN 1997; VANNUCCI 1990; VANNUCCI 1997; VOLPE 1995) have suggested the existence of a therapeutic window after resuscitation from hypoxia–ischemia, during which intervention might successfully reduce the penumbra (preferential apoptotic location) and consequently the severity of the ultimate brain damage.

In adult experimental animals and humans, the process of necrosis and apoptosis is slow and can extend to several hours or more, but in the neonate cellular destruction appears to be much more rapid, no longer than 1 or 2 h, and the therapeutic window seems to be short. Nevertheless, this obviously offers interesting possibilities for the future. Experimentally, some pharmacological agents have been used to reduce the severity of neurotoxic biochemical reactions: oxygen free radical inhibitors (LIU 1994), allopurinol (PALMER 1990), glucamate antagonists (HATTORI 1989), calcium channel blockers (GUNN 1994), monosialogangliosides (TAN 1994), glucocorticosteroids (CHUMAS 1993), and high-dose phenobarbital (HALL 1999). Nonpharmacological approaches have been proposed too, including carbon dioxide (VANNUCCI 1997), hypothermia (BONNA 1998; YAGER 1996), and hypoxic preconditioning (GIDDAY 1994).

These data explain the importance of studying cerebral arterial velocities:
- Of course, postischemic luxury perfusion has been validated as a poor prognostic sign, but an earlier hemodynamic assessment (during the first hours of life) might detect low blood flow or cerebral hypoperfusion.
- Multiplication of Doppler studies might help to determine the time for therapeutic intervention.
- Since spectroscopy detects hypoperfusion within the cortical and subcortical capillaries, ultrasound harmonic techniques with contrast injection will perhaps succeed in visualizing these microvessels and guide spectral analysis for detection of a decreased focal CBF.

- *What is the role of color Doppler in the diagnostic and prognostic evaluation of anoxic–ischemic encephalopathy?*

Compared with morphological and hemodynamic findings, color Doppler imaging seems of little interest and there are few reports in the literature concerning its role. STEVENSON (1997) has shown the appearance of luxury perfusion on power Doppler imaging during an arterial infarction.

In fact, its main role is to facilitate the location of cerebral vessels and to guide reliable Doppler analysis. In rare cases, it may demonstrate reversal of diastolic flow and suggest an increase in vascular resistance, which must be confirmed by spectral analysis (Fig. 5.25).

The color Doppler presentation of parenchymal ischemic lesions depends on the timing of the study in relation to the ischemic insult: it may show hyperemia, a sign of luxury perfusion, if performed early (Fig. 5.31), but most often (OREY 1999), ischemic lesions appear as avascular areas (Fig. 5.32), sometimes improving the visualization of the lesions' extent (Fig. 5.33).

- *Imaging correlations (US/CT/MRI) confirm that ultrasonography is accurate in locating ischemic lesions.*

Out of 82 patients with anoxic–ischemic encephalopathy that we studied sonographically, 29 newborns underwent CT (26 cases) or MRI (3 cases) between day 3 and day 30:
- Subcortical hyperechogenicity (15 cases) correlated with subcortical hypoattenuation with respect to the cortical ribbon (Fig. 5.34), on CT
- Cortico-subcortical hyperechogenicity (11 cases) correlated with diffuse hypoattenuation on CT (Fig. 5.35).
- Ultrasonography also correlated with MR in 2 out of the three cases investigated (Fig. 5.36).

This comparative study demonstrates the accuracy of ultrasonography, thanks to the use of high-frequency probes.

Although these cortical and subcortical lesions, which are located in the border zones and end fields of the anterior, middle, and posterior cerebral arteries, are fairly easily diagnosed on ultrasonography, some limitations remain evident:
- When an ultrasound study is performed too early, the ischemic or edematous lesions are not yet visible; this explains the importance of sonographic follow-up and of an early Doppler study which

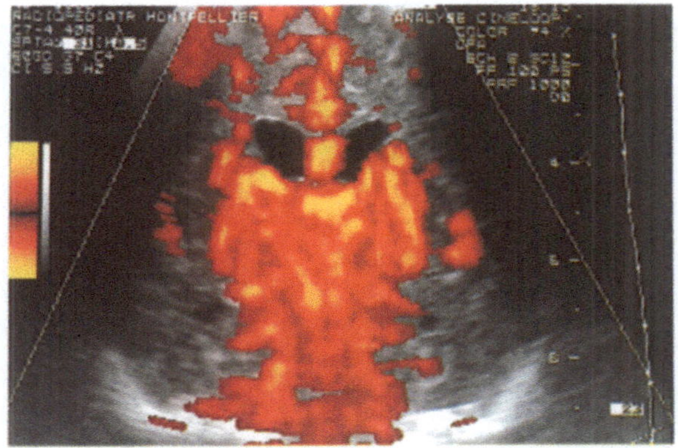

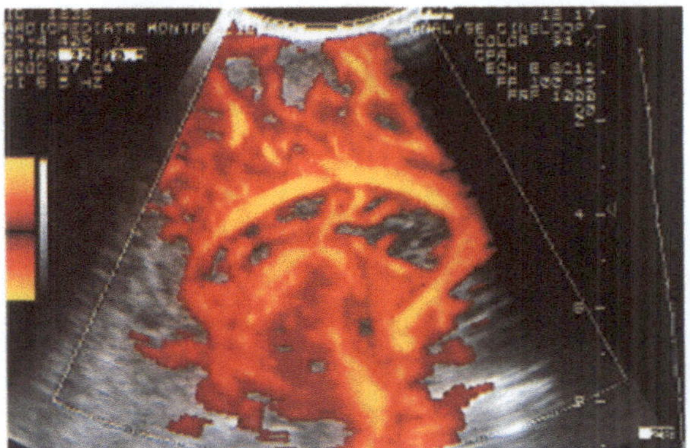

Fig. 5.31a,b. 3 months old infant. Severe dehydration. Extended cortical necrosis. On power Doppler, major hyperemia with vasodilatation of lenticulostriate, subependymal vessels (**a**) and pericallosal artery (**b**).

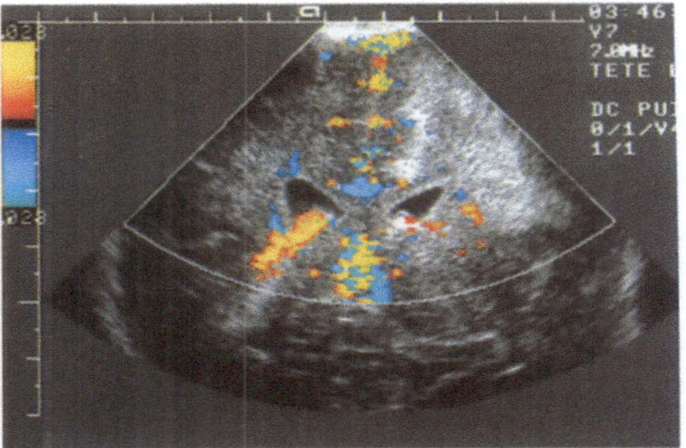

Fig. 5.32. A 4-day-old infant: *Proteus mirabilis* meningitis. Wide hyperechoic avascular area in left periventricular and subcortical location

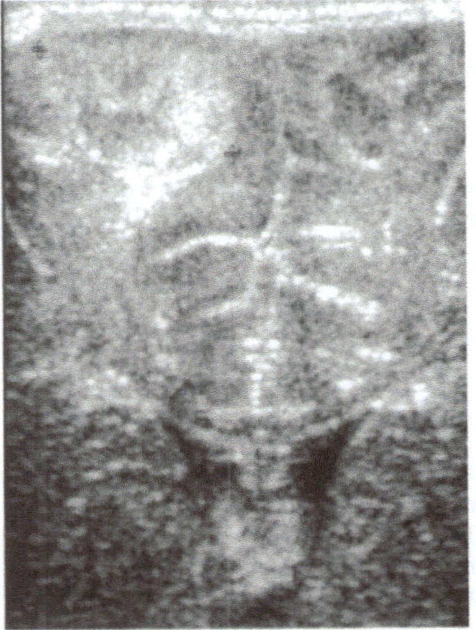

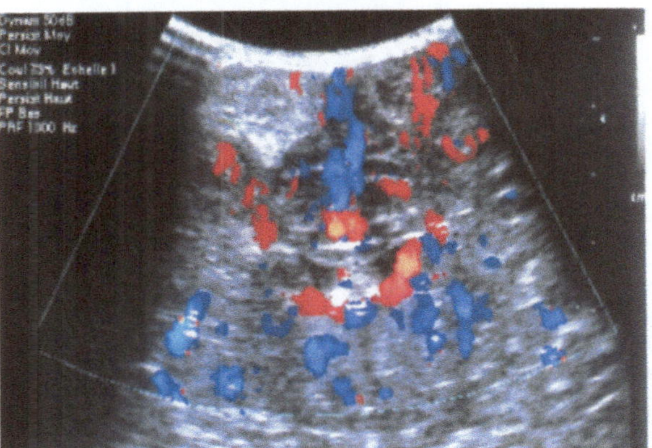

Fig. 5.33a,b. A 4-month-old baby: neurological distress. Ultrasonography (**a**) reveals cortico-subcortical lesions of different stages (hyperechoic on *right*, cystic on *left*), suggesting child abuse, which was ultimately confirmed. Color Doppler helps to detail the extent of the lesions (**b**)

may provide an immediate assessment of the prognosis (Fig. 5.37). In the same way, a late ultrasound investigation runs the risk of dreadful mistakes: the hyperechogenicity of ischemic gray or white matter may decrease early and the severity of the lesion may be underestimated, especially as hemodynamic alterations also usually disappear from day 4 to day 8 (Fig. 5.38). Ultrasound follow-up is required to show cyst formation or cerebral atrophy.

- In fact, the main difficulty is that ultrasound is unable to differentiate between reversible and irreversible ischemia by morphological examination alone. This is an acute problem when the physician is hesitating between grade II and grade III encephalopathy. Hyperechoic white matter edema has the same appearance as subcortical ischemia but is rapidly reversible. There is an obvious value in coupling the inadequate morphological imaging to an early Doppler recording which will guide the diagnosis (Fig. 5.39).

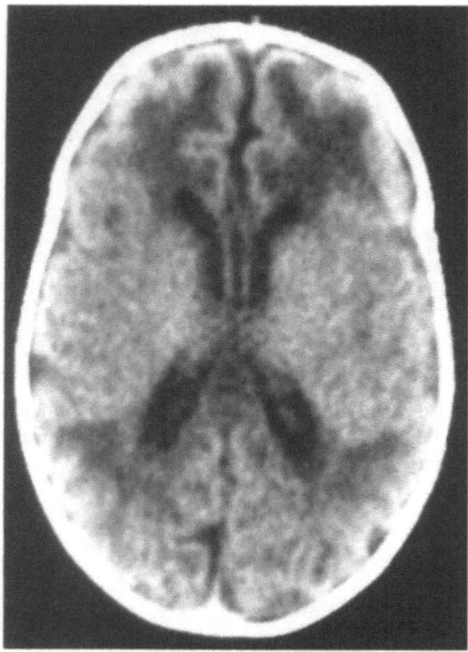

Fig. 5.34. A full-term neonate: urgent cesarean delivery (toxemia). Ultrasonography showed sub-cortical ischemia; RI=0.50. White matter damage was confirmed by CT

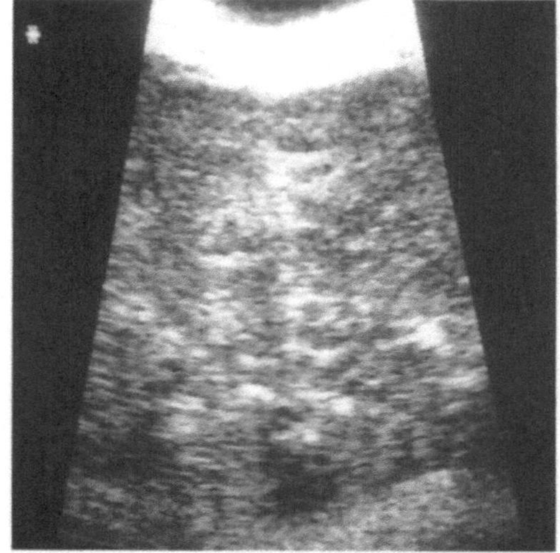

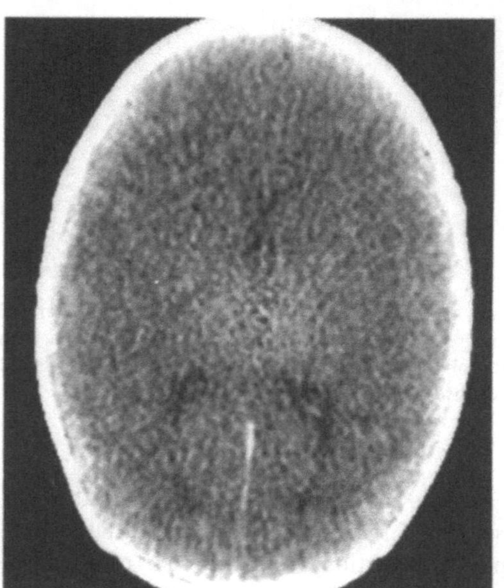

Fig. 5.35a,b. A full-term neonate: perinatal injury with neonatal seizures. Ultrasonography showed cortico-subcortical ischemic damage (**a**). On CT (**b**), there was diffuse hypoattenuation of brain parenchyma

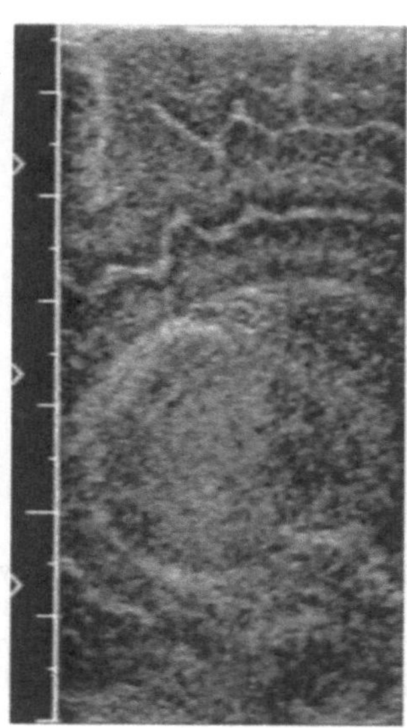

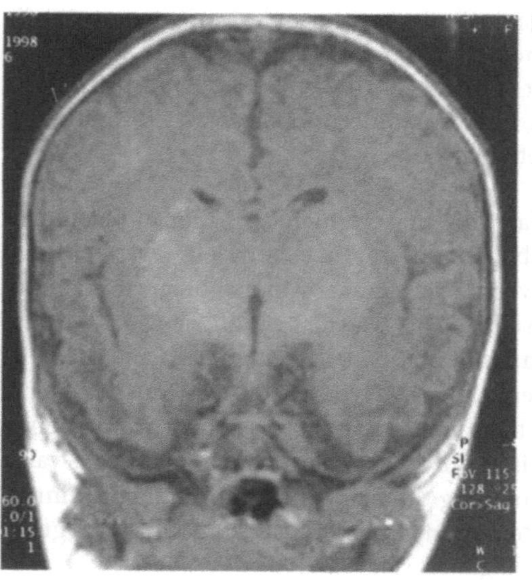

Fig. 5.36a,b. Status epilepticus after cord prolapse in a full-term newborn.
a On ultrasonography (right parasagittal plane), white matter and thalami ischemia are well seen.
b On T1-weighted MRI, the involvement was confirmed: multiple hyperintense spots are present within the lenticulostriate nuclei and thalami, and there is a diffuse decrease in the usual hypointensity of white matter and cortico-subcortical differentiation

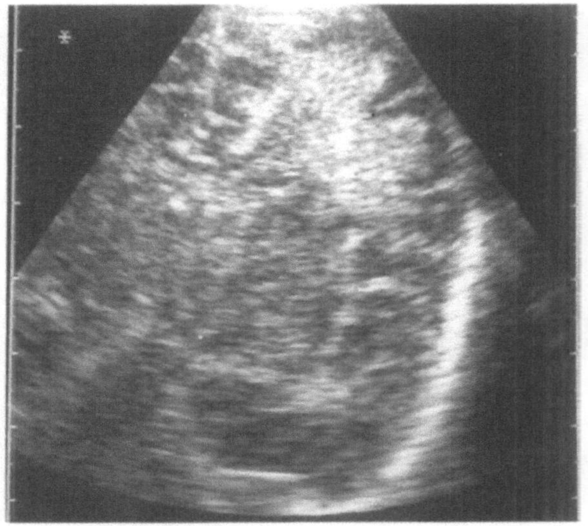

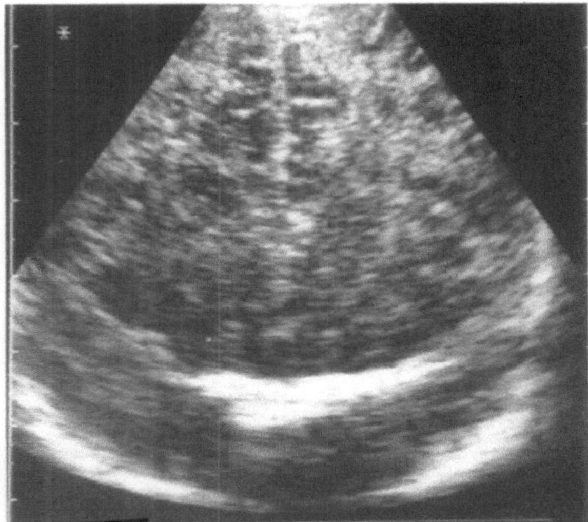

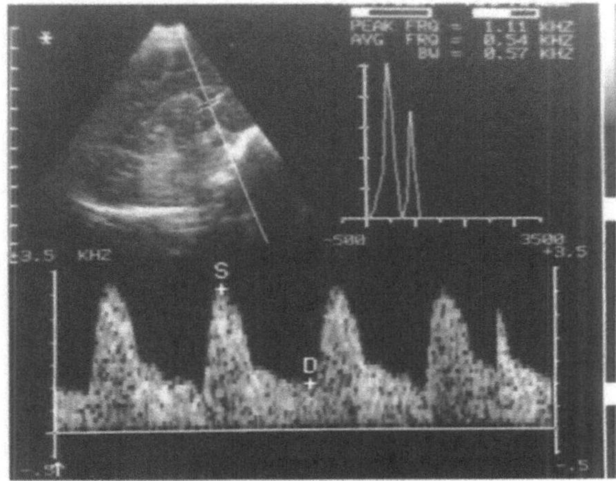

Fig. 5.37a–c. A full-term newborn: perinatal asphyxi injury. Seizures resolved with anticonvulsive drugs. Ultrasonography was performed on day 2. The morphological appearance was worrying, with hyperechoic white matter (**a,b**). By contrast, hemodynamic data were normal, with RI=0.65 in the pericallosal artery. **c** Follow-up ultrasonography showed normalization of subcortical echogenicity (probably reversible edema) while the hemodynamics remained normal. At 2 years of age, the child's psychomotor development is normal

In difficult cases, ultrasound and MRI should obviously be combined. In adults, it has now been demonstrated that diffusion-weighted MRI (GONZALES 1999) allows accurate diagnosis of acute stroke within 6 h of symptom onset. The mechanism is the decrease in water diffusion within ischemic tissue, due in part to cytotoxic edema. These new sequences seem to be promising in the early evaluation of neonatal brain ischemia (NEIL 1998).

– Ischemic brain lesions have a severe prognosis (Table 5.12). Our experience agrees with the literature since the intensity of the neonatal clinical pattern is in obvious correlation to the severity of the neurological outcome.

Among 61 patients with grade III anoxic–ischemic encephalopathy (57 newborns and four infants), 54 patients died early (88%), seven suffered motor and/or intellectual handicap; only one child had a normal development. The first ultrasound examination is essential, but sonographic follow-up of survivors is needed to show the formation of cerebral atrophy (Fig. 5.40) or porencephalic cysts (Fig. 5.26).

The long-term prognosis of grade II anoxic–ischemic encephalopathy remains uncertain, but less severe than that of grade III encephalopathy. In 21 patients, psychomotor development was evaluated for between 2 and 4 years; it was normal in 11 patients (52%), motor handicap was found in six cases, and four patients died early.

Although the clinical grading of asphyxial injury seems to provide a reliable foundation for prognosis, the severity of anoxic–ischemic encephalopathy remains difficult to appreciate. In a majority of cases,

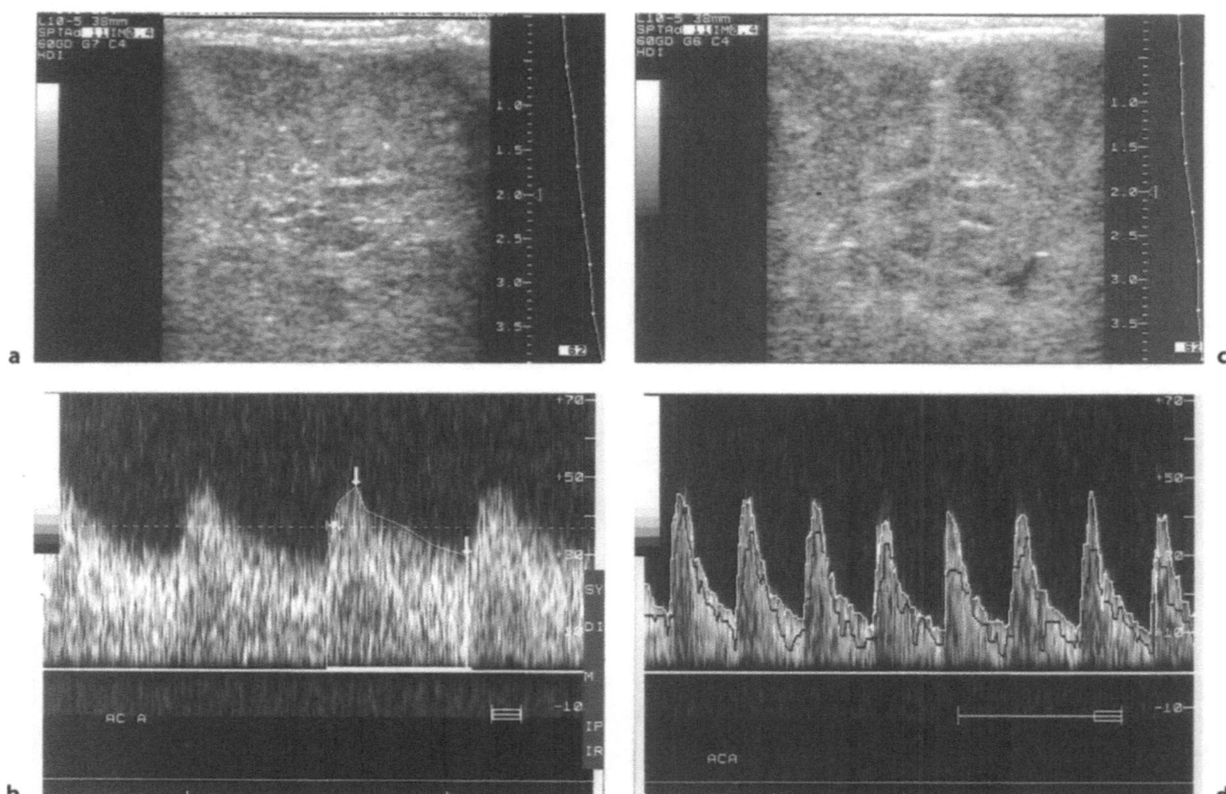

Fig. 5.38a–d. Grade III anoxic–ischemic encephalopathy. Neonatal ultrasonography confirmed the severity of the clinical pattern: cortico-subcortical ischemia (**a**), luxury perfusion (**b**), with RI=0.37 and increased velocities. On day 7, gray-scale (**c**) and pulsed Doppler imaging (**d**) showed normal findings. Reviewed at 4 years of age, the child presented with strabismus, severe psychomotor retardation, and left spastic hemiparesis

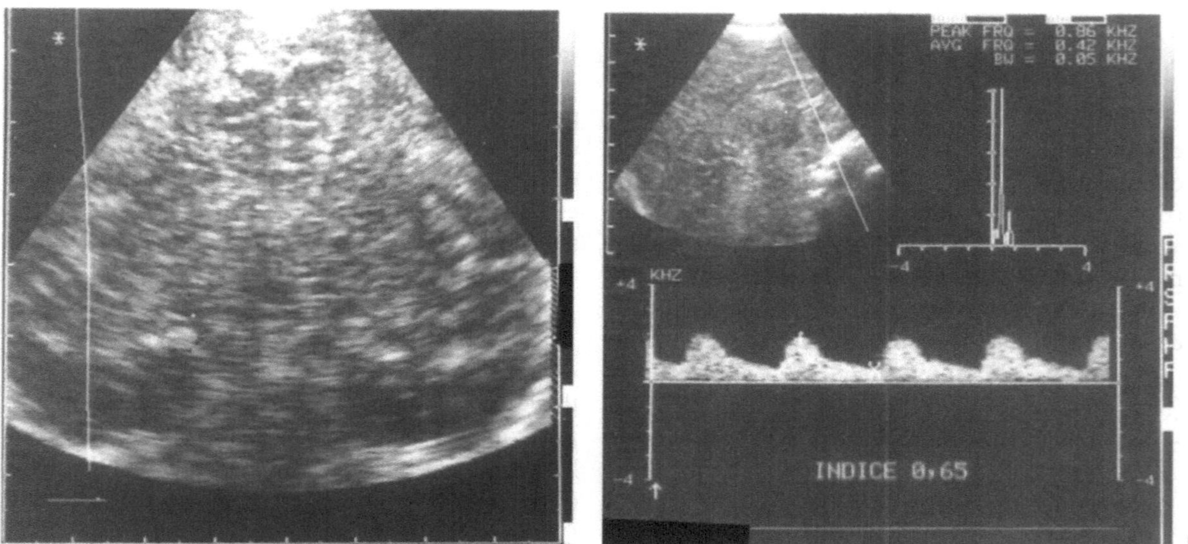

Fig. 5.39a,b. A twin gestation: seizures on day 1. The morphological appearance is worrying since hyperechoic areas are diffusely distributed within white matter (**a**). On the other hand, pulsed Doppler on anterior cerebral artery (**b**) is more reassuring: RI=0.65. The hyperechoic lesions rapidly disappeared and hemodynamic data remained normal. At 2 months of age, psychomotor development and ultrasound examination were normal

Table 5.12. Anoxic–ischemic encephalopathy Outcome (follow-up 2–23 months) in 82 patients

GRADE III	61 patients
Death	54
Sequelae	6
- Spastic tetraparesis	3
- Lower limb hypertonia	1
- Psychomotor retardation	1
- Psychomotor retardation and lower limb hypertonia	1
Normal	1

GRADE II	21 patients
Normal	11
Hypertonia	5
Death	4
Spastic diplegia	1

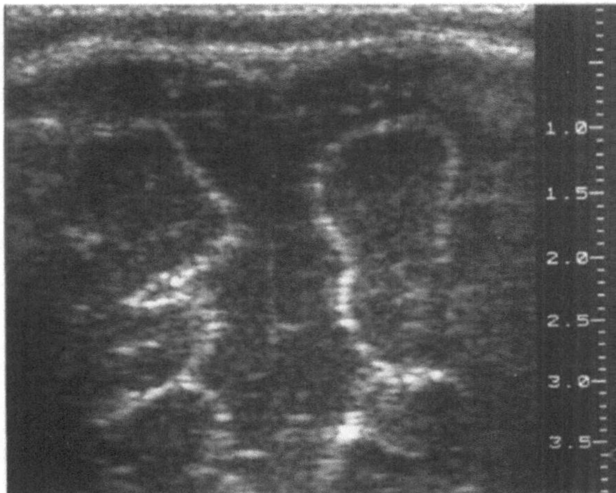

Fig. 5.40. Maternal toxemia: subcortical ischemic damage, with psychomotor retardation and repeated seizures at 5 months of life. Ultrasonography showed major cerebral atrophy with obvious enlargement of the interhemispheric fissure

asphyxia results from ante or intrapartum insult, and the severity of fetal hypoxemia and/or ischemia is difficult to specify.

Of our own 82 cases of anoxic-ischemic encephalopathy, fetal or perinatal asphyxia accounted for 82% (68 newborns). This indicates that a precise assessment of fetal acid-base status is required.

The Apgar score is known to be an inconsistently reliable criterion of ischemic damage (MARLOW 1992): first, determination of the Apgar score varies among observers, sometimes considerably; and, second, nonneurological causes (CORDERO 1971) may be responsible for a depressed score (laryngeal inhibi-

tion, maternal drug or anesthesia). In a series of 1,200 consecutive deliveries (SYKES 1982), only 20% of infants with Apgar scores lower than 7 had acidosis with pH≤7.10 (umbilical artery).

Generalized seizures constitute an indicator of poor prognosis (SCHER 1993), but subtle seizures are frequent and may be unrecognized: they include ocular phenomena such as horizontal or vertical deviation of the eyes, abnormal oral-buccal-lingual movements, swimming or rowing movements of the limbs, and apneic spells (HELMERS 1991).

These obvious difficulties in the clinical evaluation of anoxic–ischemic encephalopathy justify routine early morphological and Doppler ultrasound imaging, which seems to provide the main evidence for differential diagnosis between grade II and grade III encephalopathy. Grade II asphyxia has a favorable outcome in more than 60% of cases, whereas grade III injury is followed by early death or severe psychomotor sequelae in almost all cases.

For the last 12 years, we have performed routine ultrasonography and Doppler imaging in all patients with neonatal asphyxia:
- *In grade I encephalopathy,* morphological and hemodynamic studies and neurological outcome are normal.
- *In grade II encephalopathy,* motor or intellectual handicap occurs in 40% of cases (ARABIN 1988; ARDUINI 1989; FAVRE 1991; VYAS 1990). Gray-scale ultrasonography is most often normal, and only transient white matter hyperechogenicity may be observed, probably corresponding to brain edema. Exceptional hemodynamic disturbances are seen in individual cases, for which no plausible explanation can be proposed at present: 21 patients with grade II injury showed an increased diastolic amplitude, suggesting a poor prognosis, although psychomotor outcome was normal in 11 of them. Thus, an accurate clinical evaluation remains essential and is the main guide for neonatal resuscitation when sonographic findings are discordant. This also demonstrates the insufficiency of our knowledge of hemodynamic alterations in neonatal neurological distress. LIVES (1998) noted, during the first 12 h of life, decreased velocities in cases of moderate encephalopathy, whereas they were highly increased in grade III encephalopathy. This is in agreement with our experience, since there is a parallel relationship between the intensity of luxury perfusion and the severity of encephalopathy: diastolic velocities increase in grade II injury, but major hyperemia is only observed in severe grade III injury.

– *In grade III encephalopathy*, death or severe sequelae are the rule. Echostructural and hemodynamic alterations are constant, while subcortical and/or cortical hyperechogenicity signifies irreversible ischemic lesions.

Hemodynamic disturbances are present at birth after a prenatal insult, but are early and prolonged after a postnatal event.

– *The evaluation of a distressed fetus represents the most obvious potentiality of pulsed and color Doppler ultrasonography.*

Obviously, the axis of research should relate to the prevention of brain damage. In a distressed newborn, detection of ischemic lesions and hemodynamic alterations indicates an irreversibly damaged state: the battle has been lost. It would be important to intervene earlier, and the potential value of investigating cerebral vessels in the fetus at risk, using pulsed Doppler guided by color imaging (Fig. 5.41), is evident.

Obstetricians know the significance of hemodynamics in growth-retarded fetuses: abnormal indices in umbilical arteries constitute a valuable finding of fetal distress, and the examination of the cerebral arteries evaluates the responsiveness of fetal brain to hypoxemia. Intensive treatment or fetal extraction is decided on when blood flow redistribution is observed with cerebral vasodilatation. In acute fetal distress, the clinical conditions are different: the fetus has normal growth, but abruptly becomes asphyxial during the end of pregnancy, labor, or delivery. Predicting this insult seems to be impossible, but all efforts should be directed toward hemodynamic monitoring during the last month of high-risk pregnancy: maternal hypertension (ARBEILLE 1987), maternal diabetes (BRACERO 1986), uterine bleeding (JOUPILLA 1984), post-term continuation (BRAR 1989). In these high-risk situations, true hemodynamic monitoring should be carried out: detection of a reduced RI in fetal brain (contrasting with previously normal data) constitutes an emergency requiring immediate intervention for preserving brain parenchyma.

RIZZO (1989) has shown that a decreased pulsatility index in fetal carotid artery (below 2 deviations from the normal mean value) has good predictive value for postnatal neurological disturbances. In this author's opinion, a severe drop in cerebral RI slightly precedes the onset of an abnormal heart rate pattern in the asphyxial fetus. CYNOBER (1990) measured the diastolic index (end-diastolic velocity/peak systolic velocity) in 161 women with abnormal or a history of

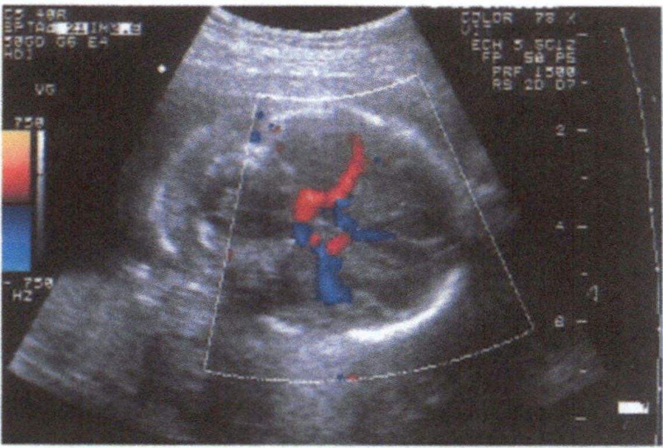

Fig. 5.41. A 24-week fetus. Color Doppler easily identifies the circle of Willis and the superficial (superior sagittal sinus) and deep (straight sinus, vein of Galen, internal cerebral vein) venous system. Thus, analysis of venous and arterial vasculature is possible in early fetal life

abnormal pregnancy. He noted that an increased carotid diastolic index may predict the delayed onset of fetal heart rate alterations or fetal death in utero.

Other authors, using different indices, have drawn the same conclusions. For example, a reverse diastolic flow in the fetal aorta or the umbilical artery indicates major blood flow disturbances and imminent fetal death (ILLYES 1988; JOUPILLA 1984).

Despite all this, the hemodynamic alterations in the distressed fetus remain poorly known. In human and experimental fetal injury, it has been demonstrated that the response to moderate hypoxemia is systemic hypertension and increased CBF with reduced distal vascular resistances (GIUSSANI 1994; DE HAAN 1993). When asphyxia persists in experimental models, cardiac contractility, arterial pressure, and CBF decrease (WILLIAMS 1990). Moreover, the hemodynamic response depends on the severity and rapidity of the asphyxial insult: BENNET (1998) reported a reduced CBF with increased vascular resistances after complete and rapid ligation of the umbilical cord in lamb fetus. These experimental data show how difficult it is to provide a clear physiopathological schema, and the human fetus does not necessarily have the same postischemic response. That is why it is important to detect and demonstrate luxury perfusion in an asphyxial fetus.

5.3
Brain Injury in the Premature Infant

Brain injury in the premature infant is mainly represented by periventricular leukomalacia and hemorrhagic infarction. Four problems predominate:

- Periventricular leukomalacia remains a severe disease, causing motor deficits and intellectual retardation. Its prevention, which is difficult, is based on suppression of all ischemia-inducing factors: systemic hypotension, hypercarbia, hypoxemia, loss of cerebral autoregulation (Fig. 5.42). Recent epidemiological studies (FINESMITH 1997; HAUTH 1995; NELSON 1999, 1996; SCHENDEL 1996) have shown that low-birth-weight preterm infants exposed antenatally to magnesium sulfate have a reduced risk of developing cystic periventricular leukomalacia.
- The diagnosis of periventricular leukomalacia relies on ultrasonography, which should be performed early, during the hyperechoic stage, not after cyst formation, which occurs too late and inconstantly.
- Color Doppler imaging helps to explain the pathogenesis of periventricular hemorrhagic infarction, but pulsed Doppler remains extremely disappointing.
- Periventricular damage is of vascular origin, but the mechanisms of ischemia are quite different from those of the term newborn, because of the immaturity of the premature brain vasculature. Periventricular leukomalacia is a consequence of intra-arterial disturbances, while hemorrhagic infarction is a venous infarct.

5.3.1
Periventricular Leukomalacia

5.3.1.1
Neuropathology and Clinical Context

Periventricular leukomalacia is defined by necrosis of white matter in a characteristic distribution (BANKER 1962) dorsal and lateral to the external angles of the lateral ventricles, involving particularly the centrum semiovale and optic and acoustic radiations (Diagram 5.3).

The lesions are usually bilateral.

The neuropathological pattern is characterized in the first 6–12 h by focal coagulation necrosis with axonal rupture and oligodendroglial loss. Over the next 24–48 h, the cellular response includes infiltration by microglia, proliferation of hypertrophic astrocytes, and endothelial hyperplasia. Macrophagic cells appear at about 5 days. The lesion evolves toward cyst formation after 1 week to 1 month (Fig. 5.43). Finally, the cavities gradually constrict, leaving a glial unmyelinized scar.

Periventricular leukomalacia is highly preponderant in premature neonates, as shown in the literature (AMATO 1987; MARRET 1998; MONSET-COUCHARD 1988; SHUMAN 1980; VOLPE 1997; ZUPAN 1996): in a study of 82 patients with periventricular leukomalacia reported by SHUMAN (1980), 88% had birth weights between 900 and 2,200 g.

Any ante-, peri-, or neonatal event able to induce a loss of cerebral autoregulation and a decrease in CBF in a fetus or a preterm neonate represents a high-risk factor for developing periventricular leukomalacia.

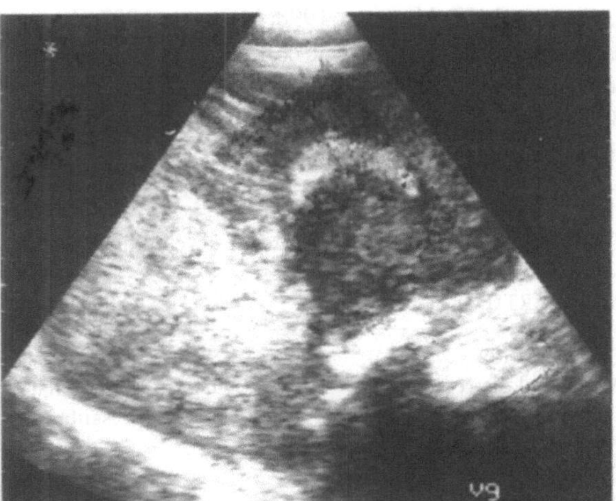

Fig. 5.42a,b. A 29-weeks' gestation premature infant: respiratory distress with mechanical ventilation and variations in arterial blood pressure. At 2 h of life, fluctuating Doppler findings characterized a loss of cerebral autoregulation (a). Seizures occurred 6 h later. Intraventricular hemorrhage and large hemorrhagic periventricular infarction occurred (b)

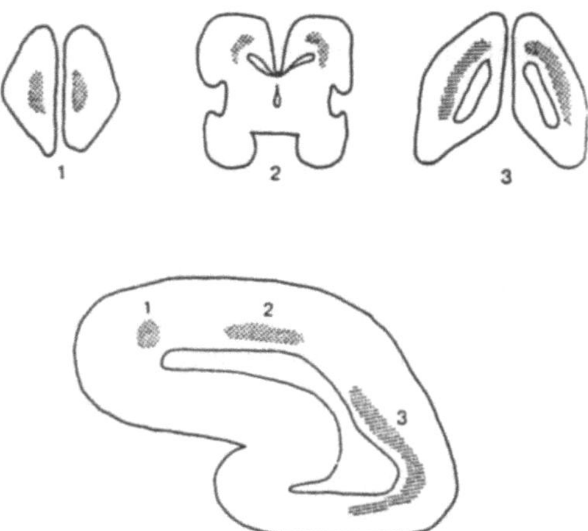

1 - Anterior
2 - Corona radiata
3 - Occipital

Diagram 5.3. Periventricular leukomalacia: preferential location (From BANKER 1962)

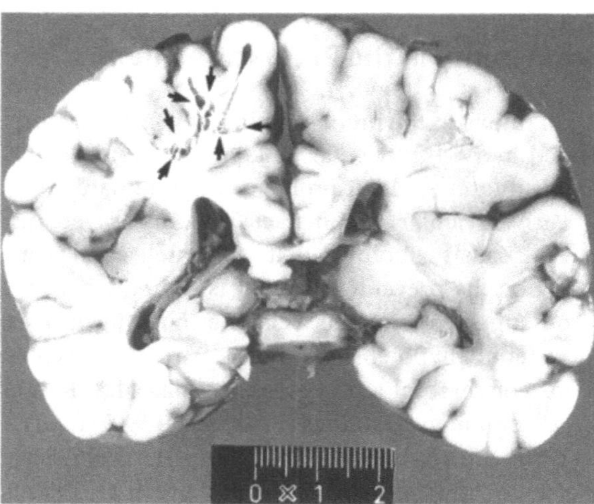

Fig. 5.43. A preterm infant with periventricular leukomalacia. Death occurred on day 15. Notice the porencephalic cysts at the lateral angle of the right ventricle (*arrows*). Microscopic specimens show liquefaction of necrotic foci. (From Drs. Fawer and Derwaz, Lausanne)

The clinical circumstances associated with this condition are multiple (Table 5.13) and, most often, interacting.

The important role of postnatal illness is apparent in all reports (AMATO 1987; BEJAR 1986; BOWERMAN 1984; CHOW 1985; KELLER 1987; MURPHY 1997; SHUMAN 1980), which highlight the significant incidence of respiratory distress. The frequency with which spastic diplegia is seen after neonatal apneic spells or severe bradycardia is well known (PERLMAN 1985).

Intrauterine infection and premature rupture of membranes correlate strongly with the occurrence of periventricular leukomalacia (ALEXANDER 1998; GRETHER 1997; MARRET 1998; MURPHY 1997; ZUPAN 1996). A prenatal infectious context is associated with leukomalacia in 22% of preterm infants (born before 32 weeks' gestation) (ZUPAN 1996). These clinical data confirm experimental studies: GILLES (1977)

reproduced periventricular white matter cystic changes after injection of endotoxin into newborn kittens. YOON (1996) created an *E. coli* chorionitis model in the pregnant rabbit, and reported that 14% of fetuses exhibited cerebral lesions similar to those in periventricular leukomalacia.

In our experience (Table 5.13), chorionitis represents approximately 20% of cases of periventricular leukomalacia.

Antepartum formation of periventricular leukomalacia is possible, as is shown by anatomical data (NAKUMURA 1986) and the detection of cystic leukomalacia at birth (SZYMONOVICZ 1985) (Fig. 5.44).

In the literature, the antecedents that are reported are ordinary: MONSET-COUCHARD (1988) notes 18 cases of threatened preterm labor, four of twin gestation, five of maternal toxemia, and 12 of premature rupture of membranes (>24 h) out of 30 patients with

Table 5.13. Brain injury. Risk factors for developing periventricular leukomalacia (103 cases)

ANTEPARTUM		INTRAPARTUM		POSTPARTUM	
Twin gestation	26	Acute cord prolapse	3	Respiratory distress	51
Acute fetal distress	8	Uterine hemorrhage	3	Infection	18
Toxemia	5	Breech presentation	2	- Group B Streptococcus	5
Hyperthermia	4			- E. coli	2
Diabetes	3			- Hemophilus influenzae	2
Placenta previa	3			Bradycardia, apnea	17
Retroplacental hematoma	3			Apparent death state	9
				Patent ductus arteriosus	3
				Hypoglycemia	1

periventricular leukomalacia. Our results are similar: 26 twin gestations, five cases of toxemia, four of maternal fever, and three of diabetes (Table 5.13). Thus, it is difficult to discern a precise pathogenesis to explain antenatal periventricular ischemia.

A history of acute placental or cord disturbances or uterine hemorrhage during labor and delivery is often encountered in periventricular leukomalacia (CALVERT 1986; WEINDLING 1985) (Table 5.13).

Finally, unexpected acute fetal distress and threatened preterm labor are obviously a frequent cause.

5.3.1.2
Pathogenesis

The pathogenesis is multifactorial, but is primarily related to the immaturity of the cerebral vasculature in premature infants. DE REUCK (1971, 1984), TAKASHIMA (1987), and RORKE (1992) have demonstrated clearly that periventricular leukomalacia occurs in areas that represent arterial border zones.

The vascular supply of the premature brain is provided by long and short penetrating arteries deriving from the middle cerebral artery and, to a lesser extent, the anterior and posterior cerebral arteries. The immediate periventricular area is supplied by the basal penetrating arteries (e.g., lenticulostriate arteries) and the choroidal arteries (Diagram 5.4).

This distribution results in arterial border and end-zones, and this vulnerable hypovascular area is more or less severely injured primarily in dependence on gestational age. At 24–28 weeks' gestation (RORKE 1992), the long penetrating arteries have few side branches and infrequent anastomoses with the short penetrating arteries. Thus, a fall in perfusion pressure and CBF will result in more severe periventricular and subcortical ischemia in a 28-week premature baby than in a 32-week baby with a more mature cerebral vasculature.

This particular vascular anatomy in the premature infant explains the periventricular location of

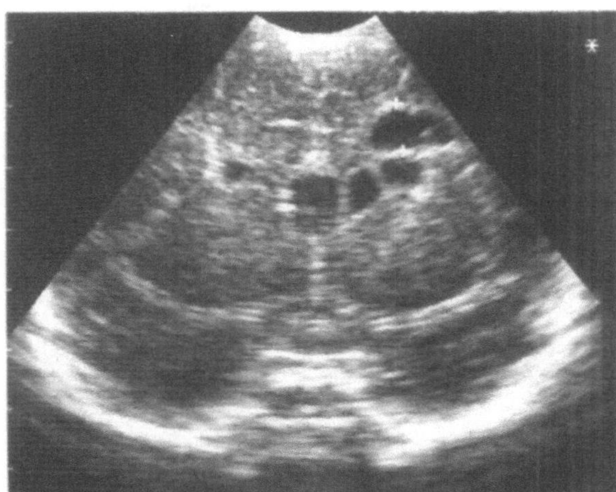

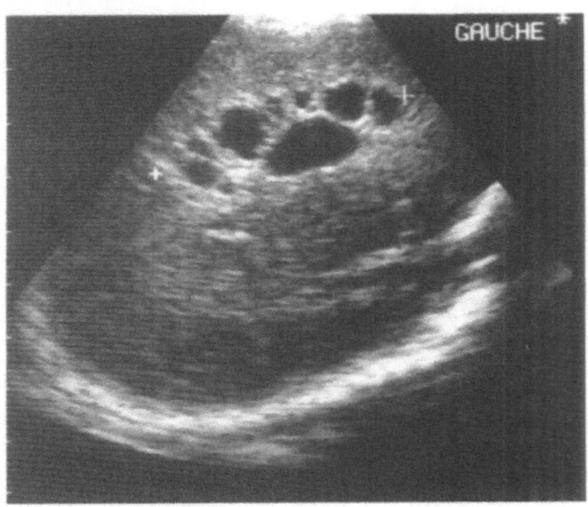

Fig. 5.44a,b. A 36-weeks' gestation preterm infant: moderate neonatal neurological distress. On day 4, ultrasonography shows paraventricular cysts (a,b), which predominate on the left, and are probably related to antenatal periventricular leukomalacia

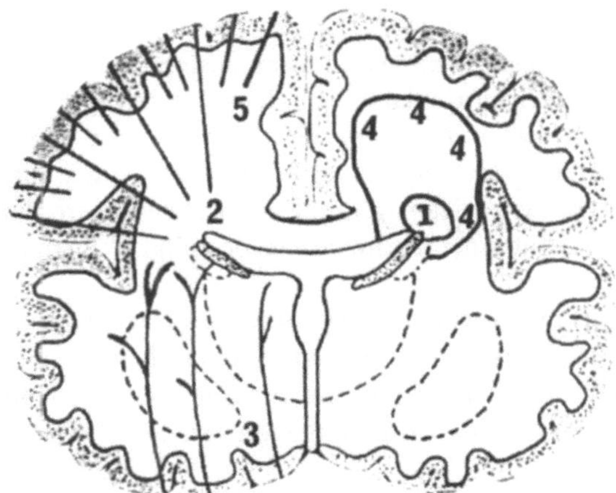

Diagram 5.4. Cerebral vascular supply in the human premature infant (from VOLPE 1997). In the premature infant, the cerebral vascular supply of the immediate periventricular region explains the occurrence of periventricular leukomalacia, which may be focal (1) where long (2) and basal (3) penetrating vessels terminate, or diffuse (4) resulting from the lack of interconnections between long (2) and short (5) penetrating vessels

the ischemic foci. The second factor is the occurrence of a pressure-passive cerebral circulation; near-infrared spectroscopy may identify this situation, which represents a high risk of developing periventricular leukomalacia, prior to the injury (VOLPE 1997).

In addition to the interaction of vascular endzones and pressure-passive cerebral circulation, factors related to an intrinsic vulnerability of white matter in the premature baby are important: there is a limited vasodilatory capacity in response to hypoxemia, hypercarbia, or hypotension (CAVAZUTTI 1982; PURVES 1969). Particular vulnerability of differentiating oligodendroglia to the action of free radicals during the ischemia–reperfusion sequence has been demonstrated (BACK 1977).

Finally, cytokines stimulated by bacterial chorionitis contribute to altering the oligodendroglial tissue and increase the incidence of periventricular leukomalacia (GILLES 1977; LEVITON 1990; PERLMAN 1996; YOON 1996).

5.3.1.3 Diagnosis

The diagnosis is, and should remain, based on ultrasonography (COUTURE 1994). The first ultrasound examination should be performed very early in the preterm asphyxial baby, in order to diagnose or rule out periventricular leukomalacia in the immediate neonatal period. Among 103 patients with periventricular leukomalacia that we studied from 1991 to 1995, the diagnosis was easily made by ultrasonography when involvement was bilateral and extensive (Table 5.14).

In 68 cases, it appeared as extensive, poorly limited, periventricular echodensities (Fig. 5.45). (FAWER 1987; GRAZIANI 1993; HASHIMOTO 1996; HOPE 1988; MURPHY 1996; ROTH 1993), either diffuse, fronto-parieto-occipital, or focalized in frontal areas, or, infrequently, in parieto-occipital white matter.

This hyperechogenicity corresponds to coagulation necrosis, sometimes with hemorrhage, and is produced by multiple sharp interfaces between areas of normal and damaged tissue (NWAESEI 1984).

In the literature, BABCOCK (1995) and others (BAARSMA 1987) report that the sensitivity of ultrasonography for diagnosing leukomalacia is only about 30%. Their explanation is that periventricular leukomalacia may be impossible to differentiate from the normal periventricular halo which is of uncertain signification: white matter immaturity, high water content of the premature brain, or increased reflec-

Table 5.14. Ultrasonographic pattern of periventricular leukomalacia (103 cases)

Extensive and Bilateral Leukomalacia 84 cases

First US		US follow-up	
Hyperechoic Pattern	68		
- Fronto parietal	31	Cysts	46
- Parieto-occipital	11	No cyst	12
- Frontal	5		
- Fronto-parieto-occipital	21	Death	10
Cystic Pattern	16	Death	2

Focal and Unilateral Leukomalacia 19 cases

First US		US follow up	
Hyperechoic Pattern	8	Cysts	5
		No cyst	3
		Death	1
Cystic Pattern	,11		

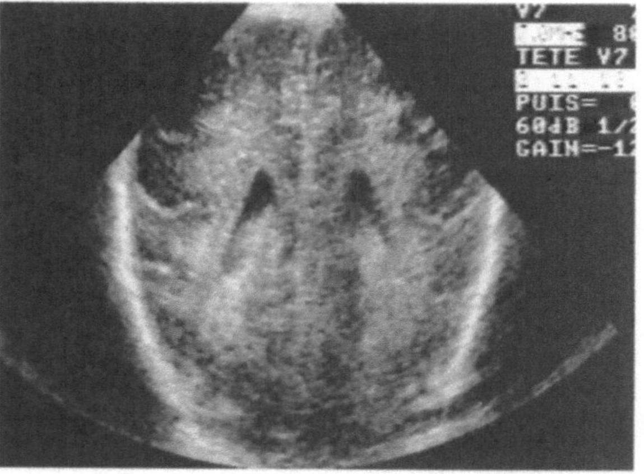

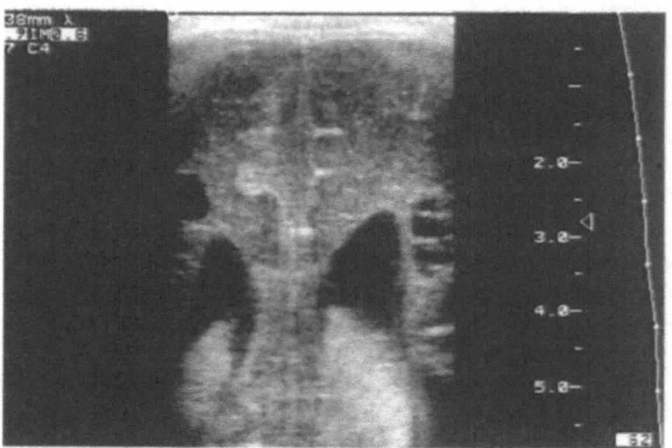

Fig. 5.45a,b. A 32-weeks' gestation premature infant with chorionitis. **a** Day 7: abnormal hyperechogenicity of periventricular white matter. **b** Day 30: development of porencephalic cysts and atrophic ventricular enlargement

tions from axons radiating outward from the ventricles.

This criticism (BABCOCK 1995) seems to be excessive, since it is based on old studies and the diagnosis may be improved by the use of newer equipment. When the examination is carried out under optimal conditions (a known clinical history, early ultrasonography utilizing high-frequency probes), it allows recognition of the leukomalacic involvement which is more extensive, more hyperechoic, and more poorly defined than normal white matter (Fig. 5.46).

This is very important since subsequent development of cysts is inconstant, as demonstrated in our series: of 68 patients with extensive bilateral leukomalacia, porencephalic cysts appeared in only 46 (69%) (Table 5.14). Thus, the diagnosis should be suspected on ultrasound study soon after birth, and should prompt MRI (BARKOVICH 1995; BATTIN 1997) if clinical and ultrasound findings are discordant.

In our experience of periventricular leukomalacia, improvement of the diagnosis and early establishment of the prognosis necessarily requires an ultrasonography protocol in neonates at risk, i.e., preterm infants born at less than 34 weeks' gestation, birth weight below 1,500 g, or neurological or asphyxial distress (Table 5.15).

Table 5.15. Periventricular leukomalacia Protocol study

Day 1 ⇒ Day 3: First US examination
Day 3 ⇒ Day 15: US every 5 days
  If normal: US at 6 weeks and 4 months
  If abnormal: US once a week

MRI:
  Early if US ineffective
  At 6 months – 1 year:
  assessment of any delay in myelination process

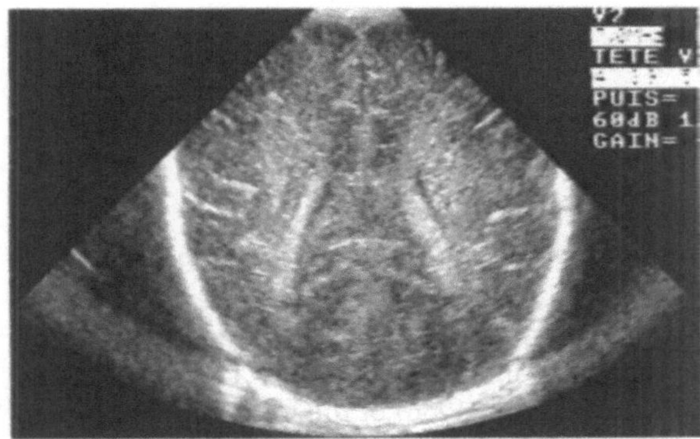

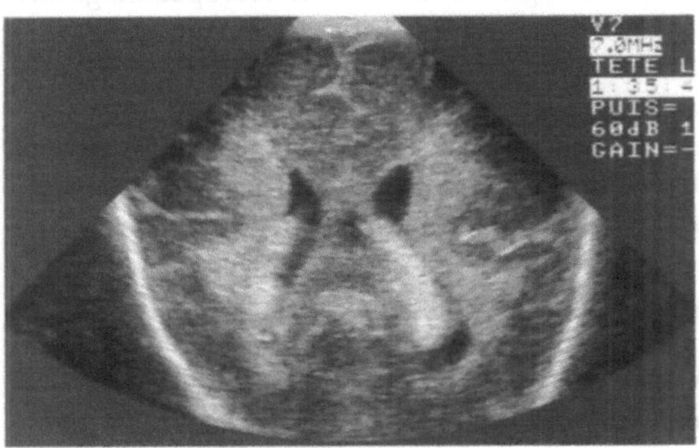

Fig. 5.46. a A 30-weeks' gestation premature infant with mild physiological periventricular hyperechogenicity. Good clinical and ultrasonographic outcome at 4 months of age. **b** A 31-weeks' gestation premature infant. The diagnosis of periventricular leukomalacia is evident. Cyst formation at 1 month of age

5.3.1.4
Pulsed and Color Doppler: What Is Their Value?

These techniques have been very disappointing in our experience. This is based on several facts:

- Leukomalacia may occur before birth, and, in our series, 16 patients had periventricular cystic changes at the first examination (Table 5.14).
- The capacity for arterial vasodilatation in periventricular areas remains moderate and poorly detectable on color Doppler imaging.
- Hemodynamic analysis does not help prevention, prediction, or early diagnosis of leukomalacia. Doppler ultrasonography of the anterior cerebral artery is worthless: the results are discordant, unreliable, and unpredictive.

Despite this disappointing verdict, attention should be paid to the recent report of BLANKENBERG (1997), who evaluated blood flow in the lenticulostriate arteries and examined 17 extremely low-birth-weight (≤1,100 g) preterm neonates during the first week after birth; five of them developed periventricular leukomalacia, germinal matrix hemorrhage, or both, and exhibited hemodynamic alterations in the form of increased and fluctuating velocities and decreased RI. In BLANKENBERG's opinion (1997), these abnormal flow velocities enable identification of preterm neonates who are at risk of developing periventricular leukomalacia, germinal matrix hemorrhage, or both during the first days of life.

This preliminary study is interesting for two reasons:
- In the distressed preterm baby, analyzing the lenticulostriate arteries makes sense as these vessels supply the periventricular white matter. The anterior cerebral artery is not relevant: it is proximal to periventricular areas, and contributes only partially to their vascularization.
- On color and power Doppler imaging, demonstration of the lenticulostriate arteries is easy and allows an accurate pulsed Doppler recording (Fig. 5.47).

There is a potential value in predicting leukomalacia (BLANKENBERG 1997), the severity of the long-term sequelae of which is known – mainly motor deficits (ROTH 1993). Among 44 babies with leukomalacia that we followed up from 8 to 36 months, we found 20 with spastic diplegia, 14 with spastic tetraparesis, one with hemiplegia, and one with moderate lower limb hypertonia, while nine had a normal outcome (Table 5.16).

Table 5.16. Periventricular leukomalacia – psychomotor development (44 cases) (Follow-up 8–36 months)

Diffuse Hyperechoic Leukomalacia 31 cases		Cystic Leukomalacia 13 cases	
Spastic diplegia	17	Diffuse	7
Spastic tetraparesis	11	- Spastic diplegia	3
Normal development	3	- Spastic tetraparesis	3
Strabismus	4	- Hemiplegia	1
Decreased visual acuity	3	Focal	6
Auditory disorders	2	- Normal development	5
Intellectual retardation	2	- Moderate hypertonia of lower limbs	1

Sonographic follow-up gives useful information on the prognosis and occurrence of ventricular dilatation, interhemispheric fissure enlargement, or cerebral atrophy (Fig. 5.48).

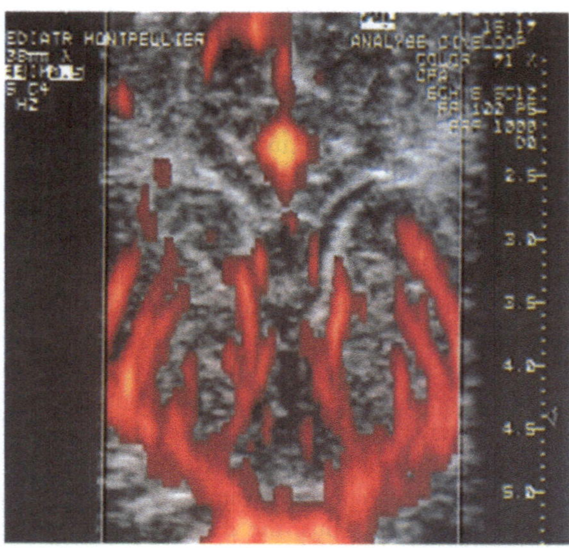

Fig. 5.47. The lenticulostriate arteries are easily identified on power Doppler. Their orientation allows a reliable hemodynamic analysis, without requiring any angle correction

5.3.2
Periventricular Hemorrhagic Infarction

This lesion of premature babies refers to hemorrhagic necrosis of periventricular white matter. It is usually wide, and invariably asymmetric.

5.3.2.1
Neuropathology and Pathogenic Hypothesis

Microscopic studies of this lesion indicate that it is a hemorrhagic infarction (GOULD 1987; GUZZETTA 1986; TAKASHIMA 1986) of the white matter, close to the lateral angle of the ventricle. Neuropathologically, it differs from periventricular leukomalacia, which is usually nonhemorrhagic and symmetric damage of periventricular white matter.

GOULD (1987) has shown that the vascular component of the infarct tends to be located where the medullary veins draining the cerebral white matter become confluent and join the terminal vein, in the subependymal region (Diagram 5.5).

These constatations are important since they provide an explanation of the pathogenesis. In the opinion of most authors (GUZZETTA 1986; VOLPE 1997), periventricular hemorrhagic infarction is directly related to an associated intraventricular and germinal matrix bleeding. The parenchymal involvement always occurs on the same side as the larger amount of hemorrhage, and develops and progresses after the occurrence of the intraventricular hemorrhage.

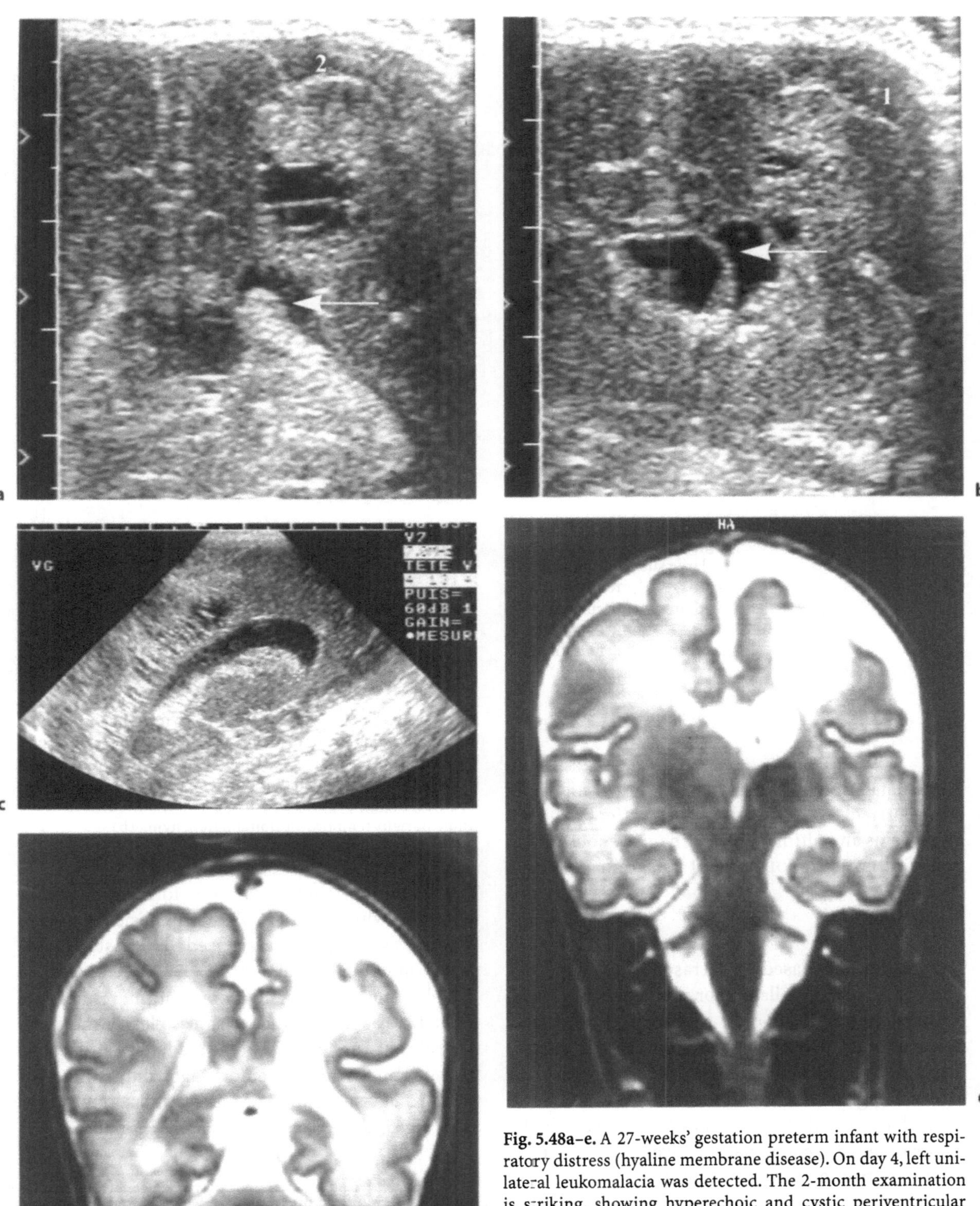

Fig. 5.48a–e. A 27-weeks' gestation preterm infant with respiratory distress (hyaline membrane disease). On day 4, left unilateral leukomalacia was detected. The 2-month examination is striking, showing hyperechoic and cystic periventricular and subcortical leukomalacia (**a,b**). There are major signs of atrophy: left ventricular enlargement (↑), frontal (1) and parietal (2) pericerebral effusion, left basal ganglial atrophy (**c**) (comparative measurements of the basal ganglia are 21.6 mm–8.7 mm on the left, 26.3 mm×17 mm on the right). T2-weighted MRI (**d,e**) confirms the sonographic results and demonstrates associated cortical damage

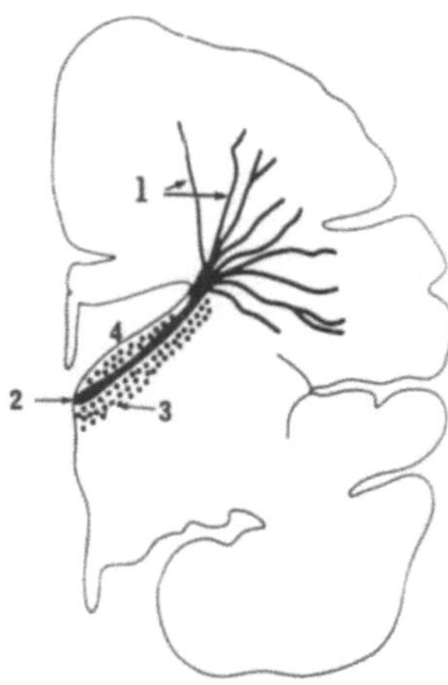

Diagram 5.5. Venous drainage of cerebral white matter (From VOLPE 1997) Medullary veins (*1*), arranged in a fan-shaped distribution, become confluent and join the terminal vein (*2*), which courses through the germinal matrix (*3*) close to lateral ventricle (*4*)

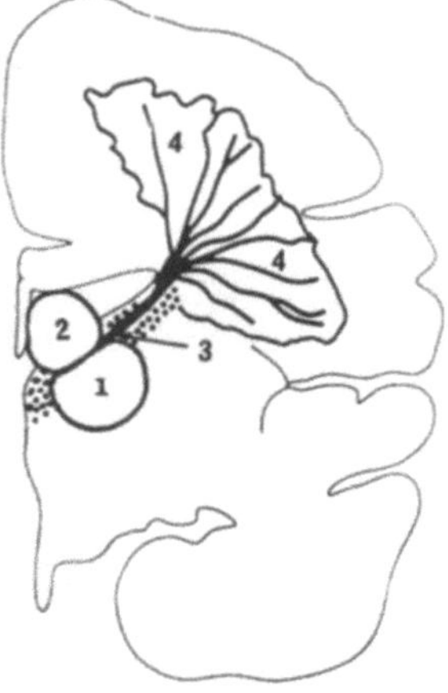

Diagram 5.6. Venous drainage of cerebral white matter A large subependymal hemorrhage (*1*), often associated with intraventricular hemorrhage (*2*), induces compression and deficient drainage of the terminal vein (*3*) and results in hemorrhagic venous infarction (*4*)

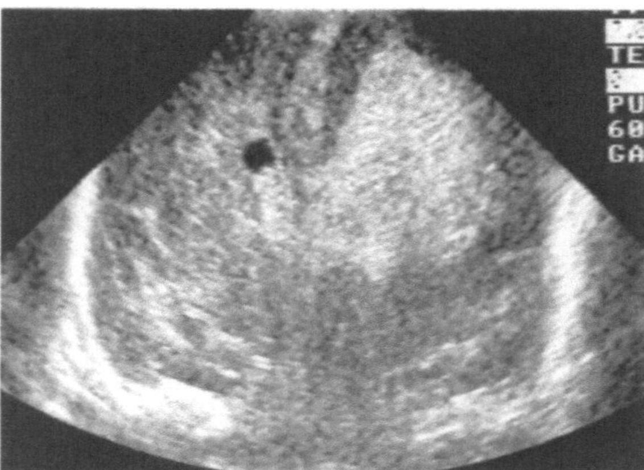

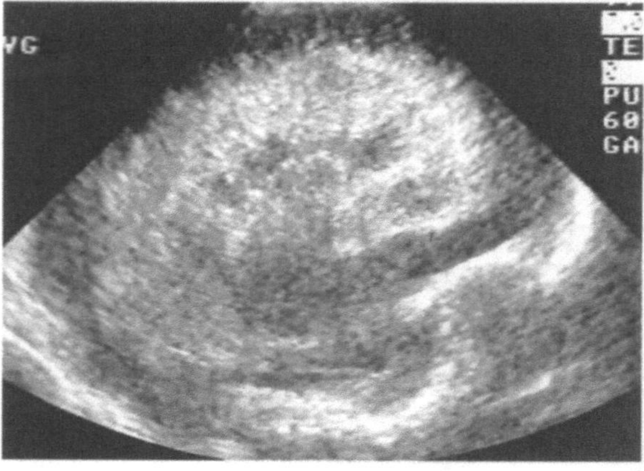

Fig. 5.49a,b. A 26-weeks' gestation premature infant: normal ultrasonography on day 3; clinical deterioration with septic shock and intravascular disseminated coagulation. Notice a large left subependymal and intraventricular hemorrhage (**a**) and a left hemispheric hemorrhagic infarct, which involves the whole parieto-temporo-occipital parenchyma (**b**)

These data strongly suggest that germinal matrix or intraventricular blood leads to obstruction of the terminal veins and ultimate hemorrhagic venous infarction (GOULD 1987; VOLPE 1989) (Diagram 5.6).

5.3.2.2 Diagnosis

The diagnosis is based on ultrasound examination. The lesion is often unilateral or, if bilateral, is invariably asymmetric. It appears as strongly hyperechoic (because of its hemorrhagic component) and is globular or fan-shaped (Fig. 5.49), radiating from the external angle of the lateral ventricle, and associated with a large germinal matrix and/or intraventricular hemorrhage. Parenchymal involvement is usually extensive (fronto-parieto-occipital).

The diagnosis of leukomalacia may be easily excluded: in hemorrhagic leukomalacia, the bleeding occurs secondarily in a pre-existing leukomalacic focus (Fig. 5.50). However, the two lesions may coexist, when an associated germinal matrix or intraventricular hemorrhage has caused a venous obstruction (Fig. 5.51).

The evolution comprises cyst formation within infarcted white matter. The prognosis is severe (GUZZETTA 1986), characterized by spastic hemiparesis and intellectual deficit.

Color Doppler imaging is of real interest (DEAN 1995; TAYLOR 1995) since it shows clearly the complete absence of flow within the medullary and terminal veins on the side of hemorrhage, contrasting with the normal visualization of these vessels on the other side (Fig. 5.52).

Fig. 5.52a–d. Multiple pregnancy, 26 weeks' gestation: immediate respiratory distress with cardiac resuscitation and mechanical ventilation. Ultrasonography at 4 h of life. **a** There is a large left hemorrhagic infarct. **b** Notice that the left terminal vein is undetected while the right vein is perfectly seen on color Doppler. **c** In this other case, flow has disappeared in the left terminal vein, which is compressed by a huge germinal matrix hemorrhage (*1*), resulting in a large hyperechoic infarction (*2*). The right terminal vein (*3*) is well visualized, its velocity is 7 cm/s (**d**)

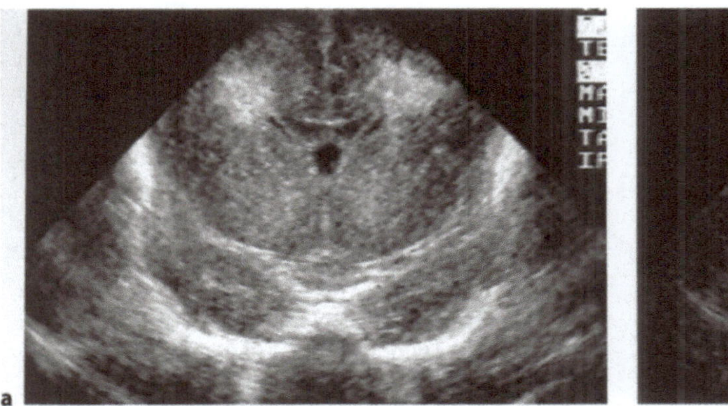
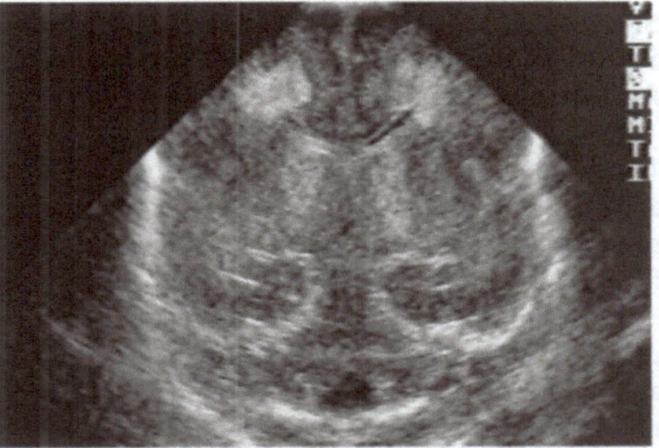

Fig. 5.50a,b. A 29-weeks' gestation premature infant: bilateral and symmetrical echodensities suggesting leukomalacia. Severe necrotizing enterocolitis occurs. Ultrasonography shows accentuation of the hyperechogenicity: periventricular leukomalacia, secondarily hemorrhagic (**a**). Bilateral ischemic lesion of thalami (**b**)

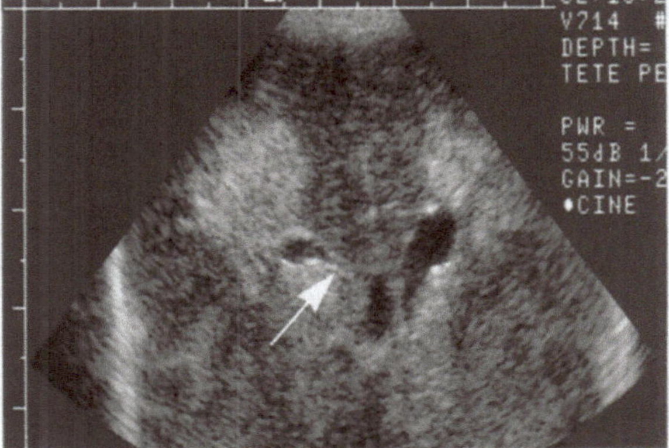

Fig. 5.51. A 30-weeks' gestation preterm infant: bilateral periventricular leukomalacia, hemodynamic deterioration. On follow-up, a large germinal matrix hemorrhage ($\uparrow$) is seen, probably associated with intraventricular bleeding on the right side. The right leukomalacic focus is replaced by a large hemorrhagic venous infarct, strongly hyperechoic

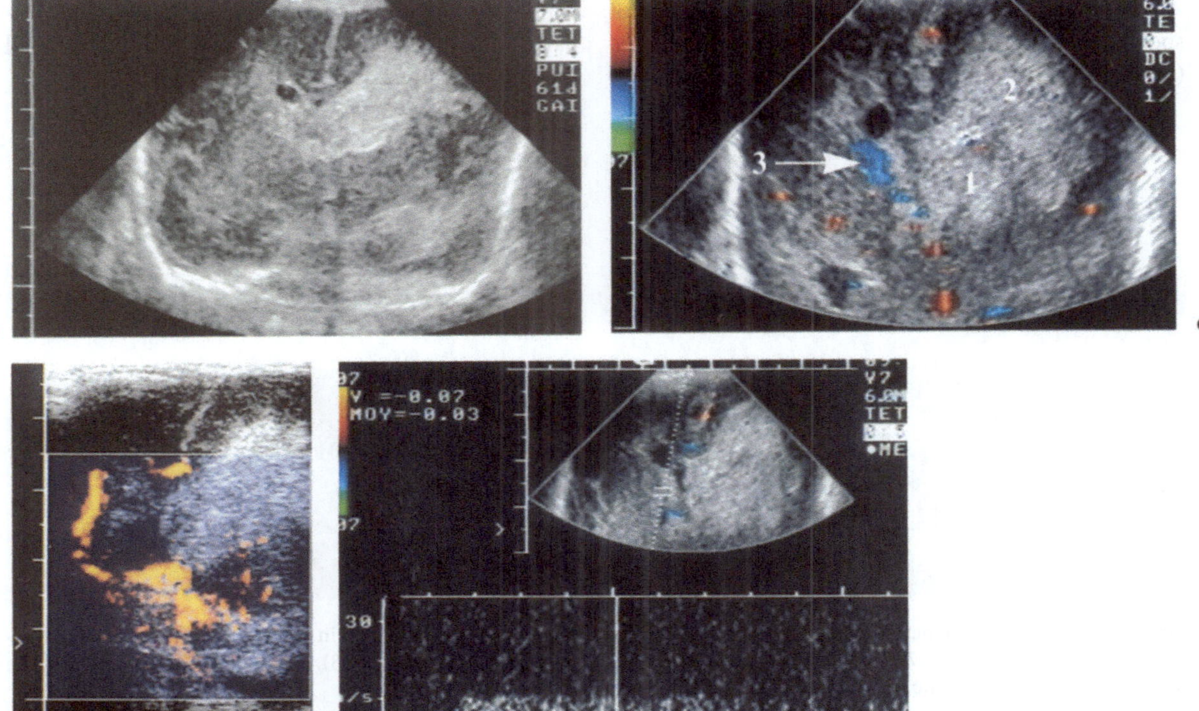

5.4
Severe Hemodynamic Alterations: A Multiplicity of Possible Openings

The frequency of brain asphyxial insult in the neonate and infant means that Doppler techniques may detect several vascular anomalies: heart rate alterations, fluctuating Doppler, low blood flow, high blood flow, hemodynamic consequences of raised intracranial pressure, disturbances in the spectral analysis curve, and absent or reverse diastolic flow. This opens up multiple exciting axes of research: assessment of brain death, evaluation of CBF during multiorgan distress, appreciation of intracranial hypertension, effect of treatments on neonatal cerebral vascularization, pulsed Doppler guidance of resuscitation, and possible prevention of acute fetal asphyxia.

5.4.1
Brain Death

Florine was a 2-month-old shaken baby. She was admitted to hospital because of sudden weakness after feeding. The neurological distress was severe, with coma and EEG silence. Morphological ultrasonography detected lesions of the white matter and basal ganglia. On color Doppler imaging, the anterior cerebral artery and proximal part of the pericallosal artery alone were visible, and showed an abnormal spectral analysis curve (Fig. 5.53).

The criteria for brain death include coma, lack of spontaneous ventilation, absence of brain stem reflexes (pupillary, corneal, pharyngeal, and tracheal) and electrocerebral silence (KOHRMAN 1993). However, these guidelines are difficult to apply in the newborn and this is why additional methods of investigation are needed to determining brain death: angiography (ASHWAL 1977; PARKER 1995; PARVEY 1976) and auditory evoked responses (LÜTSCHG 1983).

Nowadays, cranial Doppler ultrasonography should be proposed, as it is an easy, reliable, nonionizing technique (AHMANN 1987; ASHWAL 1997; BODE 1988; GLASIER 1989; JALILI 1994; MACMENAMIN 1983; MESSER 1990; POWERS 1989; QIAN 1998; RAJU 1992). MACMENAMIN (1983) was the first to describe the characteristic changes in the spectral analysis during brain death, as follows. In a first stage, diastolic velocity decreases (stage I); then a retrograde diastolic flow appears in the anterior cerebral and common carotid arteries (stage II). Systolic flow decreases (stage III), then disappears (stage IV) within the anterior cerebral artery, while remaining visible in the common carotid artery. This Doppler pattern reflects a progressive intracranial pressure increase, and when recognized always carries a poor prognosis.

Subsequent reports have confirmed these first data. GLASIER (1989) noted a highly increased RI, resulting from a reverse diastolic flow, in 8 of 9 infants aged 2 days to 11 months.

BODE (1988), examining nine older infants (age range: 2 weeks to 12 years), reported reduced flow velocities and reverse protodiastolic flow in eight; he described a pathognomonic hemodynamic pattern consisting of a short narrow systolic peak and a similarly shaped retrograde diastolic flow, correlated with clinical signs of brain death.

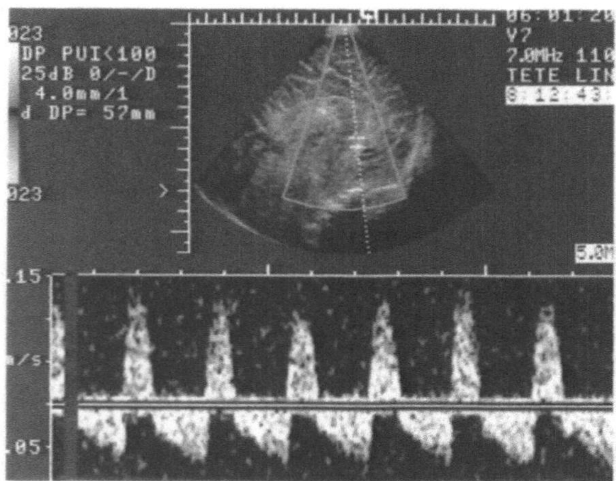
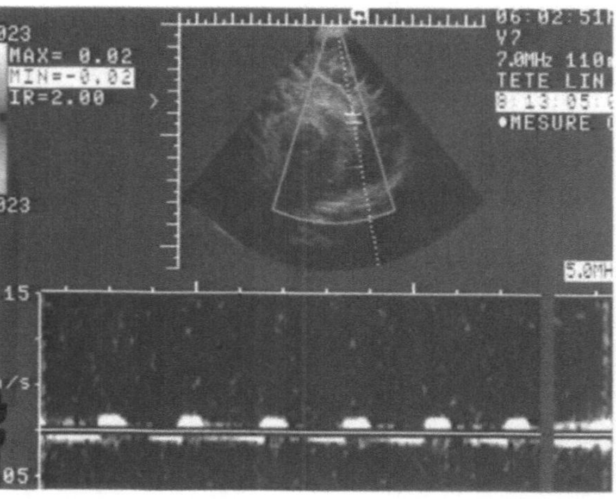

Fig. 5.53a,b. Characteristic pattern of brain death: **a** Sharp and narrow systolic peaks, drop in systolic velocity (12 cm/s), retrograde diastolic flow (EDV=−7 cm/s), drop in mean velocities (TAV=2 cm/s), high RI (=1.58). **b** In the proximal portion of the pericallosal artery, there is no progression of blood: PSV=2 cm/s, EDV=−2 cm/s, RI=2

However, the same authors (GLASIER 1989; BODE 1988) each observed one neonatal case where major basal vessels showed normal flow despite the presence of clinical and EEG criteria of brain death. BODE (1988) suggested that blood flow may be shunted through the circle of Willis and extracranial arteries, as shown by angiography (PARVEY 1976). These limitations of Doppler ultrasonography were confirmed by JALILI (1990), who found typical changes in only five of seven cases. CHIU (1994) observed a reversal of diastolic flow in a 1-month-old infant with status epilepticus who recovered without sequelae, while, by contrast, SANKER (1992) reported increased velocities despite persistent other signs of brain death in one case. This literature review tends to demonstrate the inconstancy of Doppler changes in brain death; these insufficiencies concur the clinical and EEG uncertainties (NAN-CHANG 1994; SANKER 1992).

The clinical context remains an essential element, since different pathological situations may be associated with the same Doppler pattern as irreversible cessation of intracranial flow (Fig. 5.54).

Our experience (nine patients with brain death) shows a characteristic hemodynamic pattern if compared with precise clinical findings. Four newborns and five infants (age range: 1–7 months) were examined (Table 5.17). The four neonates suffered severe neurological distress with EEG silence; of the five infants there was a severe cranial trauma in two, a near miss syndrome in two, and a cardiac arrest in one.

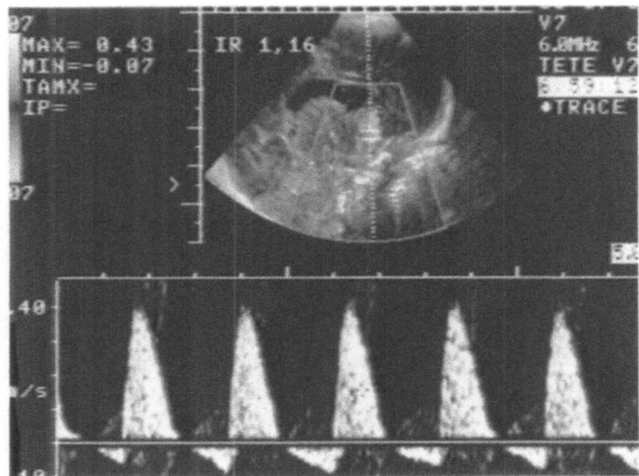

Fig. 5.54. A 27-weeks' gestation premature baby. Mechanical ventilation (hyaline membrane disease); normal brain ultrasonography. Pulsed Doppler shows retrograde diastolic flow, RI=1.16. A cardiac murmur is present. Characteristic pattern of patent ductus arteriosus

Hemodynamics are typically abnormal in all nine patients (Table 5.17):
- In six cases, peak systolic velocity was reduced (from 8 to 20 cm/s); in one 7-month-old infant, it was 40 cm/s, contrasting with a normal range above 80 cm/s. On the spectral analysis curve, the systolic peak was suggestive on the basis of its narrow shape in these seven cases.
- The main feature was the retrograde diastolic flow, the velocity of which ranged from 0 to –19 cm/s (Fig. 5.55).

Table 5.17. Brain death: clinical, US and Doppler US findings (9 patients)

Case	Age	Clinical findings	US findings	PSV	EDV	TAV	RI
1	31 Weeks of gestation	Acute fetal distress Atrio-ventricular block	White matter ischemia	8	0	2	1
2	28 Weeks of gestation	Acute fetal distress	Intraventricular hemorrhage White matter ischemia	8	–5	1	1.63
3	40 Weeks of gestation	Neonatal neurological distress	Intraventricular hemorrhage Cortical ischemia	18	–10	1	1.70
4	40 Weeks of gestation	Neonatal neurological distress	Normal	No vessel detected on color Doppler			
5	3 Months	Near miss syndrome	Basal ganglia and subcortical ischemia	20	–5	3	1.25
6	1 Month	Near miss syndrome?	Basal ganglia and subcortical ischemia	16	–4	2	1.25
7	2 Months	Battered child syndrome	Basal ganglia and subcortical ischemia	12	–7	2	1.58
8	7 Months	Cardiac arrest	Normal	40	–19	2	1.48
9	7 Months	Cranial trauma	Cerebral contusion	No vessel detected on color Doppler			

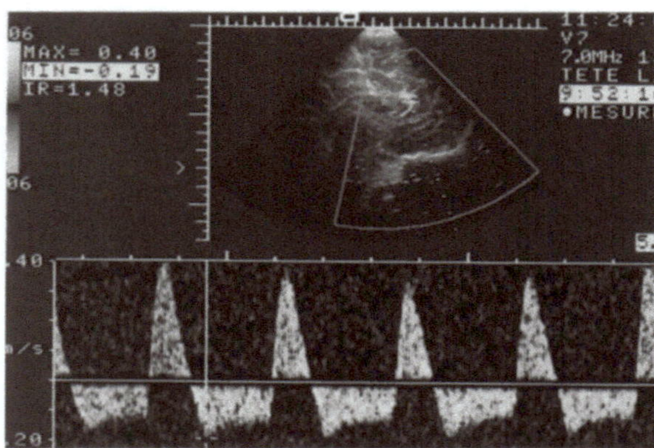

Fig. 5.55. A 7-month-old infant: cardiac arrest, areactive coma. Systolic peaks are sharp and narrow. PSV=40 cm/s (mildly decreased). Diastolic velocity is severely impaired (–19 cm/s). Grade III brain death to the classification of MacMenamin (1983)

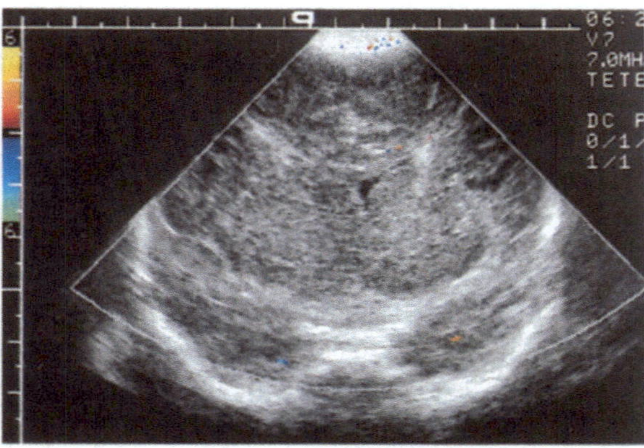

Fig. 5.56. A full-term neonate: severe neurological distress, EEG silence. Major basal vessels (carotid, anterior and middle cerebral arteries) are not identified on color Doppler. The brain is no longer supplied

– These alterations led to severely decreased mean velocities ranging from 1 to 3 cm/s.
– This resulted in a high increase in RI (range: 1–1.70).
– Finally, color Doppler was unable to detect any flow within the anterior cerebral artery, middle cerebral artery, or carotid artery in two further patients: there was a complete cessation of vascularization in the brain (Fig. 5.56). Cerebral vessels were only partially visualized in four of the seven other cases (Fig. 5.57).

Thus, according to the classification of MacMenamin, seven patients showed stage III brain death (reduced systolic velocities, absent or negative diastole, high RI) and two presented stage IV (undetectable signal on color Doppler).

The term "brain death"refers to complete irreversible cessation of brain vascularization; the physiopathology enables a clear explanation of the spectral analysis alterations. Decrease in systolic flow signifies an increase in vascular resistance, probably related to endothelial infiltration and cerebral edema; the latter mechanism certainly plays a more important role in the infant, who has less cranial compliance, than in the neonate (Fig. 5.58).

To summarize, pulsed and color Doppler provide a valuable alternative for diagnosing brain death. Of course, the clinical findings are essential, since a reverse diastolic flow may occur in other less severe circumstances such as patent ductus arteriosus, intracranial pressure rise, etc. These findings underline the value of color Doppler when cerebral vessels are undetectable (Fig. 5.59).

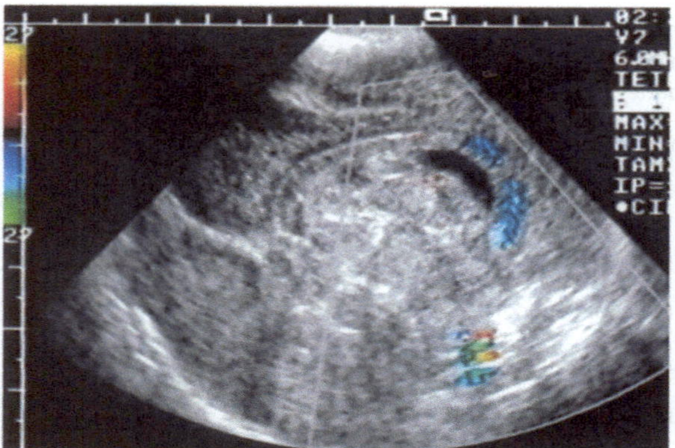

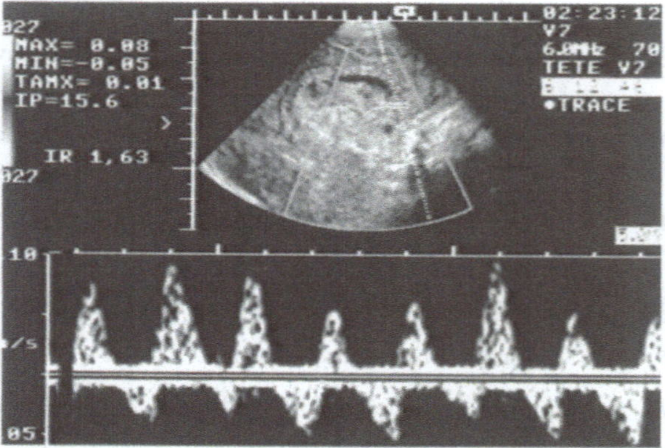

Fig. 5.57a,b. A 28-weeks' gestation premature infant: acute fetal distress, major acidosis and intravascular coagulation. Brain vessels are partially seen: the proximal part of the pericallosal artery, the basilar artery (a). Spectral analysis shows a fluctuating curve with retrograde diastolic flow and almost absent mean velocities (b)

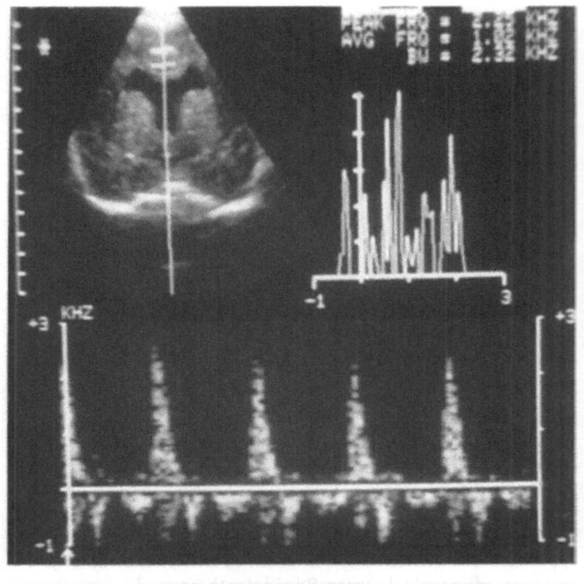

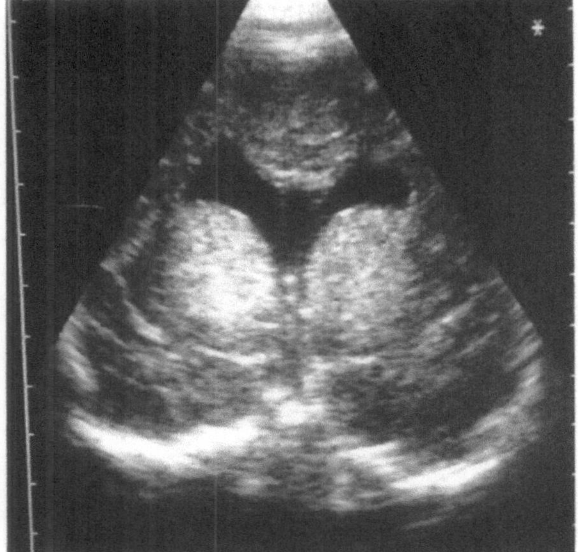

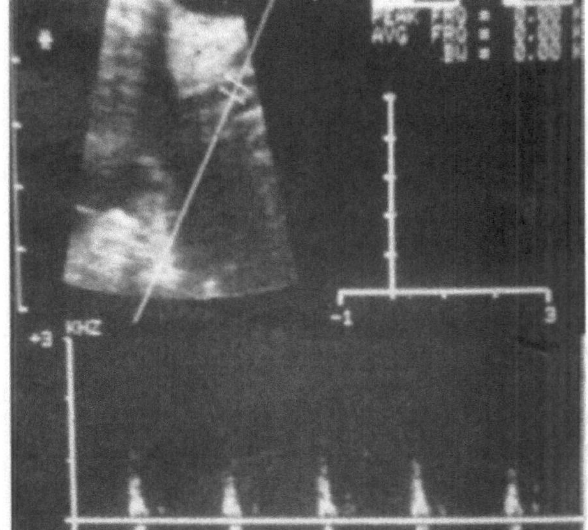

Fig. 5.58a–c. In this 7-month-old infant, ultrasonography shows cortico-subcortical ischemia and lenticulostriate hyperechogenicity after prolonged cardiac arrest. The pericallosal artery shows a reverse diastolic component (**a**). Three hours later, ischemic damage involves the whole gangliothalamic nuclei (**b**). There is no Doppler signal in the cerebral arteries. A small systolic peak is identified in the common carotid artery (**c**)

5.4.2
Alterations of Cerebral Autoregulation

Jérôme, a 4-month-old infant, was found comatose in his bed; after recovery from a prolonged circulatory arrest, his neurological status was poor, with areactive coma.

Ultrasonography was performed 3 h after the acute event. The echostructure of brain was normal, but severe hemodynamic alterations were detected: fluctuating Doppler, followed by heart rate disturbances (bigeminism and trigeminism) (Fig. 5.60). The infant rapidly died.

This observation was interesting:

- After an asphyxial insult, cell necrosis requires at least 24 h to appear on morphological ultrasonography. Diffusion-weighted MRI might probably provide an earlier morphological diagnosis (D'Arceuil 1998).
- In cases of severe asphyxia, impairment of cerebral autoregulation is immediate and the consequences of arterial blood pressure changes may be recorded on brain arteries. The heart rate alterations reflect myocardial ischemia resulting from hemodynamic deterioration (Burnard 1961; Desa 1977; Van Bel 1990).

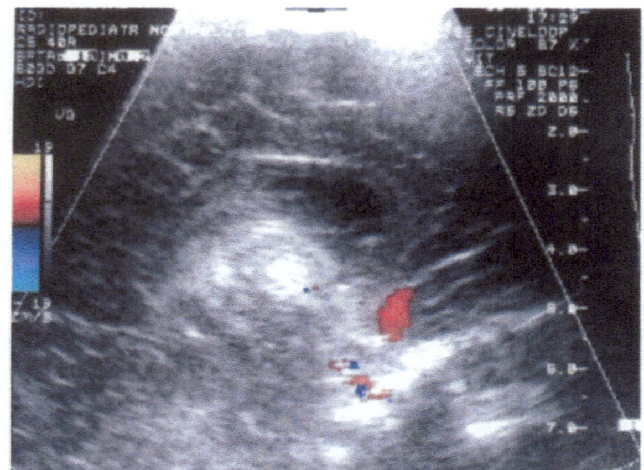

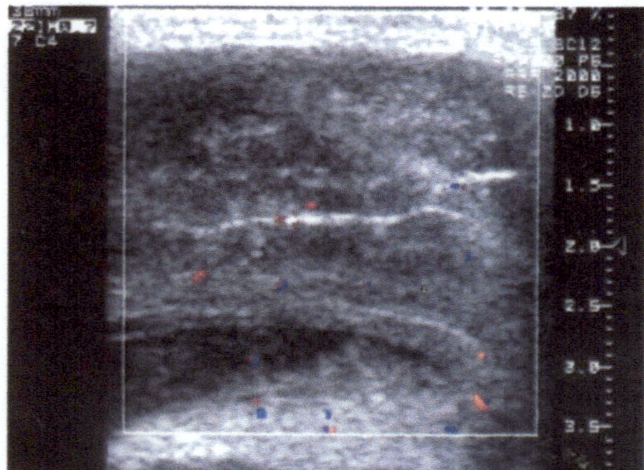

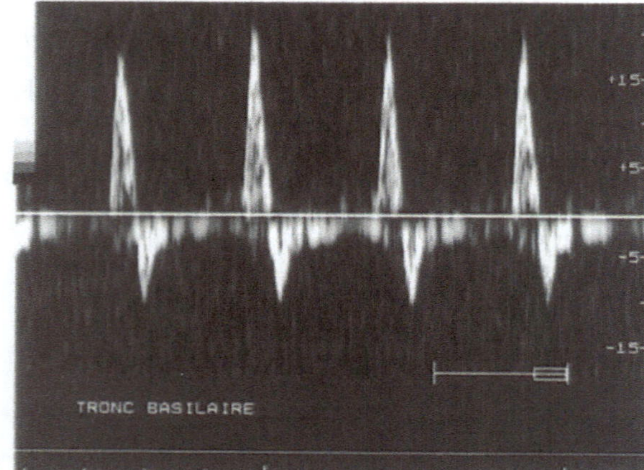

Fig. 5.59a–c. A 6-day-old neonate: severe neurological distress with major intraventricular hemorrhage and diffuse cortical ischemia. During morphological ultrasonography, arterial pulsations are absent. Color Doppler shows a very small residual flow in the anterior cerebral artery with alternative red and blue signal (**a**). Absence of hemispheric vascularization is seen (**b**). Confirmation by spectral analysis: narrow systolic peak, low systolic velocity (15 cm/s), reverse protodiastolic flow (**c**)

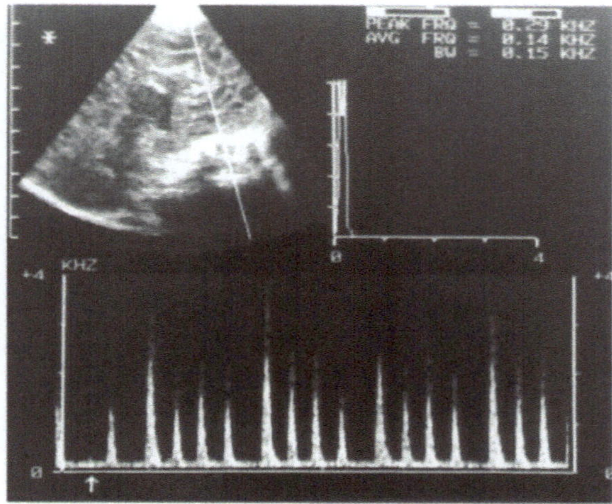

Fig. 5.60. Spectral analysis shows an irregular curve with unequal systolic peaks and absent diastolic flow. Secondary appearance of bi- and trigeminism due to myocardial ischemia and hemodynamic distress. Rapid death ensued

5.4.3
Hemodynamics and Intracranial Hypertension

Sarah's obstetrical history was severe: at 27 weeks' gestation, fetal hydrops was discovered with ascites and pericardial effusion, secondary to Rh immunization. At 28 weeks, an intrauterine blood transfusion was performed (fetal anemia, Hb=6g/l). Hydrops recurred 1 week later, with cardiac arrhythmia and failure: anemia recurred and the blood transfusion was repeated a second and a third time, the last immediately before birth, at 31 weeks. Diffuse edema and intrauterine growth retardation were obvious; Apgar score was 4 and hypertrophic myocardiopathy was confirmed. On day 1, cranial ultrasonography showed a normal brain, but Doppler imaging detected increased vascular resistance with retrograde diastolic flow. Systolic velocities were in the normal range, excluding a low blood flow. The Doppler findings were interpreted as reflectiing an acute rise in intracranial pressure, the result of severe cerebral edema (Fig. 5.61).

On day 3, oligoanuria developed, increasing the edematous syndrome. Repeated episodes of bradycardia and desaturation occurred. Ultrasonography showed the persistent hemodynamic alterations 24 h before death (Fig. 5.62).

These Doppler data demonstrate intracranial hypertension resulting from irreversible cerebral edema, as shown by the collapse of the ventricular lumen.

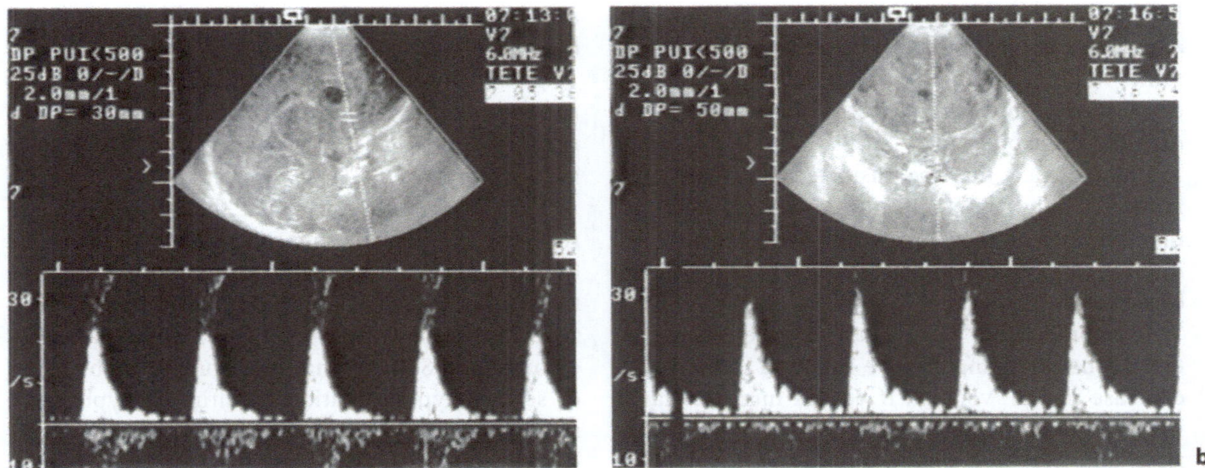

Fig. 5.61a,b. Notice the absence of diastolic flow in the anterior cerebral artery (a) and internal carotid artery (b). Indentations of the curve result from high-frequency ventilation

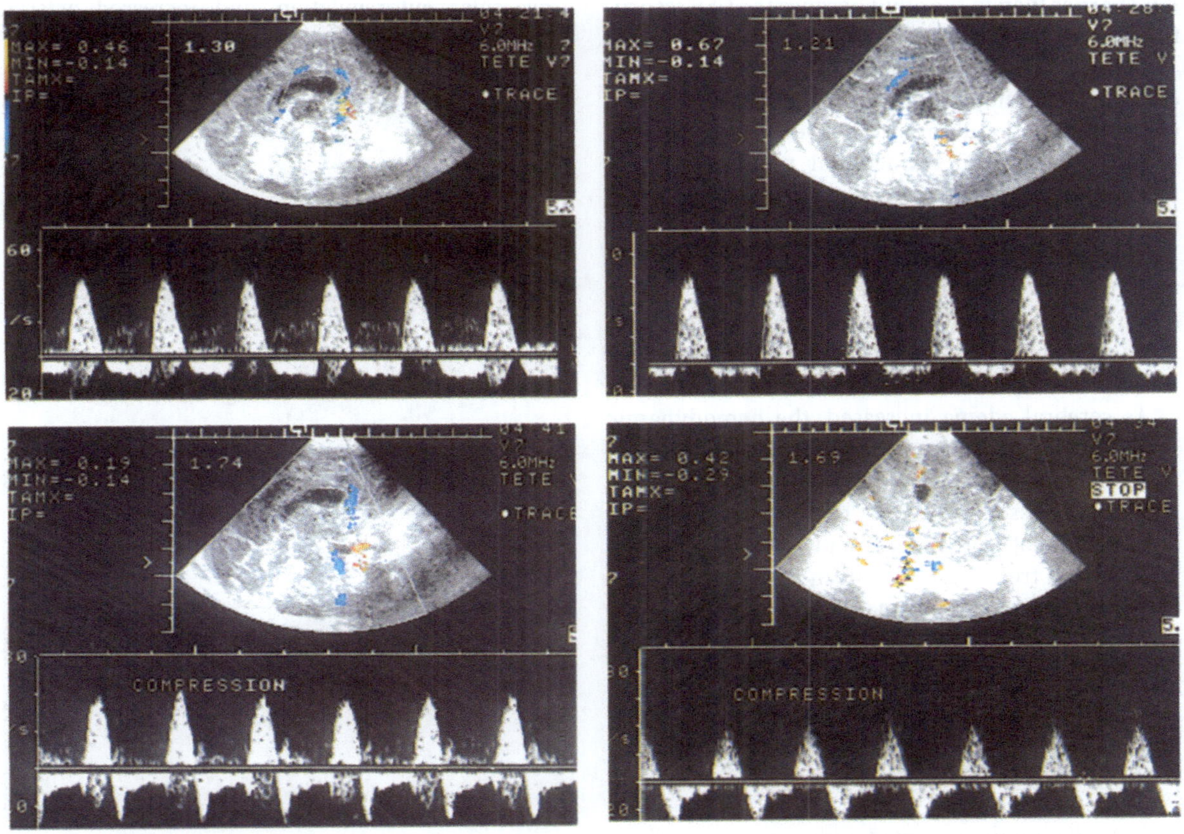

Fig. 5.62a–d. RI=1.30 in the anterior cerebral artery (a) and 1.21 in the basilar artery (b). After fontanellar compression, it reached 1.74 in the anterior cerebral artery (c) and 1.69 in the internal carotid artery (d)

Physiopathologically (ORIOT 1998), in the neonate, any change in one of the three components of intracranial volume – brain, CSF, and blood, which account for 88%, 9%, and 3% respectively – occurs at the expense of the other two.

Brain, which may be distorted but cannot be reduced, fully transmits the pressures that are imposed on it. In the neonate, one of the factors most implicated in increasing intracranial volume is cerebral edema.

"Cerebral edema" refers to an increased water content of the brain and may be balanced initially by a decrease in CSF volume. If edema increases faster than CSF volume diminishes, intracranial pressure rises and cerebral compliance is modified (ratio between changes in intracranial volume and intracranial pressure). The newborn may compensate an increased volume without increasing pressure (enlargement of fontanelles, sutures, head circumference), but when a rise in intracranial pressure occurs, it is sharper than in the adult because the CSF resorption spaces are smaller.

Finally, the effects of intracranial hypertension on cerebral circulation depend on the cerebral perfusion pressure (i.e., the difference between mean arterial pressure and mean intracranial pressure). If the intracranial pressure increases, hypoperfusion and ischemia cannot be avoided.

This physiopathogenic model provides an explanation of the case reported here:
- On the first day of life, intracranial hypertension was obvious, as shown by increased vascular resistance and the absence of diastolic flow.
- As cerebral edema increased, the hemodynamic alterations worsened: RI rose progressively (1.20–1.30). Fontanellar compression, which provides an indirect assessment of cerebral compliance, showed that compliance had altered, since RI increased from 1.20 to 1.70 (in the anterior cerebral artery) during the maneuver.

5.4.4
Hemodynamics and Seizures

At birth, Benjamin presented with a meconium ileus, and ileostomy was performed. Cystic fibrosis was confirmed.

At 1 month of age, bowel continuity was restored, but a few hours later prolonged weakness occurred, followed by several seizures. Ultrasonography was performed immediately after a seizure: morphological

imaging was normal but severe hemodynamic disturbances were observed (Fig. 5.63).

On follow-up, lenticulostriate and thalamic ischemic lesions appeared (Fig. 5.64), associated with multifocal cortical hyperechogenicities and ultimately rapid brain atrophy (Fig. 5.65).

This observation underlines the causative role of repeated seizures in the constitution of ischemic brain damage and hemodynamic adaptive response to seizures. The mechanisms by which repeated seizures may cause brain injury in the neonate have been documented. Seizures may be accompanied by apnea or serious hypoventilation, resulting in hypoxemia, sometimes cardiovascular collapse, and, in consequence, a fall in CBF. Decreases in brain ATP, glycolysis, and brain glucose levels, and an increase in excitatory amino acids contribute to ischemic brain injury.

During seizures, hypoxemia, hypercapnia, disturbances in cerebral energy metabolisms, loss of cerebrovascular autoregulation, and increased arterial

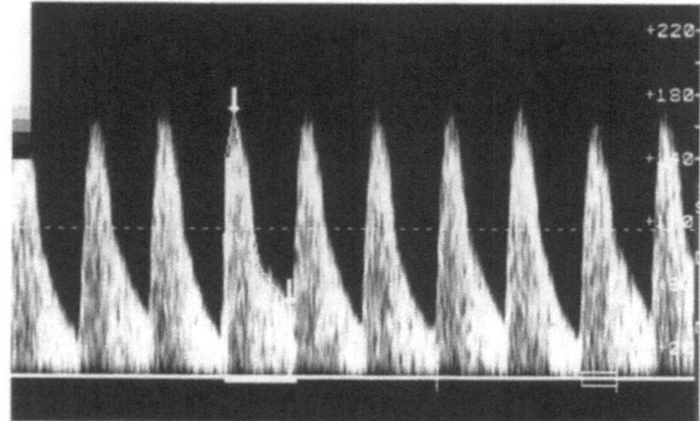

Fig. 5.63. Systolic velocities are highly increased (167 cm/s). Diastolic velocities are moderately increased (45 cm/s). RI is normal (0.71)

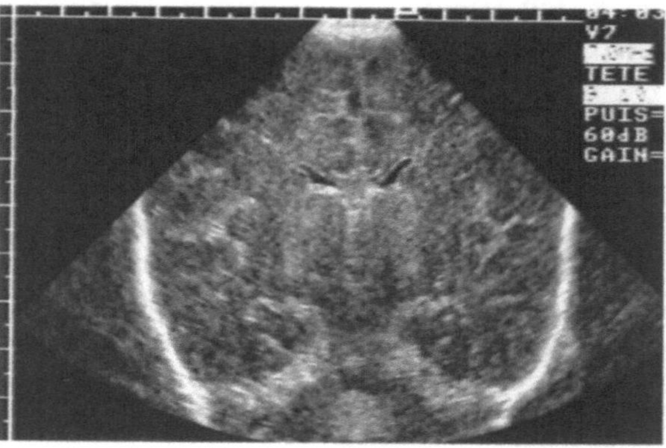

Fig. 5.64. Notice intense hyperechogenicity in the two lenticulate nuclei

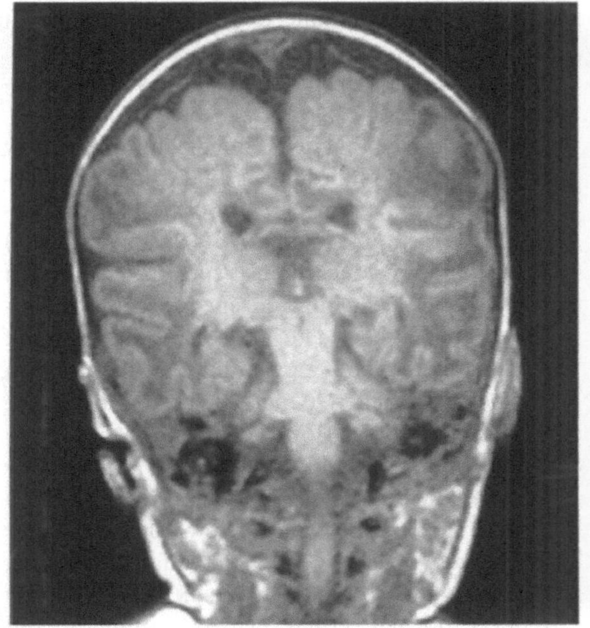

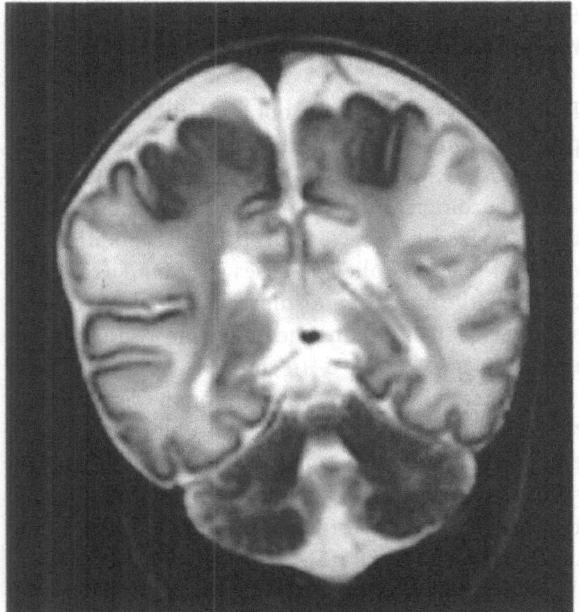

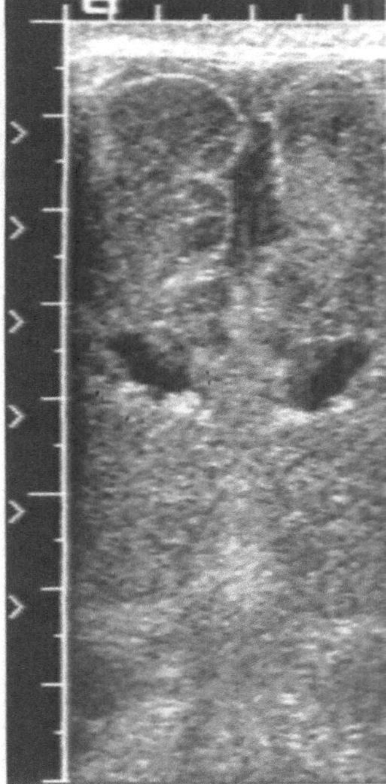

Fig. 5.65a–c. Ischemic involvement has worsened: **a** T1- and **b** T2-weighted MRI reveal cortico-subcortical damage, which predominates in the central and precentral regions. **c** On ultrasonography, the interhemispheric fissure is enlarged: cerebral atrophy

blood pressure add their effects and induce an increase in CBF. These data have been demonstrated by PERLMAN (1983), who during (or immediately after) a seizure detected an immediate rise in arterial pressure and simultaneous increase in CBF velocities in eight neonates examined by pulsed Doppler imaging.

This mechanism (BOYLAN 1999) explains in our case the high increase in systolic and diastolic velocities, contrasting with the still normal RI. This supports the idea that measurement of arterial velocities should be preferred during neonatal seizures.

To summarize, the increase in CBF refers to an initial adaptive response to the increased metabolic demand of the brain, but this response may become maladaptive in the newborn and cause rupture of the capillary bed and intraventricular bleeding or hemorrhagic infarction.

Finally, impairment of cerebral autoregulation and frequent hypotension combine to produce ischemic injury by decreasing CBF.

5.4.5
Hemodynamics and Low Blood Flow

Pulsed Doppler assessment of low CBF is obviously a progress. Our experience is based on the hemodynamic assessment and follow-up of nine neonates with neurological distress (Table 5.18). Low CBF is characterized by a severe drop in all velocities: the mean of peak systolic velocities is 17 cm/s (range 8–27 cm/s); the mean of end-diastolic velocities is 6 cm/s (range: 2–10 cm/s); the mean of time average velocities is 10 cm/s (range 6–16 cm/s).

In one case, hypoperfusion of the brain was secondary to septic shock and complicated the evolution of grade III encephalopathy. In three other cases, low blood flow initiated grade III anoxic–ischemic encephalopathy. In these four patients, luxury perfusion appeared secondarily and death was rapid (day 8–18).

In four cases, low blood flow was associated with multiorgan distress: status epilepticus after fetal distress in two (Fig. 5.66), septic shock in one, and a twin-to-twin transfusion in one (Fig. 5.67). These four patients died early.

Finally, the only survivor experienced septic shock with rapidly resolving low blood flow. Ultrasonography and CT revealed a left middle cerebral artery infarction causing right inferior limb hypertonia (at 5 months of age).

This preliminary experience leads to some conclusions:
- It is now proven that detection of a low blood flow is related to a poor prognosis. In the literature, several workers (ALTMAN 1988; BUCHER 1993; GREISEN 1997; LIPP-ZWAHLEN 1989; PRYDS 1988) using different techniques (positron emission tomography, near-infrared spectroscopy, xenon-133 clearance) have determined absolute values of CBF: from 10 ml/100g per minute in the preterm newborn, it reaches 20 mg/100g per minute in the full-term newborn. However, it is more difficult to define what threshold value of CBF is constantly associated with ischemic damage: POWERS (1985) asserts that a CBF value below 10 ml/100g per minute is observed only in infarcted tissue, whereas, by contrast, GREISEN (1987, 1989) reports normal visual evoked responses and preserved EEG activity for values as low as approximately 5 ml/100 g per minute in premature infants.

In our clinical experience, the direct part played by low blood flow in the formation of cerebral lesions (Fig. 5.68) has been impossible to assess, since

Table 5.18. Low CBF (9 cases)

CASE	CLINICAL FINDINGS	US FINDINGS	DOPPLER FINDINGS				OUTCOME
			PSV	EDV	TAV	RI	
1	Septic shock Grade III encephalopathy	Cortico-subcortical ischemia	16	2	8	0.88	Death
2	Grade III encephalopathy	Subcortical and basal ganglia ischemia	17	8	11	0.53	Death
3	Grade III encephalopathy	Subcortical and basal ganglia ischemia	8	5	6	0.37	Death
4	Grade III encephalopathy	Cortico-subcortical and basal ganglia ischemia	27	10	16	0.63	Death
5	Fetal distress Septic shock	Middle cerebral artery infarction	24	8	15	0.62	Right lower limb hypertonia
6	Fetal distress Status epilepticus	Subcortical and basal ganglia ischemia	22	8	13	0.64	Death
7	Septic shock	Normal	10	7	8	0.20	Death
8	Twin gestation Transfused twin	Normal	14	2	7	0.80	Death
9	Fetal distress Cord prolapse Status epilepticus	Subcortical and basal ganglia ischemia	15	6	8	0.74	Death

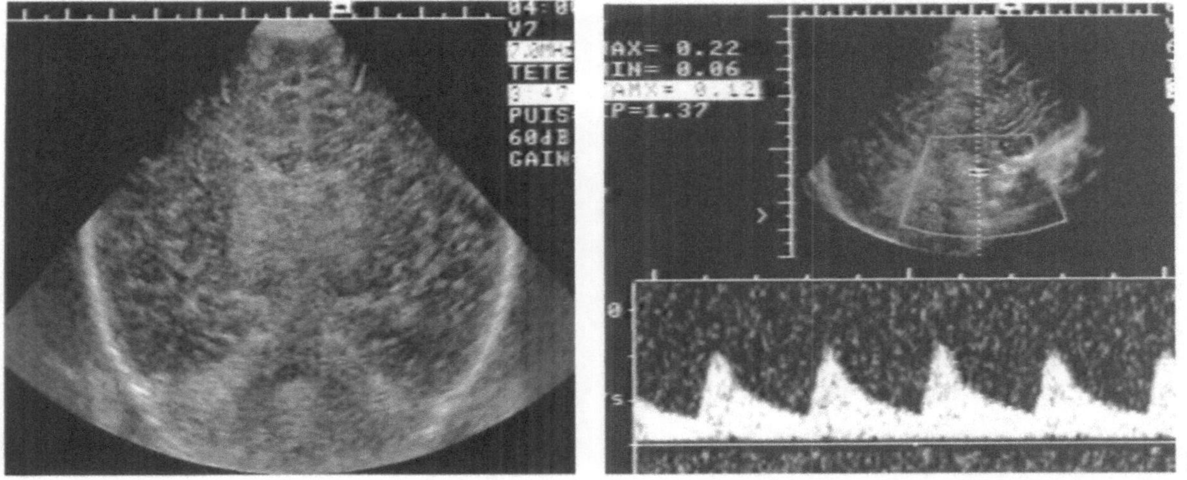

Fig. 5.66a,b. Post-term neonate: Apgar score=0, major perinatal asphyxia. **a** White matter and thalamus hyperechogenicity. **b** Low blood flow: PSV=22cm/s, EDV=6cm/s, TAV=12 cm/s. The patient died on day 6

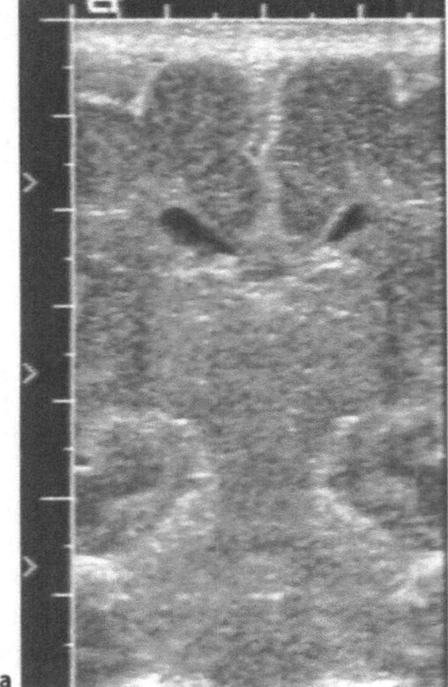

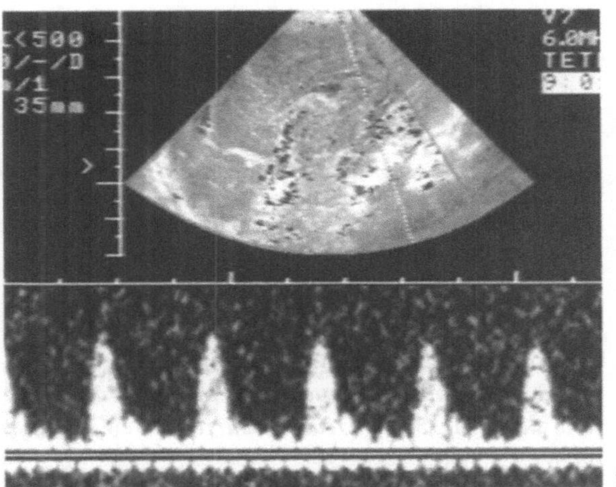

Fig. 5.67a,b. Twin pregnancy: transfused twin, perinatal hemodynamic distress. **a** Normal ultrasound examination. **b** Characteristic low blood flow: PSV=14 cm/s, EDV=2 cm/s, TAV=7 cm/s. The patient died on day 2

ischemic damage was present simultaneously with hypoperfusion in six cases. Multiple measurements of systolic, diastolic, and mean velocities should be useful for determining threshold values of brain viability.

- RI is clearly uninformative in the detection of low blood flow (Table 5.18). Its values ranged from 0.20 to 0.88 in our patients.
- Early occurrence of low blood flow should obviously prompt an assessment of hemodynamics at the time of the anoxic-ischemic injury, but this requires dedicated medical organization and availability within the intensive care unit.

5.4.6
Cerebral Perfusion and Therapeutic Interventions

Sabrina was admitted to the hospital at 2 days of life because of respiratory distress and cardiovascular collapse secondary to a severe subgaleal hemorrhage. Her clinical presentation was extremely serious, with areactive coma, bilateral myosis, extreme pallor, hypothermia, and acidosis. Doppler signal was difficult to obtain in the pericallosal artery: we found only a low systolic peak and undetectable diastolic flow.

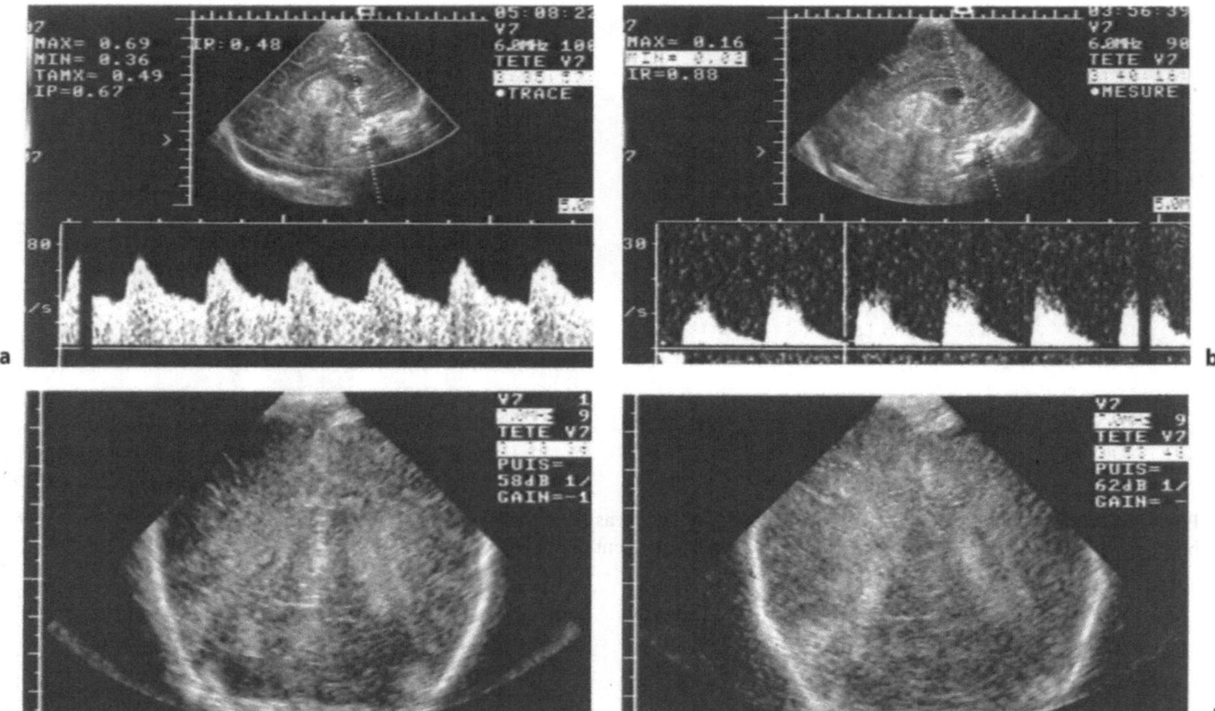

Fig. 5.68a–d. A 37-weeks' gestation premature infant: Streptococcus infection with septic shock. **a** Day 4: first ultrasound examination shows luxury perfusion and ischemic-hemorrhagic lesions of basal ganglia. **b** Day 6: low blood flow and cerebral hypoperfusion. **c** Hyperechogenic right occipito-temporal ischemic lesion. **d** Day 8: This lesion is accentuated. What part does low blood flow play in this deterioration?

Intracardiac administration of isoprenaline was followed by a transient appearance of retrograde diastolic flow (Fig. 5.69). Death occurred a few minutes later.

This observation points to exciting potentialities. Well-controlled experimental trials of specific drugs are needed to determine their effects on cerebral perfusion.

- The effects of intravenously administered indomethacin on CBF in the human newborn are well documented (EDWARDS 1990; EVANS 1987; HAMMERMAN 1995; LIEM 1994; OHLSSON 1993; PARILLA 1997). It leads to a 25%–60% reduction in CBF during the first 120 min, associated with a decrease in cerebral oxygen delivery and in cerebral oxidized cytochrome oxidase concentration, which probably reflects the reduced intracellular oxygen availability. Pulsed Doppler and near-infrared spectroscopy (LIEM 1994) show the vasoconstrictor effect of indomethacin, which increases downstream vascular resistances. It is important to take into account these consequences of the drug for CBF, especially in a preterm infant known to be highly susceptible to cerebral hypo-

perfusion. This might lead to the gradual replacement of indomethacin by ibuprofen (MOSCA 1997; VARVARIGOU 1996), which seems to be without cerebrovascular effects.

- Aminophylline is often used for preventing apnea in premature infants, and also has a vasoconstrictive action (McDONNEL 1992; GOVAN 1995).
- Surfactant therapy may (SCHIPPER 1997) induce a significant drop in mean arterial pressure and CBF in the ventilated premature baby.
- The beneficial effect of pancuronium bromide in the ventilated preterm infant with fluctuating CBF velocities has been demonstrated (CHEMTOB 1987): muscular paralysis is associated with a reduced risk of ventricular hemorrhage and brain ischemia by stabilization of arterial blood pressure and CBF.
- Several other pharmacological agents or nonpharmacological interventions have a cerebrovascular effect (Fig. 5.70), and in the future Doppler ultrasonography should will be used to analyze the consequences of these treatments on CBF and occurrence of brain ischemia.

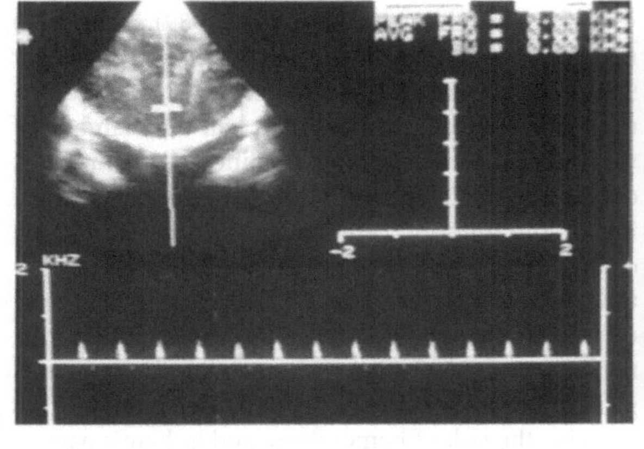

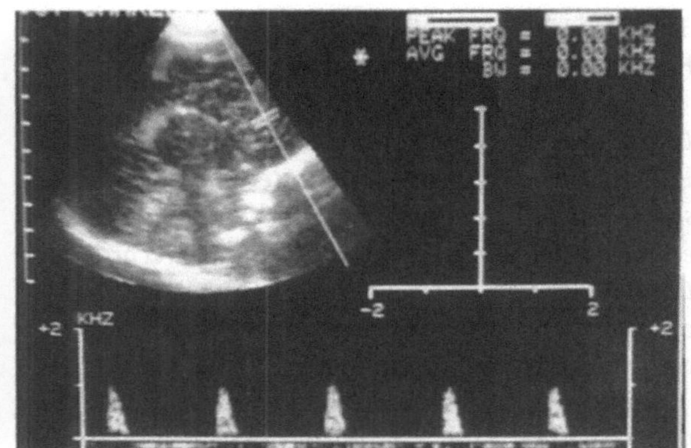

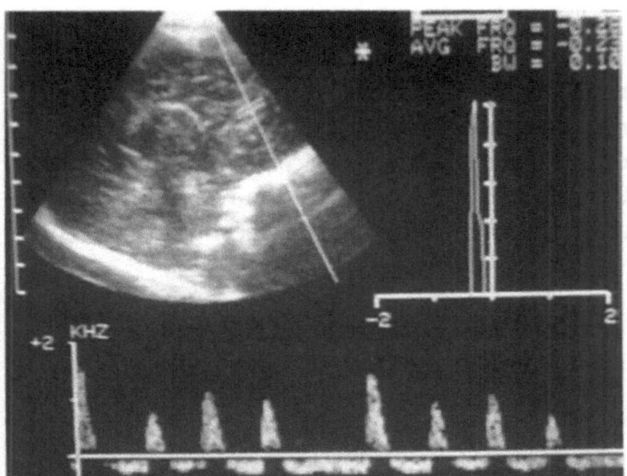

Fig. 5.69a–c. Pulsed Doppler is performed during acute hypovolemic collapse. a In the pericallosal artery, systolic peaks have low amplitude, suggesting brain death. b Forty seconds after isoprenaline administration, there is a transient improvement of the Doppler curve, increased amplitude of systolic peaks, and appearance of a retrograde diastolic component. c One minute and 30 s after treatment, an irregular curve appears with variations in peak systolic velocity. Death followed rapidly

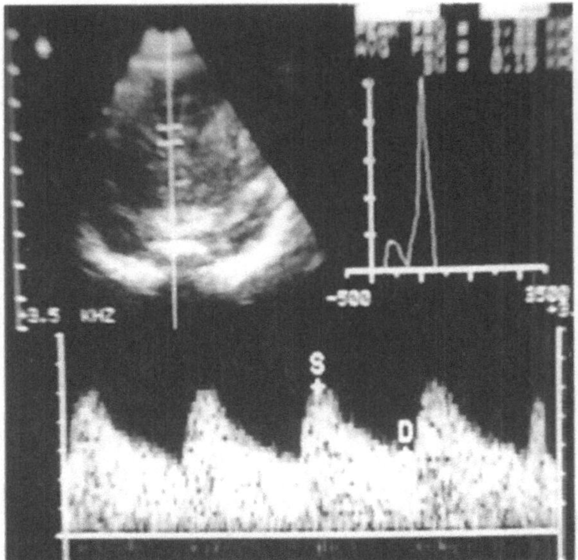

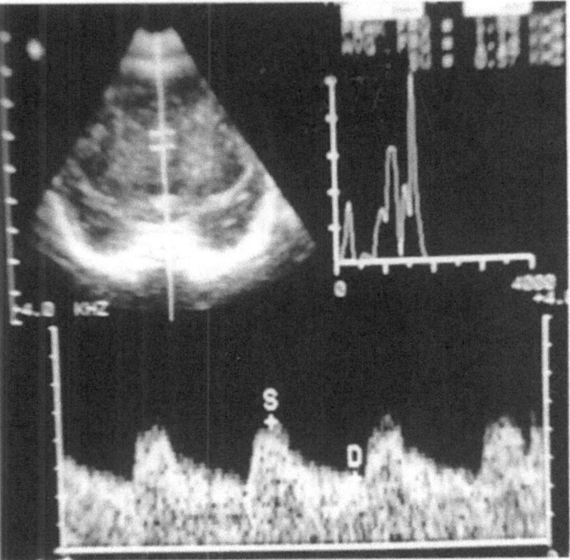

Fig. 5.70a,b. Severe neurological distress: status epilepticus with subcortical white matter and basal ganglia ischemic lesions on ultrasonography. Intense vasodilatation; RI=0.45 (a). After intravenous administration of indomethacin, the vasoconstrictive effect of which is well established, the hemodynamic alterations remain unchanged: RI=0.45 after 2, 10, and 20 min (b); this demonstrates that the vasodilatation results from acidosis and tissue necrosis as a vasoconstrictive drug has no effect

5.4.7
Hemodynamics and Endotracheal Suction

Didier was a 29-week ventilated premature infant. Pulsed Doppler imaging of the anterior cerebral artery shows normal results. During and immediately after endotracheal tube suction, a continuous recording of the Doppler signal was obtained and showed an obvious increase in vascular resistances (Fig. 5.71), which completely recovers 1 min later.

Endotracheal tube suction is a necessity in a ventilated patient and may be performed up to 6–12 times a day. The maneuver involves disconnection, sometimes fluid instillation, and suction within the tracheal tube. It changes the ventilatory conditions and induces a cough reflex, and possibly an adrenergic or vagal response.

The effects on CBF velocities are unavoidable, and in the opinion of some authors dangerous in premature babies of 30 weeks' gestation or less.

In a prospective work (MONTOYA 1989), six preterm neonates (gestational age 28–38 weeks, birth weight 940–2,000 g) were examined during tracheal tube suction (with a catheter of less than half the diameter of the tracheal tube, a drop of saline serum instilled, depression of 120 mbar for 10–15 s). Doppler recording of the anterior cerebral artery showed intense changes: decreased RI with increased diastolic amplitude in five cases, fluctuating Doppler in the sixth (Fig. 5.71). These alterations lasted at least 30 s, with a maximum of 120 s, and were more intense and prolonged in low-birth-weight premature babies. This explains the risk of hemorrhage and ischemia associated with a simple endotracheal tube suction.

One of the major consequences of tracheal suction relates to the increased arterial blood pressure that results from hypoxemia and the nociceptive stimulus of tracheal aggression. The cough reflex is elicited by the catheter in contact with the respiratory mucosa and associated with high rise in central venous pres-

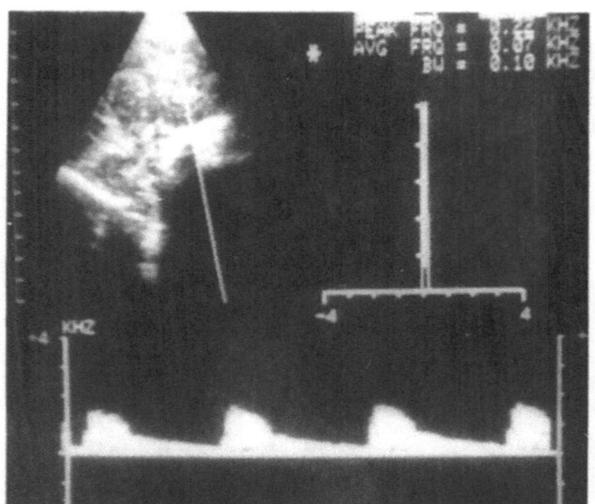

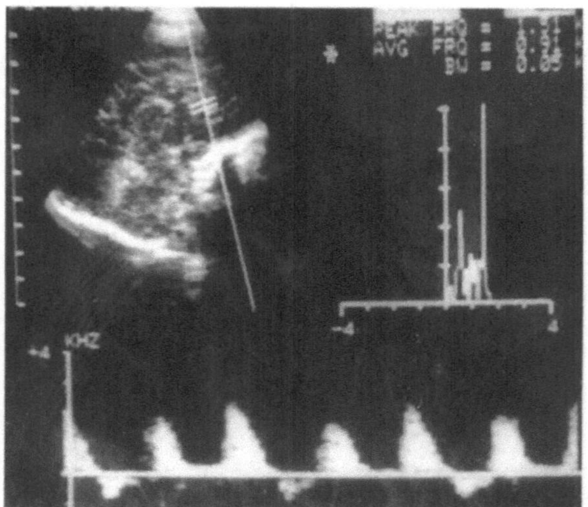

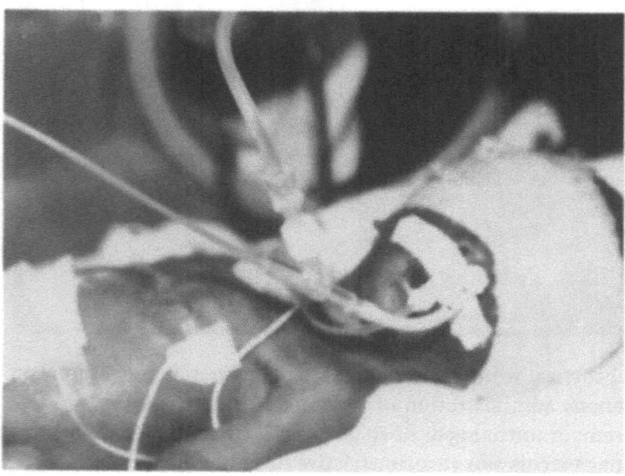

Fig. 5.71a–c. A 28-weeks' gestation premature infant, birth weight 1,000 g. Initially, the spectral analysis curve is normal, RI=0.78 (**a**). Immediately after tracheal suction, systolic and diastolic velocities change sharply (**b**). Utilization of a Y tracheal tube enables tracheal suction without changing the modality of ventilation, reducing the hemodynamic alterations in this fragile preterm infant (**c**)

sure. Finally, a frequent vagal response may cause for bradycardia.

PERLMAN (1983) studied the effects of tracheal suction on Doppler velocimetry of cerebral arteries in 35 premature infants. He reported a significant decrease in pulsatility index and an increase in intracranial pressure; he related the increased CBF to elevation of systemic arterial pressure, and the increased intracranial pressure to increased CBF and central venous pressure.

Continuous recording of the Doppler signal in cerebral arteries makes it possible to track the occurrence, the intensity, and the variability of the cerebrovascular effects of endotracheal tube suction, which is a routine maneuver in the ventilated premature infant.

Obviously, it is important to protect the cerebral vasculature from abrupt changes by utilizing a procedure which does not require changing the ventilation conditions (Fig. 5.71).

5.5
Hemodynamics and Focal or Multifocal Ischemic Brain Necrosis

The spectrum of focal and multifocal ischemic brain necrosis includes cerebral infarction, porencephaly, multicystic encephalomalacia, hydranencephaly, and complications of twin-to-twin transfusion syndrome. These lesions often have a poor prognosis (multicystic encephalomalacia, hydranencephaly); they usually form during fetal life, less frequently after a postnatal ischemic event. Pulsed Doppler provides little information on these diseases, but color imaging is increasingly helpful in understanding their pathogenesis.

5.5.1
Brain Infarction in the Arterial Distribution

Until relatively recently, neonatal cerebral infarction was thought to be uncommon, and the diagnosis was based on autopsy findings. In a neuropathological review of 592 infants (BARMADA 1979), cerebral infarcts were seen in 5.4% of infants with arterial occlusion.

Cerebral infarction is, in fact, a frequent injury in the full-term baby and infant (more than in the preterm baby), and is nowadays easily diagnosed by

modern imaging (BALCOM 1997; FUJIMOTO 1992; VANHULLE 1998; VOORHIES 1984).

Cerebral infarct of arterial origin is characterized by gray and white matter involvement, in a swollen hemisphere, often associated with secondary hemorrhages. Cavity formation is common, the shape and limits of which depend on the astroglial response to injury.

5.5.1.1
Clinical Diagnosis (KOELFEN 1995)

The clinical diagnosis of cerebral infarction is difficult since the clinical pattern lacks specificity: the infarction may be latent (MANNINO 1983) or produce few symptoms, and there may be associated hypotonia (HERNANZ-SCHULMAN 1988), sucking, or temperature control disorders (ROODHOOFT 1987), but the most prominent feature is seizure (ASO 1990; CLANCY 1985; COKER 1988; FILIPEK 1987; LANSKA 1991; MANTEROLA 1966). LEVENE (1987) reported that infarction accounted for 5% of neonatal seizures in the full-term infant.

In the literature, the clinical findings are described as disparate, often mimicking those of other conditions. Out of seven cases, BODE (1986) reported asymmetric tone in two, muscular hypertonia in two, spasticity in one, a seizure in one, and a normal examination in three. DE VRIES (1988) found no clinical or electrical signs of seizure in four premature newborns. Thus, the diagnosis is rarely suspected clinically, and although hemiplegia or hemiparesis are suggestive findings in the older infant, they are uncommon in the neonate, as noted by HILL (1983) (only two cases with hemiplegia out of six newborns examined).

These data from the literature contrast with our personal experience: out of 25 patients with ischemic infarct, hemiparesis was noted in seven and unilateral seizures in five (Table 5.19).

5.5.1.2
Predisposing Factors

Predisposing factors should be systematically sought when cerebral infarction occurs in a neonate.

Some authors (MANNINO 1983; MENT 1986; VOLPE 1995) believe that late intrauterine, intrapartum, or neonatal generalized hypoxic–ischemic events may frequently result in focal cerebral infarction.

Arterial occlusion by thrombus (polycythemia, bacterial meningitis, dehydration with hypernatremia) or embolus (congenital heart disease, placental fragments)

Table 5.19. Arterial infarction (25 cases)
(MCA: middle cerebral artery, ACA: anterior cerebral artery, PCA: posterior cerebral artery, R: right, L: left)

Case	Age	Risk factors	Clinical findings	Location of infarct
1	2 Months	Transposition of great vessels. Respiratory arrest (3 times) during surgical repair	Seizures	R MCA
2	21 Days		Right hemiparesis	L MCA
3	10 Days		Latent	R MCA – R ACA
4	3 Months		Seizures	L MCA
5	4 Months	Down syndrome. Atrioventricular canal. Severe bradycardia during catheterization	Left unilateral seizures with hemiparesis	R ACA R MCA superficial and deep
6	4 Months	Severe dehydration	Seizures	L MCA – R MCA
7	8 Months	Tetralogy of Fallot	Left hemiparesis	L MCA superficial and deep
8	7 Months	Herpes meningoencephalitis	Left hemiplegia	R MCA–R PCA
9	2 Months		Latent	L MCA
10	5 Months	Tetralogy of Fallot	Postoperative right hemiplegia	L MCA
11	2 Months		Latent	L MCA
12	1 Day		Fetal hydrocephalus	L MCA. Fetal involvement
13	6 Months	West syndrome	Latent	L MCA superficial and deep
14	3 Months	Heart rate disorders	Fetal hemiparesis	L MCA
15	6 Years	Surgical evacuation of fronto-parietal hematoma. Injury on left MCA	Right hemiplegia Prolonged coma	L MCA
16	5 Days		Unilateral seizures	L MCA
17	2 Months		Seizures Left hemiparesis	R MCA
18	10 Days		Seizures	L MCA superficial and deep
19	1 Month	Cardiac arrest during catheterization	Seizures	R MCA
20	2 Months	Surgical repair of pulmonary atresia	Hypotonia	L MCA
21	15 Days		Unilateral seizures	L MCA
22	7 Days		Unilateral seizures	L MCA
23	10 Days		Latent	L MCA
24	2 Days	Surgical repair of congenital heart disease	Latent	L MCA
25	2 Days		Latent	L MCA superficial and deep

are well documented entities (AMIT 1980; BARMADA 1979; CLANCY 1985; FUJIMOTO 1992; MANNINO 1983; PELLICER 1992; RORKE 1992; SMITH 1991).

Cerebral thrombosis secondary to hypercoagulable state has been recognized in infants with inherited deficiencies of protein C, protein S, antithrombin III and with antiphospholipid antibodies (DEVILAT 1993; SHESS 1992).

Finally, there is an increasing incidence of neurological complications after cardiac surgery (DU PLESSIS 1997; EHYAI 1984; FERRY 1987). Deep hypothermic circulatory arrest and low-flow cardiopulmonary bypass favor the usual mechanisms of ischemic infarction (microemboli, hypoxemia, cerebral hypoperfusion).

Apart from these predisposing factors, no cause is found in 30%–50% of patients (LEVY 1985; RAYBAUD 1985) and the term "idiopathic infarction" is used.

In our cohort of 25 patients, a risk factor was identified in 13 patients: this was cardiac disease in nine (surgical repair in four, cardiac catheterization in two, tetralogy of Fallot in two, heart rate disorder in one), severe dehydration in one, herpes meningoencephalitis in one, West syndrome in one, and surgery on the middle cerebral artery in one. No predisposing factor was found in the other 12 cases.

5.5.1.3 Ultrasound Examination

● *The diagnosis is made on ultrasonography or CT.* Ischemia occurs within a specific vascular distribution: a single territory was involved in 21 of our 25 patients, and two or more in the other four patients. The middle cerebral artery was affected in all cases, associated with anterior or posterior cerebral artery involvement in two cases and one case respectively (Table 5.19). This pre-eminence of middle cerebral artery involvement is reported in the literature (BARMADA 1979; LEVY 1985; MANNINO 1983; RUFF 1979; WILSON DAVIES 1983). Among 71 cases where the arterial territory was clearly identified (HERNANZ-SCHULMAN 1988), the infarction was located within the distribution of the middle cerebral artery in 56 (i.e., 71%). Approximately 80% of infarcts involved the territory of the left artery (HERNANZ-SCHULMAN 1988) – 18 cases in our own series. Finally, in our series the cortical branch was affected in 20 infants, and the main branch in five (Fig. 5.72).

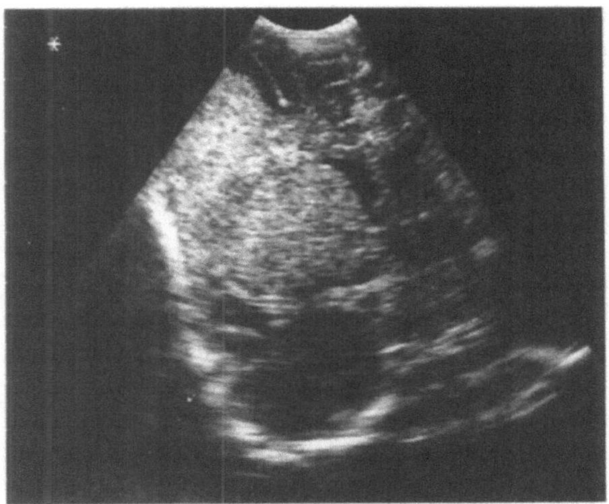

Fig. 5.72. A 4-month-old infant with Down syndrome and congenital heart disease. Marked bradycardia during cardiac catheterization. After 2 days, left-sided seizures occurred with hemiparesis. ultrasonography showed hyperechoic ischemic damage in the distribution of the main branch of the right middle cerebral artery

The infarct appears early as a hyperechoic parenchymal area, located preferentially within white matter, but also in cortical gray matter; on the basis of its shape, smooth edges, extent and topography, its vascular distribution is easy to identify (Fig. 5.73).

The early increased echogenicity of the infarct is well documented in the sonographic literature (BALCOM 1997; BODE 1986; DE VRIES 1988, 1997; HERNANZ-SCHULMAN 1988; HILL 1983), but its neuropathological basis has not been clearly established. In the opinion of most authors, this aspect is related to edema, which seems valuable since SMITH (1985) has reported a hyperechoic ring surrounding

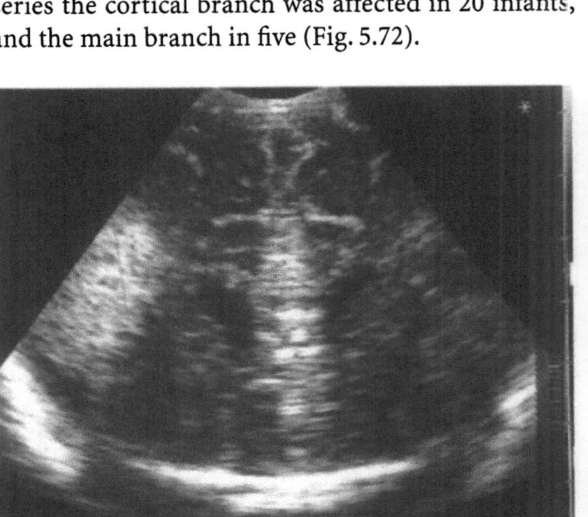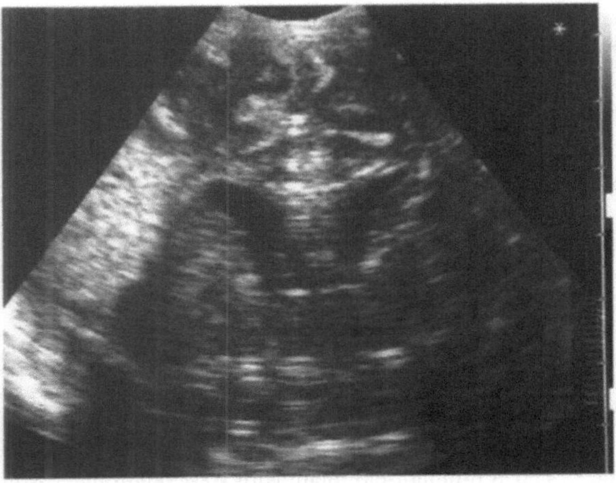

Fig. 5.73a,b. A 2-month-old infant. The sharp limits and the intense hyperechogenicity of the ischemic area allow precise identification of its topography: the territory of the right anterior (a) and middle cerebral arteries (b)

ten brain tumors, confirmed on CT and anatomic examination as edematous.

Finally, the infarct typically evolves toward cystic cavitation after 3–4 weeks (Fig. 5.74).

● *Color imaging and pulsed Doppler provide interesting information.*

Literature data are summarized by the experience of TAYLOR (1994), who found regional alterations of CBF in neonates with brain infarction. In the acute phase, apparent dilatation of veins and arterioles in the tissue surrounding the infarct was identified in five of eight infants. This hyperemia may be explained as follows: breakdown of the blood–brain barrier and neuronal disruption may cause the release of vasoactive substances (prostaglandins, excitatory aminoacids, nitric oxide) with subsequent local vasodilatation in response to the increased local metabolic demand.

The Doppler findings are likely to represent regional hyperemia in the periphery of the infarcted brain tissue: increased size of visible vessels, decreased visualization of vessels in the infarct, and highly increased arterial velocities (Fig. 5.75).

Color Doppler may explain the formation of infarction, as shown in this case.

Giovanni was a low-birth-weight preterm infant (34 weeks' gestation) born after an uneventful pregnancy. In the neonatal period, he presented with abdominal distension and necrotizing enterocolitis was suspected, but the intestinal outcome was favorable. Neurological examination was normal. Routine brain ultrasonography was performed on day 2. Color Doppler detected absence of colored signal within the left middle cerebral artery and internal carotid artery (Fig. 5.76): arterial thrombosis was diagnosed. The territory supplied by the left main middle cerebral artery was already hyperechoic, which may suggest a prenatal injury (Fig. 5.77). On pulsed Doppler, vasodilatation of the anterior cerebral artery and right internal carotid artery was noted (Fig. 5.78).

Treatment by aspirin was begun on day 3. Follow-up ultrasonography failed to show any change on day 7.

On day 9, a slight flow was detected in the left internal carotid artery (Fig. 5.79), with very low velocities on pulsed Doppler (Fig. 5.80).

On day 12, the left internal carotid flow was better seen (Fig. 5.81) but velocities were unchanged (Fig. 5.82); a colored flow was detected in the left middle cerebral artery (Fig. 5.83).

On day 18, internal carotid velocities had returned to normal and colored flow was seen in the middle cerebral artery. The infarcted territory remained hyperechoic, without cyst formation.

The neurological findings were normal throughout the course of the disease.

This observation demonstrates the mechanism of infarction and the reality of arterial occlusion. It confirms the vasodilatation in response to the ischemic event, as reported by TAYLOR (1994). It shows that hyperemia extends over much more than just the one affected region during the acute phase; luxury perfusion is, in fact, present in the contralateral internal carotid and anterior cerebral arteries.

Finally, it shows that color Doppler imaging may be used to follow vascular recovery after neonatal cerebral infarction, which is extremely slow. This is in

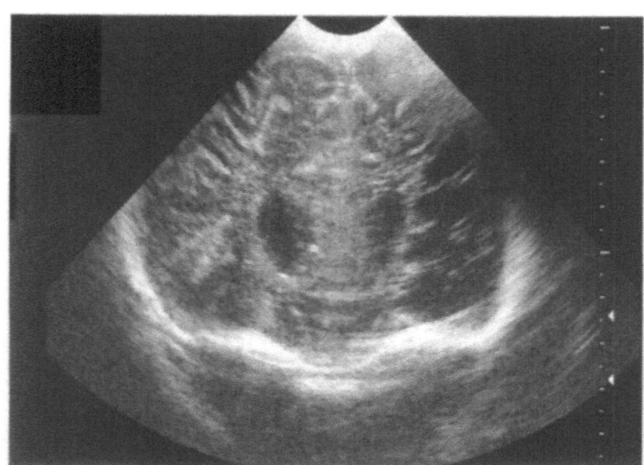

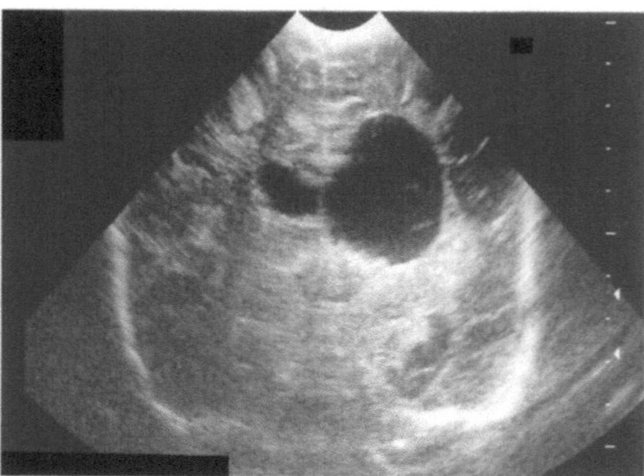

Fig. 5.74a,b. A 6-month-old infant with West syndrome. History of infarction in the territories of the left anterior and middle cerebral arteries. Several left hemispheric parenchymal cysts are present (**a**), together with ventricular enlargement of an atrophic pattern (**b**)

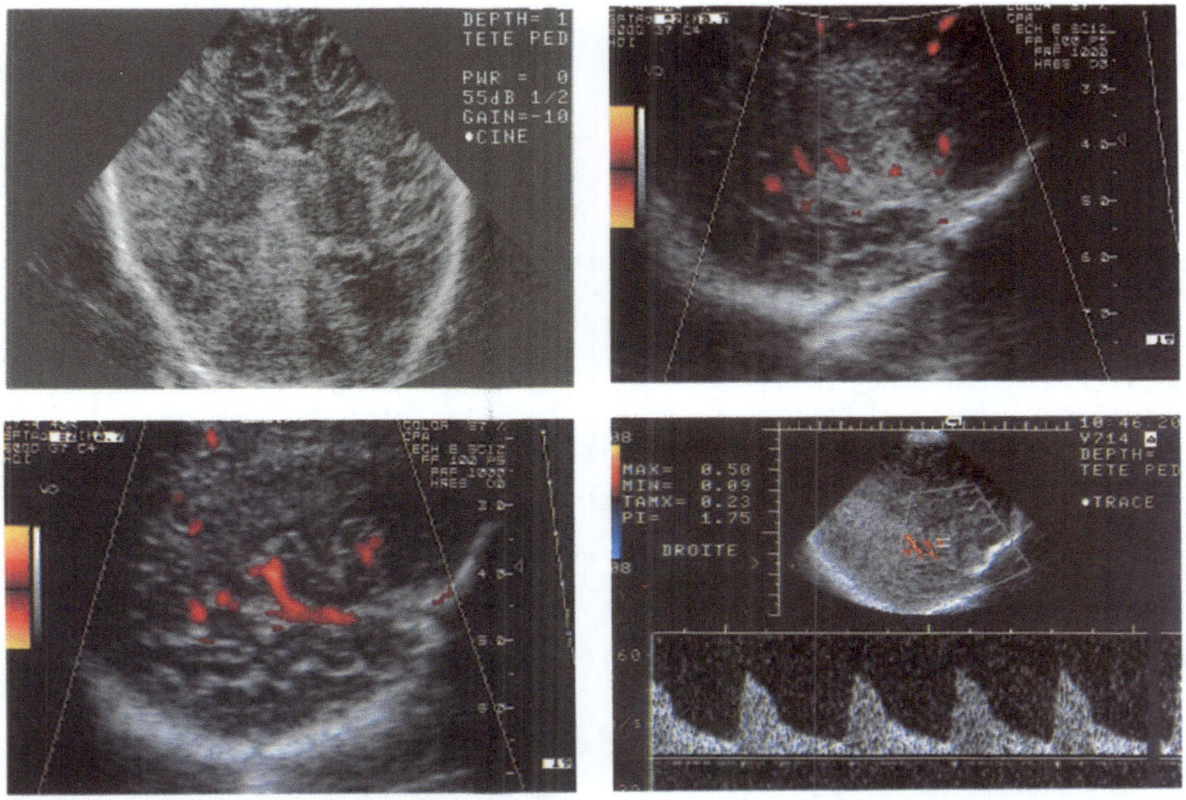

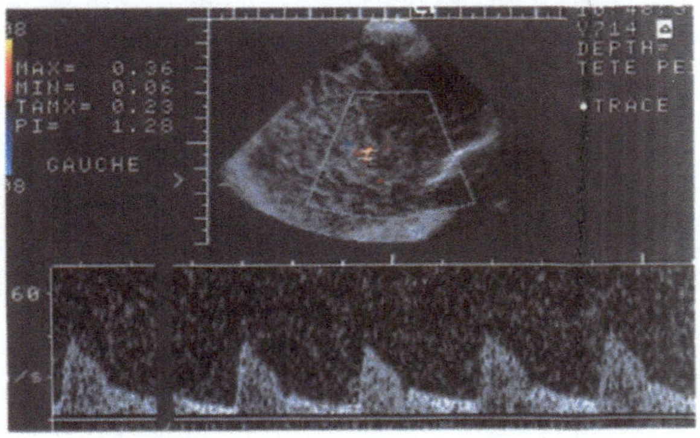

Fig. 5.75a–e. A 2-month-old infant with unilateral seizures and left hemiparesis. Hyperechoic infarct in the territory of the right middle cerebral artery (**a**) with decreased perfusion (**b**) compared with normal contralateral brain (**c**). Pulsed Doppler shows increased velocities on the side of the infarction (**d**) (PSV=50 cm/s, EDV=9 cm/s) compared with the other side (**e**) (PSV=36 cm/s, EDV=6 cm/s). This confirms the presence of hyperemia surrounding the infarcted brain tissue

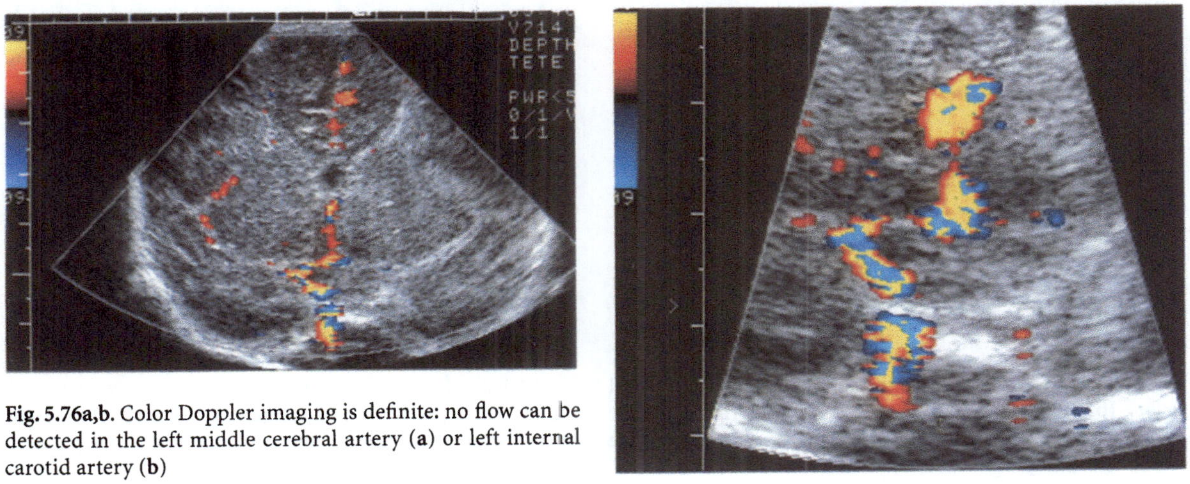

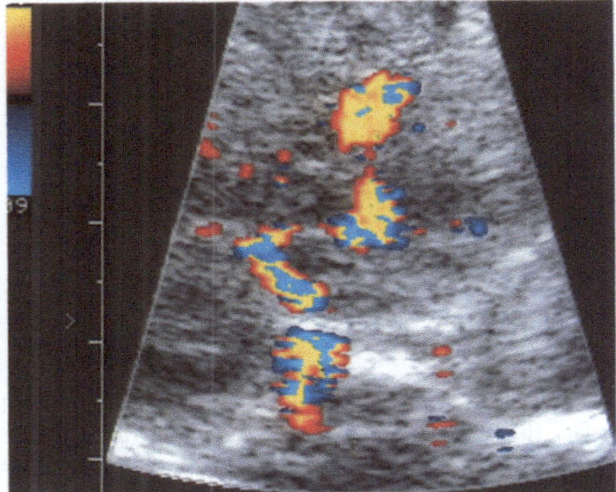

Fig. 5.76a,b. Color Doppler imaging is definite: no flow can be detected in the left middle cerebral artery (**a**) or left internal carotid artery (**b**)

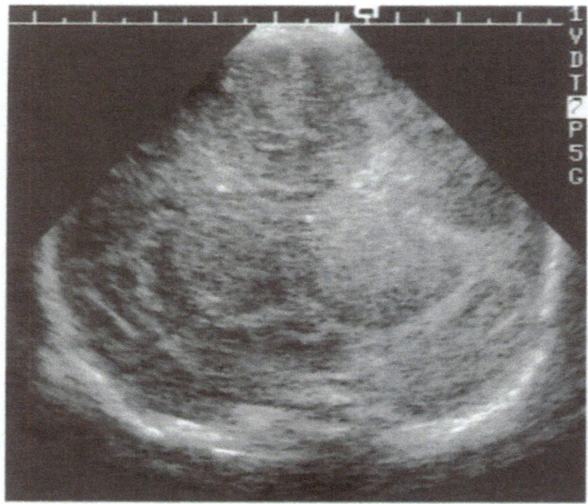

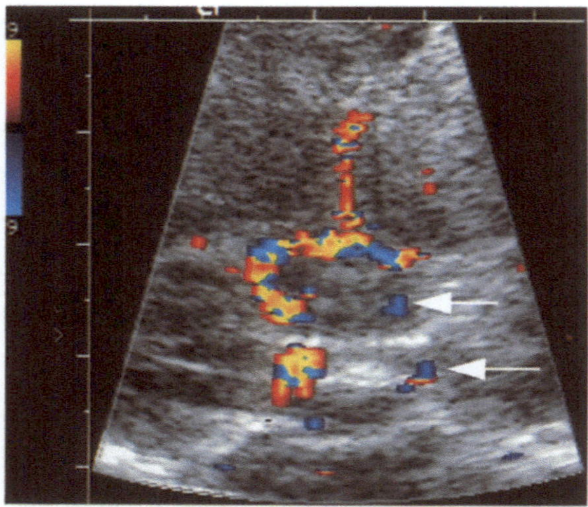

Fig. 5.77. The territory of the left middle cerebral artery is obviously hyperechoic

Fig. 5.79. Day 9. The left internal carotid artery shows a very low flow, coded blue (↑)

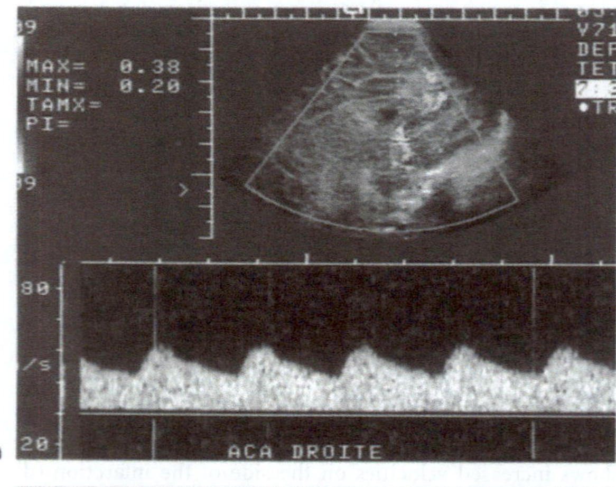

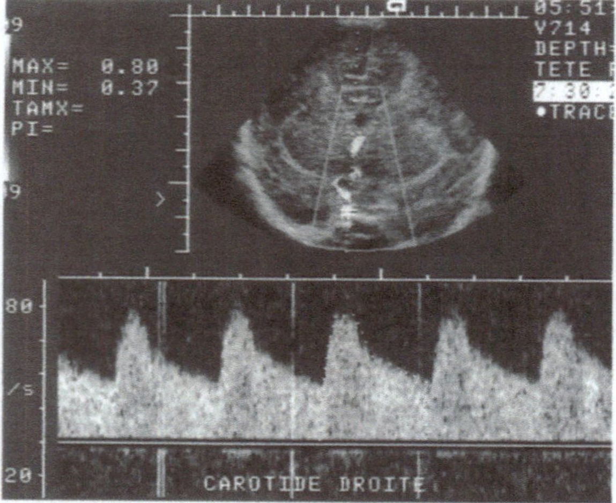

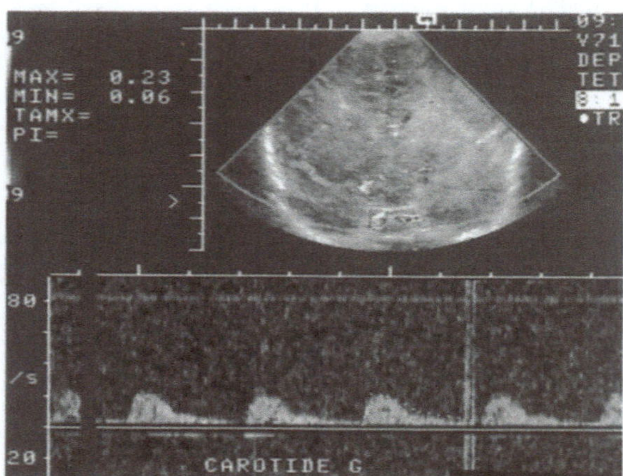

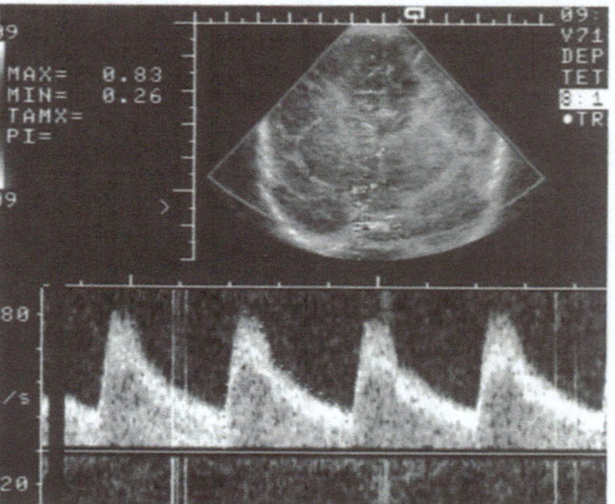

Fig. 5.78a,b. Increased velocities in the right internal carotid artery (**b**) (PSV=80 cm/s, EDV=37 cm/s) and right anterior cerebral artery (**a**) (EDV=20 cm/s). This is a sign of diffuse vasodilatory response

Fig. 5.80a,b. Left carotid artery velocities are low (**a**) (PSV=23 cm/s, EDV=6 cm/s) compared with those of the right carotid artery (**b**) (PSV=83 cm/s, EDV=26 cm/s) in hyperemic response

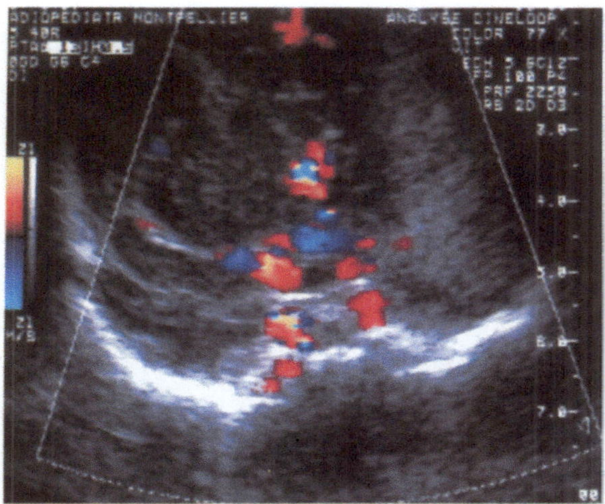

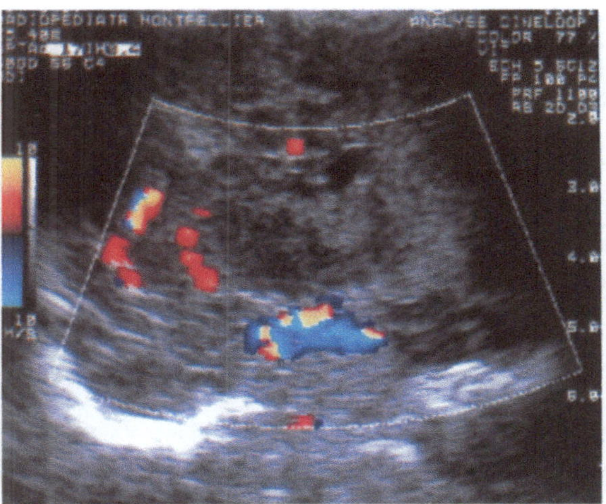

Fig. 5.81. Note almost normal visualization of the left carotid artery

Fig. 5.83. Frontal plane on color Doppler. The left middle cerebral artery remains unvisualized

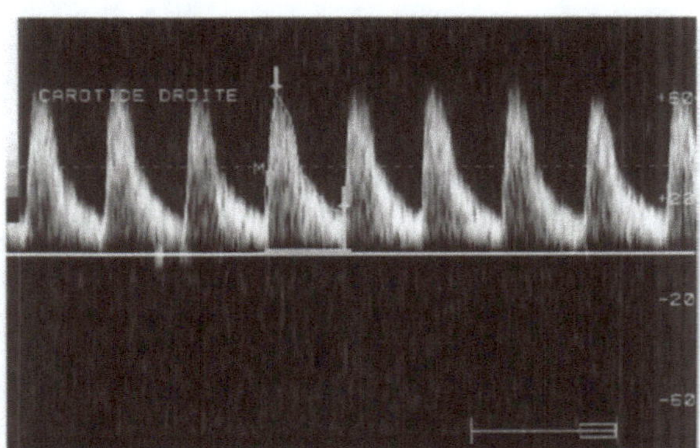

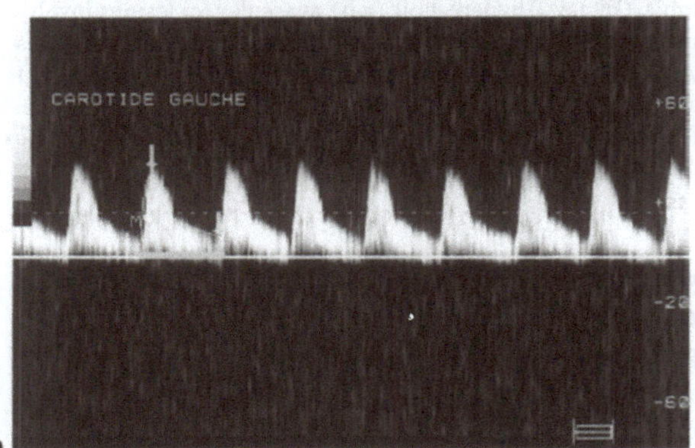

Fig. 5.82a,b. Right carotid artery (a): velocities have returned to normal: PSV=62 cm/s, EDV=15 cm/s. Left carotid artery (b): velocities remain low: PSV=33 cm/s, EDV=6 cm/s

agreement with reports of Volpe (1985): using positron emission tomography, this author demonstrated that the ischemic decrease in CBF is prolonged and extends in the whole ipsilateral hemisphere.

5.5.2
Cerebral Complications of Twin-To-Twin Transfusion Syndrome

Thromboembolic complication of twin gestation is a rare disease well described in the literature (Benirschke 1992, 1993; Caballero 1991; Filly 1990; Jung 1984; Langer 1997; Lopriore 1995; Patten 1989; Yoshioka 1979). The pathogenesis of this severe cerebral injury relates to thrombosis of cerebral arteries by emboli of infarcted necrotic placental fragments from the deceased to the surviving twin via vascular anastomosis in monochorionic placentas. More recently, a second hypothesis has been proposed: on the death of the first twin, an afflux of blood directed from the surviving to the dead twin might cause severe hypotension and irreversible cerebral damage (Benirschke 1993).

Whatever the physiopathological explanation, the developing fetal brain is highly susceptible to ischemic infarction; the damage is always severe and includes porencephaly, multicystic encephalomalacia (Fig. 5.84) (Yoshioka 1979), hydranencephaly (Jung 1984), microcephaly, and hydrocephalus (Patten 1989).

Several authors suggest premature delivery (Cabalero 1991; Patten 1989) in order to protect

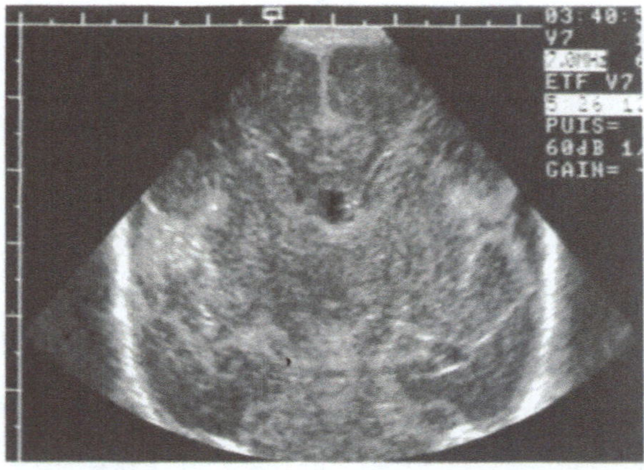

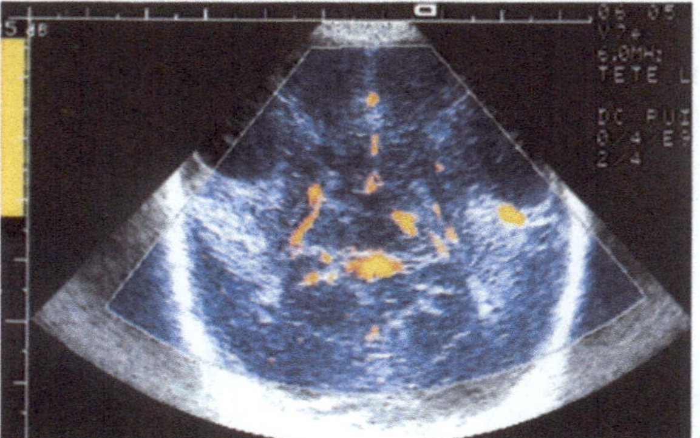

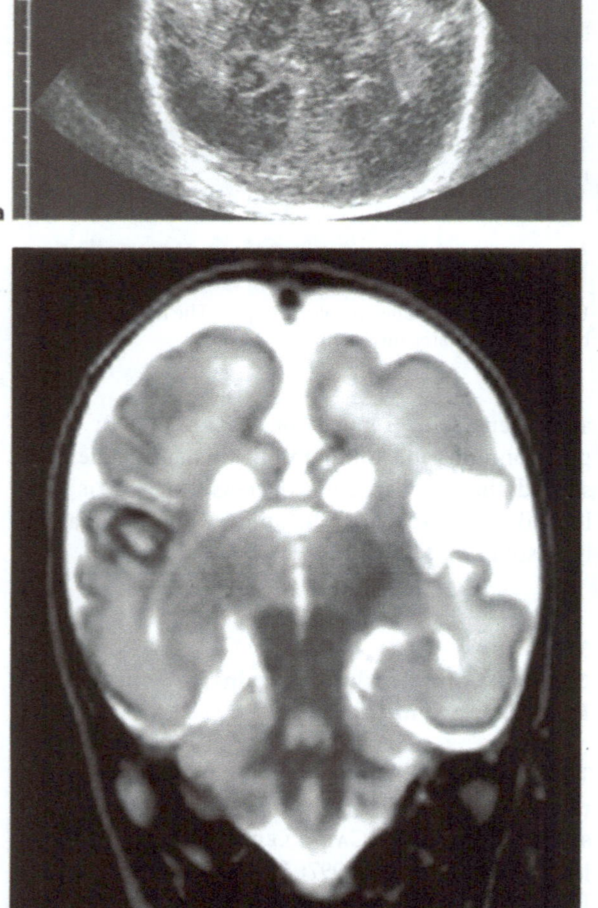

Fig. 5.84a–d. Monochorionic biamniotic twin gestation: twin-to-twin transfusion syndrome. At 28 weeks, a cesarean delivery was undertaken to preserve twin 1. Twin 2 had an extremely poor prognosis: oligoamnios, fetal weight approximately 500 g, severely disturbed Doppler indices. At birth, twin 2 died, while twin 1 had hyaline membrane disease and severe hypotonia. On day 3, hyperechoic (**a,b**), avascular (**c**) lesions involving both parieto-temporal areas close to the sylvian fissures were seen; cyst formation was observed on T2-weighted MRI at 1 month of age (**d**). Twin 1 died on day 45. To summarize: fetofetal embolization with bilateral ischemic-hemorrhagic damage

the surviving twin, but this management seems to provide only theoretical advantages, because the timing of cerebral damage and the delay between the death of one twin and ischemic injury to the surviving twin cannot be predicted (Fig. 5.85). In fact, the future appears to lie in destruction of the placental anastomosis under color Doppler guidance (VILLE 1994; VILLE 1995).

5.5.3
Antenatal Diagnosis: Present and Future Possibilities

Fetal encephalopathies result from mechanisms that mainly relate to fetal vascular supply disorders. Different lesional patterns are observed, depending on the severity and topography of fetal circulatory insufficiency: single porencephalic cyst has a good intellectual prognosis, whereas multicystic encephalomalacia and hydranencephaly have a poor neurological prognosis.

After formation of cavities, the diagnosis is always easy: ultrasonography defines the extent, location, and number of cysts in order to distinguish multicystic leu-

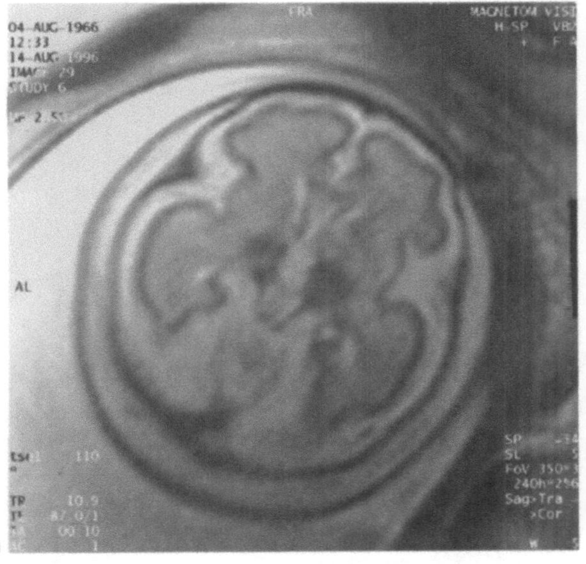

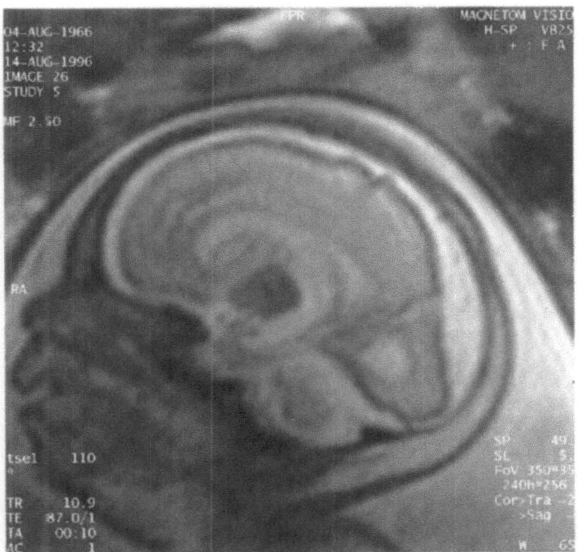

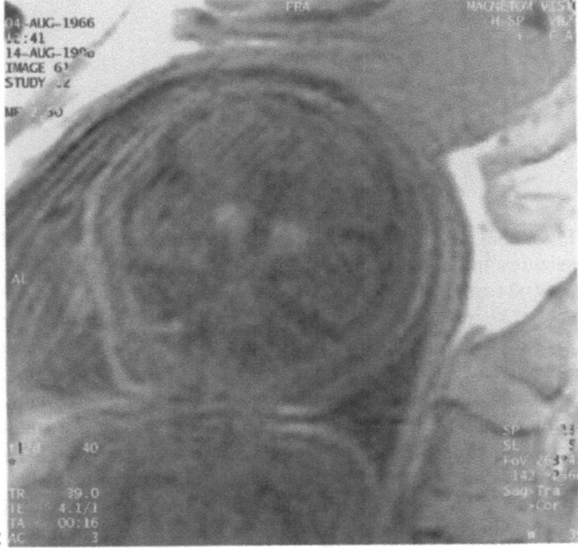

Fig. 5.85a–c. A 28-weeks' gestation fetus. Maternal anaphylactic response to bee-sting with cardiac arrest led to prolonged fetal bradycardia. Cerebral MRI is normal. At 30 weeks' gestation, on repeat MRI, thalamic ischemic lesions appear hypointense on T2 (haste sequence) (**a,b**) and hyperintense on T1 (**c**). This anatomic pattern correlates with the clinical history: ischemic injury to the basal ganglia is known to be frequent after acute total asphyxia (MYERS 1969, 1975)

komalacia from simple porencephaly. Exceptionally, the early features of parenchymal ischemia (hyperechoic) may be detected. In these conditions, fetal MRI provides remarkable information (Fig. 5.85).

The future lies in routine demonstration and analysis of the fetal cerebral vascularization by color and pulsed Doppler imaging, which will permit an understanding of the pathogenesis of hypoxic–ischemic events in the fetus.

5.6 Conclusions

Several conclusions may be drawn concerning hypoxic-ischemic brain injury in neonate.

● The diagnosis of ischemic damage (neuronal necrosis, parasagittal cerebral injury, periventricular and subcortical leukomalacia, arterial infarction, porencephaly, multicystic encephalomalacia, hycranencephaly) is based on ultrasonography and MRI: this is self-evident.

● The hemodynamic assessment (color and pulsed Doppler imaging) requires caution: this too is self-

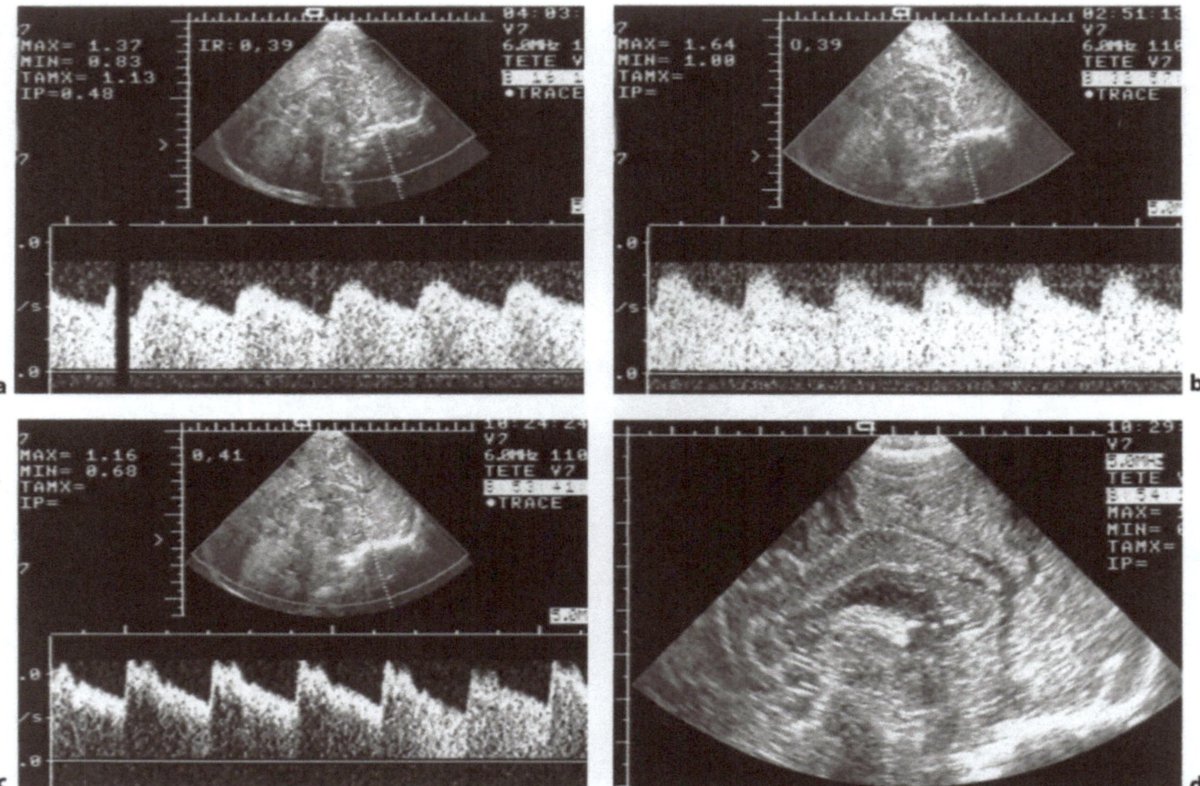

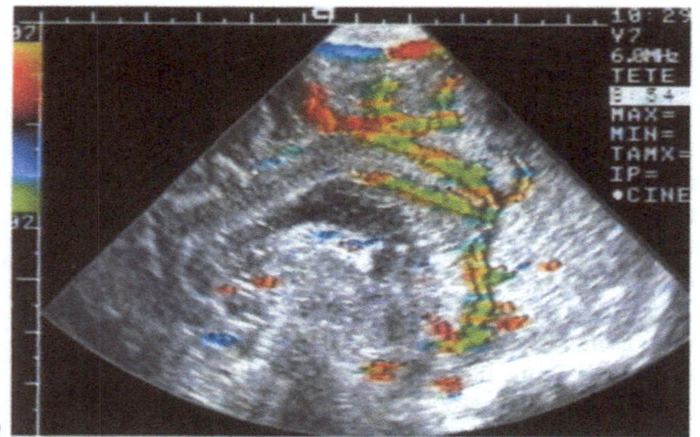

Fig. 5.86a–e. A 5-month-old infant with unexplained repeated seizures. Initial hemodynamic data are normal: PSV=71 cm/s, EDV=24 cm/s, RI=0.66. **a** Day 3. Luxury perfusion occurs: PSV=137 cm/s, EDV=83 cm/s, TAV=113 cm/s, RI=0.39. **b** Accentuation on day 4: PSV=164 cm/s, EDV=100 cm/s. **c** Day 7. Persistence of high velocities: PSV=116 cm/s, EDV=68 cm/s, TAV=89 cm/s. Parenchymal lesions are severe, with ischemic damage in basal ganglia and white matter (mainly in frontal regions). Note the striking spontaneous visualization of the anterior cerebral artery and its branches (**d**), as confirmed by color Doppler (**e**). To summarize: intense and prolonged (until day 10) luxury perfusion suggesting an extremely poor outcome. Death occurred on day 12

evident, because it reflects only a brief moment in a course where the hemodynamic alterations are changing. Despite these limitations, it nevertheless provides extremely valuable information and raises the question of having an investigator available within the intensive care unit.

● Several observations have already been validated: the relationship between postischemic luxury perfusion and poor outcome (Fig. 5.86), color Doppler detection and explanation of vascular disturbances during postnatal ischemia, and others.

● The axes of research are many:
- Detection of hypoperfusion in brain tissue
- Study of capillaries using harmonic technique and contrast medium
- Multiplication of hemodynamic data in order to differentiate grade II from grade III encephalopathy
- Early recognition of low blood flow in a neonate
- Evaluation of cerebral vessels in the fetus

● Hemodynamic assessment remains extremely disappointing in periventricular leukomalacia of the preterm infant, and we are still unable to help prevent this damage and its severe motor consequences.

References

Adams C, Hoschhauser L, Logan WJ (1988) Primary thalamic and caudate hemorrhage in term neonates presenting with seizures. Pediatr Neurol 4:175-177

Ahmann PA, Carrigan TA, Carlton D, Wyly B, Schwartz JF (1987) Brain death in children: characteristic common carotid arterial velocity patterns measured with pulsed Doppler ultrasound. J Pediatr 110:723-728

Alexander JM, Gilstrap LC, Cox SM, McIntire DM, Leveno KJ (1998) Clinical chorioamnionitis and the prognosis for very low birth weight infants. Obstet Gynecol 91:725-729

Altman DI, Powers WJ, Perlman JM (1988) Cerebral blood flow requirement for brain viability in newborn infants is lower than in adults. Ann Neurol 24:218-226

Amato M, Gambon R, Von Muralt G, Huber P (1987) Neurosonographic and biochemical correlates of periventricular leukomalacia in low birth weight infants. Pediatr Neurosci 13:84-89

Amit M, Camfield PR (1980) Neonatal polycythemia causing multiple cerebral infarcts. Arch Neurol 37:109-110

Arabin B, Siebert M, Gimenez E, Saling E (1988) Obstetrical characteristics of a loss of end diastolic velocities in the fetal aorta and/or umbilical artery using Doppler ultrasound. Gynecol Obstet Invest 25:173-180

Arbeille P, Patat F, Tranquart F, Body G, Berson M, Roncin A, Saliba E, Magnin G, Berger C, Pourcelot L (1987) Exploration Doppler des circulations artérielles ombilicale et cérébrale du foetus. J Gynecol Obstet Biol Reprod 16:45-51

Arbeille P, Roncin A, Berson M, Patat F, Pourcelot L (1987) Exploration of the fetal cerebral blood flow by duplex Doppler-linear array system in normal and pathological pregnancies. Ultrasound Med Biol 13:329-337

Archer LN, Levene MI, Evans DH (1986) Cerebral artery Doppler ultrasonography for prediction of outcome after perinatal asphyxia. Lancet 2:1116-1117

Arduini G, Rizzo G, Romanini C, Mancuso S (1989) Hemodynamic changes in growth retarded fetuses during maternal oxygen administration as predictors of fetal outcome. J Ultrasound Med 8:193-196

Arnold BW, Martin CG, Alexander BJ, Chen T, Fleming LR (1991) Autoregulation of brain blood flow during hypotension and hypertension in infant lambs. Pediatr Res 29:110-115

Ashwal S, Smith AJ, Torres F (1977) Radionucleide bolus angiography: a technique for verification of brain death in infants and children. J Pediatr 91:722-728

Ashwal S, Majcher JS, Vain N, Longo LD (1980) Patterns of fetal lamb regional cerebral blood flow during and after prolonged hypoxia. Pediatr Res 14:1104-1110

Ashwal S, Dale PS, Longo LD (1984) Regional cerebral blood flow: studies in the fetal lamb during hypoxia, hypercapnia, acidosis and hypotension. Pediatr Res 18:1309-1316

Ashwal S (1997) Brain death in the newborn. Current perspectives. Clin Perinatol 24:859-882

Aso K, Scher MS, Barmada MA (1990) Cerebral infarcts and seizures in the neonate. J Child Neurol 5:224-228

Austin NC, Pairaudeau PN, Haames TK, Hall M (1992) Regional blood flow velocity changes after indomethacin infusion in preterm infants. Arch Dis Child 67:851-854

Baarsma R., Launni RB, Baerts W, Okken A (1987) Reliability of sonography in nonhemorrhagic periventricular leukomalacia. Pediatr Radiol 17:189-191

Babcock D (1995) Sonography of the brain in infants: role in evaluating neurologic abnormalities. AJR Am J Roentgenol 165:417-423

Back SA, Volpe JJ (1977) Cellular and molecular pathogenesis of periventricular white matter injury. Mental retardation and Developmental Disabilities. Res Rev 20:96-107

Balcom TA, Redmond BG (1997) Cerebral infarction as multifocal clonic seizures in a term neonate. J Am Board Fam Pract 10:43-49

Ball RH, Espinoza MI, Parer JT (1994) Regional blood flow in asphyxiated fetuses with seizures. Am J Obstet Gynecol 170:156-161

Banker B, Larroche JC (1962) Periventricular Leukomalacia of infancy: a form of neonatal anoxic encephalopathy. Arch Neurol 7:386-410

Barkovich AJ, Sargent SK (1995) Profound asphyxia in the premature infant: imaging findings. AJNR Am J Neuroradiol 16:1837-1846

Barkovitch AJ, Westmark K, Partridge C, Sola A, Ferriero DM (1995) Perinatal asphyxia: MR findings in the first 10 days. AJNR Am J Neuroradiol 16:427-438

Barkovich AJ (1997) The encephalopathic neonate: choosing the proper imaging technique. AJNR Am J Neuroradiol 18:1816-1820

Barmada MA, Moossy J, Shuma NRM (1979) Cerebral infarcts with arterial occlusion in neonates. Ann Neurol 6:495-502

Barr LL, McCullough PJ, Ball WS, Krasner BH, Garra BS, Deddens JA (1996) Quantitative sonographic feature analysis of clinical infant hypoxia: a pilot study. AJNR Am J Neuroradiol 17:1025-1031

Battin M, Maalouf E, Counsell S, Herlihy A, Edwards AD (1997) Magnetic resonance imaging of the brain of very premature infants within a neonatal intensive care unit. Lancet 349:1741-1744

Batton DG, Hellman J, Hernandez MJ, Maisels MJ (1983) Regional cerebral blood flow, cerebral blood velocity and pulsatility index in newborn dogs. Pediatr Res 17:908-912

Bejar R, Coen RW, Merrit TA, Vaucher Y, Trice J, Centeno R, Gilles F (1986) Focal necrosis of the white matter (periventricular leukomalacia): sonographic, pathologic and electroencephalographic features. AJNR Am J Neuroradiol 7:1073-1080

Benirschke K (1992) The contribution of placental anastomoses to prenatal twin damage. Hum Pathol 23:1319-1320

Benirschke K (1993) Intrauterine death of a twin: mechanisms, implications for surviving twin, and placental pathology. Semin Diagn Pathol 10:222-231

Bennet L, Peebles DM, Edwards AD, Rios A, Hanson M (1998) The cerebral hemodynamic response to asphyxia and hypoxia in the near-term fetal sheep as measured by near infrared spectroscopy. Pediatr Res 44:951-957

Benrhagen RG, Weintraub RG, Lundstrom NR, Svenningsen NW (1998) Hypoxic-ischemic encephalopathy is associated with regional changes in cerebral blood flow velocity and alterations in cardiovascular function. Biol Neonate 73:275-286

Berhman RE, Lees MH, Peterson EN (1970) Distribution of the circulation in the normal and asphyxiated fetal primate. Am J Obstet Gynecol 108:956-969

Blankenberg FG, Norbasch AM, Lane B, Stevenson DK, Bracci PM, Enzmann DR (1996) Neonatal intracranial ischemia and hemorrhage: diagnosis with US, CT and MR imaging. Radiology 199:253-259

Blankenberg FG, Loh NN, Norbash AM, Craychee JA, Spielman DM, Person BL, Berg CA, Enzmann DR (1997) Impaired cerebrovascular autoregulation after hypoxic ischemic injury in extremely low birth weight neonates: detection with power and pulsed wave Doppler US. Radiology 205:553-568

Bode H, Strasburg HM, Pringsheim W, Kunzer W (1986) Cerebral infarction in term neonates: diagnosis by cerebral ultrasound. Child's Nerv Syst 2:195-199

Bode H, Sauer M, Pringsheim W (1988) Diagnosis of brain death by transcranial Doppler sonography. Arch Dis Child 63:1474-1478

Bona E, Hagberg H, Loberg EM, Bagenholn R, Thoresen M (1998) Protective effects of moderate hypothermia after neonatal hypoxia-ischemia: short and long term outcome. Pediatr Res 43:738-745

Boylan GB, Panerai RB, Rennie JM, Evans DH, Rabe-Hesketh S, Binnie CD (1999). Cerebral blood flow velocity during neonatal seizures. Arch Dis Child Fetal Neonatal 80:105-110

Bowerman RA, Donn SM, Di Pietro MA, D'Amato CJ, Hicks SP (1984) Periventricular leukomalacia in the preterm newborn infant: sonographic and clinical features. Radiology 231:156-161

Bracero L, Schulman H, Fleischer A, Farmakides G, Rochelson B (1986) Umbilical artery velocimetry in diabetes and pregnancy. Obstet Gynecol 68:654-658

Brann AW, Myers RE (1975) Central nervous system findings in the newborn monkey following severe in utero partial asphyxia. Neurology 25:327-328

Brar HS, Horenstein J, Medearis AL, Platt LD, Phelan JP, Paul RH (1989) Cerebral umbilical and uterine resistance using Doppler velocimetry in postterm pregnancy. J Ultrasound Med 8:187-191

Brown JK, Purvis RJ, Foriar J0, Cockburn F (1974) Neurological aspects of perinatal asphyxia. Dev Med Child Neurol 16:567-580

Brun A, Kyllerman M (1979) Clinical, pathogenic and neuropathological correlates in dystonic cerebral palsy. Eur J Pediatr 131:93-97

Bucher HU, Edwards AD, Lipp AE (1993) Comparison between near infrared spectroscopy and 133 Xenon clearance for estimation of cerebral blood flow in critically ill preterm infants. Pediatr Res 33:56-60

Burnard ED, James LS (1961) Failure of the heart after asphyxia at birth. Pediatrics 28:545-565

Caballero P, Del Campo L, Ocon E (1991) Cystic encephalomalacia in twin embolization syndrome. Radiology 178:892-893

Cabanas F, Pellicer A, Perez-Higueras A, Garcia A, Roche C, Quero J (1991) Ultrasonographic findings in thalamus and basal ganglia in term asphyxiated infants. Pediatr Neurol 7:211-215

Calvert SA, Hoskins EM, Fong KW, Forsyth SC (1986) Periventricular leukomalacia: ultrasonic diagnosis and neurological outcome. Acta Paediatr Scand 75:489-496

Cavazutti M, Duffy TE (1982) Regulation of local cerebral blood flow in normal and hypoxic newborn dogs. Ann Neurol 11:247-257

Chandran R, Serraserra V, Sellers SM (1993) Fetal cerebral Doppler in the recognition of fetal compromise. Br J Obstet Gynecol 100:139-144

Charriaut-Marlangue C, Ben Ari Y (1996) Ischémie cérébrale: la mort cellulaire est-elle de type apoptose? Arch Fr Pediatr 3:245-247

Chiamulera C, Terron A, Reggiani A (1993) Qualitative and quantitative analysis of the progressive cerebral damage after middle cerebral artery occlusion in mice. Brain Res 606:251-258

Chiu NC, Shen EY, Lee BS (1994) Reversal of diastolic cerebral blood flow in infants without brain death. Pediatr Neurol 11:337-340

Christophe C, Clercx A, Blum D, Hasaerts D, Segebarth C, Perlmutter N (1994) Early MR detection of cortical and subcortical hypoxic-ischemic encephalopathy in full term infants. Pediatr Radiol 24:581-584

Chow PP, Horgan JG, Taylor KJ (1985) Neonatal periventricular leukomalacia: real time sonographic diagnosis with CT correlation. AJNR Am J Neuroradiol 6:383-388

Chumas PD, Del Bigio MR, Drake JM (1993) A comparison of the protective effect of dexamethasone to other potential prophylactic agents in a neonatal rat model of cerebral hypoxia-ischemia. J Neurosurg 79:414-420

Clancy R, Malin S, Laraque D (1985) Focal motor seizures heralding stroke in full term neonates. Am J Dis Child 139:601-606

Clancy RR, Sladky JT, Rorke LB (1989) Hypoxic ischemic spinal cord injury following perinatal asphyxia. Ann Neurol 25:185-189

Cohn EH, Sacks EJ, Heymann MA, Rudolph AM (1974) Cardiovascular responses to hypoxemia and acidemia in fetal lambs. Am J Obstet Gynecol 120:817-824

Coker SB, Beltran RS, Myers TF (1988) Neonatal stroke: description of patients and investigation into pathogenesis. Pediatr Neurol 4:219-223

Connolly B, Kelehan P, O'brien N (1994) The echogenic thalamus in hypoxic ischemic encephalopathy. Pediatr Radiol 24:268-271

Cooke RW, Rolfe P, Howat P (1979) Apparent cerebral blood flow in newborns with respiratory disease. Dev Med Child Neurol 21:154-160

Cordero L, Hon EH (1971) Neonatal bradycardia following nasopharyngeal stimulation. J Pediatr 78:441-444

Couture A, Veyrac C, Baud C, Leboucq N, Montoya F (1987) New imaging of cerebral ischaemic lesions: high frequency probes and pulsed Doppler. Ann Radiol 30:452-461

Couture A, Veyrac C, Baud C (1994) Les lésions cérébrales anoxic–ischémiques. In: Echographie cérébrale: du foetus au nouveau-né. Imagerie et hémodynamique. Sauramps Medical. Montpellier 167-248

Couture A, Veyrac C, Baud C, Ferran JL (1996) Le Doppler cerebral en pédiatrie. JEMU 17:21-29

Cynober E, Uzan M, Uzan S, Breat G, Sureau C (1990) L'index diastolique carotidien: facteur prédictif de la souffrance foetale aiguë. J Gynecol Obstet Biol Reprod 19:53-59

D'Arceuil HE (1998) Diffusion and perfusion magnetic resonance imaging of the evolution of hypoxic ischemic encephalopathy in the neonatal rabbit. J Magn Reson Imaging 8:820-828

Dean LM, Taylor GA (1995) The intracranial venous system in infants: normal and abnormal findings on duplex and color Doppler sonography. AJR Am J Roentgenol 164:151-156

Deeg KH, Rupprecht TH, Zeilinger G (1990) Doppler-sonographic classification of brain edema in infants. Pediatr Radiol 20:509-514

De Haan HH, Van Reempts JL, Vles JS, De Haan J. Hasaart TH (1993) Effects of asphyxia on the fetal lamb brain. Am J Obstet Gynecol 169:1493-1501

Del Zoppo GJ, Schmid-Schönbein GW, Mori E, Copeland BR, Chang CM (1991) Polymorphonuclear leukocytes occlude capillaries following middle cerebral artery occlusion and reperfusion in baboons. Stroke 22:1276-1283

De Reuck J (1971) The human periventricular arterial blood supply and the anatomy of cerebral infarctions. Eur Neurol 5:321-334

De Reuck J (1984) Cerebral angioarchitecture and perinatal brain lesions in premature and full-term infants. Acta Neurol Scand 70:391-395

Desa DJ (1977) Myocardial changes in immature infants requiring prolonged ventilation. Arch Dis Child 52:138-147

De Souza SW, Richards B (1978) Neurological sequelae in newborn babies after perinatal asphyxia. Arch Dis Child 53:564-568

Devilat M, Toso M, Morales M (1993) Childhood stroke associated with protein C or S deficiency and primary antiphospholipid syndrome. Pediatr Neurol 9:67-70

De Vries LS, Regev R, Connel JA, Bydder GM, Dubowitz MS (1988) Localized cerebral infarction in the premature infant: an ultrasound diagnosis correlated with computed tomography and magnetic resonance imaging. Pediatrics 81:36-40

De Vries LS, Groenendaal F, Eken P, Van Haastert IC, Rademaker KJ, Meiners LC (1997) Infarcts in the vascular distribution of the middle cerebral artery in preterm and full term infants. Neuropediatrics 28:88-95

Duffy TE, Cavazutti M, Cruz NF, Sokoloff L (1982) Local cerebral glucose metabolism in newborn dogs: effects of hypoxia and halothane anesthesia. Ann Neurol 11:233-239

Du Plessis AJ (1997) Neurologic complications of cardiac disease in the newborn. Clin Perinatol 24:807-826

Edwards AD, Wyatt JS, Richardson C (1990) Effects of indomethacin on cerebral haemodynamics in very preterm infants. Lancet 335:1491-1495

Edwards AD, Yue X, Cox P, Hope PL, Azzopardi DV, Squier MV, Mehmet H (1997) Apoptosis in the brains of infants suffering intrauterine cerebral injury. Pediatr Res 42:684-689

Ehyai A, Fenichel G, Bender H (1984) Incidence and prognosis of seizures in infants after cardiac surgery with profound hypothermia and circulatory arrest. JAMA 252:3165-3167

Eken P, Toet MC, Groendaal F, De Vries LS (1995) Predictive value of early neuroimaging pulsed Doppler and neurophysiology in full term infants with hypoxic ischemic encephalopathy. Arch Dis Child 73:75-80

Ekert P, Perlman M, Steinlin M, Hao Y (1997) Predicting the outcome of postasphyxial hypoxic-ischemic encephalopathy within 4 hours of birth. J Pediatr 131:613-617

Ergander U, Ericksson M, Zetterstrom R (1983) Severe neonatal asphyxia. Incidence and prediction of outcome in the Stockholm area. Acta Paediatr Scand 72:321-325

Evans DH, Levene ML, Archer LN (1987) The effect of indomethacin on cerebral blood flow velocity in premature infants. Dev Med Child Neurol 29:776-782

Favre R, Schönenberger R, Nisand I, Lorenz U (1991) Standard curves of cerebral Doppler flow velocity waveforms and predictive values for intrauterine growth retardation and fetal acidosis. Fetal Diagn Ther 6:113-119

Fawer CL, Diebold P, Calame A (1987) Periventricular leukomalacia and neurodevelopmental outcome in preterm infants. Arch Dis Child 62:30-36

Fellman V, Raivio K (1997) Reperfusion injury as the mechanism of brain damage after perinatal asphyxia. Pediatr Res 41:599-606

Fenichel GM (1983) Hypoxic-ischemic encephalopathy in the newborn. Arch Neurol 40:261-266

Ferry P (1987) Neurologic sequelae of cardiac surgery in children. Am J Dis Child 141:309-312

Filipek PA, Krishnamoorthy KS, Davis KR (1987) Focal cerebral infarction in the newborn: a distinct entity. Pediatr Neurol 3:141-147

Filly RA, Goldstein RG, Callen PW (1990) Monochorionic twinning: sonographic assessment. AJR Am J Roentgenol 154:459-469

Finer NN, Robertson CM, Peters KL, Coward JM (1983) Factors affecting outcome in hypoxic-ischemic encephalopathy in term infants. Am J Dis Child 137:21-25

Finesmith RB, Roche K, Yellin PB, Walsh KK, Shen C, Zeglis M, Kahn A, Fish I (1997) Effect of magnesium sulfate on the development of cystic periventricular leukomalacia in preterm infants. Am J Perinatal 14:303-307

Foley J (1992) Dyskinetic and dystonic cerebral palsy and birth. Acta Paediatr 81:57-60

Fujimoto S, Yokochi K, Togari H, Nischimura Y, Inukai K, Futamura M, Sobajima H, Suzuki S, Wada Y (1992) Neonatal cerebral infarction: symptoms, CT findings and prognosis. Brain Dev 14:48-52

Gerard P, Verheggen P, Bachy A, Langhendries JP (1981) Intérêt de la tomodensitométrie cérébrale chez les enfants nés asphyxiés. Arch Fr Pediatr 38:591-596

Gidday JM, Fitzgibbons JL, Shah AR (1994) Neuroprotection from ischemic brain injury by hypoxic preconditioning in the neonatal rat. Neurosci Lett 168:221-224

Gilles FH, Averill DR, Kerr CS (1977) Neonatal endotoxin encephalopathy. Ann Neurol 2:49-56

Giroud M, Fayolle H, Martin D, Baudoin N, Andre N, Gouyon JB, Nivelon JL, Dumas R (1995) Late thalamic atrophy in infarction of the middle cerebral artery territory in neonates. Child's Nerv Syst 11:133-136

Giussani DA, Spencer JA, Hanson MA (1994) Fetal cardiovascular reflex responses to hypoxemia. Fetal Matern Med Rev 6:17-37

Glasier CM, Seibert JJ, Chadduck WH, Williamson SL, Leithiser RE (1989) Brain death in infants: evaluation with Doppler US. Radiology 172:377-380

Gonzales RG, Schaefer PW, Buonanno FS, Schwamm LH, Budzik RF, Rordorf G, Wang B, Sorensen AG, Koroshetz WJ (1999) Diffusion-weighted MR imaging: diagnostic accuracy in patients imaged within 6 hours of stroke symptom onset. Radiology 210:155-162

Gonzales De Dios J, Moya M, Izura V (1995) Variations in cerebral blood flow in various states of severe neonatal hypoxic-ischemic encephalopathy. Rev Neurol 23:639-643

Goplerud JM, Wagerie LC, Delivoria-Papadopoulos M (1989) Regional cerebral blood flow response during and after acute asphyxia in newborn piglets. J Appl Physiol 66:2827-2832

Gould SJ, Howard S, Hope PL (1987) Periventricular intraparenchymal cerebral haemorrhage in preterm infants: the role of venous infarction. J Pathol 151:197-202

Govan JJ, Ohlsson A, Ryan ML, Myhr T, Fong K (1995) Aminophylline and Doppler time averaged mean velocity in the middle cerebral artery in preterm neonates. J Pediatr 31:461-464

Graziani IJ, Spitzer AR, Mitchell DG (1993) Mechanical ventilation in preterm infants: neurosonographic and developmental studies. Pediatrics 90:515-522

Gray PH, Tudehope DI, Masel JP (1993) Perinatal hypoxic-ischaemic brain injury: prediction of outcome. Dev Med Child Neurol 35:965-973

Greisen G, Trojabord W (1987) Cerebral blood flow, PaCO2 changes, and visual evoked potentials in mechanically ventilated, preterm infants. Acta Paediatr Scand 76:394-400

Greisen G, Pryds O (1989) Low CBF, discontinuous EEG activity and periventricular brain injury in ill, preterm neonates. Brain Dev 11:164-168

Greisen G (1997) Cerebral blood flow and energy metabolism in the newborn. Clin Perinatol 24:531-565

Grether JL, Nelson KB (1997) Maternal infection and cerebral palsy in infants of normal weight. JAMA 278:207-211

Guzzetta F, Shackelford GD, Volpe S (1986) Periventricular intraparenchymal echodensities in the premature newborn: critical determinant of neurologic outcome. Pediatrics 78:995-1006

Gunn AJ, Williams CE, Mallard EC (1994) Flunarizine, a calcium channel antagonist, is partially prophylactically neuroprotective in hypoxic ischemic encephalopathy in the fetal sheep. Pediatr Res 35:657-663

Gupta AN, Lamba IM (1994) Neurosonographic abnormalities in neonates with hypoxic ischemic encephalopathy. Indian Pediatr 31:767-774

Hall RT, Hall FK, Daily DK (1998). High dose phenobarbital therapy in term newborn infants with severe perinatal asphyxia: a randomized prospective study with three year follow-up. J Pediatr 132:345-348

Hammerman C, Glaser J, Schimmel M, Ferber B, Kaplan M, Eidelman A (1995) Continuous versus multiple rapid infusions of indomethacin: effects on cerebral blood flow velocity. Pediatrics 95:244-248

Hammerman C, Kaplan M (1998) Ischemia and reperfusion injury. The ultimate pathophysiologic paradox. Clin Perinatol 25:757-777

Hashimoto K (1996) Diagnosis and prognosis of periventricular leukomalacia. No To Hattatsu 28:130-134

Hattori H, Morin AM, Schwartz PH (1989) Posthypoxic treatment with MK-801 reduces hypoxic ischemic damage in the neonatal rat. Neurology 39:713-718

Hauth JC, Goldenberg RL, Nelson KG (1995) Reduction of cerebral palsy with maternal MgS04 treatment in newborn weighting 500-1000 g. Am J Obstet Gynecol 172:419-427

Hellmann J, Soto G, Mackanjee H, Daneman A (1987) Doppler ultrasonography in full term hypoxic-ischemic encephalopathy. Pediatr Res 21:491-494

Helmers SL, Weiss MJ, Holmes GL (1991) Apneic seizures with bradycardia in a newborn. J Epilepsy 4:173-180

Hernandez MJ, Brennan RW, Bowman GS (1980) Autoregulation of cerebral blood flow in the newborn dog. Brain Res 185:199-202

Hernanz-Schulman M, Cohen W, Genieser NB (1988) Sonography of cerebral infarction in infancy. AJNR Am J Neuroradiol 9:131-136

Hill A, Martin DJ, Daneman A, Fitz CR (1983) Focal ischemic cerebral injury in the newborn: diagnosis by ultrasound and correlation with computed tomographic scan. Pediatrics 71:790-793

Hill A, Volpe JJ (1989) Perinatal asphyxia: clinical aspects. Clin Perinatol 16:435-457

Hill A (1991) Current concepts of hypoxic-ischemic cerebral injury in the term newborn. Pediatr Neurol 7:317-325

Holmes G, Rowe J, Hafford J (1982) Prognostic value of the electroencephalogramm in neonatal asphyxia. Electroencephalogr Clin Neurophysiol 53:60-64

Hope PL, Gould SJ, Howard S, Hamilton PA, Costello AM, Reynolds EO (1988) Precision of ultrasound diagnosis of pathologically verified lesions in the brains of very preterm infants. Dev Med Child Neurol 30:457-471

Hossmann KA (1994) Viability thresholds and the penumbra of focal ischemia. Ann Neurol 36:557-565

Huang CC, Ho MY, Shen EV (1987) Sonographic changes in a parasagittal cerebral lesion in an asphyxiated newborn. J Clin Ultrasound 15:68-70

Huppi PS, Barnes PD (1997) Magnetic resonance techniques in the evaluation of the newborn brain. Clin Perinatol 24:693-721

Illyes M, Gati I (1988) Reverse flow in the human fetal descending aorta as a sign of severe fetal asphyxia preceding intrauterine death. J Clin Ultrasound 16:403-407

Ischikawa T, Ogawa X, Kanayama M (1987) Long term prognosis of asphyxiated full term neonates with CNS complications. Brain Dev 9:48-53

Jalili M, Crade M, Davis AL (1994) Carotid blood flow velocity changes detected by Doppler ultrasound in determination of brain death in children: a preliminary report. Clin Pediatr 33:669-674

Johnson GN, Palahniuk RJ, Tweed WA, Jones MV (1979) Regional cerebral blood flow changes during severe fetal asphyxia produced by slow partial umbilical cord compression. Am J Obstet Gynecol 135:48-52

Joupilla P, Kirkinen P (1984) Umbilical vein blood flow in the human fetus in cases of maternal and fetal anemia and uterine bleeding. Ultrasound Med Biol 10:365-370

Joupilla P, Kirkinen P (1984) Increased vascular resistance in the descending aorta of the human fetus in hypoxia. Brit J Obstet Gynecol 91:853-856

Jung J, Graham J, Schultz N, Smith D (1984) Congenital hydranencephaly/porencephaly due to vascular disruption in monozygotic twins. Pediatrics 73:467-469

Karlsson BR, Grogaard B, Gerdin B, Steen PA (1994) The severity of post-ischaemic hypoperfusion increases with duration of cerebral ischaemia in rats. Acta Anesthesiol Scand 38:248-253

Keller MS, Dipietro MA, Teele RI, White SJ, Chawla HS, Curtis-Cohen M, Blane CE (1987) Periventricular cavitations in the first week of life. AJNR Am J Neuroradiol 8:291-295

Keolfen W, Freund M, Varnholt V (1995) Neonatal stroke involving the middle cerebral artery in term infants: clinical presentation, EEG and imaging studies, and outcome. Dev Med Child Neurol 37:204-212

Kohrman MH (1993) Brain death in neonates. Semin Neurol 13:116-120

Kornberg J, Williams TH (1985) The incidence and severity of post-asphyxial encephalopathy in full term infants. Early Human Dev 11:21-28

Kotagal S, Toce S, Kotagal P, Archer CR (1983) Symmetric bithalamic and striatal hemorrhage following perinatal hypoxia in a term infant. J Comp Assist tomogr 7:353-355

Kreusser KL, Schmidt RE, Shackelford GD, Volpe JJ (1984) Value of ultrasound for identification of acute hemorrhagic necrosis of thalamus and basal ganglia in an asphyxiated term infant. Ann Neurol 16:361-364

Kyllerman M, Bager B, Bensch J (1982) Dyskinetic cerebral palsy I: clinical categories, associated neurological abnormalities and incidences. Acta Paediatr Scand 71:543-549

Langer B, Boudier E, Gasser B, Christmann D, Messer J, Schlaeder G (1997) Antenatal diagnosis of brain damage in the survivor after the second trimester death of a monochorionic monoamniotic co-twin. Fetal Diagn Ther 12:286-291

Lanska MJ, Lanska DJ, Horwitz SJ (1991) Presentation, clinical course, and outcome of childhood stroke. Pediatr Neurol 7:333-341

Lassen NA (1966) The luxury perfusion syndrome and its possible relation to acute metabolic acidosis localised within the brain. Lancet 2:1113-1115

Leahy F, Cates D, McCallum M, Rigatto H (1980) Effect of CO_2 and 100% O_2 on cerebral blood flow in preterm infants. J Applic Physiol 48:468-472

Leffler CW, Busija DW, Mirro R (1989) Effects of ischemia on brain blood flow and oxygen consumption of newborn pigs. Am J Physiol 257:1917-1926

Levene MJ, Kornberg J, Williams TH (1985) The incidence and severity of postasphyxial encephalopathy in full term infants. Early Hum Dev 11:21-28

Levene MJ (1987) Asphyxia. In: Neonatal Neurology. Churchill Livingstone Edinburgh 157-200

Levene MJ (1987) Cerebral ischaemic lesions. In: Neonatal Neurology. Churchill Livingstone Edinburgh 105-130

Levene MJ, Fenton AC, Evans DH, Archer LN, Shortland DB, Gibson NA (1989) Severe birth asphyxia and abnormal cerebral blood flow velocity. Dev Med Child Neurol 31:427-434

Leviton A, Paneta N (1990) White matter damage in preterm newborns: an epidemiologic perspective. Early Hum Dev 24:1-22

Levy SR, Abroms IF, Marshall PC (1985) Seizures and cerebral infarction in the full term newborn. Ann Neurol 17:366-370

Li Y, Victor G, Jiang N (1995) Ultrastructural and light microscopic evidence of apoptosis after middle cerebral artery occlusion in the rat. Am J Pathol 146:1045-1051

Liem KD, Hopman JC, Kolle LA, Oeseburg B (1994) Effects of repeated indomethacin administration on cerebral oxygenation and hemodynamics in preterm infants: combined NIRS and Doppler ultrasound study. Eur J Pediatr 153:504-509

Linnik MD, Zobrist RH, Hatfield MD (1993) Evidence supporting a role for program cell death in focal cerebral ischemia in rats. Stroke 24:2002-2009

Lipp-Zwahlen AE, Muller A, Tuchschmid P (1989) Oxygen affinity of haemoglobin modulates cerebral blood flow in premature infants. A study with the noninvasive Xenon 133 method. Acta Paediatr Scand 360:26-32

Liu XH, Kato H, Araki T (1994) An immunohistochemical study of copper/zinc superoxide dismutase and manganese superoxide dismutase following focal cerebral ischemia in the rat. Brain Res 644:257-266

Lives P, Talvik R, Talvik T (1998) Changes in Doppler ultrasonography in asphyxiated term infants with hypoxic ischaemic encephalopathy. Acta Paediatr 67:680-684

Lopriore E, Vandenbussche F, Tiersma E, De Beaufort A, De Leeuw J (1995) Twin-to-twin transfusion syndrome: new perspectives. J Pediatr 127:657-680

Lou HC, Lassen NA, Tweed A, Johnson G, Jones M, Palahniuk RJ (1979) Pressure passive cerebral blood flow and breakdown of the blood-brain barrier in experimental fetal asphyxia. Acta Pediatr Scand 68:57-63

Lou HC, Lassen NA, Friis-Hansen B (1979) Impaired autoregulation of cerebral blood flow in the distressed newborn infants. J Pediatr 94:118-125

Lou HC, Lassen NA, Tweed A, Johnson G, Jones M, Palahniuk R (1979) Pressure passive cerebral blood flow in the distressed newborn infants. J Pediatr 94:118-125

Low JA, Galbraith RS, Muir DW (1985) The relationship between perinatal hypoxia and newborn encephalopathy. Am J Obstet Gynecol 152:256-260

Low JA (1997) Intrapartum fetal asphyxia: definition, diagnosis and classification. Am J Obstet Gynecol 176:957-959

Lütschg J, Pfenninger J, Lundin H (1983) Brainstem auditory evoked potentials and early somatosensory evoked potentials in neurointensively treated comatose children. Am J Dis Child 137:421-426

Malamud N (1950) Status marmoratus: a form of cerebral palsy following either birth injury or inflammation of the central nervous system. J Pediatr 37:610-616

Mannino FL, Trauner DA (1983) Stroke in neonates. J Pediatr 102:605-610

Manterola A, Towbin A, Yakovlev PI (1966) Cerebral infarction in the human fetus near term. J Neuropathol Exp Neurol 25:479-488

Marlow N (1992) Do we need an Apgar score? Arch Dis Child 67:765-769

Marret S, Zupan V, Gressens P, Lagercrantz H, Evrard P. (1998) Les leukomalacies périventriculaires I. Aspects histologiques et étiopathogéniques. Arch Fr Pediatr 5:525-537

Marret S, Zupan V, Gressens P, Lagercrantz H, Evrard P (1998) Les leukomalacies périventriculaires II. Diagnostic, séquelles et neuroprotection. Arch Fr Pediatr 5:538-545

Martin DJ, Hill A, Daneman CR (1983) Hypoxic ischemic cerebral injury in the neonatal brain: a report of sonographic features with computed tomographic correlation. Pediatr Radiol 13:307-313

McDonald HH, Mulligan JC, Allan AC, Taylor PM (1980) Neonatal asphyxia I. Relationship of obstetric and neonatal complications to neonatal mortality in 38 405 consecutive deliveries. J Pediatr 96:898-902

McDonnel M, Ives NK, Hope PL (1992) Intravenous aminophylline and cerebral blood flow in preterm infants. Arch Dis Child 67:416-418

McMenamin JB, Volpe JJ (1983) Doppler ultrasonography in the determination of neonatal brain death. Ann Neurol 14:302-307

McPhee AJ, Kotagal UR, Kleinman LL (1985) Cerebrovascular hemodynamics during and after recovery from acute asphyxia in the newborn dog. Pediatr Res 19:645-650

Memezawa H, Minamisawa H, Smith ML (1992) Ischemic penumbra in a model of reversible middle cerebral artery occlusion in the rat. Exp Brain Res 89:67-78

Ment LR, Duncan CC, Stewart WB (1986) Perinatal cerebral insults: hemorrhage and ischemia. Pediatr Neurosci 12:168-174

Mercuri E, Rutherford M, Cowan F, Pennock J, Counsell S, Papadimitriou M, Azzopardi D, Bydder G, Dubowitz L (1999) Early prognostic indicators of outcome in infants with neonatal cerebral infarction: a clinical, electroencephalogram and magnetic resonance imaging study. Pediatrics 103:39-45

Messer J, Burtscher A, Haddad J (1990) Contribution of transcranial Doppler sonography to the diagnosis of brain death in children. Arch Fr Pediatr 47:647-651

Monset-Couchard M, De Bethmann O, Iritz N, Relier JP (1988) Leukomalacies kystiques néonatales. Anamnèse périnatale chez 30 survivants. J Gynecol Obstet Biol Reprod 17:183-189

Montoya F (1989) Approche par Doppler pulsé du retentissement hémodynamique cérébral de l'aspiration endotrachéale chez le prématuré ventilé. JEMU 10:258-260

Mosca F, Bray M, Lattanzio M, Fumagalli M, Tosetto C (1997) Comparative evaluation of the effects of indomethacin and ibuprofen on cerebral perfusion and oxygenation in preterm infants with patent ductus arteriosus. J Pediatr 131:549-554

Mujsce DJ, Christensen MA, Vannucci RL (1989) Regional cerebral blood flow and glucose utilization during hypoglycemia in newborn dogs. Am J Physiol 256:659-666

Mulligan JC, Painter MJ, O'Donoghue PA, Donald HM, Allen AC, Taylor PM (1980) Neonatal asphyxia II: neonatal mortality and long term sequelae. J Pediatr 96:903-907

Murphy DJ, Hope PL, Johnson A (1996) Ultrasound findings and clinical antecedents of cerebral palsy in very preterm infants. Arch Dis Child 74:105-109

Murphy DJ, Hope PL, Johnson A (1997) Neonatal risk factors for cerebral palsy in very preterm babies: case control study. Br Med J 314:404-408

Myers RE (1969) Brain pathology following fetal vascular occlusion: an experimental study. Invest Ophtalmol Vis Sci 8:47-50

Myers RE, Beard R, Adamsons K (1969) Brain swelling in the newborn rhesus monkey following prolonged partial asphyxia. Neurology 19:1012-1018

Myers RE (1975) Four patterns of perinatal brain damage and their conditions of occurrence in primates. Adv Neurol 10:223-227

Myers RE (1975) Fetal asphyxia due to umbilical cord compression: metabolic and brain pathologic consequences. Biol Neonat 26:21-43

Naidich TP, Yousefzadeh DK, Gusnard DA, Naidich JB (1986) Sonography of the internal capsule and basal ganglia in infants. Part II: localisation of pathologic processes in the sagittal section through the caudothalamic groove. Radiology 161:615-621

Nakamura Y, Fukiyoshi Y, Fukuda S, Matsunaga T, Hashimoto T, Manabe A, Nakashima T (1986) Cystic brain lesion in utero. Acta Pathol J 36:613-620

Nan-chang C, Ein-Yiao S, Bo-shun L (1994) Reversal of diastolic cerebral blood flow in infants without brain death. Pediatr Neurol 11:337-340

Neil JJ, Shiran SI, McKinstry RC, Schefft GL, Snydera Z, Almli CR, Akbudak E, Aronovitz JA, Miller JP, Lee BC, Conturo TE (1998) Normal brain in human newborns: apparent diffusion coefficient and diffusion anisotropy measured by using diffusion tensor MR imaging. Radiology 209:57-66

Nelson KB, Ellenberg JH (1981) Apgar scores as predictors of chronic neurological disability. Pediatrics 68:36-44

Nelson KB, Grether JK (1995) Can magnesium sulfate reduce the risk of cerebral palsy in very low birthweight infants? Pediatrics 95:263-269

Nelson KB (1996) Magnesium sulfate and risk of cerebral palsy in very low birth weight infants. JAMA 276:1843-1844

Nwaesei CG, Pape KE, Martin DJ, Becker LE, Fitz CH (1984) Periventricular infarction diagnosed by ultrasound: a postmortem correlation. J Pediatr 105:106-110

Ohlsson A, Bottu J, Govan J, Ryan ML, Fong K, Myhr T (1993) Effect of indomethacin on cerebral blood velocities in very low birth weight neonates with a patent ductus arteriosus. Dev Pharmacol 20:100-106

Orey (d') MC, Melo MJ, Ramos I, Guimaraes H, Alves AR, Silva JS, Vasconcelos G, Costa A, Silva G, Santos BT (1999). Cerebral ischemic infarction in newborn infants. Diagnosis using pulsed and color Doppler imaging. Arch Pediatr 6:457-459

Oriot D, Nassimi A (1998) Hypertension intracrânienne de l'enfant: de la physiopathologie à la prise en charge thérapeutique. Arch Pediatr 5:773-782

O'Shea TM, Volberg F, Dillard RG (1993) Reliability of interpretation of cranial ultrasound examinations of very low birth weight neonates. Dev Med Child Neurol 35:97-101

Palmer C, Vannucci RC, Towfight J (1990) Reduction of perinatal hypoxic ischemic brain damage with allopurinol. Pediatr Res 27:332-336

Palmer C (1995) Hypoxic-ischemic encephalopathy. Therapeutic approaches against microvascular injury and role of neutrophils, PAF and free radicals. Clin Perinatol 22:481-517

Panerai RB, Kelsall AW, Rennie JM, Evans DH (1995) Cerebral autoregulation dynamics in premature newborns. Stroke 26:74-80

Papile L, Rudolph A, Heymann MA (1985) Autoregulation of cerebral blood flow in the preterm fetal lamb. Pediatr Res 19:159-165

Parisi JE, Collins GH, Kim RC, Crosley CJ (1983) Prenatal symmetrical thalamic degeneration with flexion spasticity at birth. Ann Neurol 13:94-97

Parker BL, Frewen TC, Levin SD (1995) Declaring pediatric brain death: current practice in a canadian pediatric critical care unit. Can Med Assoc J 153:903-915

Parilla B, Tamura R, Cohen L, Clark E (1997) Lack of effect of antenatal indomethacin on fetal cerebral blood flow. Am J Obstet Gynecol 176:1166-1171

Parvey LS, Gerald B (1976) Arteriographic diagnosis of brain death in children. Pediatr Radiol 4:79-82

Pasternak JF (1987) Parasagittal infarction in neonatal asphyxia. Ann Neurol 13:202-203

Pasternak JF, Piedey TA, Mickael MA (1991) Neonatal asphyxia: vulnerability of basal ganglia in term asphyxiated infant. Pediatr Neurol 7:147-149

Patten RM, Mack LA, Nyberg DA, Filly RA (1989) Twin embolization syndrome: prenatal sonographic detection and significance. Radiology 173:685-689

Pellicer A, Cabanas F, Garcia-Alix A (1992) Stroke in neonates with cardiac right to left shunt. Brain Dev 14:381-385

Perlman JM, Volpe JJ (1983) Suctioning in the preterm infant: effects on cerebral blood flow velocity, intracranial pressure and arterial blood pressure. Pediatrics 72:329-334

Perlman JM, Volpe JJ (1983) Seizures in the preterm infant: effects on cerebral blood flow velocity, intracranial pressure and arterial blood pressure. J Pediatr 102:288-293

Perlman JM, Volpe JJ (1985) Episodes of apnea and bradycardia in the preterm newborn: impact on cerebral circulation. Pediatrics 76:335-338

Perlman JM, Risser R, Broyles RS (1996) Bilateral cystic periventricular leukomalacia in the premature infant: associated risk factors. Pediatrics 97:822-827

Petito CK, Pulsinelli WA, Jacobson G, Plum F (1982) Edema and vascular permeability in cerebral ischemia: comparison between ischemic neuronal damage and infarction. J Neuropathol Exp Neurol 42:423-436

Pluta R, Lissinsky AS, Wisniewski HM, Mossakowski MJ (1994) Early blood brain barrier changes in the rat following transient complete cerebral ischemia induced by cardiac arrest. Brain Res 633:41-52

Powers AD, Graeber MC, Smith RR (1989) Transcranial Doppler ultrasonography in the determination of brain death. Neurosurgery 24:884-889

Pryds O, Greisen G, Friis-Hansen B (1988) Compensatory increase of CBF in preterm infants during hypoglycemia. Acta Paediatr Scand 77:632-637

Pryds O, Greisen G, Lou H, Friis-Hansen B (1990) Vasoparalysis associated with brain damage in asphyxiated term infants. J Pediatr 117:119-125

Purves MJ, James IM (1969) Observations on the control of cerebral flow in the sheep fetus and newborn lamb. Circ Res 25:651-667

Qian SY, Fan XM, Yin HH (1998) Transcranial Doppler assessment of brain death in children. Singapore Med J 39:247-250

Quiogue T, Keller MS, Young LW (1987) Post-asphyxial total cerebral necrosis: ultrasonographic diagnosis. Am J Dis Child 141:445-446

Raju TN (1992) Cranial Doppler applications in neonatal critical care. Crit Care Clin 8:93-111

Ramakaers VT, Casaer P (1990) Defective regulation of cerebral oxygen transport after severe birth asphyxia. Dev Med Child Neurol 32:56-62

Raybaud CA, Livet M, Jiddane M, Pinsard N (1985) Radiology of ischemic strokes in children. Neuroradiology 27:567-578

Reivich M, Brann AW, Shairo HM, Myers RE (1972) Regional cerebral blood flow during prolonged partial asphyxia. In: Meyers JS, Reivich M, Lechner H, Eichorn M. Research on the cerebral circulation. Springfield Thomas Ed. 216

Rivkin MJ (1997) Hypoxic-ischemic brain injury in the term newborn. Neuropathology clinical aspects and neuroimaging. Clin Perinatol 24:607-624

Rizzo G, Arduini D, Luciano R, Rizzo C, Tortorolo G, Romanini C, Mancuso S (1989) Prenatal cerebral Doppler ultrasonography and neonatal neurologic outcome. J Ultrasound Med 8:237-240

Robertson CM, Finer N (1985) Term infants with hypoxic-ischemic encephalopathy: outcome at 3-5 years. Dev Med Child Neurol 27:473-484

Robertson CM, Finer NN (1993) Long term follow-up of term neonates with perinatal asphyxia. Clin Perinatol 20:483-500

Roland EH, Hill A, Norman MG (1988) Selective brainstem injury in an asphyxiated newborn. Ann Neurol 23:89-92

Roland EH, Hill A (1995) Clinical aspects of perinatal hypoxic-ischemic brain injury. Semin Pediatr Neurol 2:57-71

Roodhooft AM, Parizel PM, Van Acker KJ, Depretere JR, Van Reempts PJ (1987) Idiopathic cerebral arterial infarction with paucity of symptoms in the full term neonate. Pediatrics 80:381-385

Rorke LB (1992) Anatomical features of the developing brain implicated in pathogenesis of hypoxic ischemic injury. Brain Pathol 2:211-221

Rosenberg AA, Narayanan V, Jones HD (1985) Comparison of anterior cerebral artery blood flow velocity and cerebral blood flow during hypoxia. Pediatr Res 19:67-70

Rosenberg AA (1986) Cerebral blood flow and O2 metabolism after asphyxia in neonatal lambs. Pediatr Res 20:778-782

Rosenberg AA (1988) Regulation of cerebral blood flow after asphyxia in neonatal lambs. Stroke 19:239-244

Rosenberg AA, Murdaugh E (1990) The effects of blood glucose concentration on post-asphyxia cerebral hemodynamics in newborn lambs. Pediatr Res 27:454-459

Roth SC, Baudin J, McCormick DC, Edwards A, Townsend J, Stewart AL (1993) Relation between ultrasound appearance of the brain of very preterm infants and neurodevelopmental impairment at eight years. Dev Med Child Neurol 3:755-768

Rudolph AM (1984) The fetal circulation and its response of stress. J Dev Physiol 6:11-16

Ruff RL, Shaw CM, Beckwith JB, Lozzo RV (1979) Cerebral infarction complicating umbilical vein catheterization in children. Ann Neurol 6:85-86

Ruth VJ, Raivio KO (1988) Perinatal brain damage predictive value of metabolic acidosis and the Apgar score. Br Med J 297:24-27

Rutherford MA, Pennock JM, Dubowitz LM (1994) Cranial ultrasound and magnetic resonance imaging in hypoxic-ischemic encephalopathy: a comparison with outcome. Dev Med Child Neurol 36:813-825

Rutherford MA, Pennock JM, Schwieso JE, Cowan FM, Dubowitz LM (1995) Hypoxic ischaemic encephalopathy: early magnetic resonance imaging findings and their evolution. Neuropediatrics 26:183-191

Rutherford M, Pennock J, Schwieso JE, Cowan F, Dubowitz L (1996) Hypoxic ischaemic encephalopathy: early and late magnetic resonance imaging findings in relation to outcome. Arch Dis Child 75:145-151

Saliba E, Pourcelot L, Laugier J (1996) Accidents anoxo–ischémiques du nouveau-né à terme. Modifications hémodynamiques précoces et devenir neurologique à 5 ans. JEMU 17:263-266

Sanker P, Roth B, Frowein RA (1992) Cerebral reperfusion in brain death of a newborn: case report. Neurosurg Rev 15:315-318

Sarnat HB, Sarnat MS (1976) Neonatal encephalopathy following fetal distress: a clinical and electroencephalographic study. Arch Neurol 33:696-705

Schendel DE, Berg CJ, Yeargin-Allsopp M, Boyle CA, Decoufle P (1996) Prenatal magnesium sulfate exposure and the risk for cerebral palsy or mental retardation among very low birth weight children aged 3 to 5 years. JAMA 276:1805-1810

Scher MS, Hamid MY, Steppe DA (1993) Ictal and interictal electrographic seizure durations in preterm and term neonates. Epilepsia 34:284-288

Scher MS, Aso K, Beggarly ME (1993) Electrographic seizures in preterm and full term neonates: clinical correlates, associated brain lesions and risk for neurologic sequelae. Pediatrics 91:128-134

Scherjon SA, Smoldersdehass H, Kok JH (1993) The brain sparing effect: antenatal cerebral Doppler findings in relation to neurologic outcome in very preterm infants. Am J Obstet Gynecol 169:169-175

Schipper JA, Mohammad GI, Van Straaten HL, Koppe JG (1997) The impact of surfactant replacement therapy on cerebral and systemic circulation and lung function. Eur J Pediatr 156:224-227

Scott H (1976) Outcome of very severe birth asphyxia. Arch Dis Child 51:712-716

Seibert J, McCowan TC, Chadduck WM, Adametz JR, Glasier C, Williamson S, Taylor B, Leithiser R, Connel J, Stansell C, Rodgers A, Corbitt S (1989) Duplex pulsed Doppler US versus intracranial pressure in the neonate: clinical and experimental studies. Radiology 171:155-159

Shankaran S, Woldt E, Koepke T, Bedard MP, Nandyal R (1991) Acute neonatal morbidity and long term central nervous system sequelae of perinatal asphyxia in term infants. Early Human Dev 25:135-148

Shankaran S, Kottamasu S, Kuhns L (1993) Brain sonography, computed tomography, and single photon emission computed tomography in term neonates with perinatal asphyxia. Clin Perinatol 20:379-393

Shen EV (1984) The "bright thalamus". Arch Dis Child 59:695-697

Shuman RM, Selednik LL (1980) Periventricular leukomalacia. A one year autopsy study. Arch Neurol 37:231-239

Siegel MJ, Shackelford GD, Perlman JM, Fulling KH (1984) Hypoxic-ischemic encephalopathy in term infants: diagnosis and prognosis evaluated by ultrasound. Radiology 152:395-399

Slovis TL, Shankaran S (1984) Ultrasound in the evaluation of hypoxic-ischemic injury and intracranial hemorrhage in neonates: the state of art. Pediatr Radiol 14:67-75

Smith SJ, Vogelzang RL, Marzono MI, Cerullo LJ, Gore RM, Neiman HL (1985) Brain edema: ultrasound examination. Radiology 155: 379-382

Smith CD, Baumann RJ (1991) Clinical features and magnetic resonance imaging in congenital and childhood stroke. J Child Neurol 6:263-272

Stark JE, Seibert JJ (1994) Cerebral artery Doppler ultrasonography for prediction of outcome after perinatal asphyxia. J Ultrasound Med 13:595-600

Stevenson D, John P (1997) Power Doppler ultrasound appearances of neonatal ischaemic brain injury. Pediatr Radiol 27:147-149

Sykes GS, Johnson P, Ashworth F (1982) Do Apgar scores indicate asphyxia? Lancet 1:494-496

Szymonowicz W, Yu VY (1985) Outcome of intrauterine periventricular hemorrhage and leukomalacia. Aust Paediatr 21:261-264

Szymonowicz W, Walker AM, Yu VY, Stewart ML, Cannata J, Cussen L (1990) Regional cerebral blood flow after hemorrhagic hypotension in the preterm, near term and newborn lamb. Pediatr Res 28:361-366

Takashima S, Tanaka K (1978) Development of cerebrovascular architecture and its relationship to periventricular leukomalacia. Arch Neurol 35:11-16

Takashima S, Mito T, Anto Y (1986) Pathogenesis of periventricular white matter hemorrhage in preterm infants. Brain Dev 8:25-30

Taylor G (1994) Alterations in regional cerebral blood flow in neonatal stroke: preliminary findings with color Doppler sonography. Pediatr Radiol 24:111-115

Taylor GA (1995) Effect of germinal matrix hemorrhage on terminal vein position and patency. Pediatr Radiol 25:37-40

Thomas WS, Mori E, Copeland BR, Yu JQ, Morrissey JH, Del Zoppo GJ (1993) Tissue factor contributes to microvascular defects after focal cerebral ischemia. Stroke 24:847-854

Tweed A, Cote J, Lou H, Gregory G, Wade J (1986) Impairment of cerebral blood flow autoregulation in the newborn lamb by hypoxia. Pediatr Res 20:516-519

Van Bel F, Stijnen T, Baan J, Ruys JH (1987) Cerebral blood flow velocity pattern in healthy and asphyxiated newborns: a controlled study. Eur J Pediatr 146:461-467

Van Bel F, Walther FJ (1990) Myocardial dysfunction and cerebral blood flow velocity following birth asphyxia. Acta Paediatr Scand 79:756-762

Van Bel F, Dorrepaal CA, Benders MJ, Zeeuwe PE, Van De Bor M, Berger HM (1993) Changes in cerebral hemodynamics and oxygenation in the first 24 hours after birth asphyxia. Pediatrics 92:365-372

Vanhulle C, Marret S, Parain D, Samson-Dollfus D, Fessard C (1998) Localized neonatal convulsions and cerebral arterial infarction. Arch Pediatr 5:404-408

Vannucci RC (1990) Current and potentially new management strategies for perinatal hypoxic ischemic encephalopathy. Pediatrics 85:961-968

Vannucci RC (1993) Experimental models of perinatal hypoxic-ischemic brain damage. Acta Pathol Microb Scan 10:89-95

Vannucci RC, Brucklacher RM, Vannucci SJ (1997) Effect of carbone dioxide on cerebral metabolism during hypoxia-ischemia in the immature rat. Pediatr Res 42:24-29

Vannucci RC, Perlman JM (1997) Interventions for perinatal hypoxic-ischemic encephalopathy. Pediatrics 100:1004-1014

Vannucci RC (1997) Hypoxic-ischemic encephalopathy: clinical aspects. In: Fanaroti AA, Martin RJ Eds. Neonatal prenatal Medecine IV. Philadelphia PA. Mosby-Yearbook 877-891

Varvarigou N, Bardin CL, Beharry K, Chemtob S, Papageorgiou A, Aranda JV (1996) Early ibuprofen administration to prevent patent ductus arteriosus in premature infants. JAMA 275:539-544

Ville Y, Hyett A, Vanderbussche FP, Nicolaides KH (1994) Endoscopic laser coagulation of umbilical cord vessels in twin reversed arterial perfusion sequence. Ultrasound Obstet Gynecol 4:396-398

Ville Y, Hyett J, Hecher K, Nicolaides K (1995) Preliminary experience with endoscopic laser surgery for severe twin-twin transfusion syndrome. N Engl J Med 332:224-227

Voit T, Lenborg P (1987) Damage of thalamus and basal ganglia in asphyxiated full term neonates. Neuropediatrics 18:176-181

Volpe JJ (1976) Perinatal hypoxic ischemic brain injury. Pediatr Clin North Am 23:383-397

Volpe JJ, Pasternak JF (1977) Parasagittal cerebral injury in neonatal hypoxic ischemic encephalopathy: clinical and neuroradiologic features. J Pediatr 91:472-476

Volpe JJ, Herscovitch P, Perlman JM (1985) Positron emission tomography in the asphyxiated term newborn: parasagittal impairment of cerebral blood flow. Ann Neurol 17:287-292

Volpe JJ (1987) Hypoxic-ischemic encephalopathy clinical aspects. In: Volpe JJ "Neurology of the newborn" 2nd Ed WB Saunders Company Philadelphia 236-279

Volpe JJ (1989) Current concepts of brain injury in the premature infant. AJR Am J Roentgenol 153:243-251

Volpe JJ (1995) Hypoxic-ischemic encephalopathy: biochemical and physiological aspects. In: Volpe JJ "Neurology of the newborn" 3rd EdWB Saunders Company Philadelphia 211-259

Volpe JJ (1995) Hypoxic-ischemic encephalopathy: clinical aspects. In: Volpe JJ "Neurology of the newborn" 3rd Ed WB Saunders Company Philadelphia 314-369

Volpe JJ (1995) Hypoxic-ischemic encephalopathy: neuropathology and pathogenesis. In: Volpe JJ "Neurology of the newborn" 3rd Ed WB Saunders Company Philadelphia 279-313

Volpe JJ (1997) Brain injury in the premature infant. Neuropathology, clinical aspects, pathogenesis and prevention. Clin Perinatol 24:567-587

Voorhies TM, Lipper EG, Lee BC (1984) Occlusive vascular disease in asphyxiated newborn infants. J Pediatr 105:92-95

Vyas S, Nicolaides KH, Bower S, Campell S (1990) Middle cerebral artery flow velocity waveforms in fetal hypoxaemia. Br J Obstet Gynecol 97:797-803

Weindling AM, Wilkinson AR, Cook J, Calvert SA, Fox TF, Rochefort MJ (1983) Perinatal events which precede periventricular hemorrhage and leukomalacia in the newborn. Br J Obstet Gynecol 92:1218-122

Williams CE, Gunn AJ, Synek B (1990) Delayed seizures occurring with hypoxic-ischemic encephalopathy in the fetal sheep. Pediatr Res 27:561-565

Wilson ER, Mirra SS, Schwartz JF (1982) Congenital diencephalic and brainstem damage: neuropathologic study of three cases. Acta Neuropathol 57:70-75

Wilson-Davis SL, Lo W, Filly RA (1983) Limitations of ultrasound in detecting cerebral ischemic lesions in the neonate. Ann Neurol 14:249-251

Yager JY, Asselin J (1996) Effect of mild hypothermia on cerebral energy metabolism during the evolution of hypoxic ischemic brain damage in the immature rat. Stroke 27:919-926

Yoon BH, Romero R, Yang SH (1996) Interleukin-6 concentrations in umbilical cord plasma are elevated in neonates with white matter lesions associated with periventricular leukomalacia. Am J Obstet Gynecol 174:1433-1440

Yoshioka H, Kadomoto Y, Mino M, Morikawa Y, Kasubuchi Y, Kusunoki T (1979) Multicystic encephalomalacia in liveborn twin with a still-born macerated co-twin. J Pediatr 95:798-800

Young RSK, Hernandez MJ, Yagel SK (1982) Selective reduction of blood flow to white matter during hypotension in newborn dogs: a possible mechanism of periventricular leukomalacia. Ann Neurol 12:445-448

Zhang RL, Chopp M, Chen H, Garcia JH (1994) Temporal profile of ischemic tissue damage, neurotrophil response and vascular plugging following permanent and transient middle cerebral artery occlusion in the rat. J Neurol Sci 125:3-10

Zupan V, Gonzales PTL, Lacaze-Masmonteil T, Boithias C, D Allest AM, Dehan M (1996) Periventricular leukomalacia: risk factors revisited. Dev Med Child Neurol 38:1061-1067

6 Pericerebral Fluid Collections

Corinne Veyrac

CONTENTS

For several years, transfontanellar ultrasonography has been used in the diagnosis of extracerebral collections. Two different clinical conditions are encountered:

- The first is seen in neonates and young infants with head injury or neurologic distress, hemostasis disorders, etc., in whom an acute subdural or extradural hematoma is initially suspected. In such patients, the ultrasonographic diagnosis relies on morphological analysis of the brain convexities. Color imaging does not provide significant information; pulsed Doppler helps to identify a rise in intracranial pressure.
- The second occurs in infants in the first year of life with less severe clinical symptoms, in whom a subacute or chronic pericerebral collection is discovered, sometimes complicated by acute hemorrhage. In these patients, color Doppler imaging provides very valuable diagnostic information. Only the second group is described in this chapter.

Pericerebral fluid collection is a well-known phenomenon in the infant. As early as 1914, DANDY described the association of enlarged pericerebral subarachnoid spaces with increased intracranial pressure, and defined so-called "external hydrocephalus."

C. Veyrac, MD
Service de Radiologie Pédiatrique, Hôpital Arnaud de Villeneuve, 34295 Montpellier Cedex 5, France

Since the advent of noninvasive imaging tools such as computed tomography (CT) and transfontanellar ultrasonography, a great number of pericerebral fluid collections have been diagnosed, some associated with rapid head growth, others following prematurity, meningitis, head injury, or dehydration.

6.1
Subdural or Subarachnoid Location?

● These collections have hitherto been considered as *subdural* in location. This hypothesis is supported by some of the circumstances in which they occur:
- Traumatic events, where the onset of subdural hematoma is explained by stretching and tearing of bridging veins
- Infectious diseases with inflammation of the arachnoid villi and transsudation from dilated dural capillaries
- Metabolic disorders such as hypernatremic dehydration with brain collapse and stretching of bridging veins

The intraoperative finding of *subdural membranes* (FRIEDE 1978; MARKWALDER 1981) surrounding an encapsulated hematoma is classical. The outer membrane is adherent to the dura, but cleavable, thick, and highly vascularized, while the inner membrane is described either as a thin opalescent velum, distinct from the arachnoid, or as a thicker membrane adhering to the arachnoid but cleavable. These highly vascularized membranes may explain the tendency to undergo repetitive multifocal bleeding, and may induce chronicity of the hematoma.

● However, many other arguments support a *subarachnoid* location:
- *Clinical arguments* such as the high incidence of a familial history of macrocephaly (ALVAREZ 1986; AZAIS 1992; NICKEL 1987; PALENCIA LUACES 1992), the great predominance of boys in all pub-

lished series, the classical association of macrocrania with enlarged pericerebral spaces in some genetic diseases, and the presence of enlarged fluid spaces in conditions involving increased systemic venous pressure (SAHAR 1978; PORTNOY 1978).

- *Pathological arguments* such as the finding during craniotomy in infants with external hydrocephalus of only enlarged subarachnoid spaces (ANDERSSON 1984), the description of congenital deficient dysplastic arachnoidal granulations (GILLES 1971), and the association with vitamin A deficiency, which in rat induces excessive deposition of collagen on the arachnoid villi (HAYES 1971).

- *Biological arguments*, excellently presented by STROOBANDT (1981, 1984). This author showed, by daily electrophoresis of the fluid obtained by external drainage, that the protein content diminished progressively and the fluid mimicked the profile of ventricular cerebrospinal fluid (CSF). In some cases, a ventriculoperitoneal shunt was placed, followed by disappearance of the pericerebral collection; the author confirmed the central role of CSF in the persistence and eventual recurrence of the pericerebral collection.

- *Imaging arguments*, which will be discussed later.

6.2
Clinical Data

From the clinical point of view, these subarachnoid collections occur in young infants, i.e., within a skull with open fontanelles and sutures, and thus they are not associated with an intracranial pressure increase except in cases with complications. For this reason, the term "external hydrocephalus" seems inappropriate.

Macrocrania is the most common symptom, observed in 46–72% of patients (AZAIS 1992; NICKEL 1987). There may be associated neurological findings, especially axial hypotonia or developmental retardation, but they are frequently minor and transient (GHERPELLI 1992; NICKEL 1987; NISHIMURA 1996).

However the widespread use of ultrasonography in the routine follow-up of premature infants and neonates with perinatal distress shows that widened subarachnoid spaces are often detected in these infants. Even in this population, pericerebral fluid collection is not associated with an increased risk of developmental impairment; ventricular enlargement and periventricular white matter disorders seem to be the

only significant prognostic factors (LUI 1990; VEYRAC 1994). This is why many authors prefer the denomination "benign pericerebral collection".

Nevertheless, the subarachnoid collection itself must be recognized as a risk factor for the occurrence of acute subdural hematoma (AOKI 1984; AZAIS 1992; IKEDA 1987; KAPILA 1982; MORI 1993; TSUBOKAWA 1984). These acute subdural hematomas occur after minor head injury in a young infant (less than 1 year of age) with pre-existing macrocrania and a contralateral and underlying subarachnoid collection. Finally, this hematoma contains not pure clotted blood, but a liquefied bloody fluid or a mixture of fluid and clotted blood.

Clinical manifestations are severe, with generalized tonic seizures and evidence of intracranial pressure increase.

The risk that acute subdural hematoma will occur is difficult to quantify. It could range from 8–15%, but many subarachnoid collections are probably not diagnosed, and the real risk is much lower. Nevertheless, it is very important to keep this risk in mind, because it represents the only complication of subarachnoid collection, which otherwise remains a benign condition.

Obviously, any acute subdural hemorrhage must be investigated in order to diagnose or rule out battered child syndrome. Clinical signs should be looked for, and so should ophthalmic anomalies (retinal or vitreous hemorrhage), bony lesions (by isotope scanning rather than skeletal X-ray), and ischemic damage of the brain parenchyma (axonal injury). A diagnosis of "spontaneous" acute subdural hemorrhage can be made only after child abuse has been excluded, since traumatic events are still responsible for most subdural hematomas in infants under 2 years of age (JAYAWANT 1998; MORRIS 2000; TZIOUMI 1998).

All these clinical data explain why it is important to diagnose a pericerebral collection and assess its precise location, since the two conditions differ greatly as to clinical pattern and therapeutic management and prognosis.

6.3
Anatomy of Meningeal Structures

Anatomical studies (FREDERICKSON 1991; HAINES 1993; ORLIN 1991; REINA 1998; SCHACHENMAYR 1978) have shown that subdural space does not exist under normal conditions.

The *dura* is composed of elongated, flattened fibroblasts and a copious amount of extracellular collagen variously aligned.

The *arachnoid* is made of cells grouped in three different layers: the outer barrier layer, the middle, reticular layer, and the inner, trabecular layer. It is composed of larger cells with numerous cell junctions (many tight junctions) and no extracellular space.

The *dura–arachnoid junction* is formed of flattened fibroblasts with flake-like cells stacked upon each other, long interlaced branches, and few cell junctions (SCHACHENMAYR 1978). These findings make it clear that a subdural hematoma occurs in the zone of least resistance between the dura mater and the arachnoid (FREDERICKSON 1991; ORLIN 1991) by fracture through the cytoplasm and intercellular separation, without a well-defined cleavage plane. It is a dissection of an avascular cellular plane, rather than a bleeding into a pre-existing mesothelial-lined space.
The outer layer of the arachnoid is an efficient barrier, and the subdural hematoma does not contaminate the subarachnoid space, at least at the cranial level (ORLIN 1991).

The *subarachnoid space* contains CSF traversed by a loose network of branching cells interwoven with bundles of collagen fibrils and groups of microfibrils. Fibroblasts forming the arachnoid trabeculae bridge the subarachnoid space and surround the vessels within the space as well as being attached to the pia on the surface of the brain (HAINES 1993; McLONE 1980; SCHACHENMAYR 1978). The arterial vessels are organized in compact arrangements and by bundles penetrate the cortex perpendicular to the cortical surface. The superficial veins arise on the lateral and medial surface of the hemisphere and drain toward the superior sagittal sinus through the subarachnoid space.

The *pia mater* is a flat sheet of cells reflected from the surface of the brain to form the outer coating of the meningeal vessels (McLONE 1980; HUTCHINGS 1986). Its cells are joined by junctional complexes and form a continuous sheet that separates the subarachnoid space on one side from the subpial and perivascular spaces on the other (HUTCHINGS 1986).

In the normal human, as well as in cases of recent subarachnoid hemorrhage, the pia mater functions as an effective barrier. On the other hand, in cases of purulent meningitis, a large number of inflammatory cells are encountered in the subpial perivascular and subarachnoid spaces.

It is important to know all these anatomical data because they relate to macroscopic findings that may be demonstrated by modern imaging – CT, MRI, and, above all, transfontanellar ultrasonography using high-frequency probes and color Doppler technique.

6.4
Normal Pericerebral Space: Sonographic Pattern

Several CT studies (FAN 1993; KLEINMAN 1983; PRASSOPOULOS 1995) have shown that subarachnoid spaces are more prominent and more variable in children below the age of 2 years compared with older patients. In neonates and infants, in whom transfontanellar ultrasonography may be used, normal values have been put forward. For example, the distance between the lateral wall of the superior sagittal sinus and the surface of the adjacent cerebral cortex has been measured on a coronal scan; the upper limit for a normal value is 2–3 mm (GOVAERT 1989; LIBICHER 1992).
Color imaging always depicts multiple small vessels at the cerebral surface.
- Some vessels are located on the surface of the cerebral gyrus, in the subpial space (Fig. 6.1); pulsed Doppler imaging shows them to be both arteries and veins.
- Other vessels are detached from the brain surface, within the subarachnoid space that is the only pericerebral fluid space sonographically visible in the healthy infant. Of course pulsed Doppler differentiates arteries from veins, but color Doppler alone can show the nature of these vessels (Figs. 6.2, 6.3): arterial flows are coded blue because they are directed toward the cortex and away from the transducer, while venous flows are coded red because they are directed toward the sinus and the transducer.

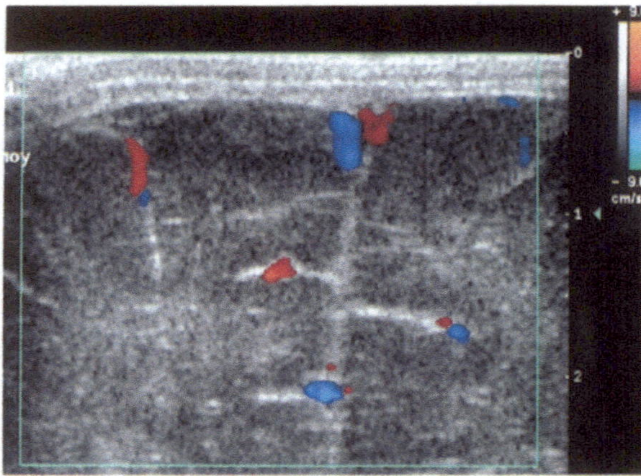

Fig. 6.1. The cortical vessels are close to the brain surface and penetrate the brain parenchyma

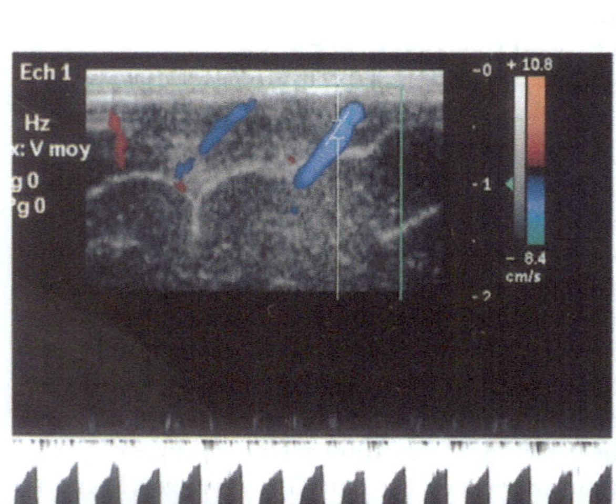

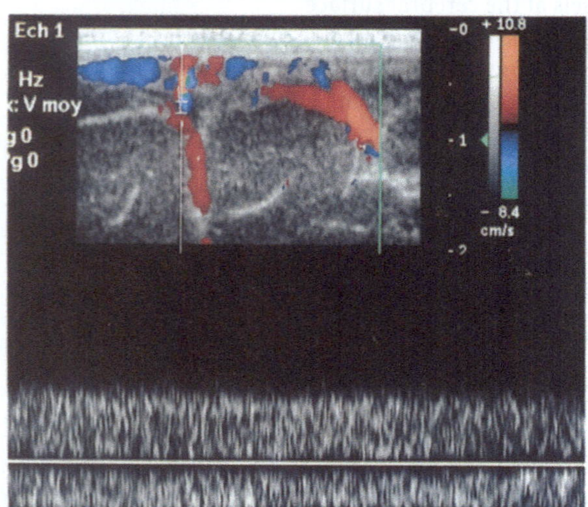

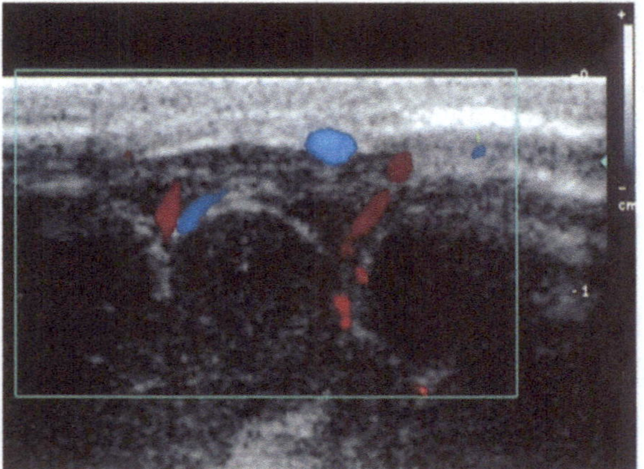

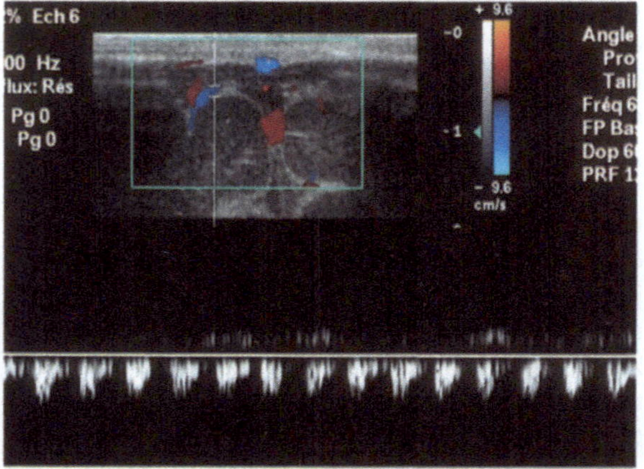

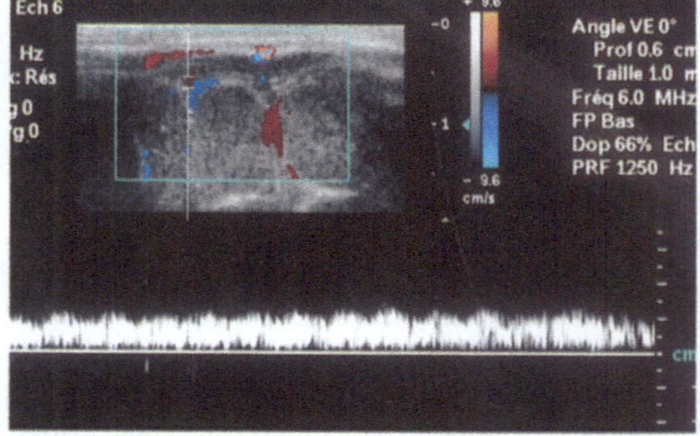

Fig. 6.2a–c. A 30-weeks' gestation preterm infant. Routine pre-discharge ultrasonography on day 23. **a** Normal arachnoid spaces contain *red* and *blue* signals. Pulsed Doppler demonstrates the respectively arterial (**b**) and venous (**c**) nature of two adjacent vessels

←

Fig. 6.3a,b. A 30-weeks' gestation preterm infant. Routine pre-discharge ultrasonography on day 45. The arterial (**a**) and venous (**b**) flows that bridge the subarachnoid spaces are not always close to each other

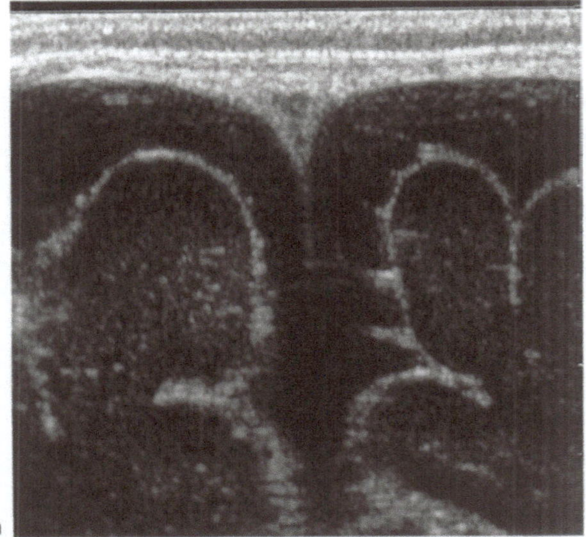

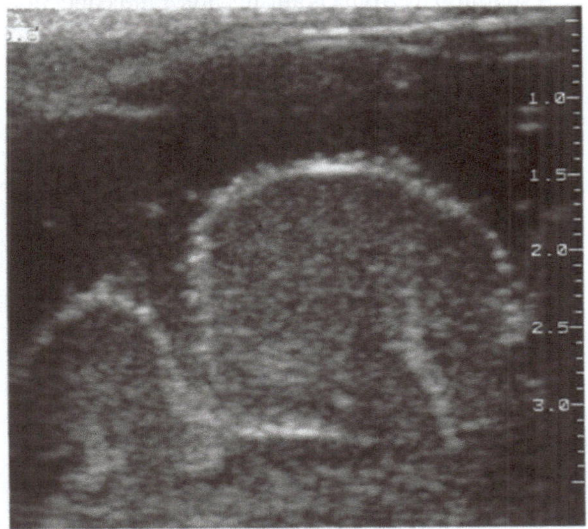

Fig. 6.4a,b. A 7-month-old infant with macrocrania (+3SD). Enlarged pericerebral fluid spaces (10 mm on the right, 13 mm on the left), widening the cerebral sulci, without mass effect. Multiple vessels are visible on the gray-scale image. Subarachnoid collection: **a** coronal plane, **b** parasagittal plane

6.5
Subarachnoid Space Enlargement

A subarachnoid collection is defined by increased volume of the subarachnoid space above normal values (TROUNCE 1985; VEYRAC 1990).

Sonographic morphological analysis confirms the subarachnoid location: the anechoic fluid penetrates and widens the sulci without any mass effect either on the brain surface or on the falx cerebri, which remains straight on the midline (Fig. 6.4). The effusion is bilateral, predominantly in the frontal regions,

thus obviously providing great sensitivity to transfontanellar ultrasonography.

Color imaging confirms the anatomic location (CHEN 1996, RUPPRECHT 1996) by showing that this enlarged fluid space is bridged by vascular flows in the same way as normal subarachnoid spaces. The multiple vessels are followed up to the bony vault (Fig. 6.5). This has been described on CT (MOROTA 1995) and MRI under the name of "cortical vein sign" (AOKI 1994; McCLUNEY 1992; WILMS 1993). Contrary to what this denomination suggests, these vessels are not only veins but also arteries; they are easily recognized on morphological imaging because of their pulsatility, and, of course, on pulsed Doppler. However, the arteries are fewer, remain closer to the brain surface, and are more difficult to record than veins.

Subarachnoid collections represent the great majority of the pericerebral collections encountered in infants. In a cohort of 171 infants (64 female and 107 male) investigated from 1985 to 1990, we demonstrated an isolated subarachnoid collection in 129 cases, against 10 acute subdural hematomas and 29 subdural hygromas (VEYRAC 1994)

6.6
Subdural Collections

A collection in a subdural location shows a quite different pattern.

The fluid collection displaces the brain surface from the cranial vault, but it is divided in *two different fluid compartments* separated by an echogenic membrane (VEYRAC 1990):

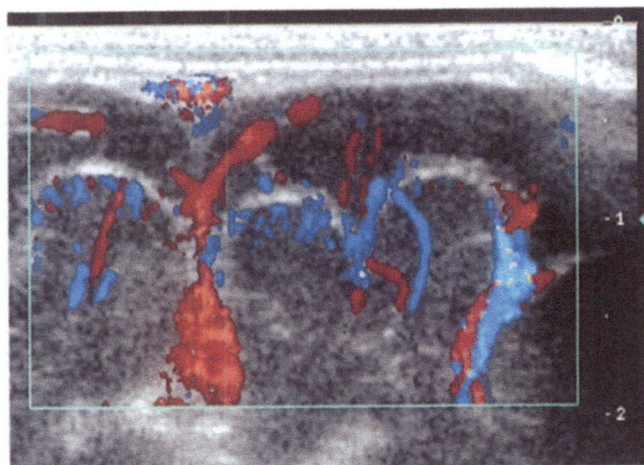

Fig. 6.5. Subarachnoid collection. Small vessels cross the enlarged fluid spaces

- The inner compartment is close to the cortex and contains small vessels that may be visualized on real-time ultrasonography and is more evident on color imaging: this is the *subarachnoid space*.
- The outer compartment does not contain any visible vessel on gray-scale real-time ultrasonography: this is the *subdural space* (Fig. 6.6).

The appearance of the subarachnoid compartment depends on the size of the subdural collection and the mass effect that it induces. When the subdural fluid is not compressive, the subarachnoid space remains quite large, the sulci are widened, and the subarachnoid vessels are still visible, detached from the brain surface (Fig. 6.7).

When, on the other hand, the subdural collection produces a mass effect, the subarachnoid space is embedded against the brain surface, the subarachnoid and subpial vessels are not distinguished, and the sulci are narrowed or even closed (Fig. 6.8).

The fluid content of the subdural space may be easily characterized by ultrasonography:
- An acute subdural hematoma is echogenic, giving multiple thin echoes, spread homogeneously; their intensity correlates quite well with the recent character of the bleeding (Fig. 6.9a).
- A subdural hygroma is an anechoic fluid collection (Fig. 6.9b).
- Subdural empyema will be further described below (Fig. 6.13).

Contrary to descriptions given in several reports (CHEN 1996; RUPPRECHT 1996), subdural collections are bridged by some vessels, well demonstrated by color Doppler. These are not multiple small arteries and veins as in the subarachnoid space, but some large veins that drain venous flow from the superficial venous network toward the superior sagittal sinus (Fig. 6.10). Because of the situation of the anterior fontanelle, they probably correspond to the posterior frontal veins, the precentral veins, the central veins, and/or the postcentral veins. Their lack of pulsatility means that they are not displayed by real-time ultrasonography, except in some cases of chronic subdural hematoma or bacterial collection. They act as guidelines for the subdural neomembranes that are classically described in surgical and anatomical-pathological reports.

Anatomic studies (FRIEDE 1978) have shown that any pathological condition inducing cleavage of tissue at the dura–arachnoid interface is followed by proliferation of dural border cells with production of neomembranes. Dural cells form multilayered tiers that vary in density and texture. The extracellular space contains collagen fibrils and elastic fibers, yet in spite of this, this tissue has little mechanical coherence because it has a loose texture and is organized in parallel sheets; moreover, there is sprouting of capillaries at the inner dural face, while the normal interface layer is characterized by an absence of blood vessels. The cleavage within the dural border leaves the arachnoid barrier layer intact. This explains the

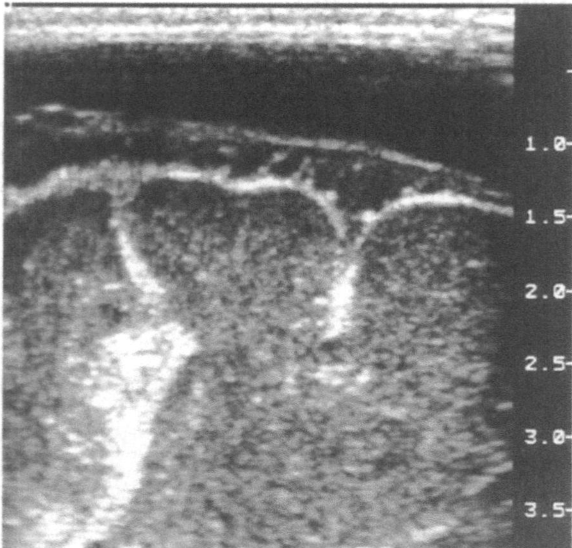

Fig. 6.6a,b. A 4-month-old infant with macrocrania and vomiting. High-frequency ultrasonography shows a mixed pericerebral collection: **a** coronal plane, **b** parasagittal plane. The subarachnoid compartment widens the sulci, contains vascular echoes, and is separated from the outer subdural compartment by a thin echogenic membrane. The subdural collection is anechoic with no mass effect, since the cerebral gyri are not flattened and the subarachnoid space remains well visualized

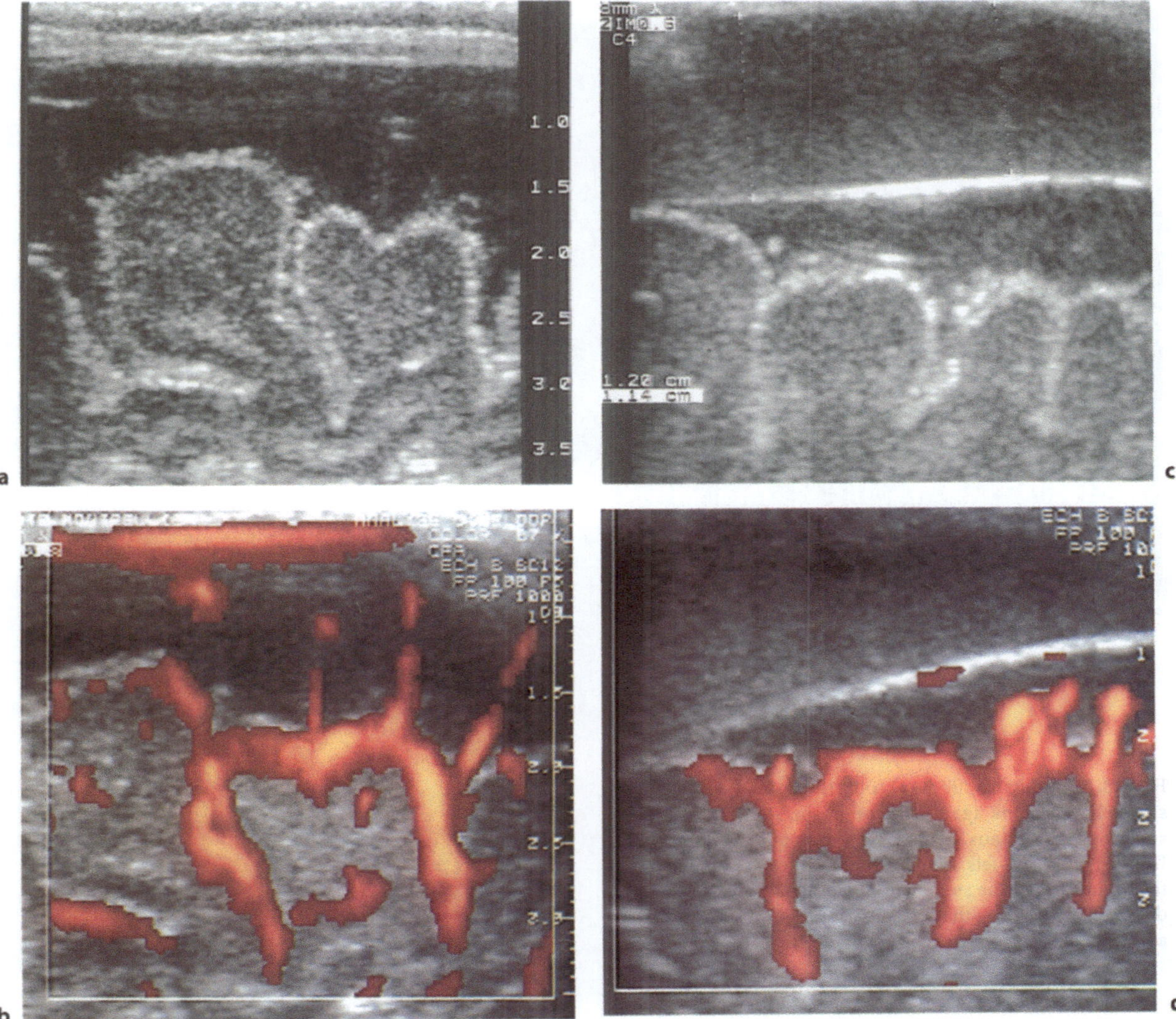

Fig. 6.7a–d. A 6-month-old infant with seizures and macrocrania. **a,b** Right parasagittal plane. Large *subarachnoid collection*, widening the sulci; several small vessels bridge the fluid space from the brain surface toward the superior sagittal sinus (a gray-scale, **b** power Doppler). **c,d** Left parasagittal plane. Large *subdural collection*, moderately compressing the subarachnoid space against the brain surface with partial narrowing of the sulci (c gray-scale). On power Doppler (**d**) vessels are only displayed within the subarachnoid space

absence of extension of the bleeding into the subarachnoid space, even if the volume of blood is large. The sprouting of capillaries in a tissue that lacks intercellular cohesion explains the tendency to repeated bleeding in these subdural collections.

On gray-scale imaging the membranes appear as echogenic structures (Fig. 6.11), that may be parallel in the subdural space and create areas of different echogenicity. One may also visualize a linear echodense structure that bridges perpendicularly the subdural space; color and pulsed Doppler demonstrate that it is centered by a venous flow (Fig. 6.12). These large veins, stretched between the subarach-

noid space and the superior sagittal sinus support the recurrence of subdural hematomas.

Certainly, these veins are also responsible for the first bleeding. They are not visualized before the subdural collection has formed, because they run close to the cranial vault; only the subarachnoid vessels may be displayed. These, however, are not involved in the bleeding process, since subarachnoid hemorrhage is not associated with subdural hematoma in this clinical condition.

The sequence of clinical events (benign enlargement of subarachnoid spaces without hemorrhage, followed by subdural hematoma without subarach-

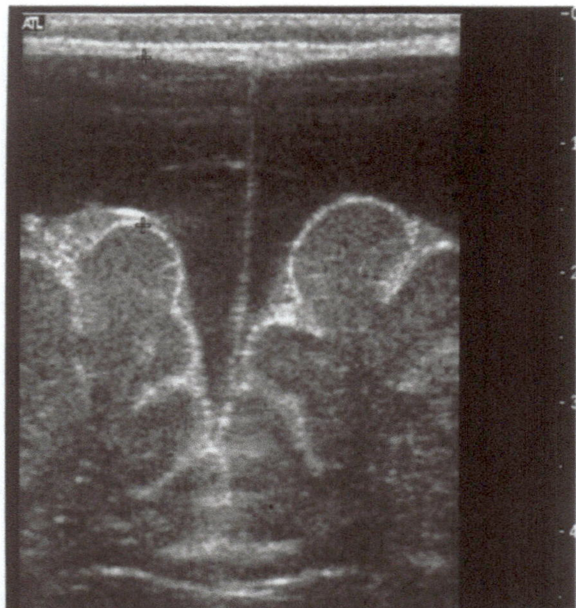

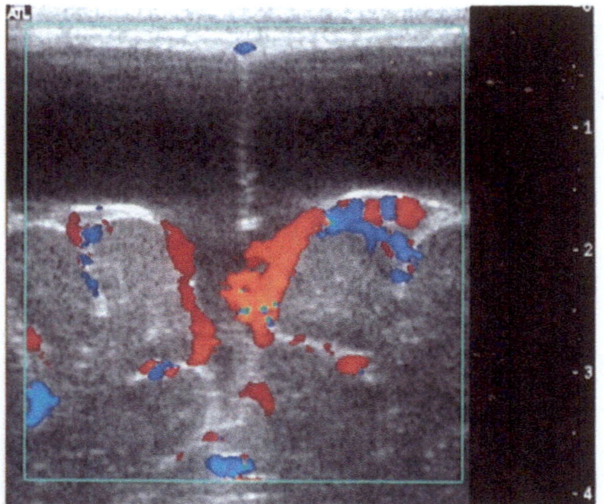

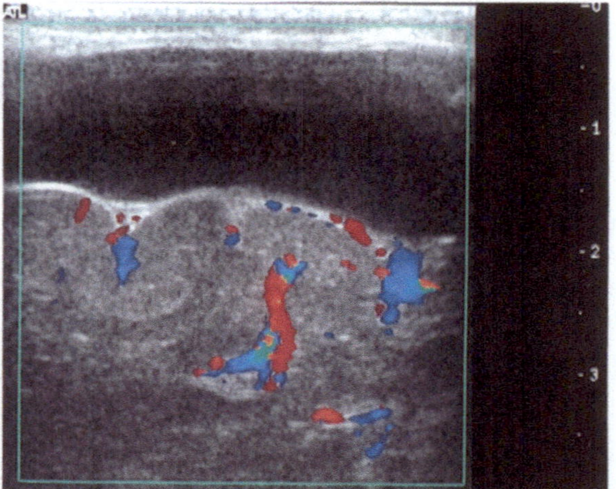

Fig. 6.8. Compressive subdural collection. **a** The subarachnoid spaces have shrunk against the brain surface. Notice that the superior sagittal sinus seems to have disappeared. **b, c** On color Doppler, many vessels are depicted but they are embedded in the brain surface; the subarachnoid and pial vessels cannot be distinguished. Notice that the superior sagittal sinus is patent. **a,b** Coronal planes, **c** parasagittal plane

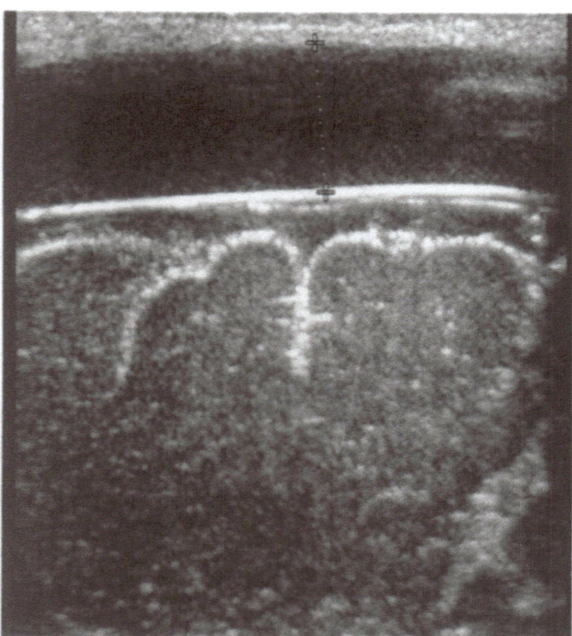

Fig. 6.9a,b. A 5-month-old infant with macrocrania and bilateral subdural collection. **a** On the *left*, anechoic subdural hygroma. **b** On the *right*, echogenic subdural hematoma

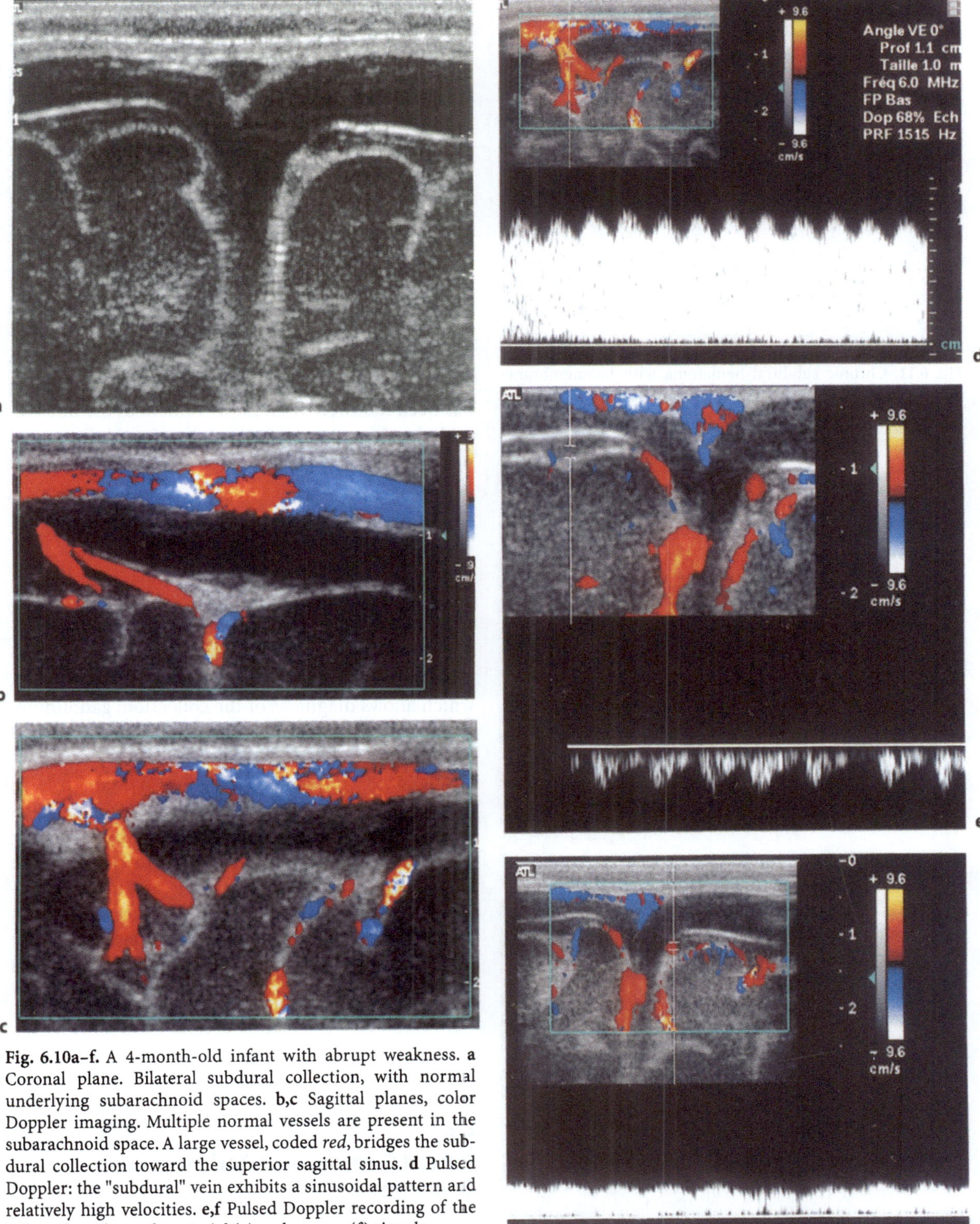

Fig. 6.10a–f. A 4-month-old infant with abrupt weakness. **a** Coronal plane. Bilateral subdural collection, with normal underlying subarachnoid spaces. **b,c** Sagittal planes, color Doppler imaging. Multiple normal vessels are present in the subarachnoid space. A large vessel, coded *red*, bridges the subdural collection toward the superior sagittal sinus. **d** Pulsed Doppler: the "subdural" vein exhibits a sinusoidal pattern and relatively high velocities. **e,f** Pulsed Doppler recording of the subarachnoid vessels: arterial (**e**) and venous (**f**) signals

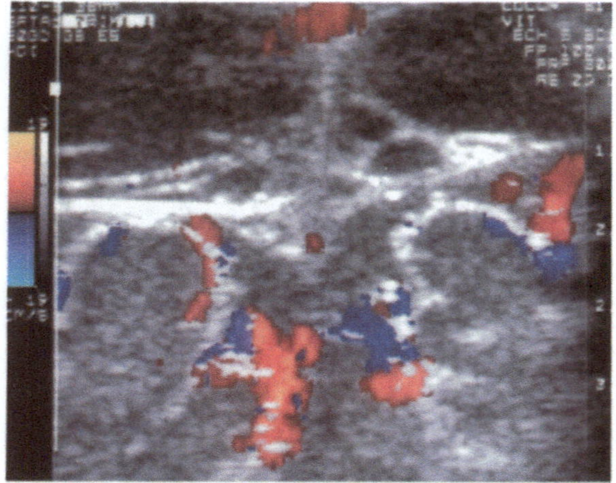

Fig. 6.11. Chronic subdural hematoma with neomembranes and multilayered appearance. No colored signal is detected within the membranes

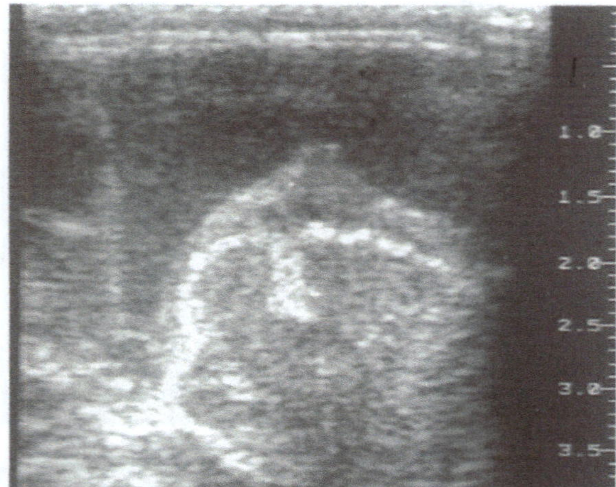

a

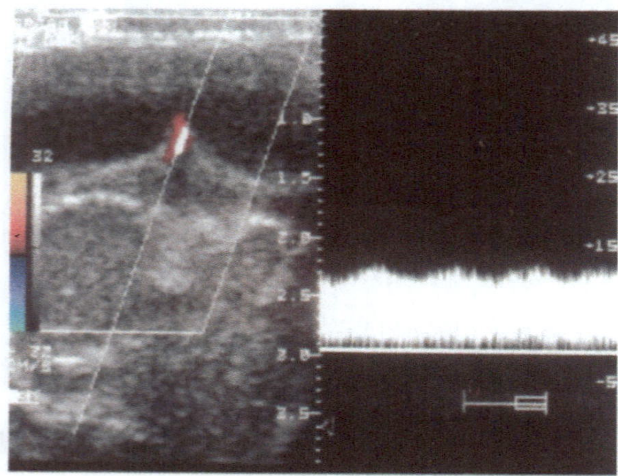

b

Fig. 6.12a,b. Subdural hematoma. Sonographic follow-up after subdural tap. **a** The arachnoid seems to be lifted and drawn toward the dura. **b** Color and pulsed Doppler depict a venous signal within this structure

noid bleeding) supports the idea that the brain and its arachnoid envelope float within the cranium and that minimal impacts or head rotation and/or translation movements may lead to an intracranial bleeding that would not have occurred if the pericerebral space had not been enlarged.

Biomechanical models have been proposed only in the adult (GENNARELLI 1982; HUANG 1999) and the 1-month-old infant (DUHAIME 1987), and they cannot prove this conception. In infants with progressive or persistent subdural collections, some authors (GUTIERREZ 1979) have proposed lowering and advancing the superior sagittal sinus with its overlying sagittal suture and performing a duraplasty in order to improve the venous drainage, to avoid angulations and stretching of the hanging veins. This technique has been followed by an improvement of the intellectual development in 50% of the infants operated upon.

6.7
Subdural Empyema

Subdural empyema is described in Chap. 8. The reference imaging modality is now MRI (OGILVY 1992), which allows diagnosis of the collection; gadolinium enhancement is more sensitive than contrast-enhanced CT.

Obviously, ultrasonography has a main role in diagnosing this complication of pyogenic meningitis in the infant (CHEN 1998). Color Doppler imaging may detect intense hyperemia in the thick wall of the collection, in its internal septations, and in the underlying brain surface (Fig. 6.13). This appearance is not seen in aseptic chronic subdural hematoma (CHEN 1996) and correlates well with pathological aspects (Chap. 8).

6.8
Pulsed Doppler and Pericerebral Collections

Although pulsed Doppler helps to characterize the vessels depicted in the pericerebral fluid space and to identify the location of the fluid collection, its main use is in assessing the effects of the collection on cerebral blood flow velocities.

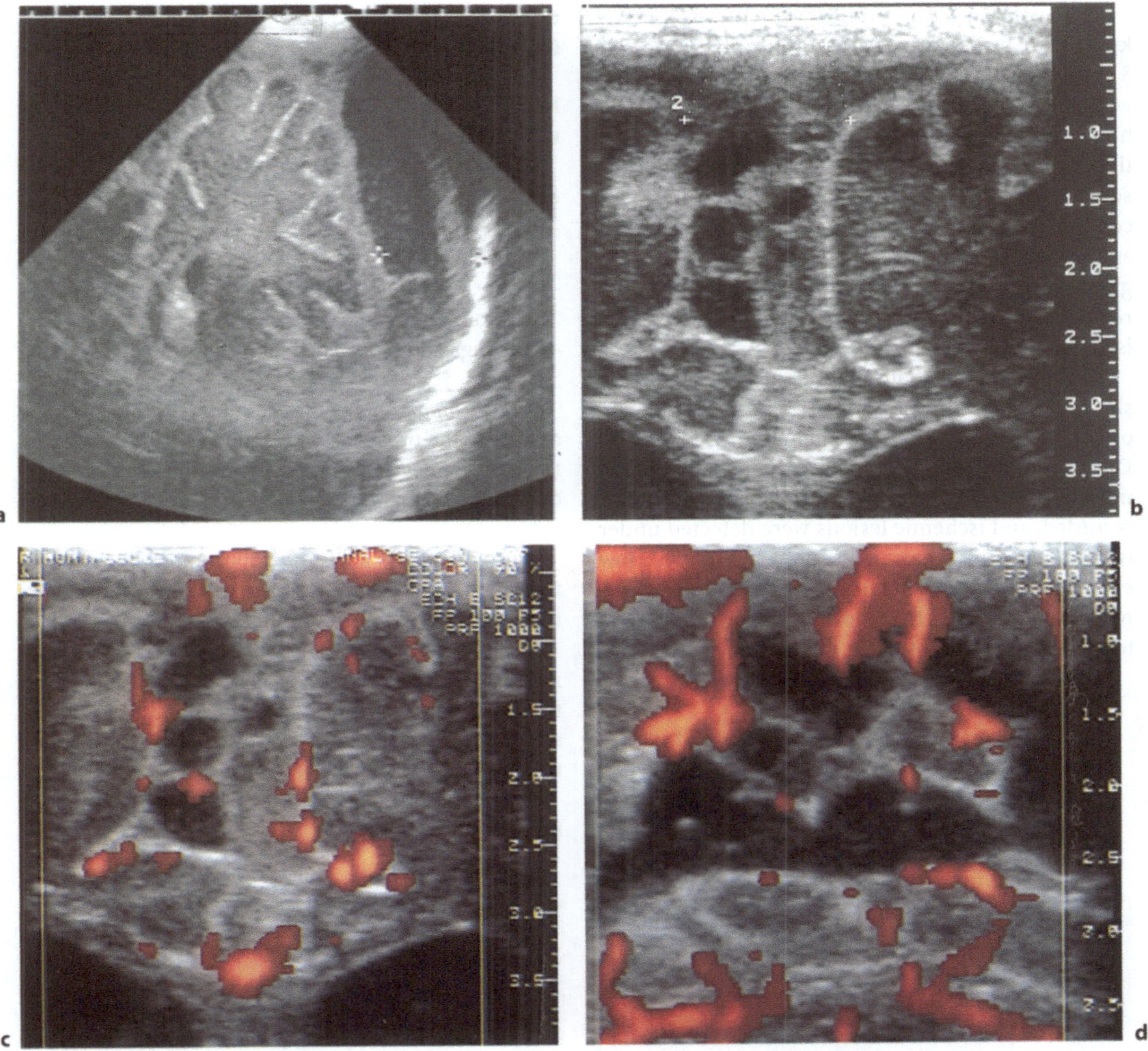

Fig. 6.13a–d. A 4-month-old infant with tonic-clonic generalized seizures and vomiting. *Salmonella enteritidis* meningitis was diagnosed. **a** Ultrasonography showed a large subdural empyema with a thick wall and hypoechoic content. A surgical drainage was placed and marked improvement followed. **b–d** Positive cultures persisted in the fluid obtained. On a coronal plane (**b**), a septated collection was detected within the interhemispheric space. Color Doppler (**c** coronal plane, **d** sagittal plane) depicted small colored spots in the echogenic septa

Flow velocities and resistive index in cases of severe head injury and subdural hematoma have been measured and the results widely reported, but only in relation to children, adolescents, and adults, i.e., to injuries sustained by a closed cranium, investigated by transcranial Doppler ultrasonography, and clinical situations with acute lateralized subdural hematoma.

The importance of measuring the intracranial pressure and following its evolution by serial examinations is well known, as is the correlation between high intracranial pressure and poor outcome (FELDMANN 1979; PAPO 1982). As a consequence, detection of a marked increase in intracranial pressure may lead to more agressive management with surgical decompression (CHO 1993).

In the infant, the resistive index may be easily determined through the anterior fontanelle, and the correlation between increased resistive index and increased intracranial pressure has been demonstrated (see Chap. 4).

The evolution of blood flow velocities is less well known. In the adult, several authors (GORAJ 1993; SANKER 1990) have reported increased velocities with increased intracranial pressure in the first few hours after head injury, and decreased velocities in the case of chronic subdural hematoma. In children, some reports (BRUCE 1979) have described increased cerebral blood flow despite decreased oxygen consumption. Experimental studies showed a decrease in global cerebral blood flow in the whole brain, and in regional blood flow within ischemic territory when ischemia occurs (KURODA 1990).

The few patients that we have been able to analyze showed decreased mean velocities in the early phase of symptomatic subdural hematoma (Fig. 6.14). During the follow-up of some patients, a pattern of intense vasodilatation (luxury perfusion) was recorded, and ischemic lesions were detected underlying the hemorrhagic collection (Fig. 6.15). However, these hemodynamic parameters (measurements of velocities) have not been assessed in a systematic prospective study.

6.9
Conclusion

Extracerebral fluid collection is a frequent finding on ultrasonography.

High-frequency gray-scale morphological analysis can:

- Differentiate subarachnoid effusion from subdural collection
- Show any mass effect induced by the subdural collection
- Distinguish between hematoma, hygroma, empyema

Color Doppler helps the diagnosis as to location by assessing the presence or absence of vessels bridging the fluid collection, and determining their appearance, situation, and direction.

Pulsed Doppler gives information on the effects of the subdural collection and determines parameters that correlate with intracranial pressure.

In most clinical situations encountered in neonates and infants, ultrasonography is sufficient for the diagnosis and decision on therapy. Only in selected cases are more invasive investigations required.

Obviously, ultrasonography can also help to monitor treatment efficacy.

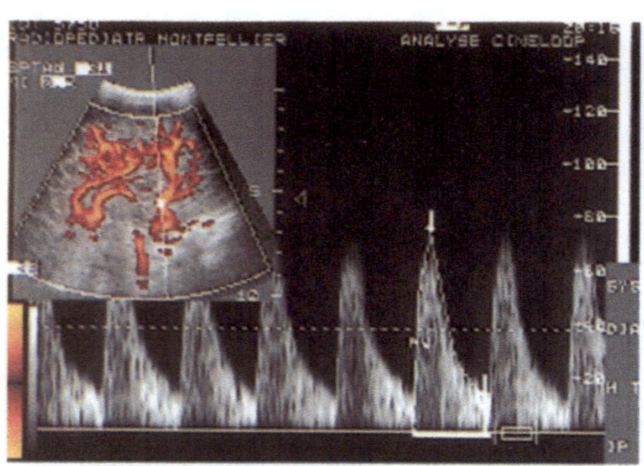
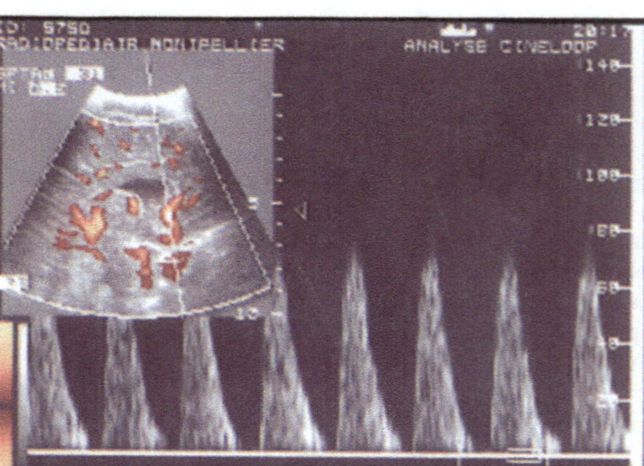

Fig. 6.14a,b. A 3-month-old infant with generalized seizures and fontanellar bulging. Ultrasonography showed a large anechoic subdural collection. Pulsed Doppler recording of the anterior cerebral artery. **a** Normal peak-systolic velocity (PSV, 73.3 cm/s), decreased end-diastolic velocity (EDV, 12.5 cm/s) and time-average velocity (TAV, 37.7 cm/s), and increased RI (0.83), indicating increased intracranial pressure. This is confirmed by fontanellar compression, which induces disappearance of diastolic flow (**b**). Resistive index (RI) = 1

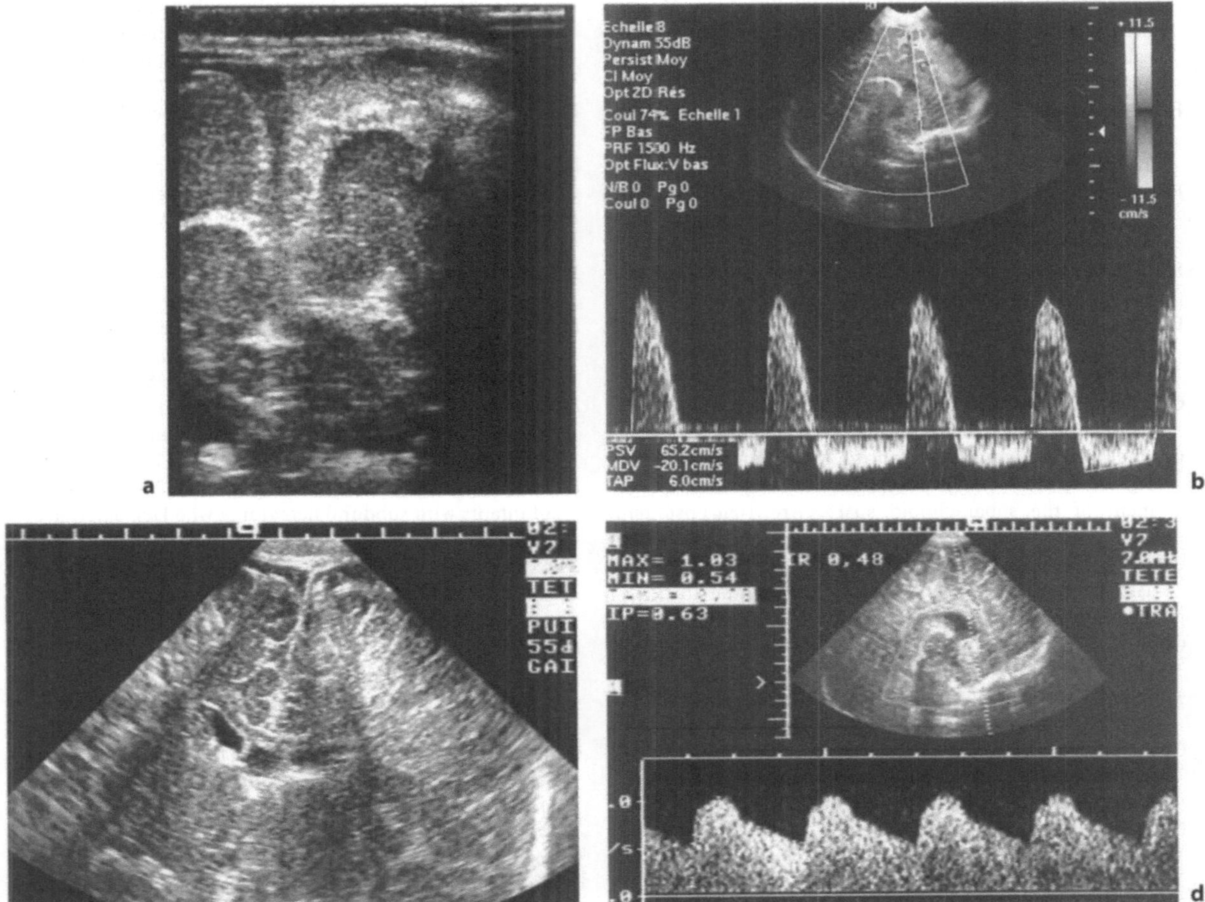

Fig. 6.15a–d. A 3-month-old girl. Focal seizure of the upper limb, clinical signs of increased intracranial pressure. Initial ultrasonography (a) detects a hyperechoic left subdural hematoma with a small anechoic right subdural hygroma. b Doppler recording of the anterior cerebral artery demonstrates a high RI (1.31) with low blood flow (TAV=6 cm/s). c Three days later, ultrasonography shows multiple ischemic corticosubcortical lesions. d Pulsed Doppler demonstrates a luxury perfusion pattern: high diastolic and mean velocities (EDV=54 cm/s, TAV=78 cm/s), low RI (0.48). CT confirms extensive corticosubcortical ischemic damage. Final diagnosis: battered child syndrome

References

Alvarez LA, Maytal J, Shinnar S (1986) Idiopathic external hydrocephalus: natural history and relationship to benign familial macrocephaly. Pediatrics 77:901-907

Andersson H, Elfverson J, Svendsen P (1984) External hydrocephalus in infants. Child's Brain 11:398-402

Aoki N (1994) Extracerebral fluid collections in infancy: role of magnetic resonance imaging in differentiation between subdural effusion and subarachnoid space enlargement. J Neurosurg 81:20-23

Aoki N, Masuzawa H (1984) Infantile acute subdural hematoma. Clinical analysis of 26 cases. J Neurosurg 61:273-280

Azais M, Echenne B (1992) Idiopathic pericerebral swelling (external hydrocephalus) of infants. Ann Pediatr 39:550-558

Bruce DA, Raphaely RC, Goldberg AI, Zimmerman RA, Bilaniuk LT, Schut L, Kuhl DE (1979) Pathophysiology, treatment and outcome following severe head injury in children. Child's Brain 5:174-191

Chen CY, Chou TY, Zimmerman RA, Lee CC, Chen FH, Faro SH (1996) Pericerebral fluid collection: differentiation of enlarged subarachnoid spaces from subdural collection with color Doppler US. Radiology 201:389-392

Chen CY, Huang CC, Chang YC, Chow NH, Chio CC, Zimmerman RA (1998) Subdural empyema in 10 infants: US characteristics and clinical correlates. Radiology 207:609-617

Cho DY, Wang YC, Chi CS (1995) Decompressive craniotomy for acute shaken/impact baby syndrome. Pediatr Neurosurg 23:192-198

Dandy WE, Blackfan KD (1914) Internal hydrocephalus: an experimental clinical and pathological study. Am J Dis Child 8:406-482

Duhaime AC, Gennarelli TA, Thibault LE, Bruce DA, Margulies SS, Wiser R (1987) The shaken baby syndrome: a clinical, pathological and biomechanical study. J Neurosurg 66:409-415

Fan YF, Chong VF, Tan KP (1993) Subarachnoid spaces in infants and young children. Ann Acad Med Singapore 22:732-735

Feldmann H, Klages G, Gartner F, Scharfenberg J (1979) The prognostic value of intracranial pressure monitoring after severe head injuries. Acta Neurochir Suppl (Wien) 28:74-77

Frederickson RG (1991) The subdural space interpreted as a cellular layer of meninges. Anat Rec 230:38-51

Friede RL, Schachenmayr W (1978) The origin of subdural neomembranes. II. Fine structures of neomembranes. Am J Pathol 92:69-84

Gennarelli TA, Thibault LE (1982) Biomechanics of acute subdural hematoma. J Trauma 22:680-686

Gherpelli JL, Scaramuzzi V, Manreza ML, Diament AJ (1992) Follow-up study of macrocephalic children with enlargement of the subarachnoid space. Arq Neuropsiquiatr 50:156-162

Gilles FH, Davidson RI (1971) Communicating hydrocephalus associated with deficient dysplastic parasagittal arachnoidal granulations. J Neurosurg 35:421-426

Goraj B, Rifkinson-Mann S, Leslie DR, Kasoff SS, Tenner MS (1993) Cerebral blood flow velocity after head injury: transcranial Doppler evaluation. work in progress. Radiology.188:137-141

Govaert P, Pauwels W, Vanhaesebrouck P, De Praeter C, Afschrift M (1989) Ultrasound measurement of the subarachnoid space in infants. Eur J Pediatr 148:412-413

Gutierrez FA, McLone DG, Raimondi AJ (1979) Physiopathology and a new treatment of chronic subdural hematoma in children. Child's Brain 5:216-232

Haines DE, Harkey HL, Al Mefty O (1993) The "subdural space": a new look at an outdated concept. Neurosurgery 32:111-120

Hayes KC, McCombs HL, Faherty TP (1971) The fine structure of vitamin A deficiency. II: arachnoid granulations and CSF pressure. Brain 94:213-224

Huang HM, Lee MC, Chiu WT, Chen CT, Lee SY (1999) Three-dimensional finite element analysis of subdural hematoma. J Trauma 47:538-544

Hutchings M, Weller RO (1986) Anatomical relationship of the piamater to cerebral blood vessels in man. J Neurosurg 65:316-325

Ikeda A, Sato O, Tsugane R, Shibuya N, Yamamoto I, Shimoda M (1987) Infantile acute subdural hematoma. Child's Nerv Syst 3:19-22

Jayawant S, Rawlinson A, Gibbon F, Price J, Schulte J, Sharples P, Sibert JR, Kemp AM (1998) Subdural haemorrhages in infants: population based study. Br Med J 317:1558-1561

Kapila A, Trice H, Spies WG, Siegel HA, Gado MH (1982) Enlarged cerebrospinal fluid spaces in infants with subdural hematomas. Radiology 142:669-672

Kleinman PK, Zito JL, Davidson RI, Raptopoulos V (1983) The subarachnoid spaces in children: normal variations in size. Radiology 147:455-457

Kuroda Y, Bullock R (1992) Failure of cerebral blood flow-metabolism coupling after acute subdural hematoma in the rat. Neurosurgery 31:1062-1071.

Libicher M, Troger J (1992) US measurement of the subarachnoid space in infants. Radiology 184:749-751

Lui K, Boag G, Daneman A, Costello S, Kirpalani H, Whyte H (1990) Widened subarachnoid space in pre-discharge cranial ultrasound: evidence of cerebral atrophy in immature infants? Dev Med Child Neurol 32:882-887

Markwalder TM (1981) Chronic subdural hematomas: a review. J Neurosurg 54:637-645

McCluney KW, Yeakley JW, Fenstermacher MJ, Baird SH, Bonmati CM (1992) Subdural hygroma versus atrophy on MR brain scans: "The cortical vein sign". Am J Neuroradiol 13:1335-1339

McLone DG (1980) The subarachnoid space: a review. Child's Brain 6:113-130

Mori K, Sakamoto T, Nishimura K, Fujiwara K (1993) Subarachnoid fluid collection in infants complicated by subdural hematoma. Child's Nerv Syst 9:282-284

Morota N, Sakamoto K, Kobayashi N, Kitazawa K, Kobayashi S (1995) Infantile subdural fluid collection: diagnosis and post-operative course. Child's Nerv Syst 11:459-466

Morris MW, Smith S, Cressman J, Ancheta J (2000) Evaluation of infants with subdural hematoma who lack external evidence of abuse. Pediatrics 105:549-553

Nickel RE, Gallenstein JS (1987) Developmental prognosis for infants with benign enlargement of the subarachnoid spaces. Dev Med Child Neurol 29:181-186

Nishimura K, Mori K, Sakamoto T, Fujiwara K (1996) Management of subarachnoid fluid collection in infants based on a long term follow-up study. Acta Neurochir (Wien) 138:179-184

Ogilvy CS, Chapman PH, McGrail K (1992) Subdural empyema complicating bacterial meningitis in a child: enhancement of membranes with gadolinium on MRI in a patient without enhancement on CT. Surg Neurol 37:138-141

Orlin JR, Osen KK, Hovig T (1991) Subdural compartment in pig: a morphologic study with blood and horseradish peroxidase infused subdurally. Anat Rec 230:22-37

Palencia-Luaces R, Aldana Gomez J, Tresierra Unzaga F (1992) Hidrocefalia externa idiopatica en la infancia y macrocefalia familiar. An Esp Pediatr 36:186-188

Papo I, Caruselli G, Luongo A (1982) Intracranial pressure in children and adolescents with severe head injuries. J Neurosurg Sci 26:193-198

Portnoy HD, Croissant PD (1978) Megalencephaly in infants and children: the possible role in increased dural sinus pressure. Arch Neurol 35:306-316

Prassopoulos P, Cavouras D, Golfinopoulos S, Nezi M (1995) The size of the intra- and extraventricular CSF compartments in children with idiopathic benign widening of the frontal subarachnoid space. Neuroradiology 37: 418-421

Reina MA, Lopez Garcia A, De Andres JA, Villanueva MC, Cortes L (1998) Does the subdural space exist? Rev Esp Anestesiol Reanim 45:367-376

Rupprecht T, Lauffer K, Storr U, Hofbeck M, Wenzel D, Bowing B (1996) Extracerebral intracranial fluid collections in childhood: differentiation between benign subarachnoid space enlargement and subdural effusion using color-coded duplex ultrasound. Klin Padiatr 208:97-102

Sahar A (1978) Pseudo hydrocephalus-megalocephaly, increased intracranial pressure and widened subarachnoid space. Neuropadiatrie 9:131-139

Sanker P, Terhag D, Richard KE, Frowein RA (1990) Cerebral blood flow velocity. A prognostic factor following severe craniocerebral trauma? Aktuelle Traumatol 20:152-156

Schachenmayr W, Friede RL (1978) The origin of subdural

neomembranes. I. Fine structure of the dura-arachnoid interface in man. Am J Pathol 92:53-68

Stroobandt G, Evrard P, Thauvoy C, Laterre C (1981) Les épanchements pericérébraux du nourrisson à localisation sous-durale ou sous-arachnoidienne. Neurochirurgie 27:49-57

Stroobandt G (1984) De l'épanchement sous dural à l'hydrocéphalie sous-arachnoidienne du nourrisson. Med Infant 91:89-96

Trounce JQ, De Vries L, Levene MI (1985) External hydrocephalus-diagnosis by ultrasound. Br J Radiol 58:415-417

Tsubokawa T, Nakamura S, Satoh K (1984) Effect of temporary subdural-peritoneal shunt on subdural effusion with subarachnoid effusion. Child's Brain 11:47-59

Tzioumi D, Oates RK (1998) Subdural hematomas in children under 2 years. Accidental or inflicted? A 10-year experience. Child Abuse Negl 22:1105-1112

Veyrac C, Couture A, Baud C (1990) Pericerebral fluid collections and ultrasound. Pediatr Radiol 20:236-240

Veyrac C (1994) Les collections extra-cérébrales. In: Couture A, Veyrac C, Baud C: Echographie cérébrale: du foetus au nouveau-né. Sauramps Medical, Montpellier pp 249-266

Wilms G, Vanderschueren G, Demaerel PH, Smet MH, Van Calenbergh F, Plets C, Goffin J, Casaer P (1993) CT and MR in infants with pericerebral collections and macrocephaly: benign enlargement of the subarachnoid spaces versus subdural collections. Am J Neuroradiol 14:855-860

7 Cerebral Venous Thrombosis

ALAIN COUTURE and CORINNE VEYRAC

CONTENTS

Cerebral venous thrombosis is rarely described and poorly known in the infant (BAILY 1931; BYERS 1933) and discovered only on anatomical investigation, until recently; their diagnosis and treatment have greatly benefited from modern imaging. In this disease, which has been unknown rather than uncommon, angiography was the gold standard of diagnostic imaging before the advent of CT and MRI/ MR angiography. Several recent reports (BEZINQUE 1995; DEAN 1995; GOVAERT 1992; LAM 1995; PEDESPAN 1996) have highlighted the value of color Doppler in the diagnosis of cerebral venous thrombosis in neonates.

Our experience agrees with the literature data, as is shown by this case report:

Vincent was born at 39 weeks of gestation, after cesarean delivery. He quickly developed respiratory distress syndrome, due to meconium aspiration, which required mechanical ventilation for 6 days.

On day 1, brain ultrasonography demonstrated a minimal white matter echodensity and a normal Doppler spectrum on the anterior cerebral artery. Color imaging of the superior sagittal sinus was normal.

On day 8, clinical evolution was normal. Routine transfontanellar ultrasonography detected a complete

thrombosis of the superior sagittal sinus and transverse sinuses (Fig. 7.1).

Twenty-four hours later, MRI confirmed the thrombosis, which involved the superior sagittal sinus, torcular, and transverse sinuses (Fig. 7.2).

The deep venous system (internal cerebral vein, vein of Galen, straight sinus) remained patent. There was no hemodynamic sign of increased intracranial pressure since resistive index (RI=0.75) and peak-systolic (PSV) and end-diastolic velocities (EDV) were normal in the anterior cerebral artery. No ischemic-hemorrhagic parenchymal damage was seen on either ultrasonography or MRI.

Heparin therapy was initiated, but quickly stopped because thrombocytopenia appeared on the second day.

On day 10, the superior sagittal sinus was still thrombosed. Color Doppler imaging showed normal flow direction in the internal cerebral vein, vein of Galen, and straight sinus, as well as normal mean velocity in the internal cerebral vein (8 cm/s) (Fig. 7.3).

On day 14, the superior sagittal sinus and transverse sinuses were unchanged.

At 3 weeks of life, the clinical examination was normal. The superior sagittal sinus thrombosis persisted, but the transverse sinuses had recovered patency (Fig. 7.4).

At 5 weeks, Vincent showed only moderate hypotonia; on ultrasonography the brain had a normal appearance and the superior sagittal sinus had become recanalized (Fig. 7.5).

This case provides physiopathological, etiological, and clinical data for discussion, and demonstrates that ultrasonography, especially color Doppler imaging, provides imaging tools of quality for diagnosis and follow-up of cerebral venous thrombosis.

A. COUTURE, MD; C. VEYRAC, MD
Service de Radiologie Pédiatrique, Hôpital Arnaud de Villeneuve, 371 av. Doyen Gaston Giraud, 34295 Montpellier Cedex, France

7.1
Physiopathological Data

We know that cerebral venous flow is influenced by several factors.

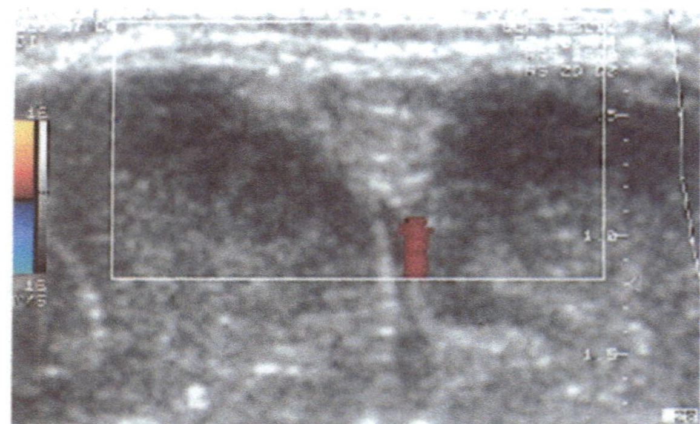

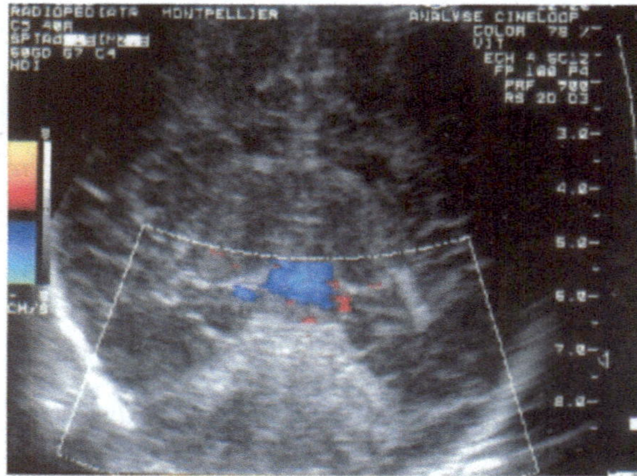

Fig. 7.1a,b. Day 8. **a** Superior sagittal sinus appears as a wide hyperechoic triangular image, without colored signal. **b** Blood flow is well seen in the straight sinus, but absent in the lateral sinuses

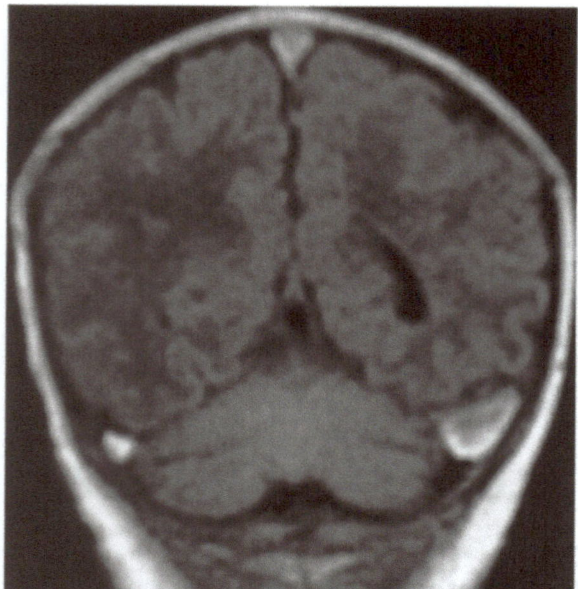

Fig. 7.2. Day 9. On MRI, the T1-weighted sequence confirms the sonographic diagnosis by showing a hyperintense signal in the superior sagittal sinus and lateral sinuses

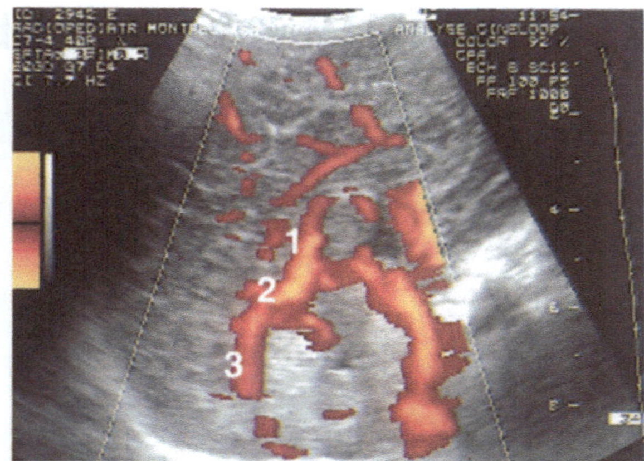

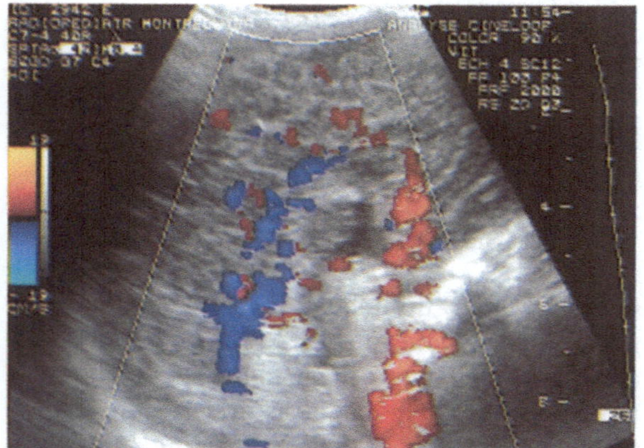

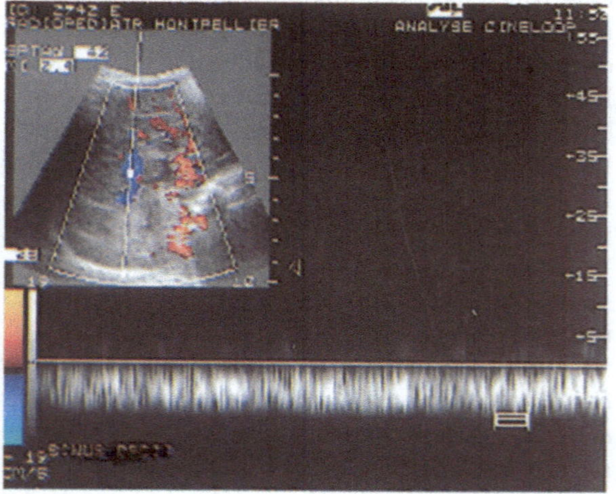

Fig. 7.3a–c. The deep venous system is normally patent: internal cerebral vein (*1*), vein of Galen (*2*) , straight sinus (*3*) are free (**a**), with flow coded in blue (**b**). Normal velocity in the internal cerebral vein (**c**): 8 cm/s

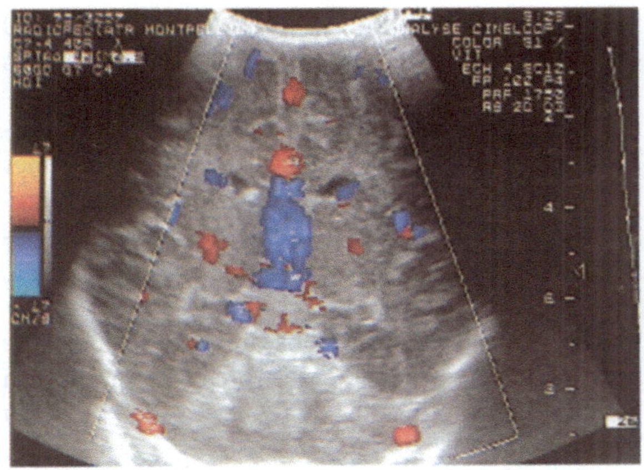

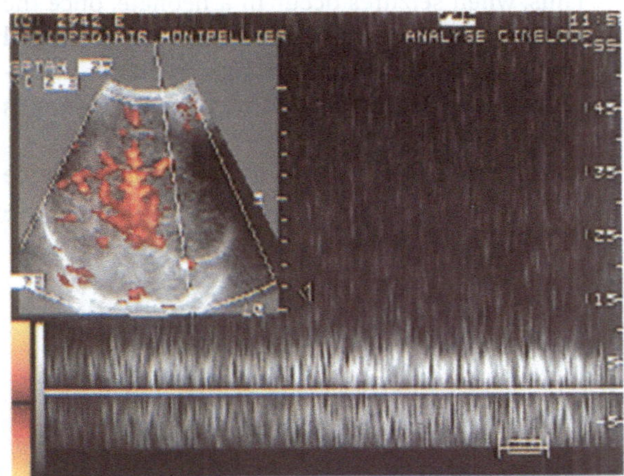

Fig. 7.4a,b. The two lateral sinuses (a) are perfectly displayed on color Doppler; velocity in the left lateral sinus is normal (b)

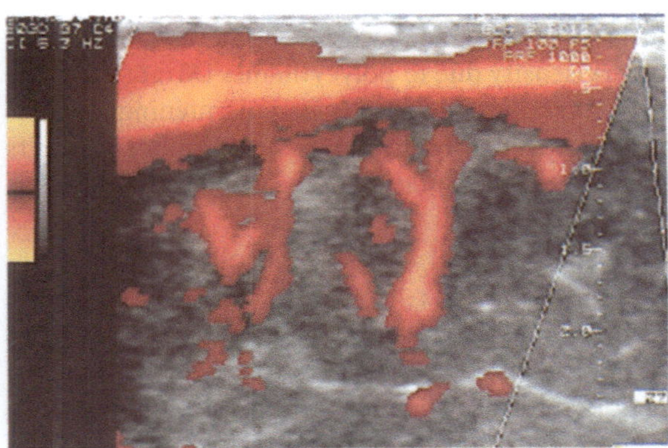

Fig. 7.5. Day 37. Superior sagittal sinus has recovered normal patency

It may change during some physiological events such as crying or head rotation (WATSON 1974). For example, COWAN (1983) showed that a 60° head rotation may produce complete occlusion of the internal jugular vein. FENTON (1991) reported that velocities may be reduced by 50% in the vein of Galen when there is moderate compression of the jugular veins.

In the neonate, multiple pathological conditions may severely affect the cerebral venous flow. In the preterm infant with acute respiratory distress and mechanical ventilation, intrathoracic pressures are increased and cerebral venous flow return is disturbed (GOVAERT 1992). Instability of arterial blood pressure, acute sepsis, posthemorrhagic hypovolemia, and complications of congenital heart disease, are all conditions that considerably disturb cerebral blood flow, especially venous flow. Patent ductus arteriosus is known to decrease venous flow (WRIGHT 1988). Finally, hypercoagulable state (congenital or acquired), hemoconcentration, and poly-

cythemia may obviously be responsible for venous thrombosis.

All these data demonstrate how preterm and full-term resuscitated neonates are at high risk of intracerebral thrombosis.

When these pathological conditions are combined, venous flow becomes intermittent, producing stasis and subsequent thrombosis. The superior sagittal sinus and superficial veins (CURE 1995) are the most commonly involved. The clot progressively organizes, then spontaneously disappears and the vein recovers its patency after a delay varying from weeks to months. The consequences of the venous thrombosis are well known: meningeal damage (subarachnoid hemorrhage, subdural hemorrhage) and parenchymal damage (capillary congestion, edema, hemorrhage, ischemia, necrosis).

7.2
Etiological Data

Several conditions may lead to cerebral venous thrombosis. Otitis/sinusitis and acute dehydration predominated until introduction of appropriate antibiotic treatment and intravenous rehydration, and improved control of systemic hypotension.

In patients with dehydration, thrombosis has a multifactorial mechanism: hemoconcentration, systemic collapse, anemia, and infection. Acute severe hypernatremic dehydration is always involved (AICARDI 1973), and the original location of the thrombosis is the superior sagittal sinus.

Congenital heart disease (tetralogy of Fallot, transposition of great vessels) favors cerebral thrombosis through anoxia, venous stasis, and blood hyperviscosity due to polycythemia (MILLER 1981).

In infectious diseases (pyogenic meningitis, subdural empyema, brain abscess), thrombosis results from direct inflammation of the venous walls (FRIEDE 1973).

Finally, perinatal asphyxia is an obvious causal factor (KONISHI 1987; VOORHIES 1984; WONG 1987). Among six asphyxiated neonates with diffuse hypodense lesions on CT, VOORHIES (1984) detected angiographically a venous thrombosis in five, associated with arterial thrombosis in two of them. The pathogenesis was uncertain: in addition to arterial ischemic injury, intense changes in venous vascularization occurred (cause or consequence?), resulting in intricate ischemic lesions and venous thrombosis.

Other less common situations may be encountered with cerebral vein thrombosis: Sturge-Weber disease (CURE 1995), nephrotic syndrome (FOFAH 1997), or coagulation disturbances such as antithrombin III (AMBRUSO 1980) or protein C deficiency (MARCINIAK 1985; WINTZEN 1985). Finally, HURST (1989) reported the case of a thrombosis involving the superior sagittal sinus, straight sinus, torcular, and transverse sinuses, associated with placement of a right subclavian-jugular catheter in a dehydrated infant. Several mechanisms have been discussed: retrograde infusion of solute disturbing the intracranial venous flow, propagation of a clot from the internal jugular vein, or a possible role of the preceding dehydration.

In addition to these conditions associated with the risk of developing venous sinus thrombosis, it is important to know that the thrombosis may occur spontaneously, without recognizable cause in 25% of cases (BARRON 1992; RIVKIN 1992). For example, RIVKIN (1992) reported seven neonates with idiopathic venous thrombosis.

The etiologies determined in our six cases confirm the literature data: sepsis was noted in two cases, a traumatic delivery in two, severe neonatal asphyxia in one case, and a combination of several factors in one case (acute respiratory distress syndrome, mechanical ventilation, and hemodynamic disorders).

7.3
Clinical Data

Seizures are the most frequent presentation of a cerebral venous thrombosis in neonate or infant (BARRON 1992; KONISHI 1987; LEE 1995; MEDLOCK 1992; RIVKIN 1992; SHEVELL 1989). LEE (1995) observed initial seizures in all of 8 cases, and SHEVELL (1989) in 15 of 17 newborns. In a recent literature study, VOLPE (1995) found seizures in 31 of 47 neonates.

The seizures may be tonic or clonic, focal or multifocal, and partial or generalized, but focal ones appear the most frequent (BARRON 1992; MARTINEZ-MENENDEZ 1992). Muscle tone disorders are frequently observed in the newborn, mainly hypotonia, sometimes with lethargy.

The clinical manifestations probably relate to the intracranial pressure increase, which is common with cerebral venous thrombosis (KONISHI 1987; RIVKIN 1992).

Thus, when seizures occur in a neonate, once the more common causes have been excluded (perinatal asphyxia, intracranial hemorrhage, infection, metabolic disturbances), one should search for a venous thrombosis.

The clinical presentation of our six cases agree with these data: three patients experienced initial seizures and two, hypotonia.

7.4
Imaging

7.4.1
CT and MRI

For over 15 years, the diagnosis of cerebral vein thrombosis in the neonate and infant has been made on CT (BARRON 1992; EDWARDS 1987; GOVAERT 1992; HOROWITZ 1995; HURST 1989; KONISHI 1987; LAM 1995; LEE 1995; MEDLOCK 1992; PEDESPAN 1998; RIVKIN 1992; SCHUBIGER 1982; SHEVELL 1989; WONG 1987), and more recently on MRI (BARAM 1988; BARRON 1992; CURE 1994; EDWARDS 1987; GOVAERT 1992; HANIGAN 1986; HURST 1989; LAM 1995; LEE 1995; MEDLOCK 1992; PEDESPAN 1996; RIVKIN 1992; SHEVELL 1989).

CT provides suggestive information: the spontaneous high attenuation of a clot within the superior sagittal sinus (Fig. 7.6), straight sinus, or cortical veins is a valuable finding (BARRON 1992; SHEVELL 1989; HURST 1989; PEDESPAN 1996). However, this is an inconstant sign (BARRON 1992) that disappears early (PEDESPAN 1996) and is of uncertain reliability: KRISS (1998) reported absence of thrombosis in 10 out of 11 patients with hyperdense venous sinuses (color Doppler: 7, MRI: 4). He proposed two explanations: first, the neonatal lack of myelination leads to decreased attenuation of brain parenchyma and relative hyper-

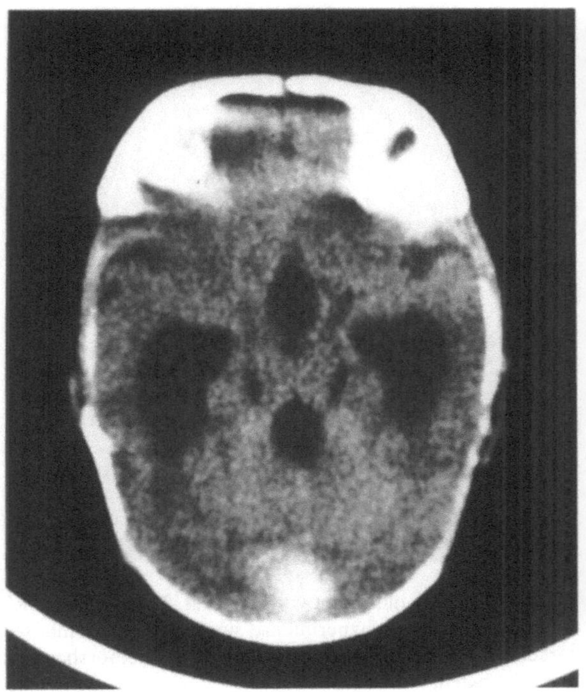

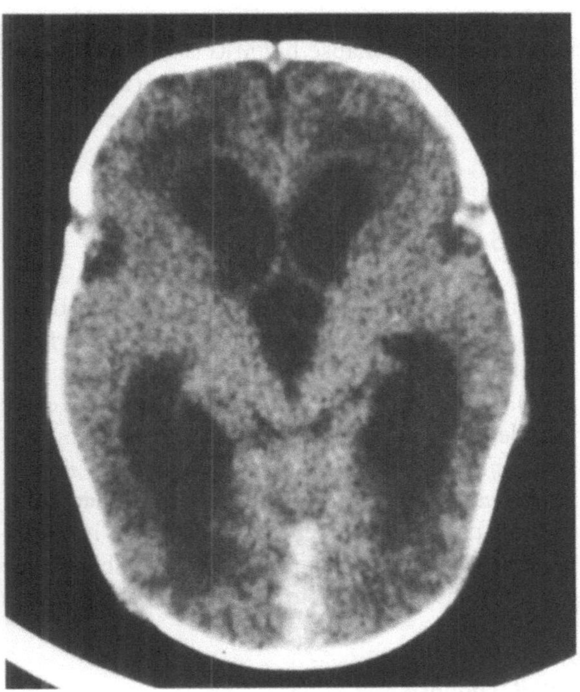

Fig. 7.6a,b. A 3-week-old infant who showed abrupt weakness with altered consciousness. The superior sagittal sinus appeared thrombosed on color Doppler imaging. The diagnosis was confirmed by CT, which revealed a large, hyperdense sagittal sinus (a, b). (Dr. J.F. Chateil, Bordeaux)

attenuation of the falx and sinuses; second, elevated hematocrit in the neonate increases sinusal density. In fact, hyperdensity in the straight sinus or superior sagittal sinus is observed in 20% of infants without sinus thrombosis (KIM 1986; VIRAPONGSE 1987). In the opinion of VIRAPONGSE (1987) such hyperdensity may be significant only if associated with sinusal bulging and convex walls.

The "empty delta sign" refers to direct visualization of the clot, which produces a rim of enhanced attenuation and a core of decreased attenuation. It is a classical CT feature but little reported in the pediatric literature (DAVIES 1994; SEGALL 1982), because it is a source of multiple errors: bony artifact, septated sinus, arachnoid granulation, and so on.

MRI is now the gold standard for diagnosing cerebral venous thrombosis (PEDESPAN 1996; RIVKIN 1992). Its advantages are direct visualization of the thrombus and its phase of evolution, and accurate delineation of associated ischemic-hemorrhagic parenchymal damage (GOVAERT 1992; GROSSMAN 1993; KHURANA 1996; LEE 1995; MEDLOCK 1992; PEDESPAN 1996). In the acute phase, MRI is able to demonstrate deoxyhemoglobin (PEDESPAN 1996) better than CT demonstrates the high density of blood proteins. In the subacute phase, the diagnosis is easy: the thrombus is hyperintense on T1-weighted

sequences because of the transformation of deoxyhemoglobin into methemoglobin (Fig. 7.7). Finally, postcontrast MRI and MR angiography (LEE 1995; MEDLOCK 1992) allow equivocal cases to be elucidated.

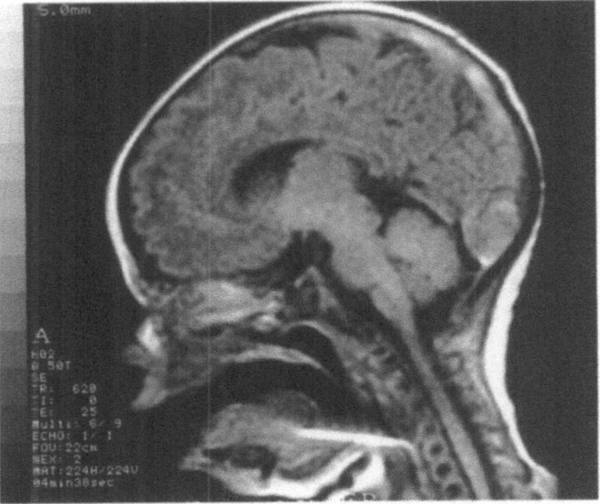

Fig. 7.7. An 8-day-old infant without clinical symptoms but with thrombosis of the superior sagittal sinus revealed on color Doppler imaging. MRI, T1-weighted sequence in a sagittal plane, shows characteristic hyperintense signal in the posterior part of the superior sagittal sinus and torcular

CT may demonstrate cerebral edema and associated ventricular collapse, but MRI is the procedure of choice for detecting hemorrhagic (Fig. 7.8) or ischemic (Fig. 7.9) parenchymal damage.

7.4.2
Ultrasonography

Recently, Doppler techniques have demonstrated their great value for this diagnosis (BEZINQUE 1995; DEAN 1995; GOVAERT 1992; LAM 1995; PEDESPAN 1996). LAM (1995) documented the accuracy of color Doppler imaging in three patients with superior sagittal sinus thrombosis, and highlighted its noninvasiveness. PEDESPAN (1996) reported that color Doppler provided a correct initial diagnosis in 6 of 11 patients with superior sagittal sinus thrombosis. Our experience is in agreement with the literature data.

7.4.2.1
Initial Diagnosis

In all cases the initial diagnostic assessment was by ultrasonography (Table 7.1).

The diagnosis was first suggested by subtle morphological features: the thrombosed superior sagittal sinus appeared as a large hyperechoic triangle with convex walls (Fig. 7.10).

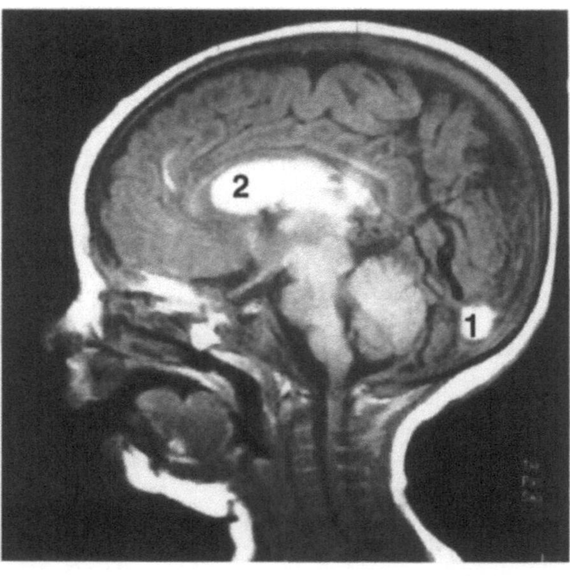

Fig. 7.8. A 21-day-old infant with seizures. T1-weighted MRI, sagittal plane, shows hyperintense signal of the thrombosed torcular (1) associated with third ventricular hemorrhage (2) (Dr. J.F. Chateil, Bordeaux)

In contrast, this feature was not observed in our only case of lateral sinus thrombosis (Fig. 7.1). EDWARDS (1987) described, in two neonates investigated by transfontanellar ultrasonography, an enlarged echodense torcular in one, and a hyperechoic distension of the superior sagittal sinus and

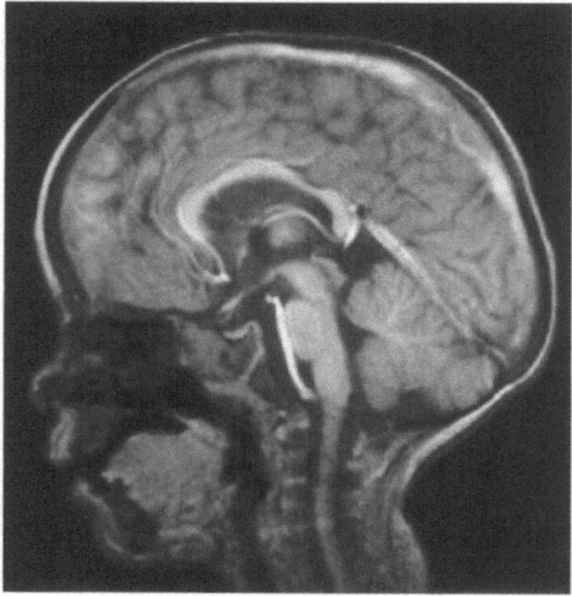
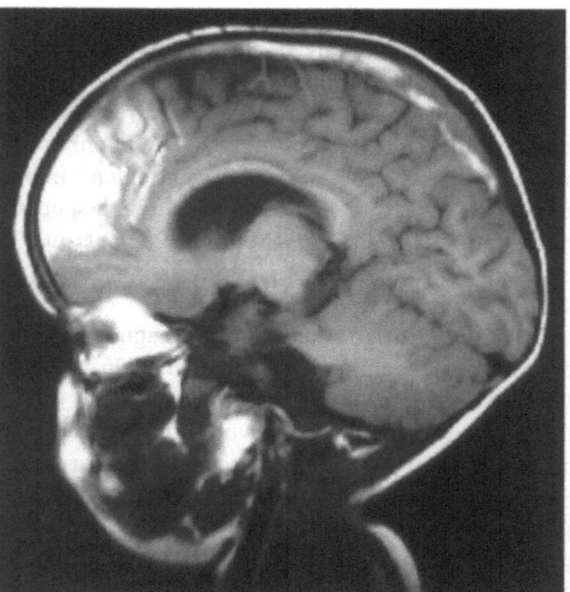

Fig. 7.9a,b. An 11-month-old infant with clonic seizures of the right upper limb. CT and MRI demonstrate thrombosis of the superior sagittal sinus and straight sinus (a). There is an ischemic lesion in the frontal corticosubcortical parenchyma (b). (Dr. J.F. Chateil, Bordeaux)

Table 7.1. Sonographic pattern of cerebral venous thrombosis (6 cases)

	Diagnosis	Location	Size	Collateral circulation	Evolution	Resolution Size of SSS
Case 1	Day 18	SSS	5×6 mm	–	Good outcome Partial recanalization day 35	D50 3×3 mm
Case 2	Day 6	SSS	8.5×7.5 mm	D10	Good outcome Partial recanalization day 36	D150 4×3.5 mm
Case 3	Day 15	SSS	6×6 mm	–	Good outcome	D60 3.5×3.2 mm
Case 4	Day 8	SSS	5×6 mm	D14	Good outcome	D37 3×4 mm
Case 5	Day 11	SSS – TS	6×6 mm	D21	Good outcome	D60 3×4 mm
Case 6	Day 8	SSS	7×5 mm	–	Corticosubcortical ischemic damage. Death day 13	

TS: Transverse sinus   SSS: Superior sagittal sinus

torcular in the other case; sinusal thrombosis was suspected and confirmed by CT and MRI.

Thus, especially in the superior sagittal sinus, there is a direct sign of intraluminal anomaly: the hyperechoic thrombus changes the appearance of the affected sinus (Fig. 7.10) because of its volume.

Thrombosis of the superior sagittal sinus is easily definitively confirmed by color and pulsed Doppler (Bezinque 1995; Dean 1995; Pedespan 1996). Absence of colored signal and of detectable flow permitted diagnosis of a thrombosis of the superior sagittal sinus in our six patients, extending to the lateral sinus in one (Fig. 7.11). In three patients it was confirmed with CT (2 cases) or MRI (1 case). In the other three infants, ultrasonography constituted the only imaging modality for the diagnosis and follow-up of the disease.

The sonographic pattern invites a change in diagnostic strategy:

● In the routine daily experience of transfontanellar ultrasonography, the superior sagittal sinus is always well depicted by color Doppler and recorded by pulsed Doppler (Dean 1995; Pfannschmidt 1989) in the healthy neonate and infant. If it is impossible to obtain a colored signal and the Doppler spectrum is always abnormal (Bezinque 1995, Dean 1995, Pedespan 1996), sinusal thrombosis is diagnosed.

Morphological findings are valuable: a normal sinus appears as an anechoic, small-sized triangle with straight or concave walls, that expands when the baby cries. By contrast to this, a widened sinus with convex walls that does not enlarge with crying suggests the presence of sinusal thrombosis (Fig. 7.12).

Two pitfalls must be avoided: a residual flow may persist within the proximal anterior part of the sinus (Fig. 7.13); and despite complete total thrombosis, the anterior part of the sinus remains smaller than the posterior part (Fig. 7.13). Thus, the posterior portion of the sinus should be always analyzed by angulating the transducer backward along the midline sagittal plane. Finally, high-frequency imaging is required for diagnostic reliability (Fig. 7.14).

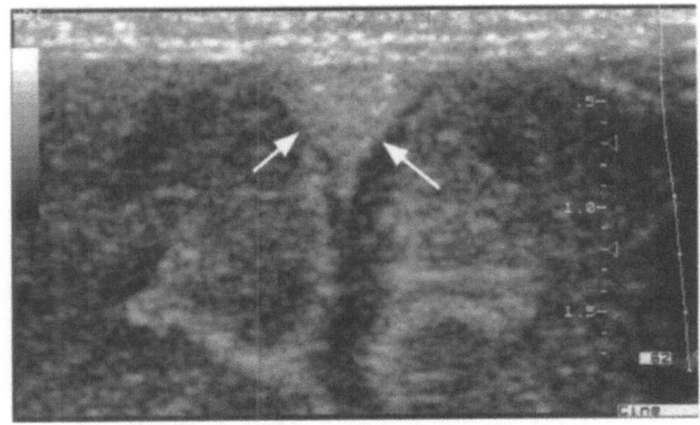

Fig. 7.10. A 15-day-old infant with hypotonia. High-frequency ultrasound, frontal plane. The superior sagittal sinus is widened (6 mm × 6 mm) with convex walls (*arrows*)

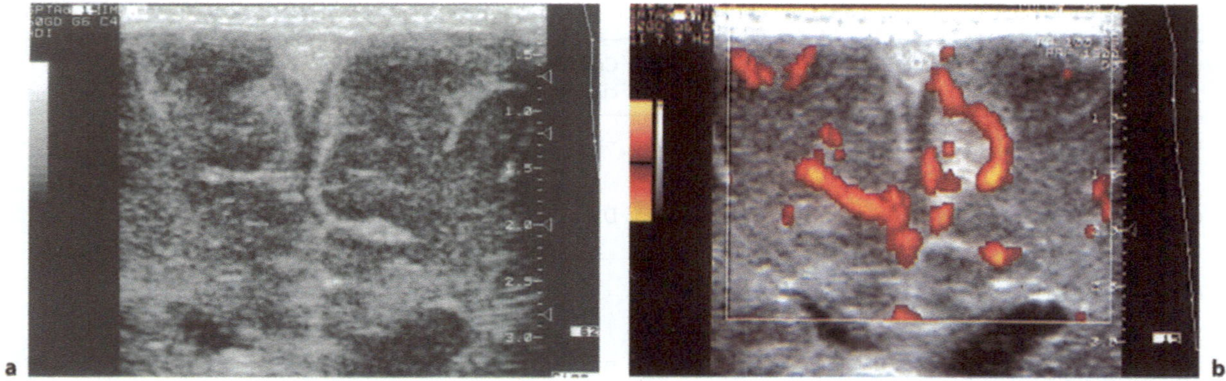

Fig. 7.11a,b. Seizure at 4 days of life. Sonographic investigation on day 15 showed a hyperechogenic superior sagittal sinus with convex walls (**a**). The diagnosis of thrombosis was confirmed by color Doppler, which failed to reveal any colored signal within it (**b**)

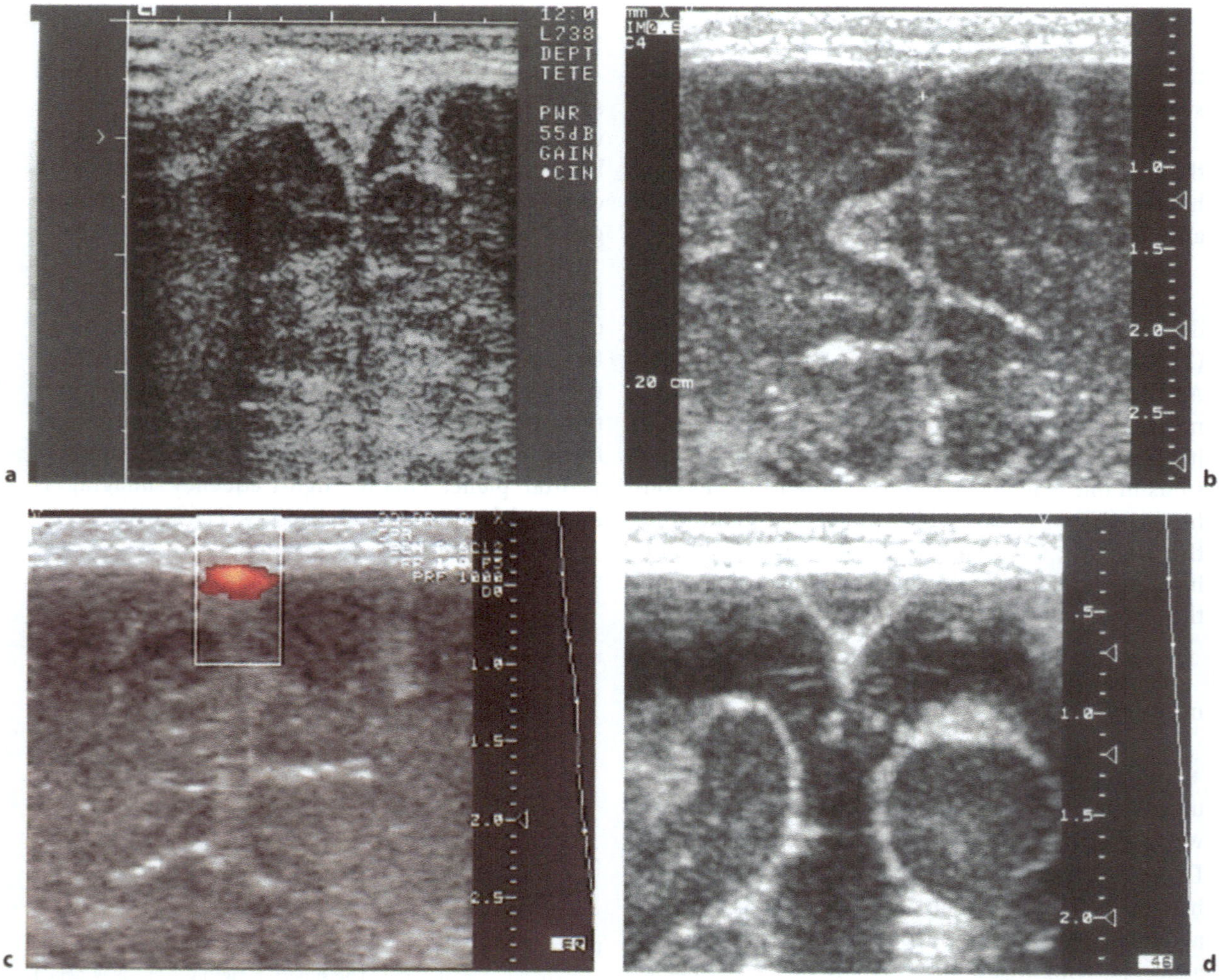

Fig. 7.12a–d. a Thrombosis of the superior sagittal sinus. **b–d** In the healthy newborn, the sinus is small (2 mm) and hypoechoic (**b**), with a colored flow on color Doppler (**c**); its lumen enlarges and becomes echofree when the baby cries (**d**)

Fig. 13a–c. A 4-day old neonate with ischemic brain damage. The superior sagittal sinus in incompletely thrombosed: its posterior part (*arrows*) shows no flow (**a**), while its anterior part (*arrow*) demonstrates a normal colored signal (**b**). **c** In this other patient with superior sagittal sinus thrombosis, the volume of the clot is much greater in the posterior (*single arrow*) than in the anterior portion of the sinus (*double arrows*)

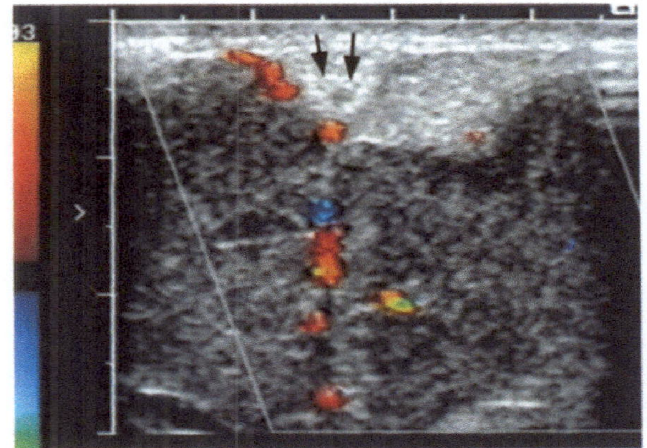

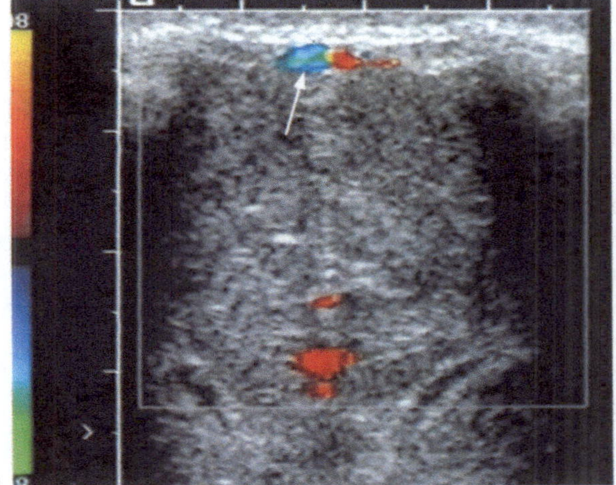

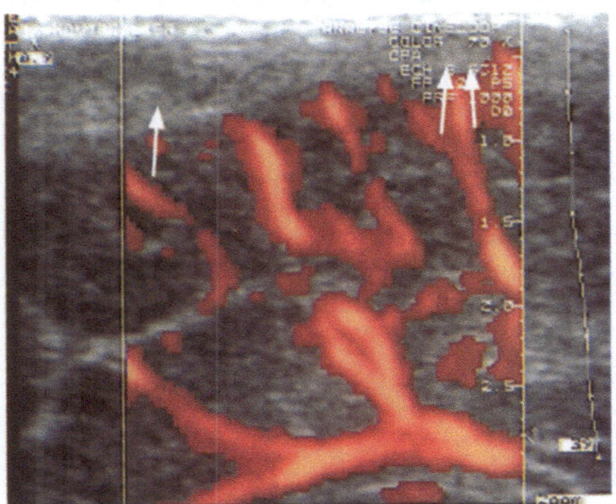

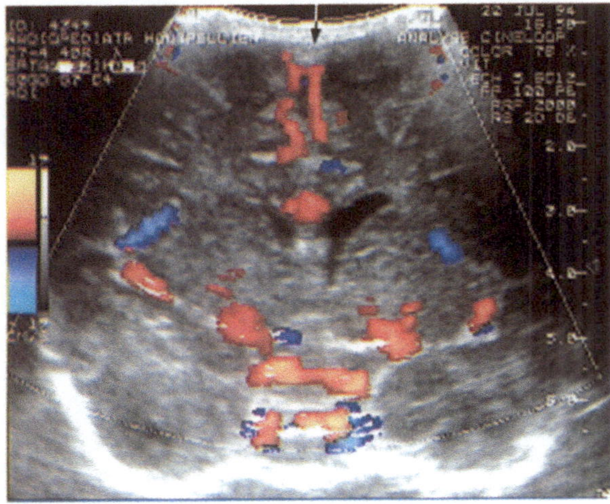

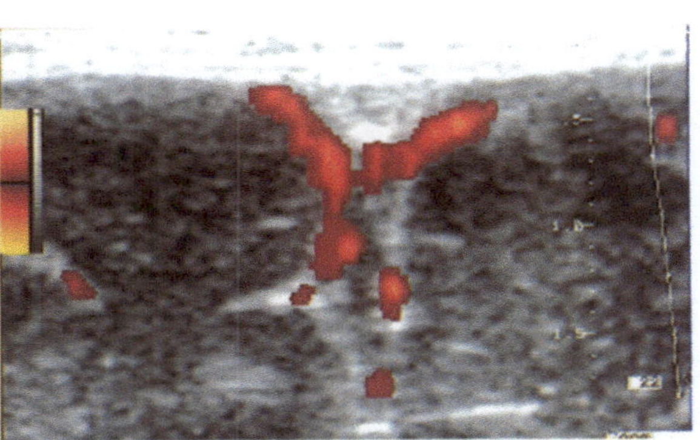

Fig. 7.14a,b. A 15-day-old infant. The superior sagittal sinus thrombosis (*arrow*) is difficult to detect with a 5-MHz transducer (**a**), but is evident with a high-frequency probe (**b**)

A well-established point is the high incidence of superior sagittal sinus involvement: 85% of venous thrombosis affect this dural sinus (DEVEBER 1993; KHURANA 1996; VOLPE 1995). VOLPE (1995) reported that the superior sagittal sinus was involved in 34 of 40 neonates.

● What about Doppler ultrasonography to diagnose thrombosis in the other sinuses and intracranial veins? The situations where this is relevant are rare, since most authors (KHURANA 1996; VOLPE 1995) consider that involvement of cerebral veins, especially the lateral sinuses and torcular, represents extension of the thrombotic process from the superior sagittal sinus. Less frequently, the deep venous system (internal cerebral vein, vein of Galen, straight sinus) is the first affected (HURST 1989; KHURANA 1996).

Morphological ultrasonography provides no information because the veins and sinuses are too small and too deeply located; everything relies on color Doppler.

During routine examination of a healthy newborn, the internal cerebral veins and vein of Galen are always excellently assessed by color and pulsed Doppler (Fig. 7.1). The only difficulty relates to the straight sinus, which is well depicted in the normal preterm and full-term newborn but may not (for technical reasons) be detected in the older infant. Finally, in contrast to CT and MRI, color Doppler imaging is unable to detect thrombosis of the cortical veins.

Among our six patients, color Doppler showed thrombosed lateral sinuses in one case and normal patency of the internal cerebral veins and vein of Galen in all six. The straight sinus was not detected in two cases.

7.4.2.2
Follow-Up

When venous thrombosis is diagnosed, follow-up becomes important. It is based on Doppler imaging (color and pulsed), which provides irreplaceable information relating to evolution, prognosis, and therapy.

● Follow-up ultrasonography shows morphological changes on the site of the thrombosis. In the five of our cases where serial examinations could be performed, the intraluminal thrombus constantly reduced in size (Fig. 7.15). Clot echogenicity remained unchanged in two cases, increased in one, and decreased in the other two (Fig. 7.16).

Although the echogenicity is variable and uninformative, progressive decrease of the clot volume is always a sign of favorable evolution and precedes recanalization of the sinus. Color Doppler demonstrated the development of collateral circulation around the sinus in three cases, appearing 4–10 days after the onset of disease (Fig. 7.17). It corresponds to dilated collateral veins (BEZINQUE 1995) within the superior sagittal sinus wall, and to the "empty delta sign" of CT.

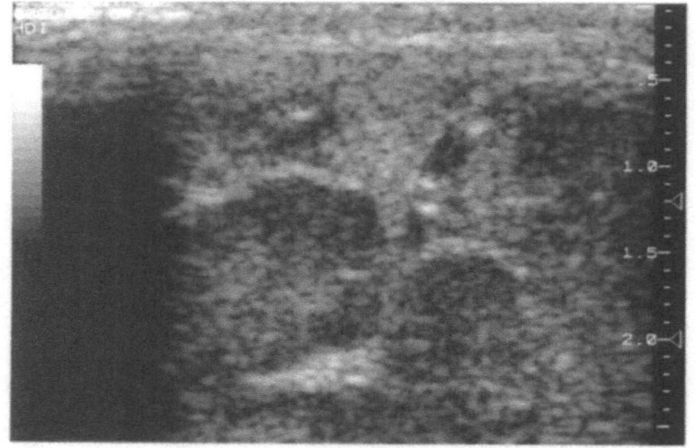

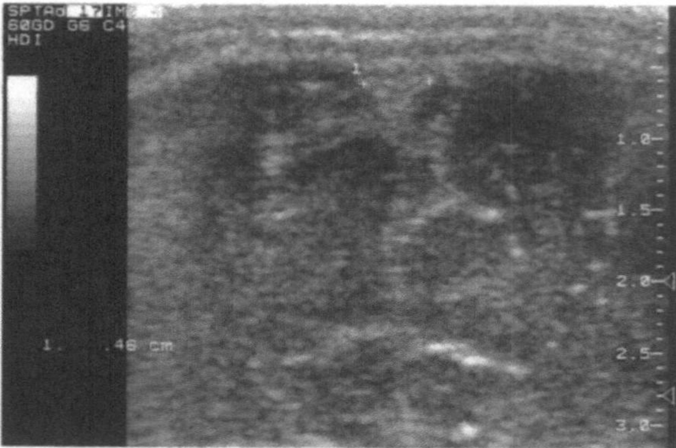

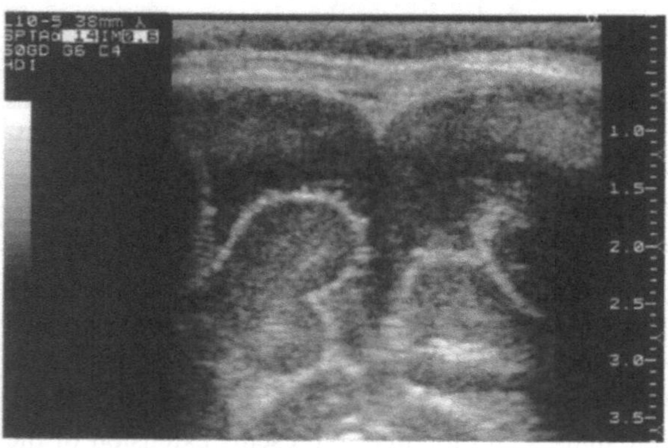

Fig. 7.15a–c. Thrombosis of the superior sagittal sinus.
a Day 5: the thrombosed sinus measures 8.5×7.5 mm.
b Day15: the sinus measures 5×4 mm. c Day 110: the sinus has recovered normal patency and measures 4×3.5 mm

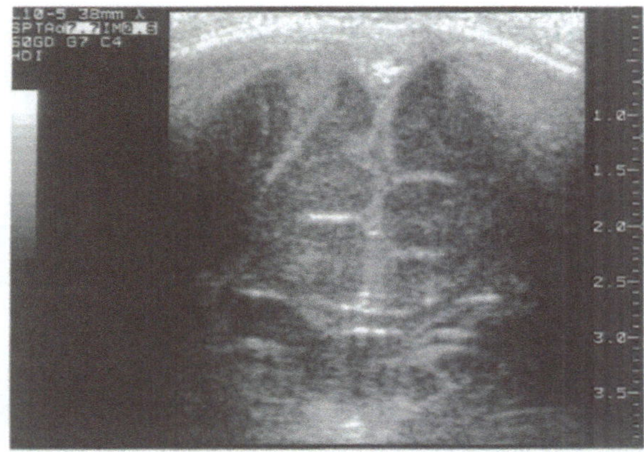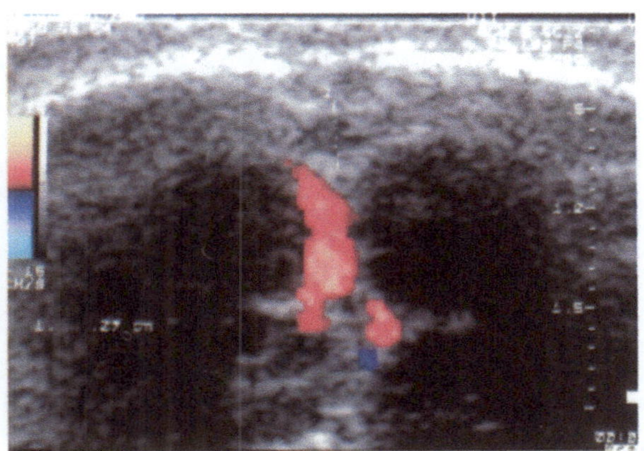

Fig. 7.16a,b. a A 3-week-old infant with pyogenic meningitis and superior sagittal sinus thrombosis. Hyperechoic punctuations are visible within the thrombosed sinus. b A 6-day-old neonate with superior sagittal sinus thrombosis. On day 15, the sinus takes on a misleading hypoechoic aspect, but color Doppler confirms persistence of the thrombosis

● The complications of cerebral venous thrombosis are well known and worsen the prognosis when present. They may be shown by ultrasonography (PEDESPAN 1996): small size of the lateral ventricles relates to cerebral edema; enlargement of the pericerebral spaces shows disturbed CSF resorption due to obstruction of venous flow return; while an increased resistive index and decreased diastolic velocity result from a rise in intracranial pressure.

In our cohort, transient acute intracranial hypertension was observed in one case (Fig. 7.18) and a pericerebral collection discussed in another case (Fig. 7.19).

However, obviously, ischemic and/or hemorrhagic brain injury constitute the most deleterious damage. Hemorrhagic venous infarction is located in the subcortical white matter: paramedian, bilateral frontal infarcts are strongly suggestive of superior sagittal sinus thrombosis. The deep white matter is less frequently involved. A common association is deep vein thrombosis with thalamic ischemic–hemorrhagic lesion (GOVAERT 1992).

A characteristic appearance with multiple rounded echodense nodes (VEYRAC 1994) may be observed. Although these lesions have been widely described in the literature (BARRON 1992; GOVAERT 1992; PEDESPAN 1996; VOLPE 1995), their mechanism remains unclear and the responsibility of vein thrombosis in the constitution of ischemic brain lesions is still uncertain.

– In several neonatal circumstances, ischemic damage may be either the cause or the consequence of cerebral venous thrombosis (PEDESPAN 1996). A preterm or full-term infant with neonatal distress (acute respiratory distress with disturbed cerebral venous flow return, arterial blood pressure instability, hypovolemia, severe neonatal asphyxia) is obviously susceptible to venous thrombosis, and

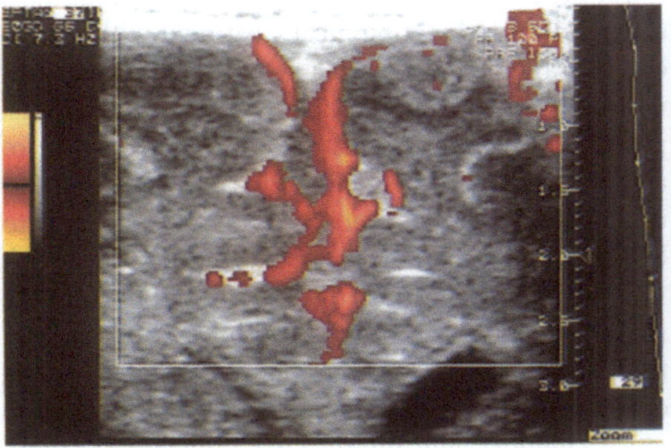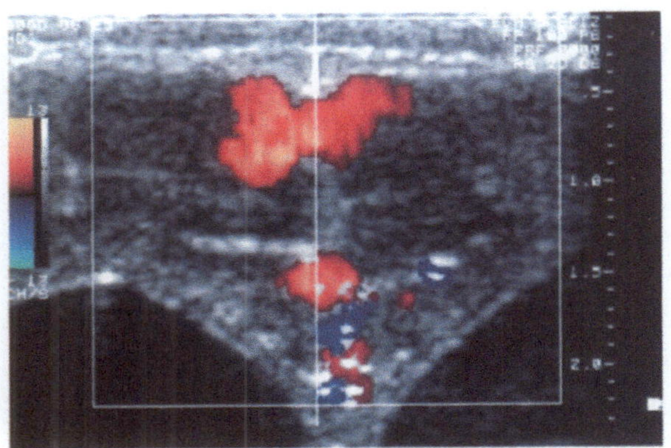

Fig. 7.17a,b. In these two cases of superior sagittal sinus thrombosis, the sinus walls appear moderately (a) or intensely (b) hyperemic

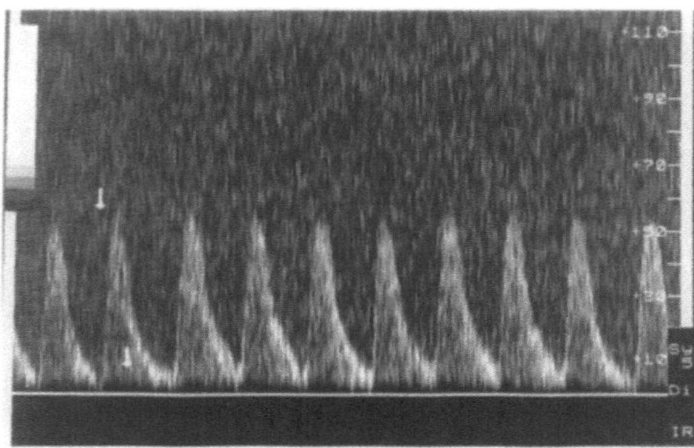 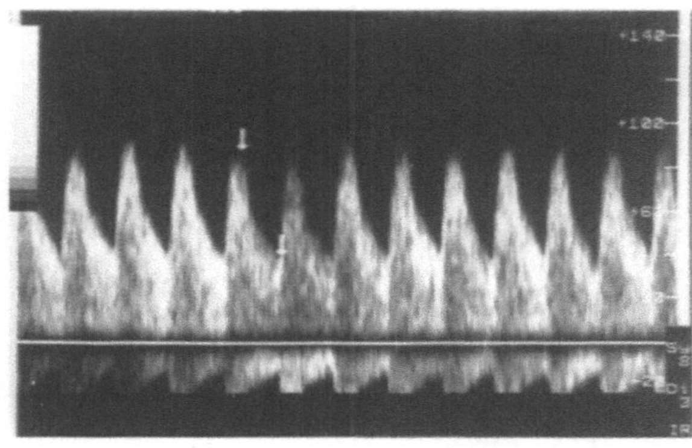

a   b

Fig. 7.18a,b. Purulent meningitis with superior sagittal sinus thrombosis. At 29 days of life, the Doppler spectrum of the anterior cerebral artery appears altered (**a**): normal PSV (57 cm/s), lowered EDV (7 cm/s), increased RI (0.88). This is probably related to an intracranial pressure rise that is moderate, latent, and transient; on day 38 (**b**) velocities and RI have returned to normal values

the first event is difficult to assess. This highlights the value of serial sonographic investigations (Fig. 7.20).

– In the opinion of most authors, the combination of venous thrombosis with ischemic brain damage is infrequent. VOLPE (1995) notes that the most common pattern of cerebral vein thrombosis is the absence of infarction. Despite this infrequency, there is an apparent correlation between the site of thrombosis and the location of ischemic–hemorrhagic lesions: parasagittal infarct and superior sagittal sinus involvement (VOLPE 1995), for example.
Several authors (BARRON 1992; GOVAERT 1992) consider that there is a real risk of gangliothalamic ischemia with deep vein thrombosis; the caudate nucleus and dorsal part of the thalamus are drained into the internal cerebral veins, and their

occlusion may obviously induce a deep hemorrhagic infarct.

– These uncertainties explain the high variability in evolution of neonatal cerebral thrombosis, the prognosis of which is poorly defined in the literature. The seven newborns reported by RIVKIN (1992) experienced a good outcome, but on the other hand MEDLOCK (1992) observed severe disorders of psychomotor development in four preterm infants. In the literature (BARAM 1988; HANIGAN 1986; RIVKIN 1992; SHEVELL 1989; VOLPE 1995) , more or less intense psychomotor retardation was seen in 11 (28%) of 40 patients studied. In a general manner, a more severe prognosis correlates with thrombosis occurring early with perinatal asphyxic injury (MEDLOCK 1992; PEDESPAN 1996; SHEVELL 1989). In our cohort, five patients had a favorable outcome and one patient died after severe hemodynamic distress.

As prognostic data are difficult to define, treatment is a subject of controversy in the literature (DE VEBER 1998; HIGASHIDA 1989; HOROWITZ 1995; MARCINIAK 1985). Some therapeutic interventions are not disputed – etiological treatment with antibiotic therapy or rehydration, symptomatic treatment with antiedematous, anticonvulsive medications, prevention of high-risk situations – but the role of any anticoagulant or fibrinolytic treatment remains undefined. Several authors report a given therapy to be useless or even dangerous, while others consider it to have value. HOROWITZ (1995) studied fibrinolytic treatment: in 12 newborns, urokinase infusion into the thrombosed sinus was followed by a favorable outcome in 10 cases, although 4 of them had previously a hemorrhagic infarct. DE VEBER (1998), studying 22 patients, showed that anticoagulant therapy, especially with low-molecular-weight heparin, may

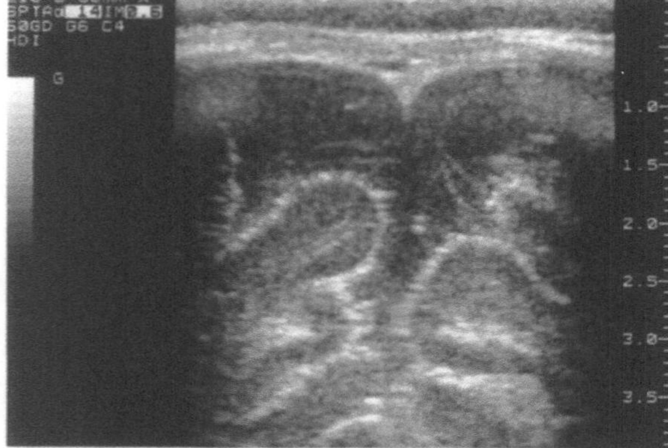

Fig. 7.19. Neonatal thrombosis of the superior sagittal sinus. On day 110, the last ultrasound examination showed resolution of the thrombosis and detected a pericerebral collection

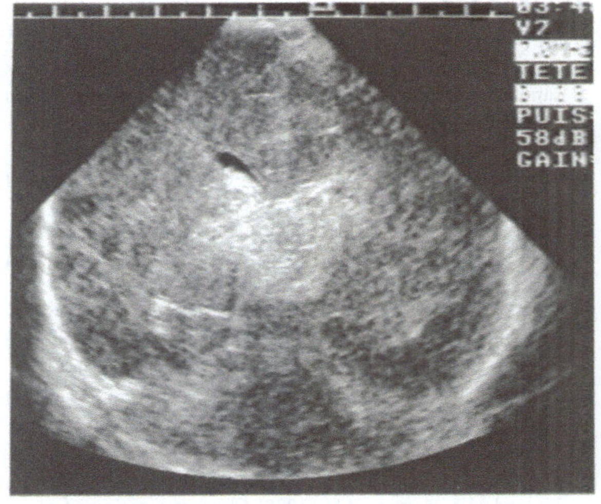

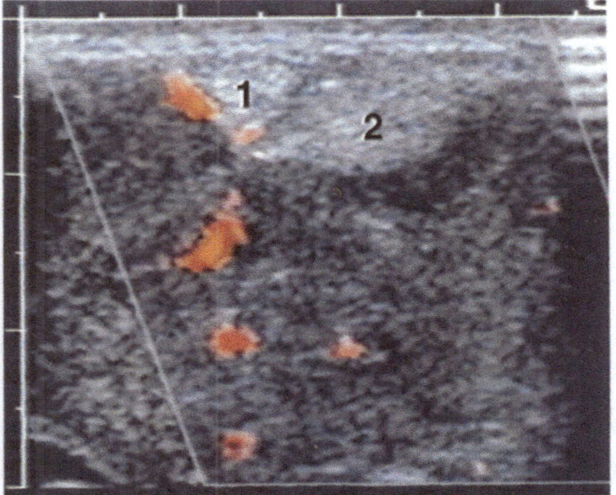

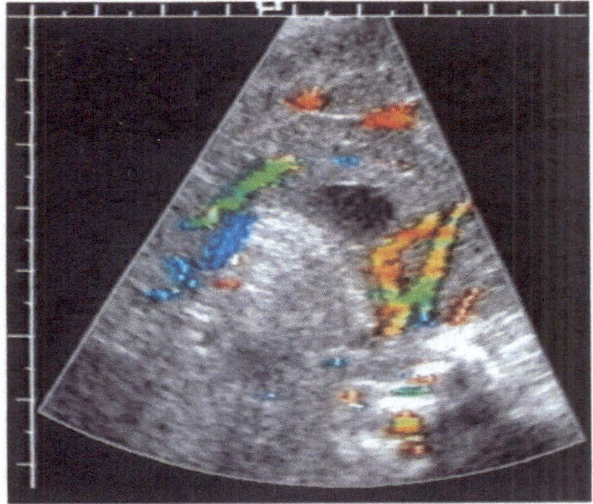

Fig. 7.20a–c. A 37-weeks' gestation infant with maternofetal sepsis and severe instability of arterial blood pressure. Ultrasonography (a,b) detects intraventricular hemorrhage, thalamic ischemic injury, superior sagittal sinus thrombosis (*1*), and an adjacent corticosubcortical hyperechoic lesion (*2*). Since the deep cerebral veins appear normally patent (c), the thalamic ischemia may be considered a result of the neonatal distress and the corticosubcortical lesion a post-thrombotic venous infarct

contribute to a good prognosis for cerebral venous thrombosis. In fact, between these two extreme positions, therapeutic intervention might be decided on the basis of imaging data: isolated sagittal sinus thrombosis might not require any treatment, whereas extensive or deep veins thrombosis might tend to indicate a specific treatment because of the risk of gangliothalamic ischemic injury.

7.4.2.3
Demonstration of Resolution of Thrombosis

It is important to demonstrate when a thrombosis has resolved. Some authors propose using MR angiography (CURE 1995; LEE 1995; MEDLOCK 1992; PEDESPAN 1996; WASENKO 1995). Our experience shows that color imaging is reliable for assessment of vessel recanalization, especially the superior sagittal sinus (Fig. 7.21) and lateral sinuses (Fig. 7.1).

7.5
Conclusion

Ultrasonography provides important information for diagnosing cerebral venous thrombosis:

- In the neonate, venous thrombosis is often unrecognized, especially because of its clinical latence. A color Doppler study in every neonatal brain ultrasonography might determine the true incidence of this disease. Color Doppler is obviously required in cases of unexplained seizure.
- Ultrasound diagnosis of superior sagittal sinus thrombosis is easy; detection of extensive or deep vein thrombosis (internal cerebral vein, vein of Galen, straight sinus) is possible. After 1 month of age, since a normal straight sinus may not be displayed, MRI is required for a complete evaluation.
- Despite the uncertainties in the evolution of the cerebral venous thrombosis, some factors are

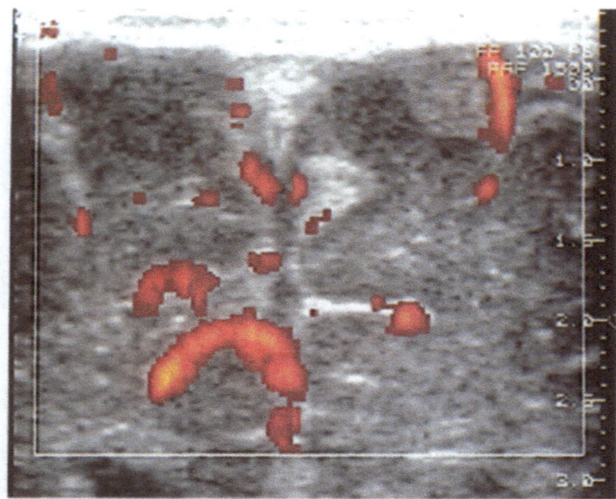

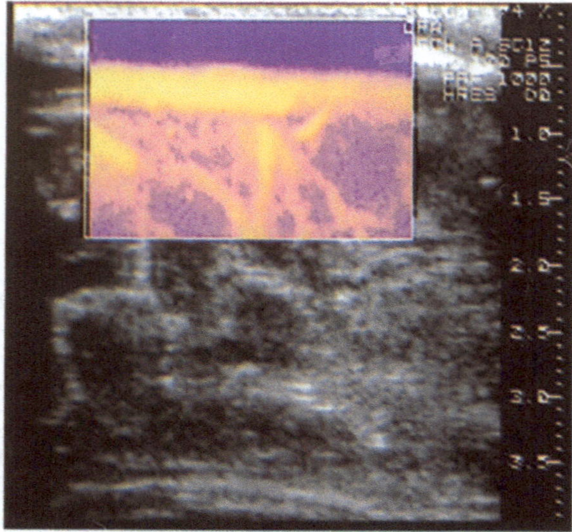

Fig. 7.21. a A 15-day-old infant with thrombosis of the superior sagittal sinus. **b** Recovery of normal intrasinusal flow at 2 months of age

important to determine. The pattern and severity of seizures do not tell very much, but a more severe outcome is observed in the case of the very young infant with secondary venous thrombosis. The main indicators are provided by imaging (ultrasound and MRI): a parenchymal ischemic injury is pejorative, while an extensive thrombosis carries the risk of gangliothalamic ischemia and probably requires specific treatment (GOVAERT 1992).
- The follow-up, detection of complications (intracranial hypertension, pericerebral collection), and confirmation of complete resolution are based on ultrasonography.
- In sum, detection of a cerebral venous thrombosis in neonates relies on ultrasonography, often complemented by MRI, while ultrasonography is the mainstay of follow-up.

References

Aicardi J, Goutieres F (1973) Les thromboses veineuses intracrâniennes. Complication des déshydratations aiguës du nourrisson. Arch Fr Pediatr 30:809-830

Ambruso DR, Jacobson LJ, Hataway WE (1980) Inherited antithrombin III deficiency and cerebral thrombosis in a child. Pediatrics 65:125-131

Baily OT, Hass GM (1931) Dural sinus thrombosis in early life: the clinical manifestations and extent of brain injury in acute sinus thrombosis. J Pediatr 11:755-771

Baram TZ, Butler IJ, Nelson MD, McArdle CB (1988) Transverse sinus thrombosis in newborns: clinical and magnetic resonance imaging findings. Ann Neurol 24:792-794

Barron TF, Gusnard DA, Zimmerman RA, Clancy RR (1992) Cerebral venous thrombosis in neonates and children. Pediatr Neurol 8:112-116

Bezinque SL, Slovis TL, Touchette AS, Schave DM, Jarski RW, Bedard MP, Martino AM (1995) Characterization of superior sagittal sinus blood flow velocity using color flow Doppler in neonates and infants. Pediatr Radiol 25:175-179

Byers BK, Hass GM (1933) Thrombosis of the dural venous sinuses in infancy and in childhood. Am J Dis Child 5:1161-1183

Cowan F, Thoresen B (1985) Changes in superior sagittal sinus blood velocities due to postural alterations and pressure on the head of the newborn infant. Pediatrics 75:1038-1047

Cure JK, Holden KR, Van Tassel P (1995) Progressive venous occlusion in a neonate with Sturge-Weber syndrome: demonstration with MR venography. AJNR Am J Neuroradiol 16:1539-1542

Davies RP, Slavotinek JP (1994) Incidence of the empty delta sign in computed tomography in the paediatric age group. Aust Radiol 38:17-19

Dean LM, Taylor GA (1995) The intracranial venous system in infants: normal and abnormal findings on duplex and color Doppler sonography. AJR Am J Roentgenol 164:151-156

De Veber G, Chan A, Monagle P, Marzinotto V, Armstrong D, Massicotte P, Leaker M, Andrew M (1998) Anticoagulation therapy in pediatric patients with sinovenous thrombosis: a cohort study. Arch Neurol 55:1533-1537

Edwards MK, Kuharik MA, Cohen MD (1987) Sonographic demonstration of cerebral sinus thrombosis. AJNR Am J Neuroradiol 8:1153-1155

Fenton AC, Papathoma E (1991) Neonatal cerebral venous flow velocity measurement using a color flow Doppler system. J Clin Ultrasound 19:69-72

Fofah O, Roth P (1997) Congenital nephrotic syndrome presenting with cerebral venous thrombosis, hypocalcemia and seizures in the neonatal period. J Perinatal 17:492-494

Friede RL (1973) Cerebral infarcts complicating neonatal leptomeningitis. Acta Neuropathol 23:245-248

Govaert P, Achten E, Vanhaesebrouck P, De Praeter C, Van Damme J (1992) Deep cerebral venous thrombosis in thalamo-ventricular hemorrhage on the term newborn. Pediatr Radiol 22:123-127

Govaert P, Voet D, Achten E, Vanhaesebrouck P, Van Rostenberghe H, Van Gysel D, Afschrift M (1992) Non invasive diagnosis of superior sagittal sinus thrombosis in a neonate. Am J Perinatol 9:201-204

Grossman R, Novak G, Patel M (1993) MRI in neonatal dural sinus thrombosis. Pediatr Neurol 9:235-238

Hanigan WC, Rossi LJ, McLean JM, Wright RM (1986) MRI of

cerebral vein thrombosis in infancy a case report. Neurology 36:1354-1356

Higashida RT, Helmer E, Van Halbach V, Hieshima GB (1989) Direct thrombolytic therapy for superior sagittal sinus thrombosis. AJNR Am J Neuroradiol 10:1-6

Horowitz M, Purdy P, Unwin H, Carstens G, Greenlee R, Hise J, Kopitnik T, Batjer H, Rollins N, Samson D (1995) Treatment of dural sinus thrombosis using selective catheterization and urokinase. Ann Neurol 38:58-67

Hurst RW, Kerns SR, McIlhenny J, Park TS, Caill WS (1989) Neonatal dural venous sinus thrombosis associated with cerebral venous catheterization: CT and MR studies. J Comput Assist Tomogr 13:504-507

Khurana DS, Buonanno F, Ebb D, Krishnamoorthy KS (1996) The role of anticoagulation in idiopathic cerebral venous thrombosis. J Child Neurol 11:248-250

Kim KS, Walczak TS (1986) Computed tomography of deep cerebral venous thrombosis. J Comput Assist Tomogr 10:386-390

Konishi Y, Kuriyama M, Sudo M, Konishi K, Hayakawa K, Ishii Y (1987) Superior sagittal sinus thrombosis in neonates. Pediatr Neurol 3:222-225

Kriss VM (1998) Hyperdense posterior falx in the neonate. Pediatr Radiol 28:817-819

Lam AH (1995) Doppler imaging of superior sagittal sinus thrombosis. J Ultrasound Med 14:41-46

Lee WT, Wang PJ, Young C, Shen YZ (1995) Cerebral venous thrombosis in children. Chung Hua Min Kuo Hsiao Erh Ko I Hsueh Hui Tsa Chih 36:425-430

Marciniak E, Wilson D, Marlar RA (1985) Neonatal purpura fulminans: a genetic disorder related to the absence of protein C in blood. Blood 65:15-20

Martinez-Menendez B, Sempere AP (1992) Cerebral venous thrombosis as a cause of neonatal focal clonic seizures. J Neurol 239:294

Medlock MD, Olivero WC, Hanigan WC, Wright RM, Winek SJ (1992) Children with cerebral venous thrombosis diagnosed with magnetic resonance imaging and magnetic resonance angiography. Neurosurgery 31:870-876

Miller GM, Black VD, Lubchenco LD (1981) Intracerebral hemorrhage in a term newborn with hyperviscosity. Am J Dis Child 137:377-380

Pedespan JM, Chateil JF, Pedespan-Joly L, Fontan D, Demarquez JL, Guillard JM (1996) Thromboses du sinus longitudinal superieur chez l'enfant au cours de la première année de vie: aspects cliniques, imagerie et évolution. Arch Fr Pediatr 3:561-565

Pfannschmidt J, Jorch G (1989) Transfontanelle pulsed Doppler measurement of blood flow velocity in the internal jugular vein, straight sinus, and internal cerebral vein in preterm and term neonates. Ultrasound Med Biol 15:9-12

Rivkin MJ, Anderson ML, Kaye EM (1992) Neonatal idiopathic cerebral venous thrombosis: an unrecognized cause of transient seizures or lethargy. Ann Neurol 32:51-56

Schubiger G, Schubiger O, Tonz O (1982) Superior sagittal sinus thrombosis in the newborn. Diagnosis by computed tomography. Helv Paediatr Acta 37:193-199

Segall HD, Ahmadi J, McComb JG, Zee CS, Becker TS, Han JS (1982) Computed tomographic observations pertinent to intracranial venous thrombotic and occlusive disease in childhood. Radiology 143:441-449

Shevell ML, Silver K, O'Gorman AM, Watters GV, Montes JL (1989) Neonatal dural sinus thrombosis. Pediatr Neurol 5:161-165

Veyrac C, Couture A, Baud C (1994) Echographie cérébrale du fœtus au nouveau-né: imagerie et hémodynamique. Sauramps Médical, Montpellier, pp 371-392

Virapongse C, Cazenave G, Quisling R, Sarwar M, Hunter S (1987) The empty delta sign: frequency and significance in 76 cases of dural sinus thrombosis. Radiology 162:779-785

Volpe JJ (1995) Neurology of the newborn, 3rd edn. Saunders, Philadelphia, pp 279-313

Voorhies TM, Lipper EG, Lee BC, Vannucci RC, Auld PA (1984) Occlusive vascular disease in asphyxiated newborn infants. J Pediatr 105:92-96

Wasenko JJ, Holsapple JW, Winfield JA (1995) Cerebral venous thrombosis. Demonstration with magnetic resonance angiography. Clin Imaging 19:153-161

Watson GH (1974) Effect of head rotation on jugular vein blood flow. Arch Dis Child 49:237-239

Wintzen AR, Broekmans AW, Bertina RM, Briet E, Briet PE, Zecha A, Vielvoye GJ, Bots GT (1985) Cerebral hemorrhagic infarction in young patients with hereditary protein C deficiency: evidence for spontaneous cerebral venous thrombosis. Br Med J 290:350-352

Wong VK, Lemesurier J, Franceschini R (1987) Cerebral venous thrombosis as a cause of neonatal seizures. Pediatr Neurol 3:235-237

Wright LL, Baker KR, Hollander DI, Wright JH, Nagey DA (1988) Cerebral blood flow velocity in term newborn infants: changes associated with ductal flow. J Pediatr 112:768-773

8 Intracranial Infections

CORINNE VEYRAC

CONTENTS

8.1
Bacterial Meningitis

Purulent meningitis remains a severe disease in the neonate, with a high death rate (ranging from 19% to 50%) and common neurodevelopmental sequelae (in up to 30% of survivors). This potential severity is related to the frequency of complications and irreversible brain damage.

Ultrasound has a major place in the detection of complications (VEYRAC 1994), since clinical symptoms are often latent and mostly nonspecific (fever, irritability, vomiting, poor feeding, lethargy, bulging fontanelle, focal cerebral signs).

Complications depend in part on the infecting agent. In recent years, Group B *Streptococcus* has been commonly encountered, with its high risk of ischemic injury; *Escherichia coli* and *Listeria* tend to be responsible for ventriculitis, and *Proteus mirabilis* for brain abscess, while *Streptococcus pneumoniae*, *Haemophilus influenzae*, and *Neisseria meningitidis*, more usually observed in the older infant, may lead to ischemic damage and subdural collections.

C. VEYRAC, MD
Service de Radiologie Pédiatrique, Hôpital Arnaud de Villeneuve, 371 av. Doyen Gaston Giraud, 34295 Montpellier Cedex, France

The severity of the brain disease is due to impairment of the cerebral perfusion as a consequence of meningitic infection. This is why it is important to study hemodynamics in a newborn with pyogenic meningitis.

8.1.1
Physiopathogenic Phenomena

MINNS (1989) reported increased intracranial pressure as a common accompaniment of pyogenic meningitis. It may be due to an increase in any intracranial compartment (TUREEN 1990), including CSF; SHELD (1980) demonstrated increased resistance to CSF outflow, probably due to dysfunction of the arachnoid membrane.

Increased brain water content as a consequence of brain edema may also contribute, and may be aggravated by inappropriate ADH secretion. However, some authors have shown that antiedematous effect of some drugs did not correlate with a decrease in intracranial pressure (TAÜBER 1987; TUREEN 1987).

In a rabbit model with experimental pneumococcal meningitis, TUREEN (1990) demonstrated that intracranial pressure changed in parallel with cerebral blood flow, although this phenomenon was not observed in controls. He noted that cerebral edema may result in loss of brain compliance, which may be responsible for increased sensitivity to small changes in intracranial blood volume. Finally, he observed a loss in cerebral autoregulation, as shown by a correlation between changes in cerebral blood flow and systemic arterial pressure. This phenomenon was not present in controls.

Impairment of the normal mechanism for matching cerebral perfusion with metabolic demand leaves the brain at risk of significant hypo- or hyperperfusion. Cerebral perfusion is known to be a critical determinant of short- and long-term neurodevelopmental outcome. Thus, GOITEIN and TAMIR (1983) found that low cerebral perfusion pressure correlated strongly with death or neurological injury. Increased intracranial pressure associated with increased mean arterial pressure should not indicate a poor prognosis unless the arterial pressure elevation is injurious by causing a spike in intracranial pressure.

It appears that there is probably a narrow range of cerebral perfusion pressure required for adequate cerebral blood flow without aggravating intracranial hypertension.

It is important to know these different physio-pathogenic data that lie behind cerebral injury in neonatal purulent meningitis, because some of them may be easily assessed by pulsed Doppler imaging.

An increased resistive index (RI) has been shown to be significantly related to increased intracranial pressure. MacMenamin and Volpe (1984) reported that the degree of intracranial hypertension was not usually severe enough to raise the possibility of impaired cerebral perfusion except in infants older than newborns. In these cases, they described increased RI and decreased mean flow velocities. In 17 children, aged between 8 days and 6 years, and including 4 newborns, Goh and Minns (1993) observed a significant increase in RI at hospital admission, associated with decreased end-diastolic velocity. In their 16 survivors, they noted a gradual decrease in this index under treatment, a significant correlation between RI and intracranial pressure, RI and cerebral perfusion pressure, and mean flow velocity and cerebral perfusion pressure. In contrast to this, they did not demonstrate any significant correlation between RI and mean arterial pressure, or between mean flow velocity and mean arterial pressure. Finally, in the three patients in whom Doppler studies were correlated with mannitol infusions, the authors observed a decrease in RI after mannitol administration. During the course of the disease, RI normalization was due to a significant increase in end-diastolic velocity, with no significant change in the peak-systolic velocity. In the only neonate who died, they noticed a correlation between cerebral blood flow velocities and systemic mean arterial pressure, following a pressure-passive pattern, suggesting loss of cerebral autoregulation. Thus, this is important for management, since close attention to maintaining normal systemic blood pressure should be required when a pressure-passive response is shown in a newborn with pyogenic meningitis.

Determination of cerebral blood flow requires the use of stable xenon computed tomography (Ashwal 1990), but mean velocity changes reflect CBF variations. Therefore, it is useful to detect situations with markedly decreased mean flow, because they correlate with poor outcome (brain death, severe ischemic damage, shunted hydrocephalus).

In our experience of 20 cases of meningitis studied using Doppler imaging, we noted an increased RI on hospital admission in all cases, except for three newborns in whom it was normal. Two of these developed an *Escherichia coli* ventriculitis but recovered without ventriculoperitoneal shunting, while the third had a subdural collection that resolved spontaneously with normal outcome. Complications occurred in all the other infants who had a markedly increased index: shunted postventriculitis hydrocephalus, multifocal abscesses, severe ischemic lesions, and subdural collections with neurological sequelae.

8.1.2
Ventriculitis

Ventriculitis is a common feature of neonatal meningitis, and, on anatomic examination, overt ventriculitis is present in 65%–100% of brains (Berman 1986; Daum 1978). It is particularly frequent after *E. coli* meningitis, and different reports have recorded frequencies ranging from 14% to 50% of all complications (in our experience the frequency was 38%).

Ultrasonography has demonstrated excellent reliability for this diagnosis. The main feature is the presence of more or less dense echoes, moving within the ventricular lumen (Fig. 8.1), or fluid-fluid levels, or thin membranes, or thick strands septating the ventricles.

Color Doppler provides valuable new data when it demonstrates a colored flow within the sylvian aqueduct (Fig. 8.2).

This pattern has been described and detailed in Sect. 3.1.2. It means that the CSF contains an abnormal concentration of scattering particles, sufficient to enable color detection of a to-and-fro motion of CSF through the ventricular system; this appears on scanning as an area of red and blue, best observed in the aqueduct of Sylvius, the narrowest point of the ventricular system.

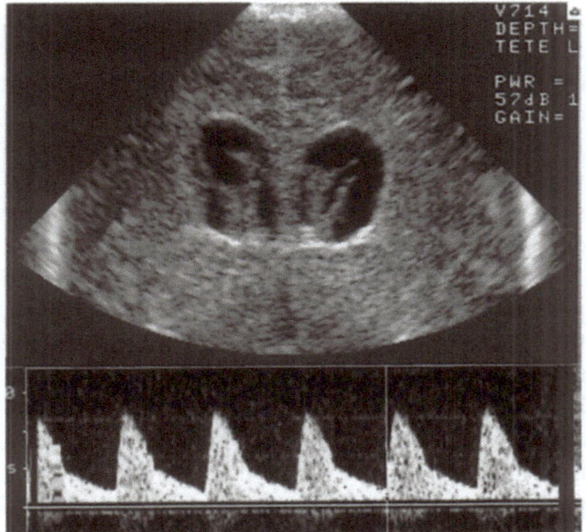

Fig. 8.1. An 11-day-old neonate with tonic-clonic seizures. *Escherichia coli* meningitis. First ultrasonography, at admission, showed the presence of thin membranes within dilated ventricles. Pulsed Doppler was performed on the anterior cerebral artery. Increased RI: 0.84; normal peak-systolic velocity: 50 cm/s

First described by WINKLER (1992) in infected neonates, it was observed by TATSUNO (1993) in two of eight cases of meningitis with ventricular involvement. These two infants presented signs of ventriculitis and eventually required ventriculoperitoneal shunt, while the other six neonates demonstrated normal findings in four and a transient subdural effusion in two. Among eight patients with ventriculitis that we studied in the last years, a colored flow was detected in seven when it was investigated. The only negative case was that of a 3-month-old infant whose lateral ventricles were already septated at first ultrasonography, 2 days after clinical onset of the disease.

In all our cases, intraluminal echoes were simultaneously detected, but in two infants, only very thin echoes were found, close to the medial wall of the left ventricle and difficult to differentiate from technical artifacts. In the literature (TATSUNO 1993), a colored flow has been described as detected earlier than intraventricular echoes, confirming the great value of this feature for early diagnosis of ventriculitis.

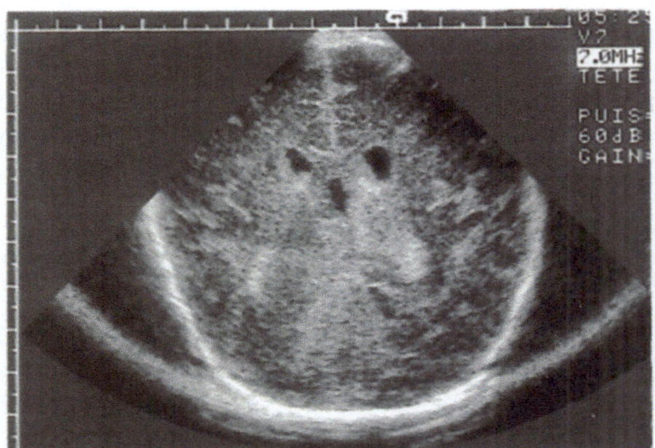

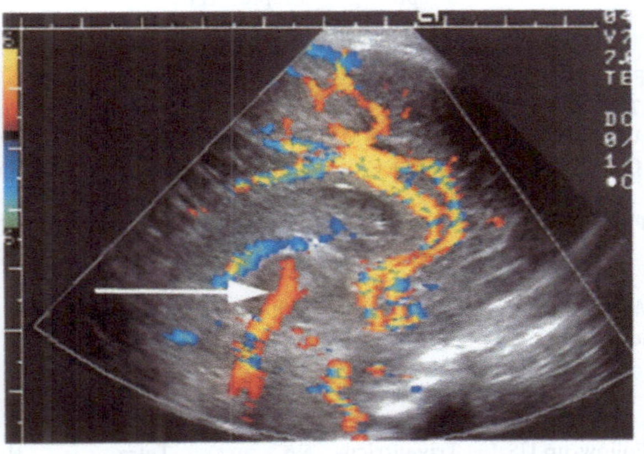

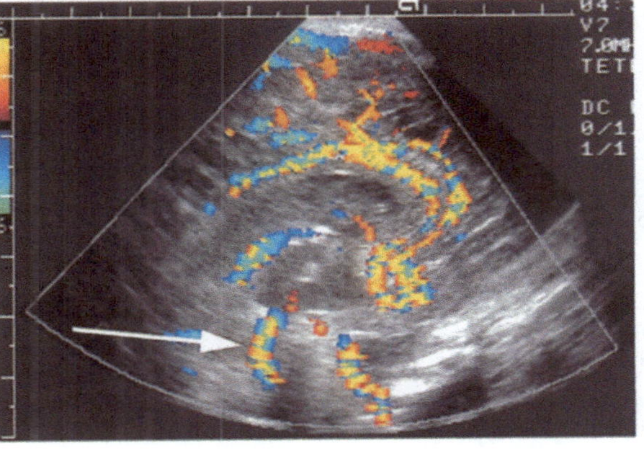

Fig. 8.2a–c A 4-day-old newborn with fever and seizures. *Escherichia coli* meningitis. On day 1, the sonogram was normal. Routine follow-up on day 4. **a** Small thin echoes, in the left ventricle, close to the medial wall: the diagnosis of ventriculitis is doubtful. **b,c** Color Doppler on the medial line (sagittal plane). Colored signal, alternating *red* and *blue*, within the aqueduct of Sylvius (*straight arrow*): ventriculitis is confirmed

In our series, demonstration of a colored signal in CSF did not correlate with a worse prognosis: two patients had a normal outcome, three required a ventriculoperitoneal shunt, and three died (two with diffuse ischemic lesions and one with a severe myelomeningocele) / (Table 8.1).

Of course, this finding lacks specificity: it is a common sign of ventricular hemorrhage. We also detected it in a patient with Down syndrome and congenital leukemia (3×10^5 leukoblasts in CSF), and in a neonate with chylothorax (another case is described by WINKLER 1992).

Theoretically, this sign should be useful to confirm persistent patency of the sylvian aqueduct. In the same way, detection of similar flow within the foramina of Lushka and Magendie would be valuable, but requires a transcranial examination (WINKLER 1992). In fact, in clinical practice, colored signal rapidly disappears with effective treatment, even in a patent aqueduct.

The second great usefulness of Doppler imaging in ventriculitis is to diagnose raised intracranial pressure when ventricular dilatation develops. This was detailed in Chap. 4.

In our patients with ventriculitis, when RI and peak systolic velocities were measured on admission, they had higher values in neonates who eventually required a shunt placement (except those with ischemic lesions), than in those who did not. However, this is based on a too small number of cases and needs to be confirmed before it can be regarded as a prognostic indicator.

Table 8.1. Ventriculitis (8 patients)

	Patient 1	Patient 2	Patient 3	Patient 4	Patient 5	Patient 6	Patient 7	Patient 8
Clinical data Age at symptoms	Maternal infection No symptoms	Septic shock Day 2	Seizures Day 4	Seizures Day 11	Septic shock Day 3	Seizures Day 15	Seizures Day 18	Status epilepticus 3 months
Infecting agent	Group B Strepto- coccus	Group B Streptococcus	E. coli	E. coli	E. coli	E. coli	E. coli	Neisseria meningitidis
First US Time of disease US finding[a] Color Doppler[b]	Day 1 Echoes + Flow +++	Day 11 Echoes +++ Flow ++	Day 6 Echoes + Flow ++	Day 1 Echoes +++ Flow +++	Day 4 Echoes ++ Flow ++	Day 1 Echoes ++ Non searched flow	Day 1 Echoes ++ Flow +++	Day 2 Septations + No flow
Pulsed Doppler	RI: 0.60 PSV: 35	RI: 0.64 PSV: 34	RI: 0.60 PSV: 45	RI: 0.80 PSV: 50	RI: 0.80 PSV: 45	RI: 0.71 PSV: 57	RI: 0.80 PSV: 55	RI: 0.60 PSV: 72
Associated lesions		Ischemia +++				Sagittal sinus thrombosis		Ischemia +++ Subdural collection
Follow-up US	Triventricular dilatation Days 4→15 Regression Days 20→30	No dilatation	Tetra- ventricular dilatation Days 12→27 Regression after D30	Highly progressive dilatation VP Shunt at D26	Highly progressive dilatation	Highly progressive dilatation VP Shunt at day 23	Highly progressive dilatation VP shunt at day 34	Highly progressive dilatation
Clinical outcome	Macro- crania Torticollis No shunt	Died	Normal No shunt	Deafness Hypotonia Retardation	Died (myelome- ningocele)	Normal	Normal	Died

[a] Presence of intraventricular echoes.
[b] Presence of colored flow within Sylvian aqueduct.
RI: resistive index
PSV: peak systolic velocity (cm/s)

8.1.3
Ischemic Complications

In neonatal pyogenic meningitis, aseptic ischemic lesions are characterized by their frequency (approximately 30% of complications according to FRIEDE 1973, 33% in our recent series), and their severe neurodevelopmental prognosis (VOLPE 1987). Several lesional patterns are encountered:

1. Venous infarcts are caused by multiple thrombi occluding leptomeningeal and cortical veins, which are encompassed or/and directly infiltrated by dense inflammatory exudates. Most often, the infarcts are located within cortical gray matter and underlying white matter, although subependymal and deep white matter damage is not uncommon. These lesions are frequently hemorrhagic (characteristic of venous infarcts). They may appear as intensely hyperechoic nodules, tending to be cortical or subcortical in location (Fig. 8.3a,b).

Color Doppler imaging shows these nodules distorting the small adjacent vessels, which remain patent (Fig. 8.3c,d). In other cases, it may demonstrate the disappearance of flow in larger veins, such as the terminal vein which drains the cerebral white matter through the medullary veins; terminal vein thrombosis may result in secondary white matter hemorrhagic infarction.

2. Major arterial occlusions are more usually observed in infants with *Streptococcus pneumoniae* or *Haemophilus influenzae* meningitis. The arteritis is manifested by inflammatory cells in the adventitia, although involvement of the intima is not uncom-

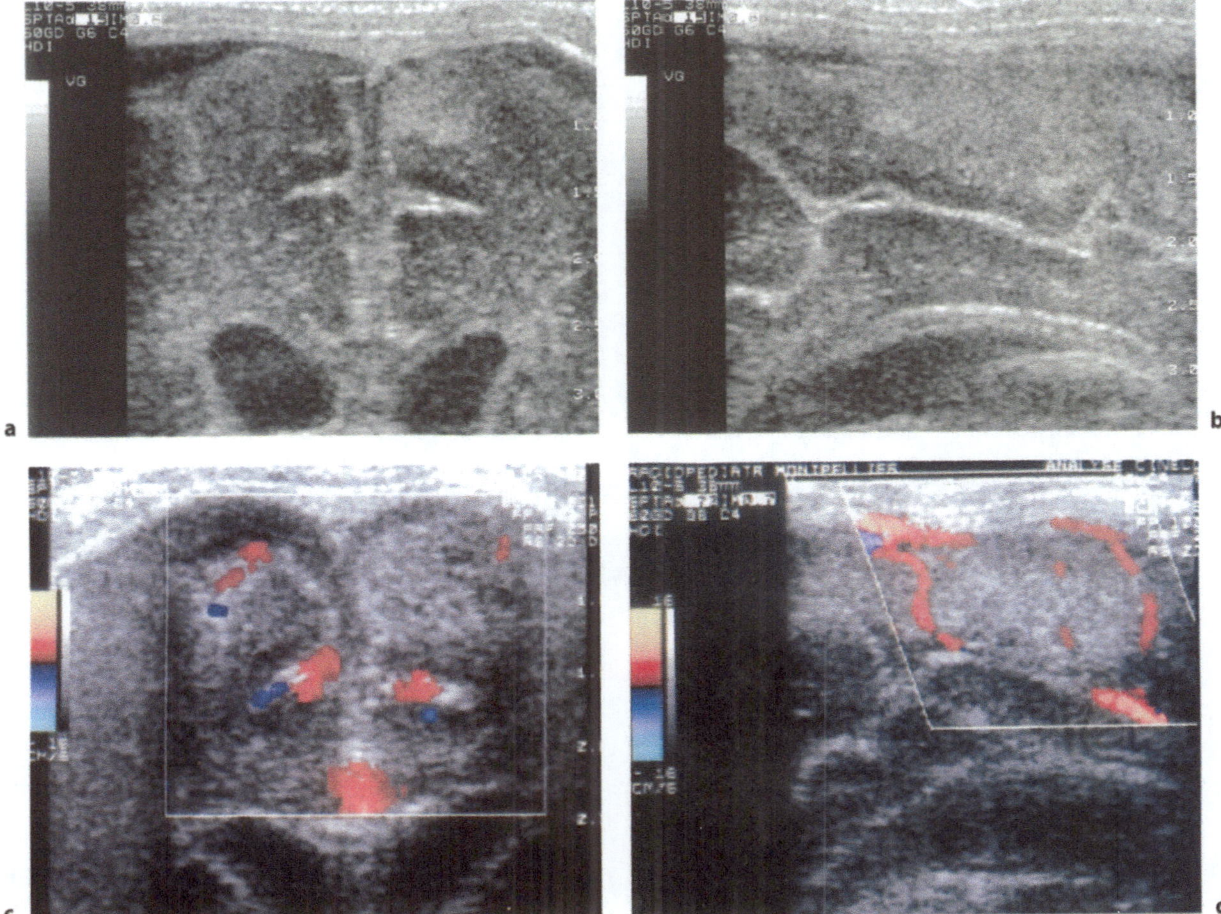

Fig. 8.3a–d A 36-hour-old neonate with septic shock and seizures. Group B *Streptococcus* meningitis. Ultrasonography on day 13 (**a,b**) shows cortical echogenic nodules, suggesting venous infarcts. **a** Coronal scan, **b** parasagittal scan. On color Doppler imaging (**c,d**), there is absence of flow within the nodule, compression of adjacent vessels, which are arcuate and displaced forward backward and outward, but a normal situation of the underlying sulcus. **c** Coronal scan, **d** parasagittal scan

mon (RAIMONDI 1979). In contrast to venous involvement, arterial wall thickening leads to secondary narrowing of the lumen, only rarely is complete occlusion observed. Segmental vasospasm close to the inflammatory area certainly plays an additional role. Post-mortem studies frequently fail to detect a thrombus or embolus within an artery that was occluded at the time of angiography. RAIMONDI (1979) suggested a combination of factors such as intimal hyperplasia, compression of the arteries by thickened meninges and exudates, spastic constrictions of the arteries, and increased intracranial pressure. This results in an infarction of arterial distribution, and cystic evolution.

In these cases, color Doppler imaging of major cerebral arteries show asymmetric flow with disappeared signal on one side. Hemodynamic study confirms either the complete absence of signal, or accelerated flow velocity within the damaged cerebral artery, as has been described by transcranial Doppler (BORNKE 1996). The recovery of arterial patency may also be demonstrated and followed-up by color and pulsed Doppler (Fig. 8.4a,b). Most vasospasms are not long and intense enough to produce ischemic damage.

3. Ischemic lesions are similar in their topography and evolution to hypoxic ischemic encephalopathy, of which we have previously described the risk factors and modalities of occurrence. Pulsed Doppler is of great value and can provide some critical findings:

- It can detect high-risk situations of severe ischemia by showing markedly decreased systolic and mean flow velocities, indicating low cerebral blood flow; it is associated with either an increased RI, a sign of marked intracranial hypertension (Fig. 8.11c), or a low RI, a sign that ischemic lesions are already patent (Fig. 8.5c).
- It can detect loss of cerebral autoregulation by demonstrating fluctuations in blood flow velocities correlated with systemic arterial pressure changes (Fig. 8.11b).

The main limitation of Doppler analysis is that it corresponds to a brief recording; any treatment interacting on cerebral hemodynamics should rely on Doppler monitoring.

In our experience, ischemic injury appears very early in the course of meningitis, and in most cases the lesions are already visible on admission to hospital.

Color Doppler shows distorted small vessels close to the hyperechoic ischemic lesion, confirming its edematous character, and absence of colored signal within it.

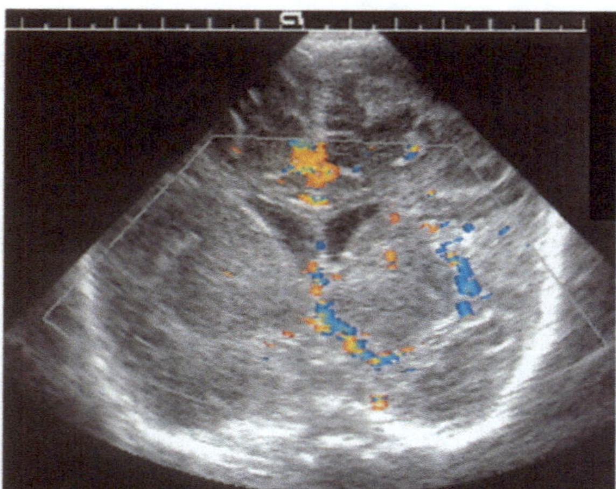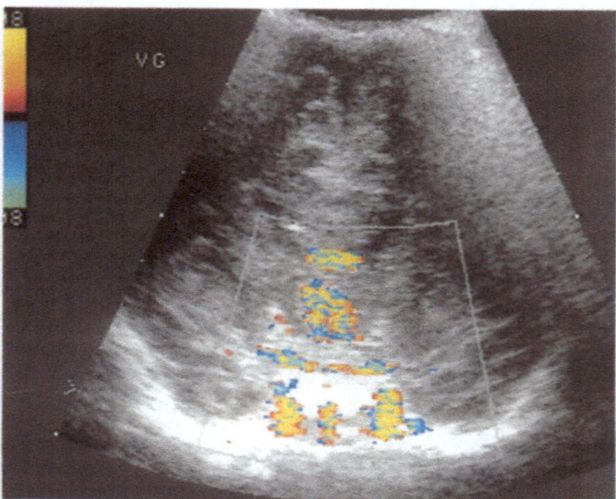

Fig. 8.4a,b. A 3-month-old infant with unilateral left seizures and paralysis of left cranial nerves (III, VI, VII). *Streptococcus pneumoniae* meningitis with ethmoiditis. **a** Day 1. Color Doppler. No flow was visualized in the right internal carotid and right middle cerebral arteries; otherwise the examination was normal. **b** Two days later, there was normal and symmetric visibility of carotid flow, without infarction. Clinical outcome was normal at 15 months. The probable explanation is vasospasm of the major basal vessels of the brain

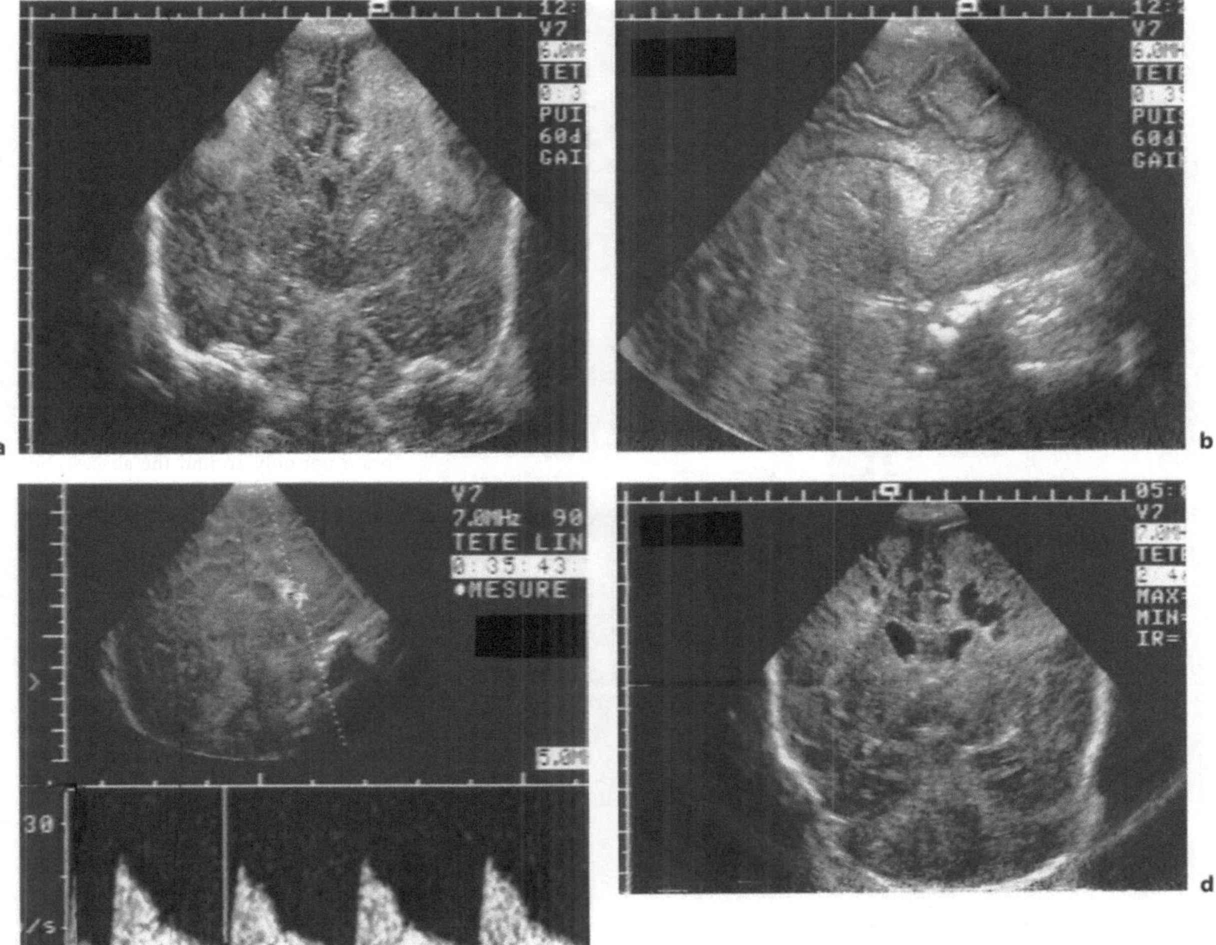

Fig. 8.5a–d. A 4-day-old newborn with fever, bulging fontanelle, abnormal behavior, and seizures on EEG. *Proteus mirabilis* meningitis. a–c First ultrasonography on admission shows extensive hyperechogenicity of subcortical white matter. Pulsed Doppler on the anterior cerebral artery (c) shows increased RI (0.77) and low PSV (22 cm/s) and time-average velocity (10 cm/s): low blood flow with intracranial pressure increase. d Five days later, cysts have formed within the lesions

8.1.4
Brain Abscess

This uncommon complication is associated with a poor neurodevelopmental prognosis, and a high mortality rate. The clinical features are ambiguous and not very suggestive, meaning that a systematic sonographic examination is required for early diagnosis.

The causative organisms are *Proteus mirabilis*, but also *Serratia, Citrobacter, Staphylococcus aureus*, and others. Brain abscesses are commonly multifocal (SUTTON 1983), located at the cortico-subcortical junction, usually in frontal (50%) and parietal (parieto-occipital or parieto–temporal) lobes.

Nowadays, they are often detected at the stage of cerebritis, before being collected (ENZMAN 1982); the lesion is hyperechoic, smooth-edged, unwalled, and located at the cortico-subcortical junction (Fig. 8.6).

Color Doppler does not show any signal in the lesion (since it corresponds to infected necrotic tissue, FOREMAN 1984), and only small peripheral vessels are visualized, which remain distant from the lesion (Fig. 8.6a).

Very quickly, the lesion becomes circumscribed, round in shape, with a hypoechoic heterogeneous center and an hyperechoic rim. Vessels that appear on color Doppler are close to the collected lesion, running around it. Early perilesional hyperemia may also be found (Fig. 8.6g).

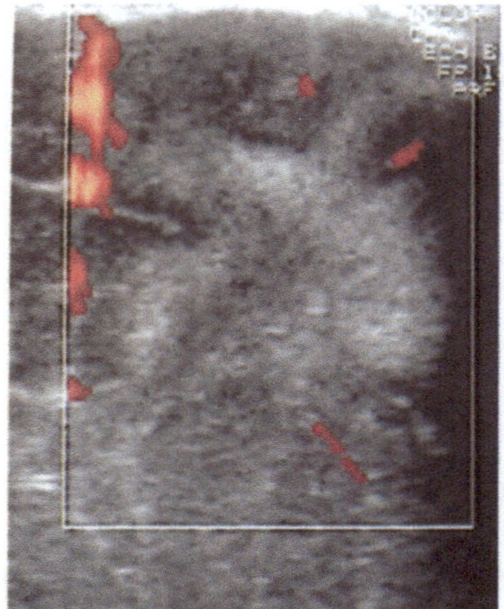

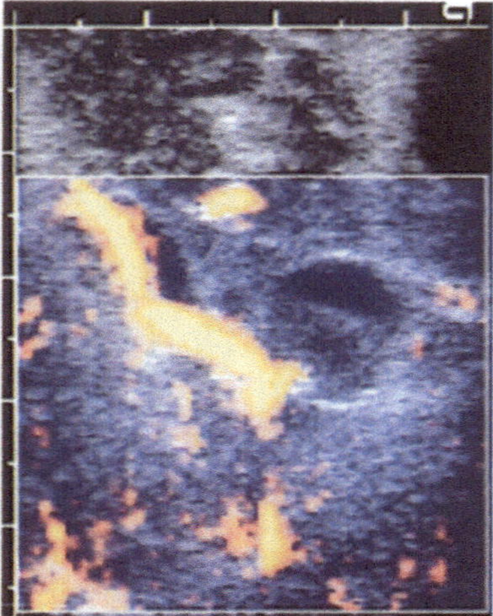

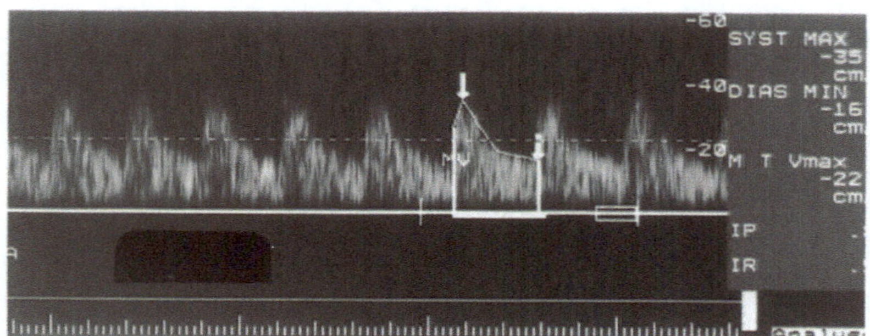

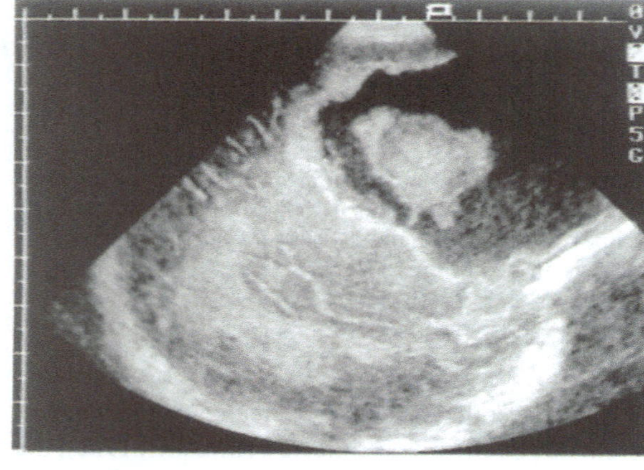

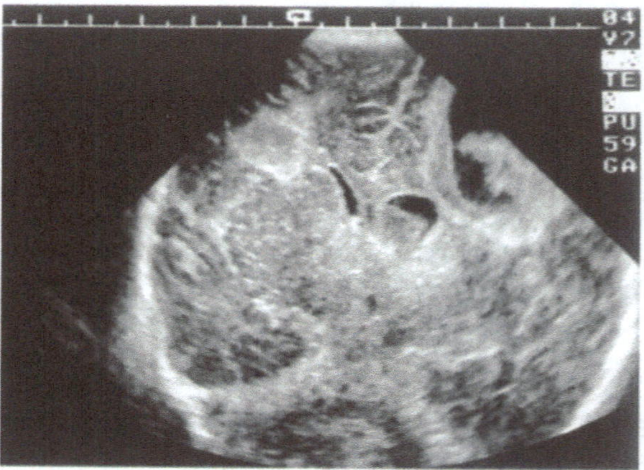

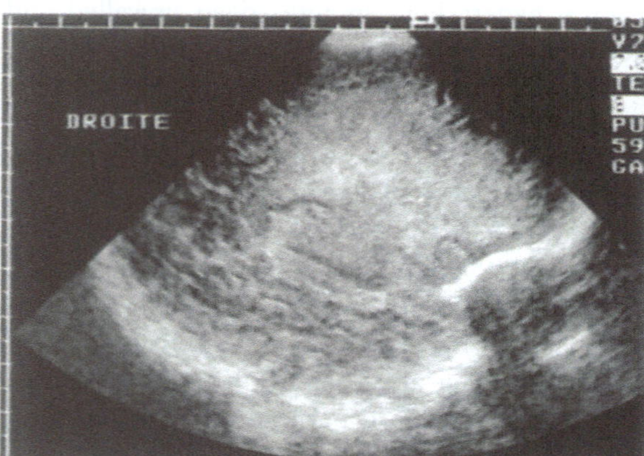

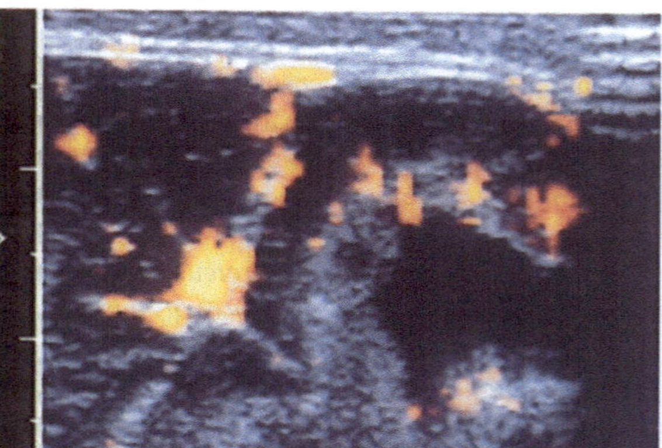

Fig. 8.6a–g. A 9-day-old newborn with fever and subtle seizures. *Proteus mirabilis* meningitis. **a,b** First ultrasonography on admission. **a** Coronal scan, high-frequency probe, power Doppler. A finger-shaped hyperechoic area is present at the cortico-subcortical junction of the left frontal lobe: cerebritis. Small peripheral vessels remain distant from the lesion. **b** Pulsed Doppler on the anterior cerebral artery. PSV and RI are rather low, 35 cm/s and 0.53 respectively. This pattern suggests more severe damage. This is confirmed by US follow-up. On day 9 (**c,d**), the left frontal lesion has become abscessed (**c** left parasagittal scan), with hyperechogenicity of brain not only around the abscess, but also in the left occipitotemporal white matter (**c**) and right frontal lobe (**d** right parasagittal scan). **e** Power Doppler, coronal scan. Left intraventricular echoes, indetectable flow in the left terminal vein (in contrast to the right). **f** Left abscess with ventriculitis, basal ganglia infarction, and right paraventricular lesion. **g** Power Doppler, coronal scan, multiple signals are seen between microcystic areas surrounding the abscess. All lesions confirmed on MRI (at day 15). The infant died

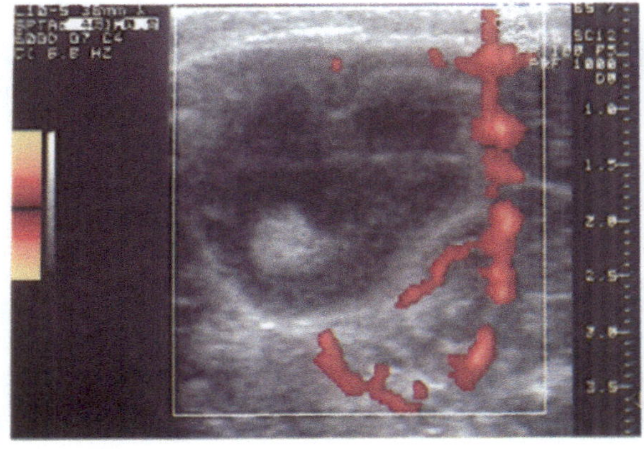

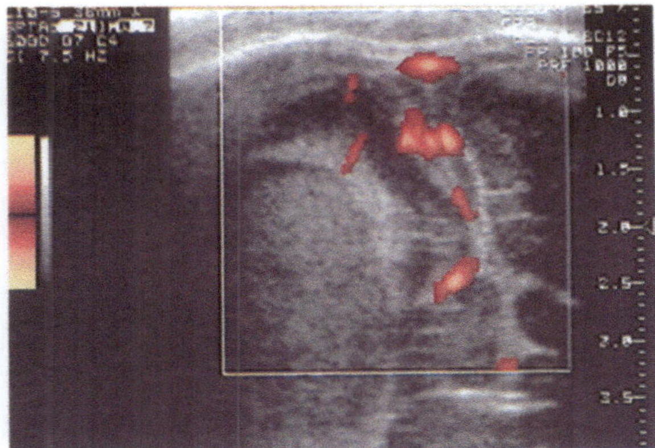

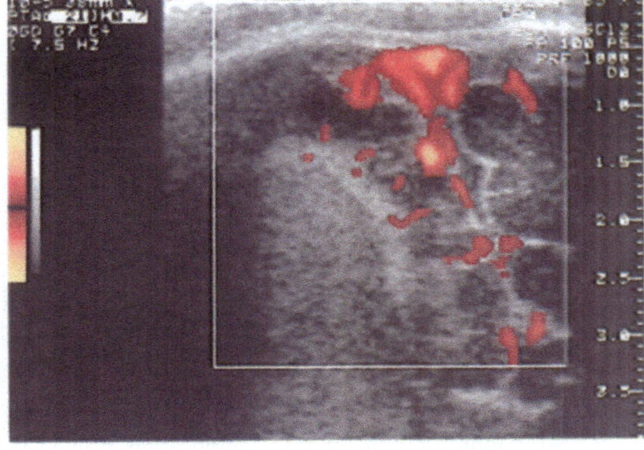

Fig. 8.7a–c. Evolution of brain abscess on power Doppler imaging. **a** At 8 days there is a necrotic, thin-walled collection; adjacent vessels close to the abscess are displaced. **b,c** At 1 month, aseptic puriform echogenic content is shown, with a thicker wall, shadowed external edges, and colonized by small vessels

As the abscess wall gradually thickens, small peripheral vessels penetrate and colonize it (Fig. 8.7).

Doppler ultrasonography may also help in detecting associated complications:

- Hypoxic-ischemic encephalopathy, suspected on the basis of a low blood flow on pulsed Doppler.
- Ventriculitis, suspected when a colored signal is identified within the sylvian aqueduct on color Doppler.
- Severe intracranial hypertension, revealed by an increased RI.

8.1.5
Subdural Collections

Pericerebral effusions are frequent in the course of neonatal pyogenic meningitis (Stroobandt 1983); they are usually aseptic fluid effusions, located in the subarachnoid or subdural space. These conditions are described in Chap. 6.

Subdural empyema is extremely uncommon in the neonate, and rare in the infant; it is usually caused by *Haemophilus influenzae* or *Streptococcus pneumoniae* meningitis. Detection is based on transfontanellar US (Chen 1998) and CT or MR, but early diagnosis, prompt surgical drainage, and appropriate antibiotic therapy are necessary to obtain a favorable outcome (Jacobson 1981).

Cerebral hemodynamics can be studied by pulsed Doppler for an appreciation of the consequences of extra-axial collection, and the occurrence of intracranial hypertension detected by determining the RI.

Color Doppler shows vessels with a venous pattern spectrum in septa and membranes that develop within the subdural space in response to infection (Fig. 8.8); the brain surface is also intensely hyperemic with high cortical venous velocities (Fig. 8.9).

The hyperemia appears early, as early as the 2nd day of the disease, while peripheral enhancement on CT or MRI is observed later (1–3 weeks). This pattern characterizes subdural empyema, and is not observed in the case of simple aseptic subdural collection.

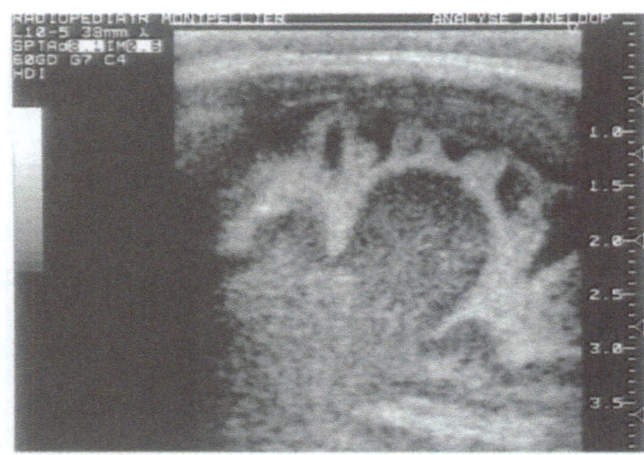

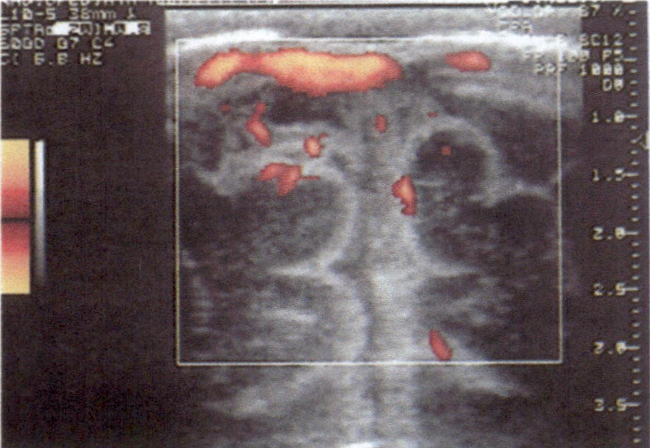

a · b

Fig. 8.8a,b. A 5-month-old infant with fever, nuchal rigidity and seizures. *Streptococcus pneumoniae* meningitis. Ultrasonography was performed on the 3rd day of the disease. Coronal scan, high-frequency probe. **a** Pericerebral collection with thick hyperechogenic arcuate strands close to the brain surface. On power Doppler (**b**), multiple colored signals are recognized within the septa

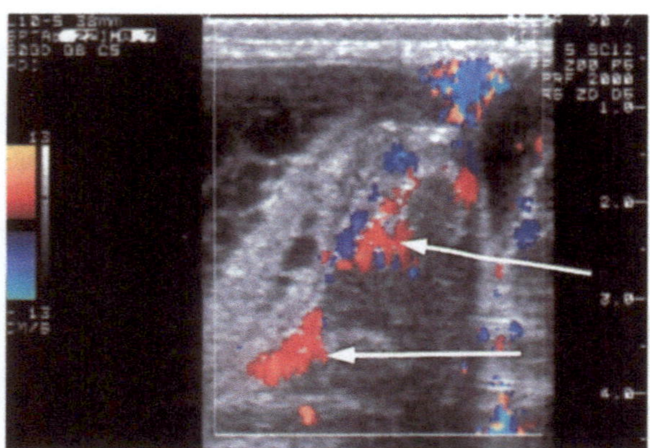

Fig. 8.9. An 8-month-old infant with complication of infected ventriculoperitoneal shunt. Large compressive subdural empyema with septations. There is intense hyperemia of cerebral parenchyma, close to the collection. Color Doppler, high-frequency probe, coronal scan

8.1.6
Dural Sinus Thrombosis

A classical complication of neonatal pyogenic meningitis, dural sinus thrombosis is explained by the usual risk factors for intracranial sinus thrombosis (intracranial hypertension, blood pressure instability induced by septic shock; see also Chap. 7, associated with direct involvement of venous walls by inflammatory and infectious processes. The clinical pattern is not specific, the most common features being seizures or lethargy. Thus, a color Doppler assessment of the venous network should be routinely performed during US examination of purulent meningitis. Most frequently, the superior sagittal sinus is involved (Fig. 8.10), but thrombosis may affect the deep veins of the galenic system and induce hemorrhagic infarction, especially within the basal ganglia. In our experience, the diagnosis is first made on ultrasonography, subsequently confirmed by CT or MRI. In fact thrombosis of the sagittal sinus is easily detected if only it is looked for: the sinus appears hyperechoic (Fig. 8.10a), without any detectable signal on color Doppler (Fig. 8.10b). Complete evaluation of the venous system is required (more difficult on ultrasonography alone) and infarcts must be investigated because they will determine the neurodevelopmental prognosis. Whatever treatment is given (anticoagulant therapy or not), the thrombosis can be followed up on color Doppler: several small cortical and dural veins appear close to the thrombosed sinus, with variable delays (day 4 to day 15 in our cases) (Fig. 8.10c,d). Recovery of intraluminal flow may be monitored (day 20 to day 30 in our cases).

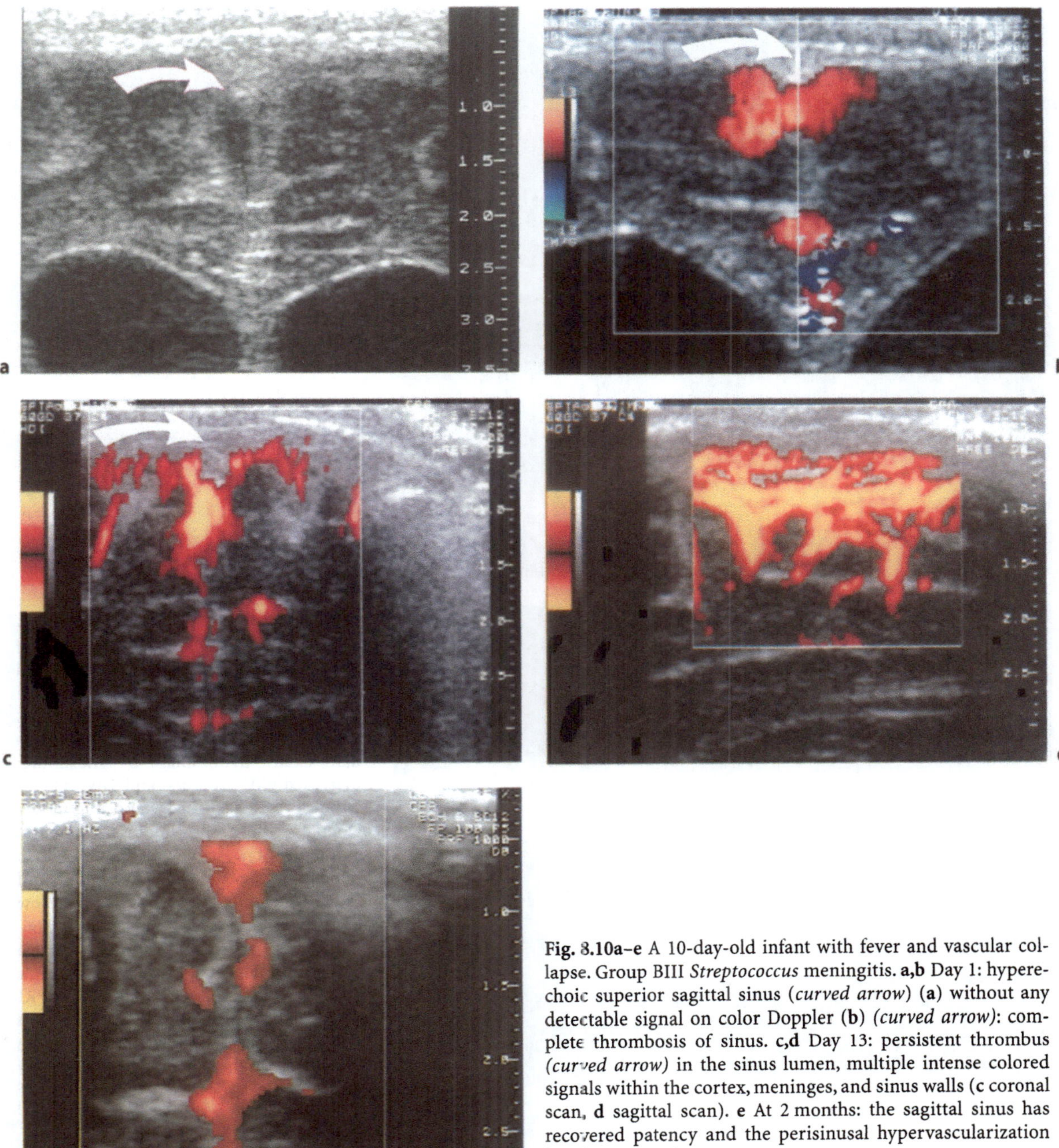

Fig. 8.10a–e A 10-day-old infant with fever and vascular collapse. Group BIII *Streptococcus* meningitis. **a,b** Day 1: hyperechoic superior sagittal sinus (*curved arrow*) (**a**) without any detectable signal on color Doppler (**b**) (*curved arrow*): complete thrombosis of sinus. **c,d** Day 13: persistent thrombus (*curved arrow*) in the sinus lumen, multiple intense colored signals within the cortex, meninges, and sinus walls (**c** coronal scan, **d** sagittal scan). **e** At 2 months: the sagittal sinus has recovered patency and the perisinusal hypervascularization has disappeared

8.1.7
Conclusion

In a neonate with pyogenic meningitis, ultrasonography should be used to analyze the cerebral hemodynamics by pulsed Doppler and search (Fig. 8.11) for signs of:
- Severe intracranial hypertension: increased RI

- Cerebral hypoperfusion: decrease in peak-systolic and mean flow velocities
- Loss of cerebral autoregulation: fluctuating Doppler curve

Color Doppler should be used to study the major cerebral arteries, dural sinuses, deep veins, and the ventricular system.

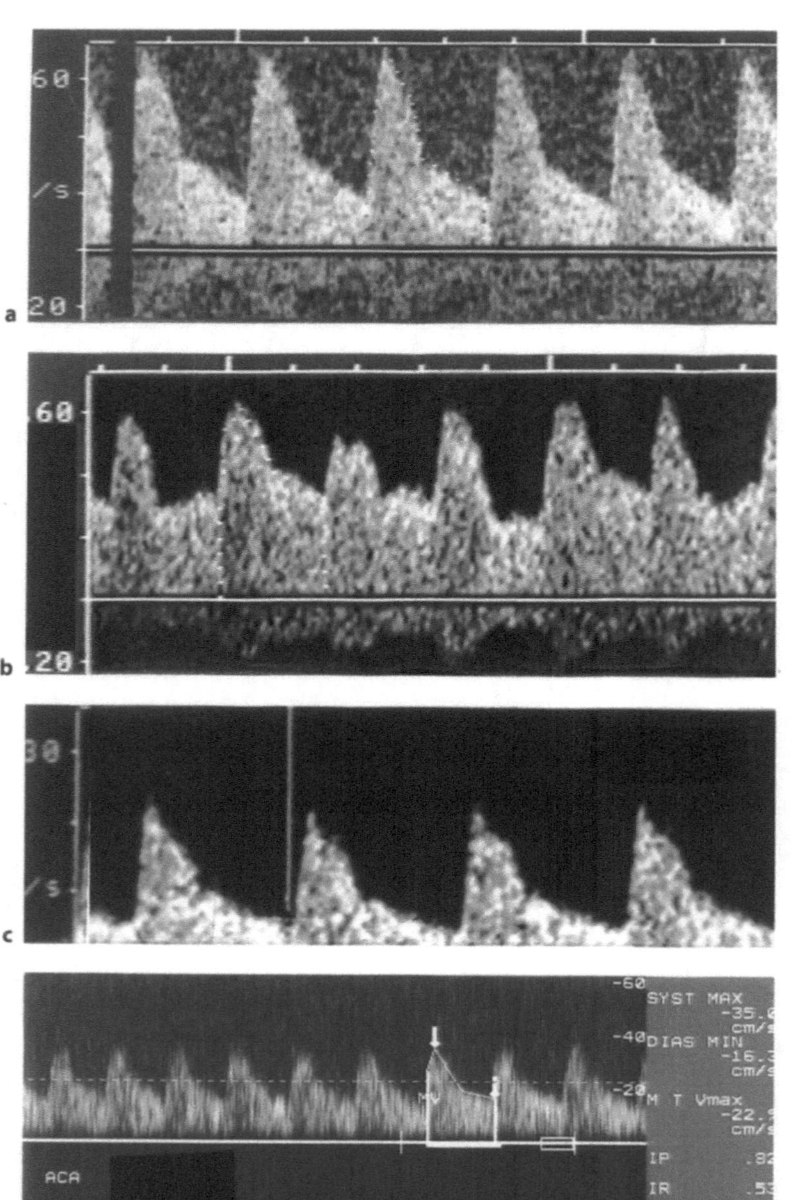

Fig. 8.11a–d. Different hemodynamic patterns encountered in the acute phase of pyogenic meningitis. a Sarah: increased PSV (70 cm/s), TAV (38 cm/s), and RI (0.73): a good hemodynamic situation. There is no parenchymal damage. Residual axial hypotonia. b Alexandre: increased PSV (61 cm/s) and TAV (44 cm/s) but low RI (0.40--0.47) and fluctuating Doppler pattern, showing loss of cerebral autoregulation. He died 48 h after birth. c Benjamin: very low PSV (22 cm/s) and TAV (10 cm/s) and increased RI (0.77): low blood flow with intracranial hypertension. Extensive destructive brain damage occurred, followed by death. d Nathan: low PSV (35 cm/s), TAV (23 cm/s), and RI (0.53), indicating low blood flow with reduced vascular resistance. Extensive destructive brain damage was followed by death

8.2
Viral and Protozoan Infections

A rich imaging pattern has been described in TORCH infections (*t*oxoplasmosis, *o*thers – e.g., syphilis and HIV –, *r*ubella, *c*ytomegalovirus, *h*erpes simplex) following either intrauterine or postnatal contamination (SHAW 1993; BARKOVITCH 1994). Manifestations include microcephaly, polymicrogyria and other disturbances of neuronal migration, cerebellar hypoplasia, encephaloclastic parenchymal damage, delays in myelination, hemorrhagic or leukomalacic areas, periventricular or/and cortical calcifications, subependymal cysts, and lenticulostriate vasculopathy. This last lesion is only detectable on ultrasonography, except when it is calcified. It appears as branched, candlestick-shaped echodensities, located within the basal ganglia. Sometimes only hyperechoic punctuations in the same site may be visualized.

Color Doppler confirms the vascular or perivascular situation of these lesions (CABANAS 1994; RIES 1990) by showing that they are superimposed or in close contact with pulsatile flows, which are demon-

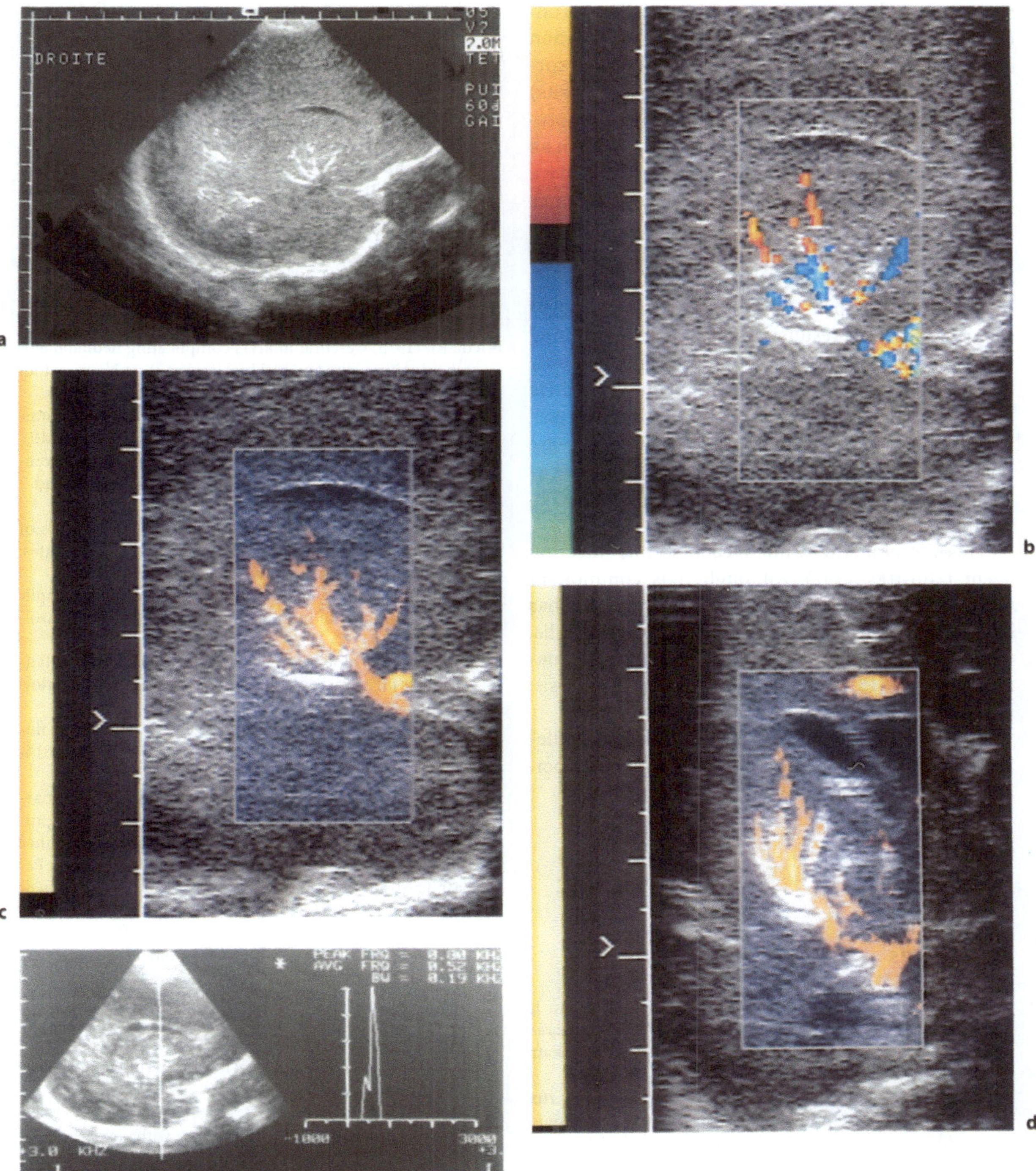

Fig. 8.12a–e. Maternofetal CMV infection with systemic clinical features. a Candlestick echodensities in lenticulostriate nuclei (parasagittal scan). b,c Same scan on color Doppler (b) and power Doppler (c), with excellent visibility of intraluminal flow. d Coronal power Doppler scan of right basal ganglia. e Pulsed Doppler scan of lenticulostriate arteries

strated on pulsed Doppler as an arterial spectrum (BEN AMI 1990). The neuropathological explanation is unclear. In the opinion of TEELE (1988), they correspond to mineralization (calcic or ferric deposits) and hypercellularity of arterial walls. They have previously been described by RORKE (1969) and VOLPE (1987) in different infections, but other authors have not found the same histological characteristics (HUGHES 1991).

In our experience, color Doppler visualizes a persistent flow within lenticulostriate vessels despite the hyperechoic stripes (Fig. 8.12). WANG (1995) reported different results: of 34 neonates exhibiting these anomalies, he detected a colored signal in only 3, whereas he showed it in 100% of normal infants. He suggested that lenticulostriate arteries supplying germinal matrix that is active in cell proliferation are obstructed or stenosed in the fetus, resulting in neuronal migration disturbances, such as are observed in cytomegalovirus (CMV) infection.

This vasculopathy is not specific to one infecting agent (HUGHES 1991). Although it is common in CMV (TEELE 1988) and rubella (RORKE 1969), it has been described in other perinatal infections (syphilis, toxoplasmosis, HIV disease), chromosome anomalies (trisomy 13), lysosomal disorders (sialidosis, etc.), neonatal asphyxia, and others.

Finally, when the only feature detected is candlestick echodensities, this does not seem to be associated with a poor developmental outcome.

References

Ashwal S, Stringer W, Tomasi L, Schneider S, Thompson J, Perkin R (1990) Cerebral blood flow and carbon dioxide reactivity in children with bacterial meningitis. J Pediatr 117:523-530

Barkovich AJ, Lindan CE (1994) Congenital cytomegalovirus infection of the brain: imaging analysis and embryologic considerations. AJNR Am J Neuroradiol 15:703-715

Ben-Ami T, Yousefzadeh D, Backus M, Reichman B, Kessler A, Hammerman-Rozenberg C (1990) Lenticulostriate vasculopathy in infants with infections of the central nervous system. Sonographic and Doppler findings. Pediatr Radiol 20:575-579

Berman PH, Banker BQ (1966) Neonatal meningitis: a clinical and pathological study of 29 cases. Pediatrics 38:6-24

Bornke C, Buttner T, McMonagle U, Przuntek H (1996) Secondary cerebral vasculitis in suppurative meningitis. Clinical aspects and findings in color-coded transcranial duplex ultrasound. Fortschr Med 114:104-106

Cabanas F, Pellicer A, Morales C (1994) New pattern of hyperechogenicity in thalamus and basal ganglia studied by color Doppler flow imaging. Pediatr Neurol. 10:109-116

Chen CY, Huang CC, Chang YC, Chow NH, Chio CC, Zimmerman RA (1998) Subdural empyemas in 10 infants: US characteristics and clinical correlates. Radiology 207:609-617

Daum RS, Scheifele DW, Syriopoulou VP, Averill D, Smith AL (1978) Ventricular involvement in experimental Hemophilus influenzae meningitis. J Pediatr 93:927-930

Enzman DR, Britt RH, Lyons R, Carroll B, Wilson DA, Buxton J (1982) High resolution ultrasound evaluation of experimental brain abscess evolution: comparison with CT and neuropathology. Radiology 142:95-102

Foreman SD, Smith EE, Ryan NJ, Hogan GR (1984) Neonatal citrobacter meningitis. Pathogenesis of cerebral abscess formation. Ann Neurol 16:655-659

Friede RL (1973) Cerebral infarcts complicating neonatal leptomeningitis: acute and residual lesions. Acta Neuropathol 23:245-253

Goh D, Minns RA (1993) Cerebral blood flow velocity monitoring in pyogenic meningitis. Arch Dis Child 68:111-119

Goitein KJ, Tamir I (1983) Cerebral perfusion pressure in central nervous system infections of infancy and childhood. J Pediatr 103:40-43

Hughes P, Weinberger E, Shaw DWW (1991) Linear areas of echogenicity in the thalami and basal ganglia of neonates: an expanded association. Radiology 179:103-105

Jacobson PL, Farmer TW (1981) Subdural empyema complicating meningitis in infants: improved prognosis. Neurology 31:190-193

McMenamin JB, Volpe JJ (1984) Bacterial meningitis in infancy: effects on intracranial pressure and cerebral blood flow velocity. Neurology 34:500-504

Minns RA, Engleman HM, Stirling H (1989) Cerebrospinal fluid pressure in pyogenic meningitis. Arch Dis Child 64:814-820

Pedespan JM, Chateil JF, Pedespan-Joly L, Fontan D, Demarquez JL, Guillard JM (1996) Thromboses du sinus longitudinal supérieur chez l'enfant au cours de la première année de vie: aspects cliniques, imagerie et évolution. Arch Fr Pediatr 3:561-565

Raimondi AJ, Di Rocco C (1979) The physiopathogenetic basis for the angiographic diagnosis of bacterial infections of the brain and coverings in children. I. Leptomeningitis. Child's Brain 5:1-13

Ries M, Deeg KH, Heininger U (1990) Demonstration of perivascular echogenicities in congenital CMV infection by color Doppler imaging. Eur J Pediatr 150:34-36

Rorke LB, Spiro AJ (1967) Cerebral lesions in congenital rubella syndrome. J Pediatr 70:243-255

Scheld WM, Dacey RG, Winn HR, Walsh JA, Sande MA (1980) CSF outflow resistance in rabbits with experimental meningitis. J Clin Invest 66:243-253

Shaw DWW, Cohen WA (1993) Viral infections of the CNS in children: imaging features. AJR Am J Roentgenol 160:125-133

Stroobandt G, Belpaire-Dethiou MC, Thauvoy C, Evrard P (1983) Les épanchements péricérébraux postméningitiques du nourrisson. Neurochirurgie. 29:247-253

Sutton DL, Ouvrier RA (1983) Cerebral abscess in the under 6 month age group. Arch Dis Child 58:901-905

Tatsuno M, Hasegawa M, Okuyama K (1993) Ventriculitis in infants: diagnosis by color Doppler flow imaging. Pediatr Neurol 9:127-130

Täuber MG, Khayam-Bashi H, Sande MA (1985) Effects of ampicillin and corticosteroids on brain water content, CSF pressure and CSF lactate levels in experimental pneumococcal meningitis. J Infect Dis 151:528-534

Teele RL, Hernanz-Schulman M, Sotrel A (1988) Echogenic vasculature in the basal ganglia of neonates: a sonographic sign of vasculopathy. Radiology 169:423-427

Tureen JH, Stella FB, Clyman RI, Mauray F, Sande MA (1987) Effect of indomethacin on brain water content, CSF white blood cell response, and prostaglandin E2 levels in CSF in experimental pneumococcal meningitis in rabbits. Pediatr Infect Dis J 6 (suppl):1151-1153

Tureen JH, Dworkin RJ, Kennedy SL, Sachdeva M, Sande MA (1990) Loss of cerebral autoregulation in experimental meningitis in rabbits. J Clin Invest 85:577-581

Veyrac C, Couture A, Baud C (1994) La pathologie infectieuse. In: Echographie cérébrale du foetus au nouveau-né. Couture A, Veyrac C, Baud C (eds). Sauramps Medical, Montpellier, pp 371-392

Volpe JJ (1987) Bacterial and fungal intracranial infections. In: Neurology of the newborn. 2nd Ed Saunders, Philadelphia

Wang HS, Kuo MF, Chang TC (1995) Sonographic lenticulostriate vasculopathy in infants: some associations and a hypothesis. AJNR Am J Neuroradiol 16:97-102

Winkler P (1992) Color-coded echographic flow imaging and spectral analysis of CSF in meningitis and hemorrhage. Part I. Clinical evidence. Pediatr Radiol 22:24-30

Yoshioka H, Yoshioka H (1982) Arterial occlusion in purulent meningitis and multicystic encephalomalacia. Eur J Pediatr 139:303-305

9 Neonatal and Fetal Brain Malformations

ALAIN P. COUTURE

CONTENTS

Ultrasound constitutes the basis for the neonatal diagnosis of brain malformations (COUTURE 1994), although it is frequently and efficiently complemented by MRI (BARKOVICH 1989, 1990, 1992; GEORGY 1993; KALIFA 1987). A decisive step forward has been that these abnormalities may be often detected early and reliably in the fetus (BENNET 1996; KOMARNISKI 1990; VAN ZALEN-SPROCK 1995); in this diagnostic situation fetal MRI is being increasingly used to confirm and improve the results of ultra-

A. COUTURE, MD
Service de Radiologie Pédiatrique, Hôpital Arnaud de Villeneuve, 371 av. Doyen Gaston Giraud, 34295 Montpellier Cedex, France

sound investigation (HILL 1988; LEVINE 1997; MATTISON 1988; OKAMURA 1993; RYPENS 1996; SONIGO 1996, 1998). Thus, in both fetus and neonate, the diagnostic evaluation of most cerebral malformations requires morphological ultrasound and an MRI study.

What, then, is the role of pulsed and color Doppler in these situations?

- Their first role is in showing the vascular nature of an intracranial malformation: the diagnosis is suspected on the basis of morphology, and is confirmed by pulsed and color Doppler. Such vascular malformations are rare and mainly relate to vein of Galen aneurysm. They are easily diagnosed by color Doppler in fetus and neonate, and the new challenge is to assess the fetal prognosis. The size of the developmental complex (feeding vessels, mode of communication with vein of Galen, appearance of venous drainage) is analyzed by color imaging and spectral analysis; the search for ischemic brain damage is based on MRI; while, finally, fetal heart examination evaluates the secondary cardiac manifestations. Thus, Doppler techniques obviously play a main role in diagnostic and prognostic evaluation of a galenic aneurysmal malformation.

- It is more difficult to assess the role of Doppler in improving the diagnosis of nonvascular malformations. Ultrasound coupled to MRI allows the diagnosis and complete evaluation of all brain abnormalities in the neonate, but hesitations and diagnostic errors remain frequent: in corpus callosum abnormalities, in some cases of holoprosencephaly, in disorders of neuronal migration, and schizencephaly, especially with closed-lip clefts. In these situations, color Doppler shows specific findings that may provide new, reliable diagnostic information.

9.1
Vascular Malformations

9.1.1
Aneurysm of Vein of Galen

For a long time, aneurysm of the vein of Galen has been associated with a disastrous prognosis in the literature: JOHNSTON (1987) reports mortality in 91.4% of 80 newborns and EIRAS (1985) in 100% of neonates with cardiac failure.

Today, thanks to progress in treatment (endovascular embolization), this pessimistic feeling is giving way to relative optimism, so long as the neonates and fetuses are evaluated according to a strict clinical and radiological protocol. This underlines the importance of imaging in the advances in management. Fetal and neonatal diagnosis has become easy since the arrival of color imaging. Evaluation of the prognosis in the fetus is also based on ultrasonography (fetal heart, arterial supply to the malformation) and MRI (brain parenchyma). Angiography no longer has a place in the neonatal diagnosis.

Galenic arteriovenous fistula is defined as a deep vascular malformation, draining into a more or less ectatic vein of Galen, in the region of the velum interpositum. It is usually supplied by myriad vessels, especially posterior choroidal arteries and, less frequently, thalamo-perforating vessels and a distal branch of the anterior cerebral arteries. This shunt gradually induces galenic dilatation and increases cerebral venous pressure, leading to heart failure and hydrocephalus. This definition, although accurate, is obviously too simplistic, and recent publications (BRUNELLE 1997; LASJAUNIAS 1997; QUISLING 1989; RAYBAUD 1989) have documented the great complexity of this arteriovenous malformation.

9.1.1.1
Analysis of Angiogram

Angiography reveals more mysteries than it resolves (RAYBAUD 1989): there is great polymorphism in arterial feeding and venous drainage.

In the opinion of RAYBAUD (1989), arterial supply usually involves the posterior choroidal arteries, branches of the posterior cerebral arteries. Frequently, a distal branch of the anterior cerebral arteries contributes to the malformation (Fig. 9.1).

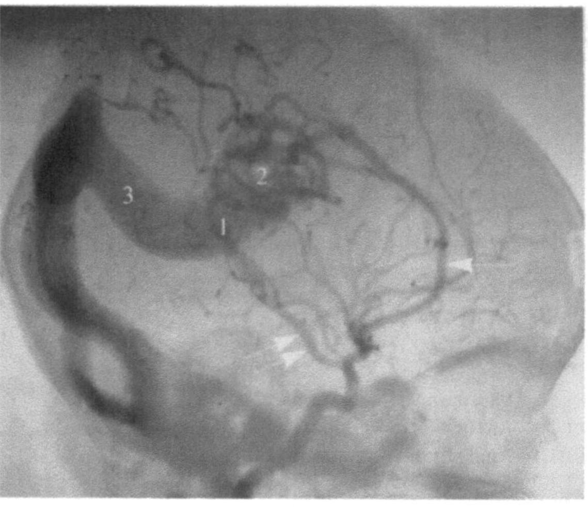

Fig. 9.1. Severe neonatal congestive heart failure. Angiography shows a massive aneurysm of the vein of Galen. Note dilatation of the anterior cerebral artery (*arrow*) and posterior cerebral arteries (*double arrow*), which supply the malformation via the posterior choroidal arteries (*1*) and distal branches of the anterior cerebral arteries (*2*). The vein of Galen drains into an aberrant dural sinus, located high above the tentorium (*3*)

BRUNELLE (1997) records the proportion of feeding by each artery: posterior choroidal arteries supply the galenic malformation in 100% of cases, while the distal branch of the anterior cerebral arteries (trigonal branch of pericallosal artery) is recruited in 69% of cases, and the transmesencephalic artery arising from the basilar artery in 30% of cases. Other arteries may, very rarely, supply the aneurysm, such as the middle cerebral arteries, anterior choroidal arteries, and lenticulostriate arteries.

These vessels constitute arteriovenous fistulas within the wall of the aneurysmal sac, either directly from an arterial branch (most often the distal part of the anterior cerebral artery) or through an interposed arterial network (most often choroidal vessels).

QUISLING (1989) grades galenic malformations using angiographic criteria, according to the size and complexity of their angiomatous matrix:

- Category I is characterized by a small matrix (less than 1 cm) and fewer than five feeding vessels.
- Category II is characterized by a larger matrix (1–2 cm in size) supplied mainly by thalamo-perforating arteries.
- Category III is characterized by a matrix greater than 2 cm in size and many feeding vessels (choroidal and anterior cerebral arteries) (HOUDART 1993; RAYBAUD 1989).

Obviously, the severity of hemodynamic disturbances and the prognosis depend on the number of the supplying vessels.

For a long time (AUBE 1975; LITTVAK 1960; ROOSEN 1986) galenic aneurysm was considered to be a dilatation of the cerebral vein, straight sinus, and torcular. In fact, this anatomic arrangement is far from the rule, and dural anomalies are common: the galenic–sinus junction may be narrowed, the straight sinus may be less dilated than the vein of Galen, and most often the straight sinus is absent.

RAYBAUD (1987) observed nonopacification of the straight sinus in 13 of 29 cases (i.e., 45%). In the series reported by BRUNELLE (1997), the straight sinus was absent or thrombosed in 56% of patients. In cases of agenesis of the straight sinus, the collateral circulation forms the bridge between the galenic pouch and the torcular, the lateral sinus, or the superior sagittal sinus: the latter arrangement is the one most frequently encountered [14 out of 29 cases reported by RAYBAUD (1987)] and corresponds to a persistent embryonic sinus, the so-called falcine sinus (BRUNELLE 1997; LASJAUNIAS 1997; RUCHOUX 1987; YOKOTA 1978). For LASJAUNIAS (1997), the presence of dural venous obstructions and anomalies is the rule: agenesis or stenosis may be located at any level of the venous system (Fig. 9.2).

In the case of an obstruction along the skull base, the only possible drainage is via the cavernous sinus, emissary veins of the superior sagittal sinus, and sigmoid sinus.

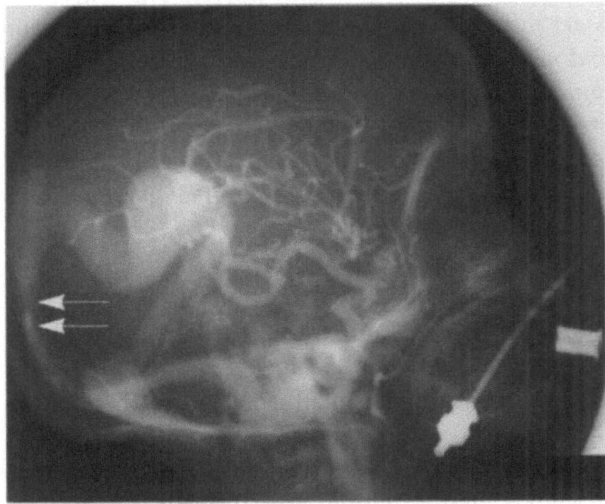

Fig. 9.2. Neonate with aneurysm of the vein of Galen. Stenosis of the transverse part of a lateral sinus (*arrows*). Note that the vein of Galen drains into an aberrant dural sinus

Venous dural obstructions (or developmental defects) are most often seen in older patients. Since spontaneous thrombosis has been described in vivo (RAYBAUD 1987), these anomalies probably correspond to an evolving process.

In contrast to this, in the neonate, venous drainage may be abnormal (into an aberrant sinus, especially a falcine sinus), but it is always patent, directed toward the jugular veins.

Finally, in both the human neonate (BRUNELLE 1997; REICHMAN 1993) and the animal (PILE-SPELLMAN 1986), histological examination shows myointimal proliferation in the galenic vein walls: this arterialization of the vein develops in response to increased flow pressure and turbulence.

9.1.1.2
Consequences of Arteriovenous Aneurysm

The consequences of arteriovenous aneurysm relate to the progressive ectasia of the vein of Galen and to the increase in cerebral venous pressure (QUISLING 1989). Such venous ectasia is commonly attributed to a combination of increased blood volume delivered through the shunt, and increased venous pressure, due in part to arterial pressures transmitted through the shunt and in part to obstruction of venous outflow (LASJAUNIAS 1997). Elevated pressure within the dural venous sinuses contributes to elevated pressure in the cerebral veins, ultimately disturbing the hemodynamic balance by narrowing the arteriovenous pressure differential.

QUISLING (1989), studying cerebral venous pressure via transtorcular catheterization in 15 patients, reported valuable data relating to the pathogenesis. He found that venous pressure appeared to be constantly increased and did not significantly differ across age groups; moderate ectasia of the aneurysmal complex (vein of Galen and straight sinus) correlated to moderately increased venous pressure, while marked ectasia correlated to higher venous pressure. However, in cases with disproportionate ectasia (dilated galenic vein but normal or narrowed straight sinus) a pressure gradient was exhibited across the stenotic straight sinus (with minimal venous pressure elevation in the torcular).

The physiopathological implications are obvious: 9 out of the 15 patients showed dural obstructions, but none of them presented in overt failure.

YUVAL (1997) confirmed the hypothesis of QUISLING (1989), describing a 38-weeks' gestation fetus without heart failure, in whom the straight sinus appeared stenotic with a minimal flow. The postnatal outcome was favorable. On the other hand, cardiac failure was severe in the six patients without venous obstruction. This anatomical-clinical pattern is characteristic of the neonate and reflects the severity of the malformation. Low venous resistance obviously induces high flow through the shunt, resulting in rapid cardiac decompensation.

9.1.1.3
Embryologic Development of Cerebral Vascular Malformations Remains Unknown

According to RAYBAUD (1989), the development of the CNS vasculature may be divided into three major periods.

During the extraembryonal phase, the neural tube is nourished by the amniotic fluid, the brain parenchyma is supplied by diffusion through the highly vascularized meninx primitiva, and at this time choroid plexuses develop within the ventricles. In the beginning, the vascular network is not differentiated into arteries, veins, and capillaries. Primary circulation is gradually established while the heart function develops and blood pressure in the arteries increases.

During the 5th week, the choroidal and quadrigeminal arteries develop markedly. On the roof of the diencephalon, the choroid plexus expansion is accompanied by differentiation of a dorsal vein that drains the choroid plexus. This vein, the so-called medial prosencephalic vein, probably plays an important role in the constitution of a galenic aneurysm.

The normality of arterial supply that is already determined by the 8th week, and the persistence of a medial vein that normally regresses after the 12th week, allow the supposition that an accident occurring during the 3rd month of gestation is responsible for the formation of an aneurysm on the vein of Galen. However, there is still no information to suggest a specific cause. Vein of Galen aneurysm may be the consequence of an arteriovenous malformation involving the choroidal arteries and this medial prosencephalic vein that at this stage is the major venous drainage of the third ventricle choroid plexus.

9.1.1.4
Advances in Imaging

Obviously, progress in imaging has improved both diagnosis and the evaluation of the prognosis.

Myriam's birth was uneventful (weight 4150 g, head circumference 36 cm). On day 4, tachypnea, *intercostal retraction, and liver enlargement necessitated her admission to hospital. She suffered congestive heart failure, with tachycardia (180/min) and systolic murmur. Arterial blood pressure was normal, femoral pulsations were present. Chest X-rays showed severe cardiomegaly and normal pulmonary vascularity. Digitalic and diuretic treatment failed to improve her clinical status significantly. Vomiting occurred, and her head circumference quickly increased (3 cm in 10 days).*

The newborn was transferred to our hospital. Brain ultrasonography was performed immediately and showed moderate triventricular dilatation and outward displacement of the left ventricle by a rounded, anechoic mass, almost 3 cm in diameter, located at the posterior part of the thalamus (Fig. 9.3).

Clinical examination reveals a continuous cranial bruit. These sonographic and clinical findings suggest the diagnosis of galenic aneurysmal malformation. Various investigations confirm this diagnosis:
- *Besides the massive cardiomegaly, chest X-rays show a widened superior mediastinum and a retrosternal density with posterior displacement of the trachea, while a lateral view of the neck shows a retropharyngeal mass (Fig. 9.4).*
- *Cerebral angiography demonstrated a complex vascular malformation with early arteriovenous shunt; very high flow drained, from the first second, into an extremely dilated galenic pouch. The malformation was mainly supplied by the two posterior cerebral arteries, and also by accessory vessels from anterior cerebral arteries. Finally, there was a complex abnormality of venous dural sinuses (Fig. 9.5).*

The clinical state gradually altered. The congestive heart failure failed to respond to medical treatment and neurological status worsened with raised intracranial pressure. Embolization was rejected because of the vascular architecture of the lesion, and surgical reduction of the vascular pedicle was decided on. The infant died during surgery (cerebral hemorrhage and cardiac arrest) at 2 months of age.

This case report, published in 1981 (COUTURE 1981), already demonstrates the value of ultrasonography, which was just beginning at this period, in diagnosing malformation of the vein of Galen.
- Twenty years ago, detection of a cerebral arteriovenous malformation was difficult. Of course, major cardiomegaly and intracranial hypertension were suggestive but this was a rare association; cardiac failure might so predominate that

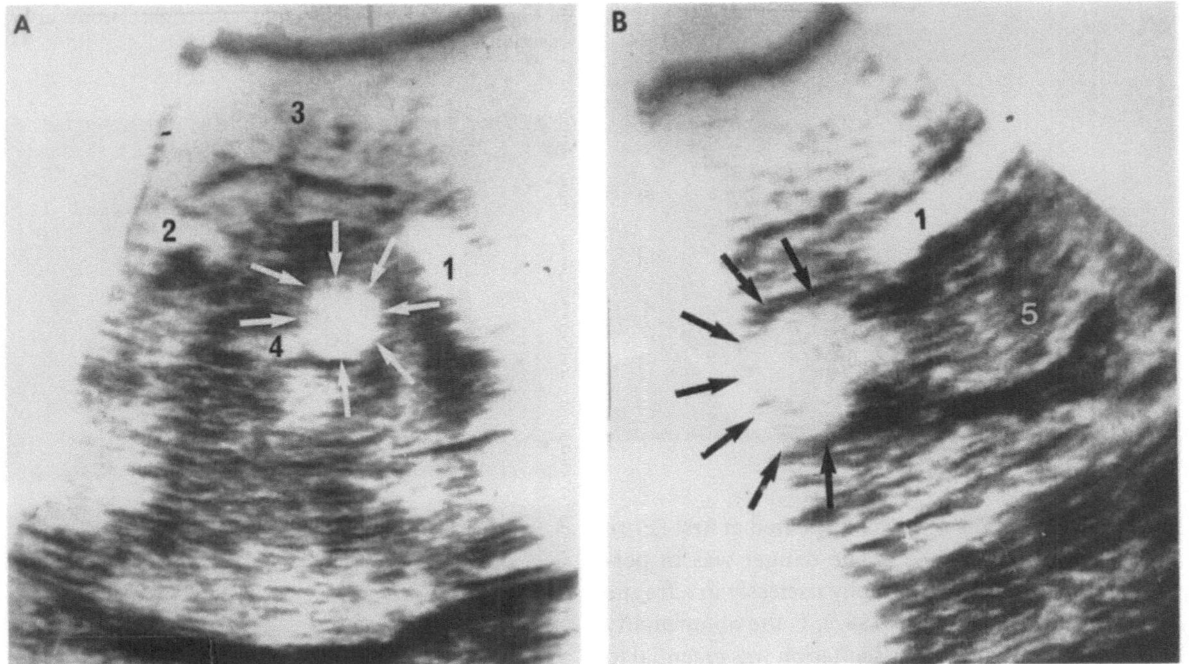

Fig. 9.3. a Posterior frontal plane ultrasonography detects a rounded, anechoic image (*arrows*) displacing the left ventricle (*1*). Right ventricle (*2*) and interhemispheric fissure (*3*) remain in normal place. Notice a feeding vessel or a draining vein (*4*). b On a right paramedial sagittal plane, the echofree image is retrothalamic (*5*)

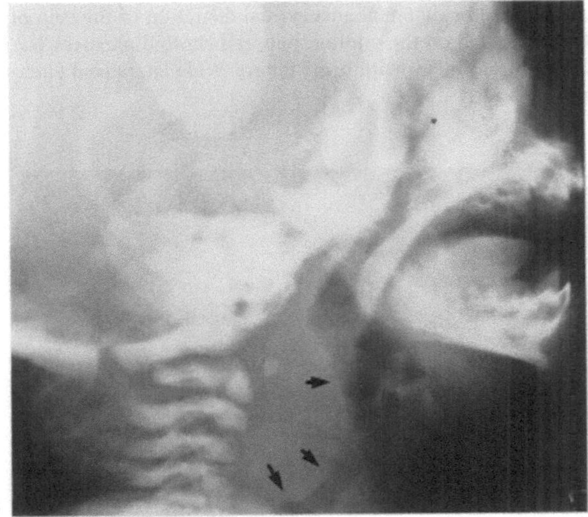

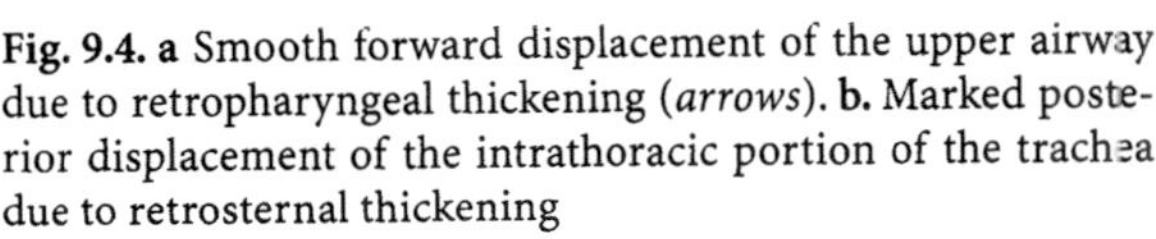

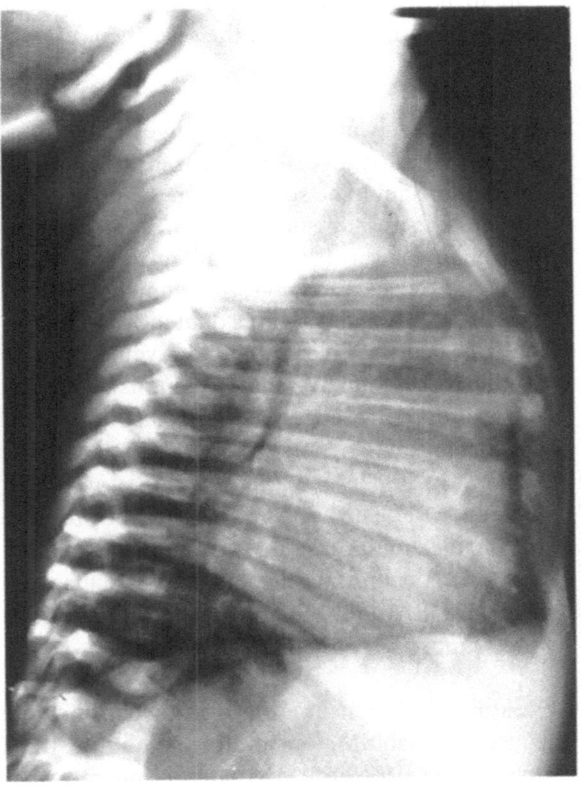

Fig. 9.4. a Smooth forward displacement of the upper airway due to retropharyngeal thickening (*arrows*). b. Marked posterior displacement of the intrathoracic portion of the trachea due to retrosternal thickening

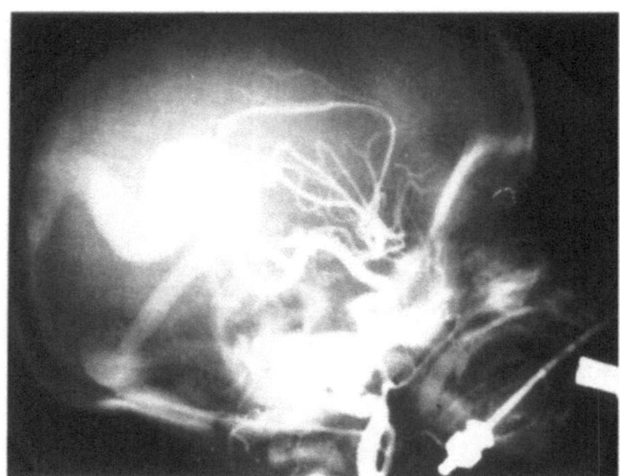

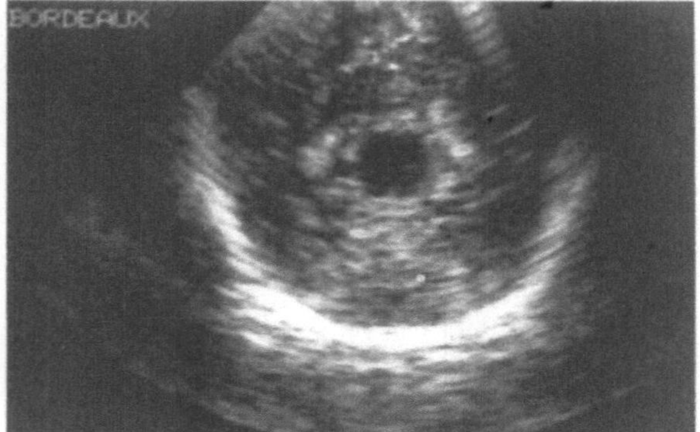

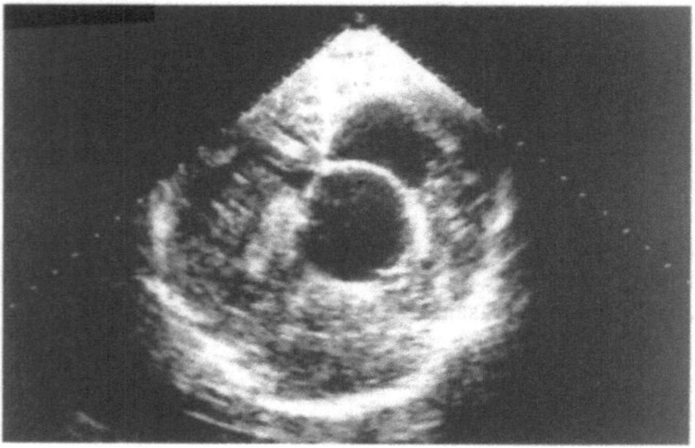

← **Fig. 9.5.** Cerebral angiography after right carotid artery injection

Fig. 9.6. a A 1-month-old infant with minimal macrocrania and intracranial bruit. Small aneurysmal dilatation of the vein of Galen, located on the midline, between choroid plexuses. **b** A 3-month-old infant with heart failure. Wide lateralized aneurysmal pouch

primary heart disease was suspected at first (EIDE 1978; KACHANER 1977). The danger was in performing cardiac angiography uselessly in a fragile newborn (PELLEGRINO 1987). If the abnormality was suspected cranial auscultation was essential to detect an intense, continuous bruit (BOUVAIST 1998; VINTZILEOS 1986). However, as is well known (GLATT 1960; GOMEZ 1963), this intracranial bruit may be absent or intermittent even when arteriovenous fistula is confirmed on anatomical investigation. Thus, at this period, invasive complementary investigations were often required and had to be chosen among the neuroradiological possibilities, depending on the severity of presentation.

- Chest and cervical X rays (Fig. 9.4). were useful. If cardiomegaly and vascular congestion suggest congenital heart disease, a cerebral vascular malformation should be suspected in the presence of a widened superior mediastinum, posterior displacement of the trachea, and retropharyngeal thickening. These changes, as shown by SWISCHUK (1977) are due to large dilated vessels, especially brachiocephalic and jugular veins.

- In those years, many reports demonstrated that ultrasonography enabled diagnosis of galenic malformation (COUTURE 1981; CUBBERLEY 1982; MULLAART 1982; NEWLIN 1981; SIVAKOFF 1982; SNIDER 1981). The basic findings are the presence of an anechoic, rounded structure, most often located in the midline, displacing ventricular cavities (Fig. 9.6) and widely communicating with one or more vessels (Fig. 9.3).

Anatomic relationships were defined: either the aneurysmal dilatation was midline behind the third ventricle (Fig. 9.7), or it was lateral and retrotha-

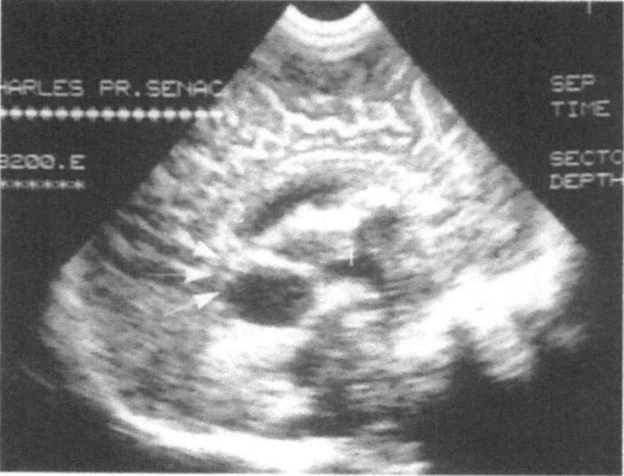

Fig. 9.7. A 2-month-old infant with aneurysm of the vein of Galen. The vascular pouch (*arrows*) is located behind and below the third ventricle (*1*) before the splenium of corpus callosum (*2*). This location is suggestive because it corresponds to the normal situation of the vein of Galen, easily demonstrated by color Doppler imaging

lamic. The diagnosis was easier when drainage into a more or less dilated, more or less tortuous straight sinus could be demonstrated (Fig. 9.8).

Finally, in the absence of pulsed and color Doppler imaging, enhanced CT and angiography were required (Fig. 9.9).

Nowadays, everything has changed. Improved knowledge about the malformation, the improvement of pediatric radiologists in ante- and postnatal imaging, and the arrival of new technologies (pulsed, color, and power Doppler) enable a precise, reliable diagnosis, in any circumstances and at any time (fetal or neonatal). The main difficulty now is estimating the prognosis, as demonstrated in the following case report.

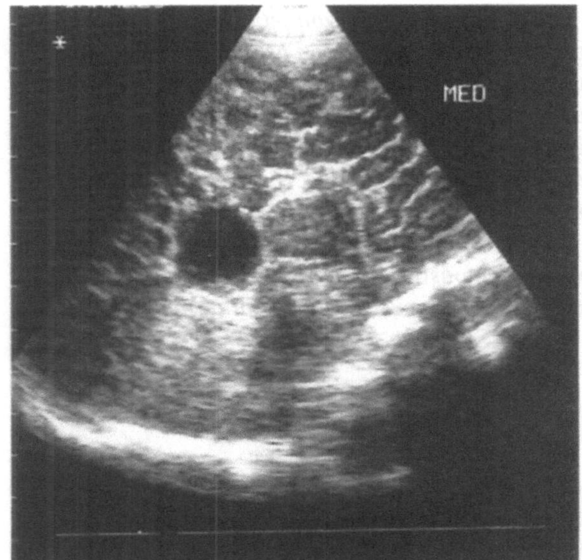

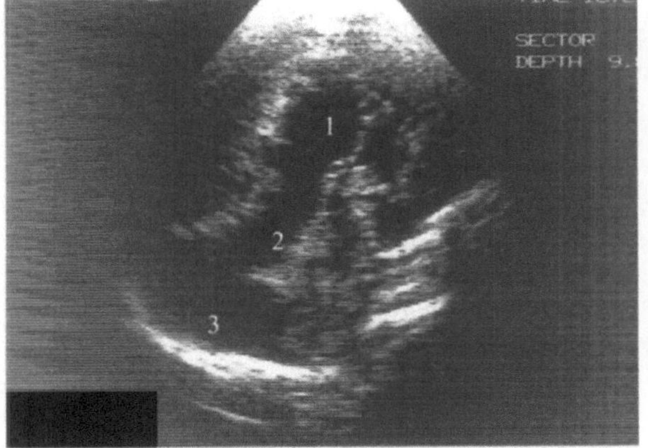

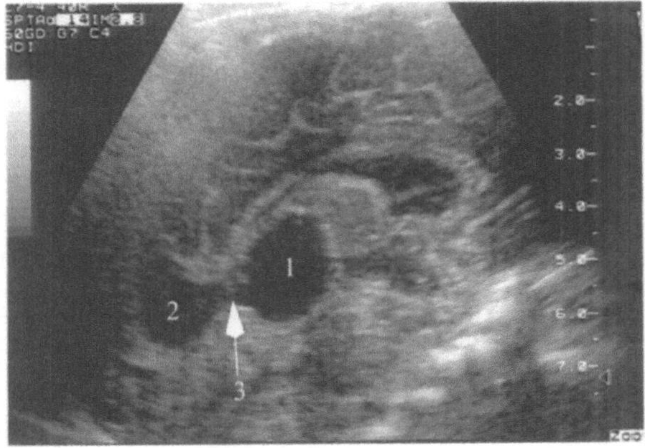

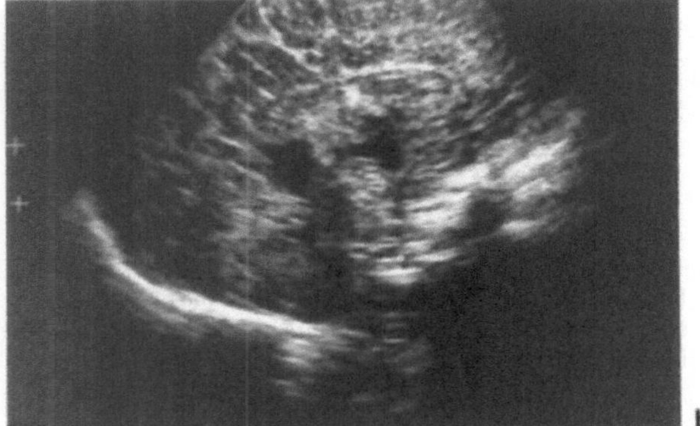

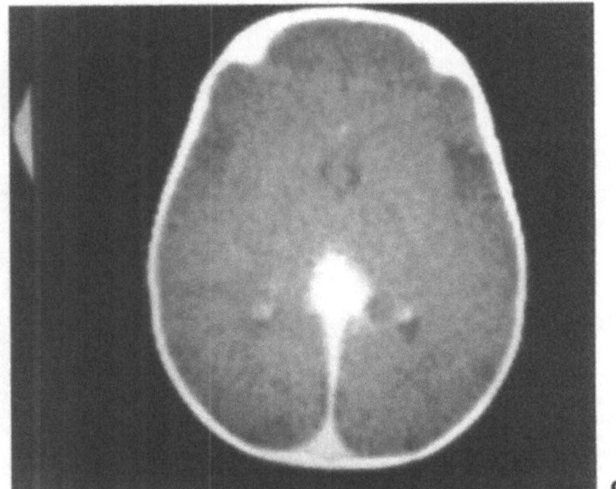

Fig. 9.8. a A 3-day-old newborn with major cardiomegaly, severe heart failure, and intracranial bruit. The infant died on day 6. A huge galenic aneurysm (*1*) drains in a markedly dilated straight sinus (*2*) that joins the torcular Herophili (*3*): irreducible heart failure is the logical consequence. b An 18-day-old newborn. Antenatal color Doppler and MRI diagnosis of ectatic vein of Galen. Normal cardiovascular status. Marked venous stenosis (*3*) between dilated vein of Galen (*1*) and straight sinus (*2*). Absence of hemodynamic disturbances is a natural consequence

Fig. 9.9. a Routine ultrasonography detected a fluid mass behind the third ventricle. Final diagnosis: incisural cyst with posterior partial agenesis of corpus callosum. b A 1-month-old infant with macrocrania. A rounded, midline, echo-free structure was located behind the third ventricle and above the tentorium. In the absence of pulsed Doppler, several etiologies were suspected: supratentorial arachnoid cyst, vascular malformation, isolated cisternal dilatation. c Postcontrast CT affirmed the vascular nature of the lesion

In a 37-weeks' gestation fetus, brain ultrasonography revealed a cystic lesion behind the third ventricle, the vascular nature of which was shown by color Doppler. Only two feeding vessels were detected, originating from the vertebrobasilar vasculature. A galenic aneurysm was diagnosed (Fig. 9.10). ECG was normal.

Ultrasonography was complemented by MRI, which demonstrated the rounded lesion, hypointense on HASTE sequence, draining into a normal straight sinus and ending in the superior sagittal sinus, as a fan-shaped structure. A stenosis between the enlarged vein of Galen and straight sinus was suspected. Brain parenchyma remained normal (Fig. 9.11).

Taken together, the morphological data suggested an aneurysm of the vein of Galen with a reasonably favorable prognosis: a small number of feeding arteries, no sonographic features of heart failure, no MRI signs of ischemic brain damage.

At term, delivery was uneventful; Anthony exhibited minimal cardiac enlargement; atrial communication and ductus arteriosus quickly closed after birth. At 1 week of life, clinical examination showed a normal baby (weight 3200 g, head circumference 34 cm, normal neurological and cardiovascular status). Brain ultrasonography showed the abnormality:

– The galenic aneurysmal dilatation appeared as an anechoic midline cavity, located in the area of the velum interpositum (Fig. 9.12).

– Color Doppler reproduced the results of fetal MRI, showing a vascular mass followed by a small straight sinus that widened in its distal portion, becoming fan-shaped. Despite this suggestive appearance, a straight sinus stenosis could not be confirmed. Feeding vessels were easily demonstrated: the basilar artery was slightly enlarged, while the two posterior cerebral arteries and the two posterior choroidal arteries were widely dilated before they join the aneurysmal lumen. The ante-

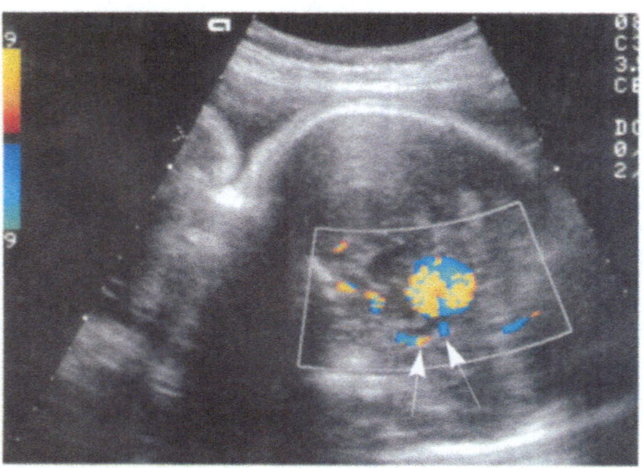

Fig. 9.10. On color Doppler imaging, one of the two vessels that supply the galenic pouch (posterior choroidal artery) is easily identified (arrows) (Dr. Deschamps, Montpellier)

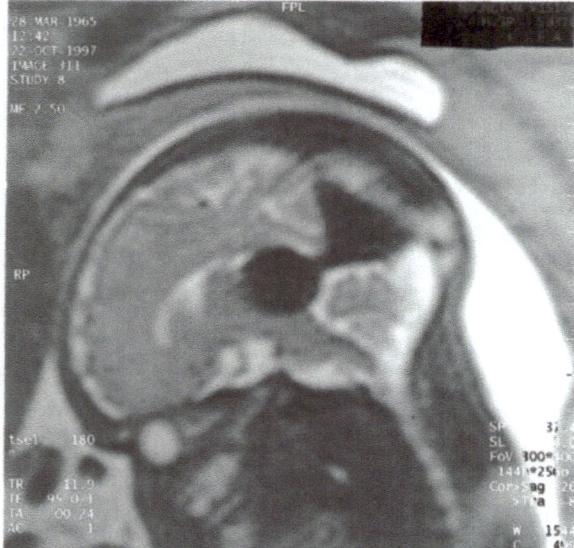
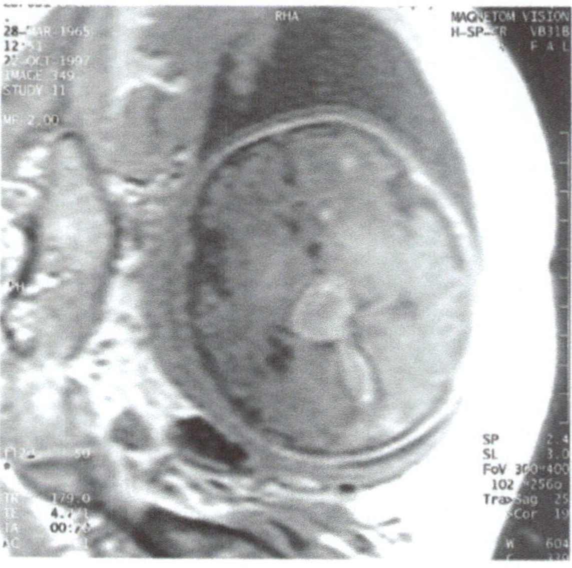

Fig. 9.11a,b. MRI in a 37-weeks' gestation fetus. **a** T2 HASTE sequence, sagittal plane. Markedly hypointense signal from a galenic malformation and probable proximal stenosis of the straight sinus. **b** T1-weighted sequence. The aneurysmal sac, straight sinus, and superior sagittal sinus are moderately hyperintense

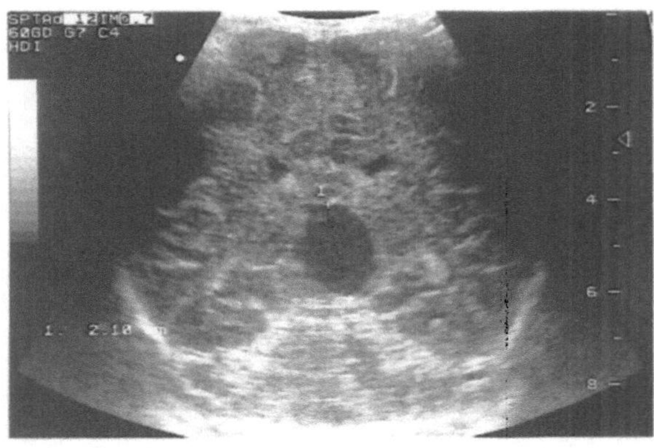
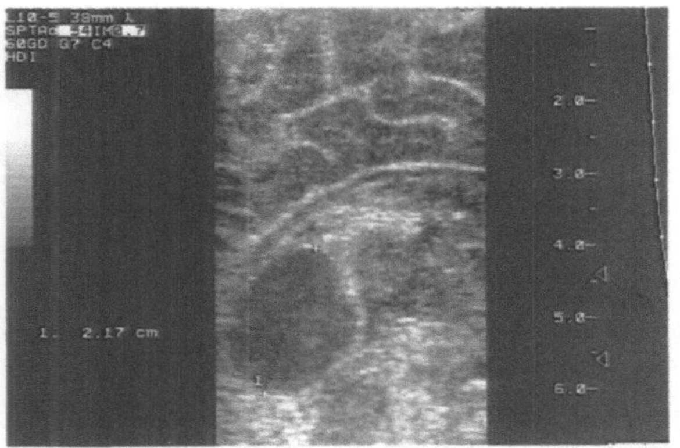

Fig. 9.12a,b. Galenic ectasia appears as a midline anechoic pouch located behind the third ventricle and below the splenium of corpus callosum; it measures 21 mm in diameter

rior cerebral arteries and pericallosal arteries, on the other hand, were normal in diameter and did not form part of the malformation (Fig. 9.13).

- These data were confirmed by pulsed Doppler. In all vessels that contributed to the abnormality (basilar, posterior cerebral, and posterior choroidal arteries), peak-systolic (PSV), end-diastolic (EDV), and time-average velocities (TAV) were markedly increased and downstream resistance decreased, with a very low resistive index (RI) (Fig.9.14). By contrast, hemodynamic data were normal (velocities and RI) in the arteries not involved in the malformation (internal carotid, anterior cerebral, and pericallosal arteries) (Fig. 9.15).

- Within the aneurysmal pouch, velocities were highly increased, with an arterial spectrum, contrasting with the draining straight sinus where velocities were only moderately increased. This appearance seemed to confirm that a protective stenosis followed the aneurysm. In the same way, the hemodynamics in the superior sagittal sinus and transverse sinuses revealed that venous pressure was only slightly increased (Fig. 9.16).

In sum, the sonographic neonatal evaluation showed that this galenic malformation should have a good outcome: it was supplied only by choroidal arteries, there was a protective stenosis of the straight sinus, no congestive heart failure, and a normal parenchymal echostructure.

Sonographic follow-up was decided on and a transarterial embolization planned when the patient reached 5 months of age.

- At 3 weeks of life, some mobile echoes were detected within the aneurysmal sac, and gradually increased. At 2 months, pulsed Doppler imaging revealed a marked decrease in straight sinus veloc-

ities, suggesting that the venous ectasia and the draining vein were thrombosing (Fig. 9.17).

- In parallel to this, abnormal flow velocities were moderately decreased in the feeding arteries. However, at 2 months, the basilar artery and posterior cerebral arteries remained wider than the anterior cerebral artery, and only the right posterior choroidal artery supplied the aneurysm.

- In fact, the onset of progressive triventricular dilatation (Fig. 9.18) and the increase in volume of the aneurysm with compression of the third ventricle led to earlier performance of embolization (at 2.5 months).

- Pretreatment MRI confirmed the sonographic findings: ventriculomegaly and a large, partially thrombosed galenic aneurysm, compressing the sylvian aqueduct (Fig. 9.19). Angiography (Fig. 9.20) showed the galenic vein, supplied by the right posterior choroidal artery, and the absence of venous drainage (thrombotic straight sinus).

The two pedicles of the posterior choroidal artery were embolized using butylcyanoacrylate mixed with Lipiodol and glue. Post-treatment MRI revealed that the arteriovenous malformation was almost completely thrombosed and residual flow was minimal.

At 3 months of life, ventriculomegaly was still progressive and the galenic aneurysm still very large (31 mm×34 mm); it was partly thrombosed and fed by the right posterior choroidal artery (Fig. 9.21). The hemodynamic situation had obviously improved, since peak-systolic and end-diastolic velocities had almost normalized in the basilar artery.

- At 3.5 months of age, the infant presented with repeated vomiting and bulging fontanelle, signs of an intracranial pressure increase that required a

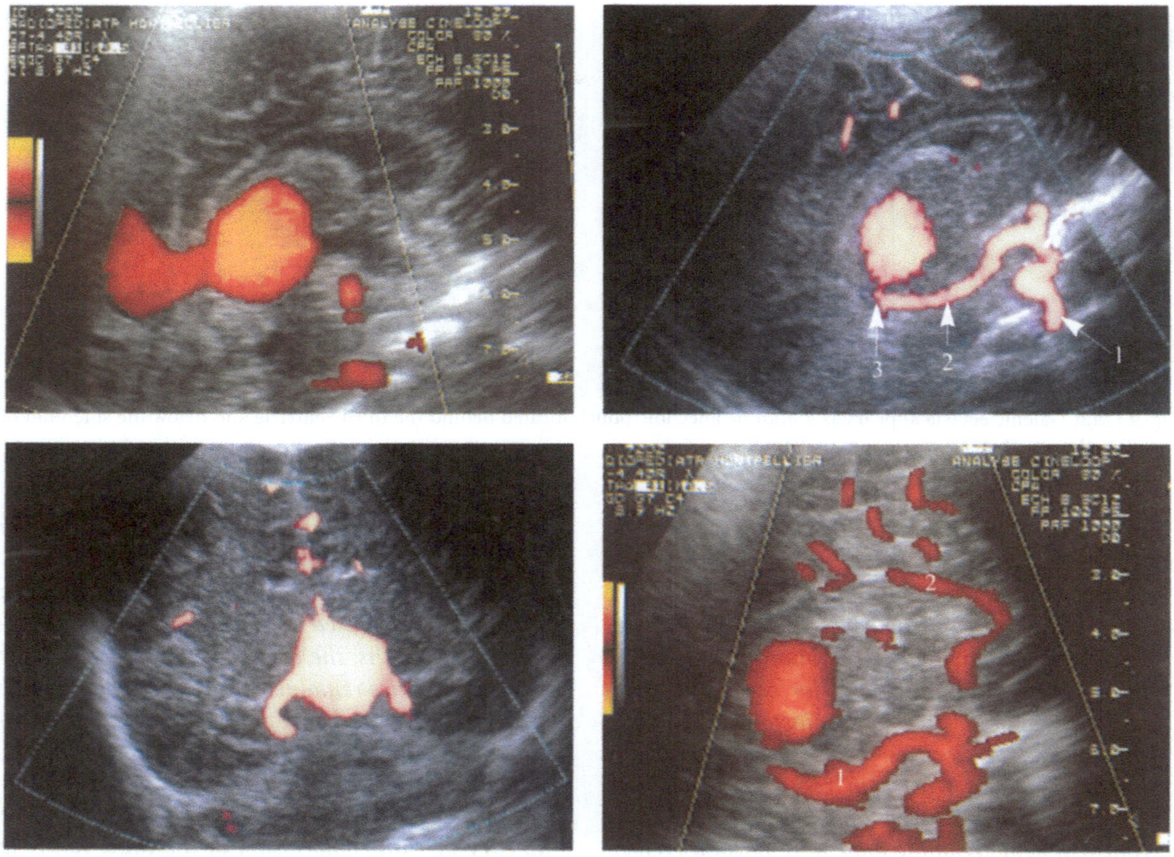

Fig. 9.13. a Power Doppler evaluation in the midline sagittal plane. There is perfect agreement between fetal MRI and neonatal color Doppler (**b**): the aneurysmal sac is fed by the basilar artery (*1*), posterior cerebral artery (*2*), and posterior choroidal artery (*3*). **c** The two posterior choroidal arteries drain entirely into a venous ectasia. **d** The diameters of the posterior choroidal artery (*1*) (5.4 mm) and the pericallosal artery (*2*) (2.9 mm) are obviously different

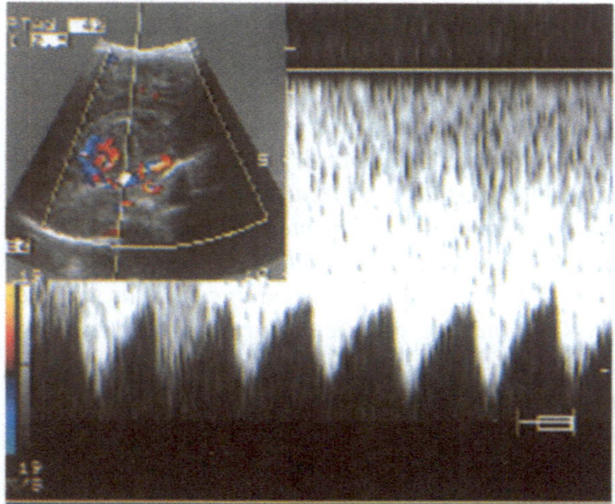

Fig. 9.14. Day 2. Spectral analysis of the right posterior choroidal artery. Velocities are markedly increased: PSV=166 cm/s, EDV=124 cm/s, RI=0.34

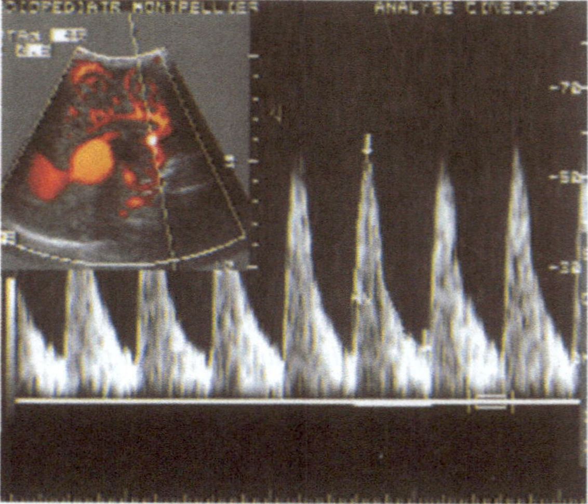

Fig. 9.15. The anterior cerebral artery (like the internal carotid artery) does not contribute to the malformation. Its velocities are normal for a 10-day-old infant: PSV=54 cm/s, EDV=10 cm/s, TAV=26 cm/s, RI=0.80

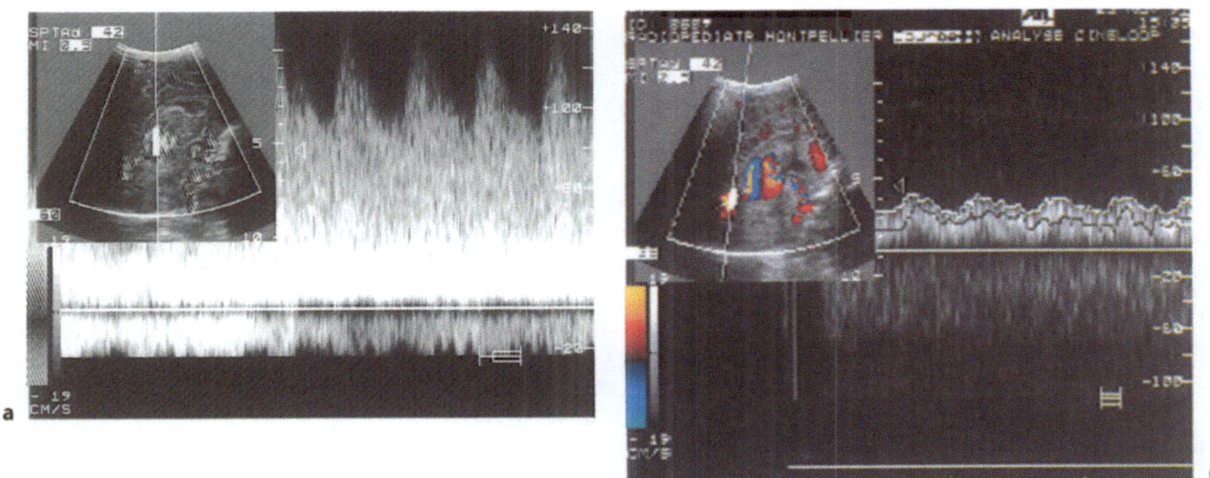

Fig. 9.16. a Spectral analysis of the aneurysmal pouch: arterial spectrum with highly raised velocities; PSV=140 cm/s. **b** In straight sinus, moderately increased velocities (40 cm/s) confirm the hypothesis of a protective stenosis and mild venous hyperpressure

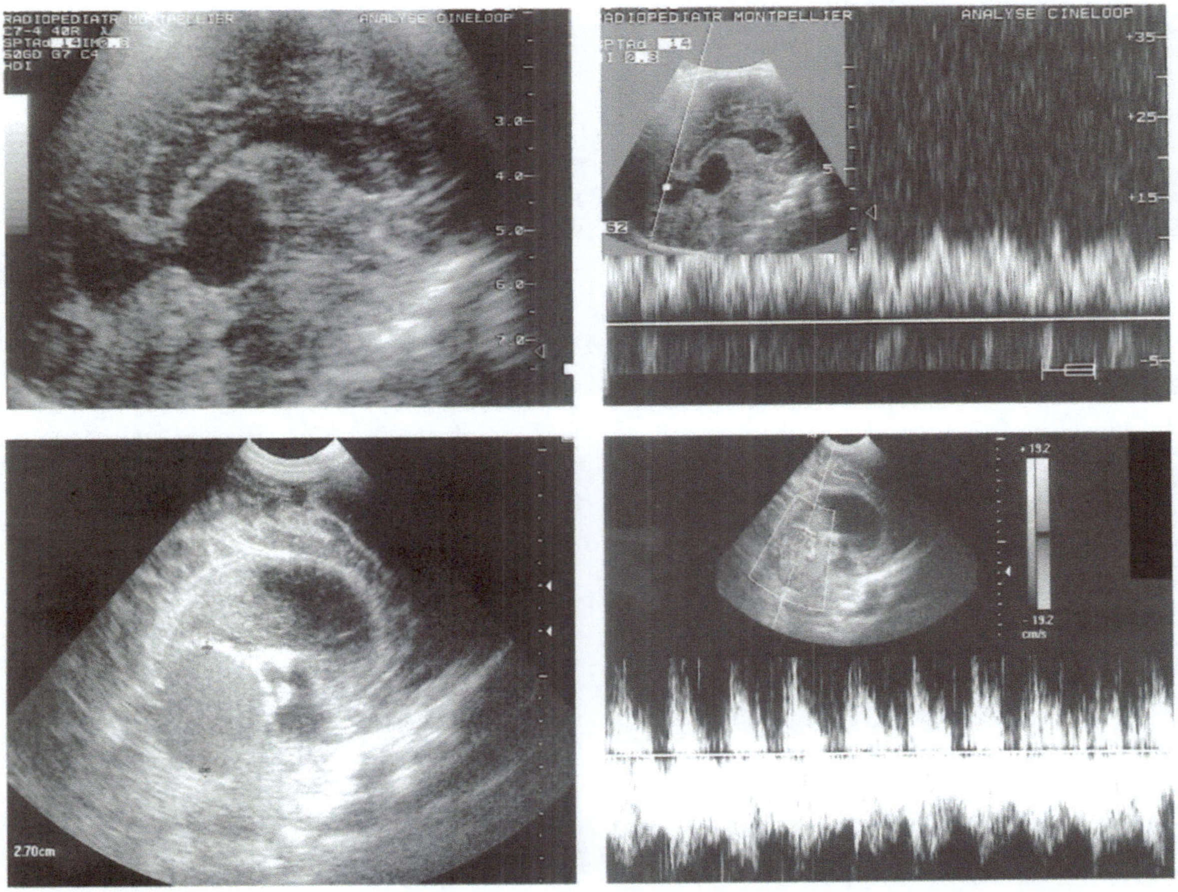

Fig. 9.17. a Day 19. Some echoes appear within the aneurysm and straight sinus; however, straight sinus flow remains present, with low velocities (less than 15 cm/s) (**b**). **c** Day 67: the huge aneurysm is full of echoes, the straight sinus is no longer visible and is definitely thrombosed. Velocity in the galenic ectasia is markedly reduced: 20 cm/s (**d**)

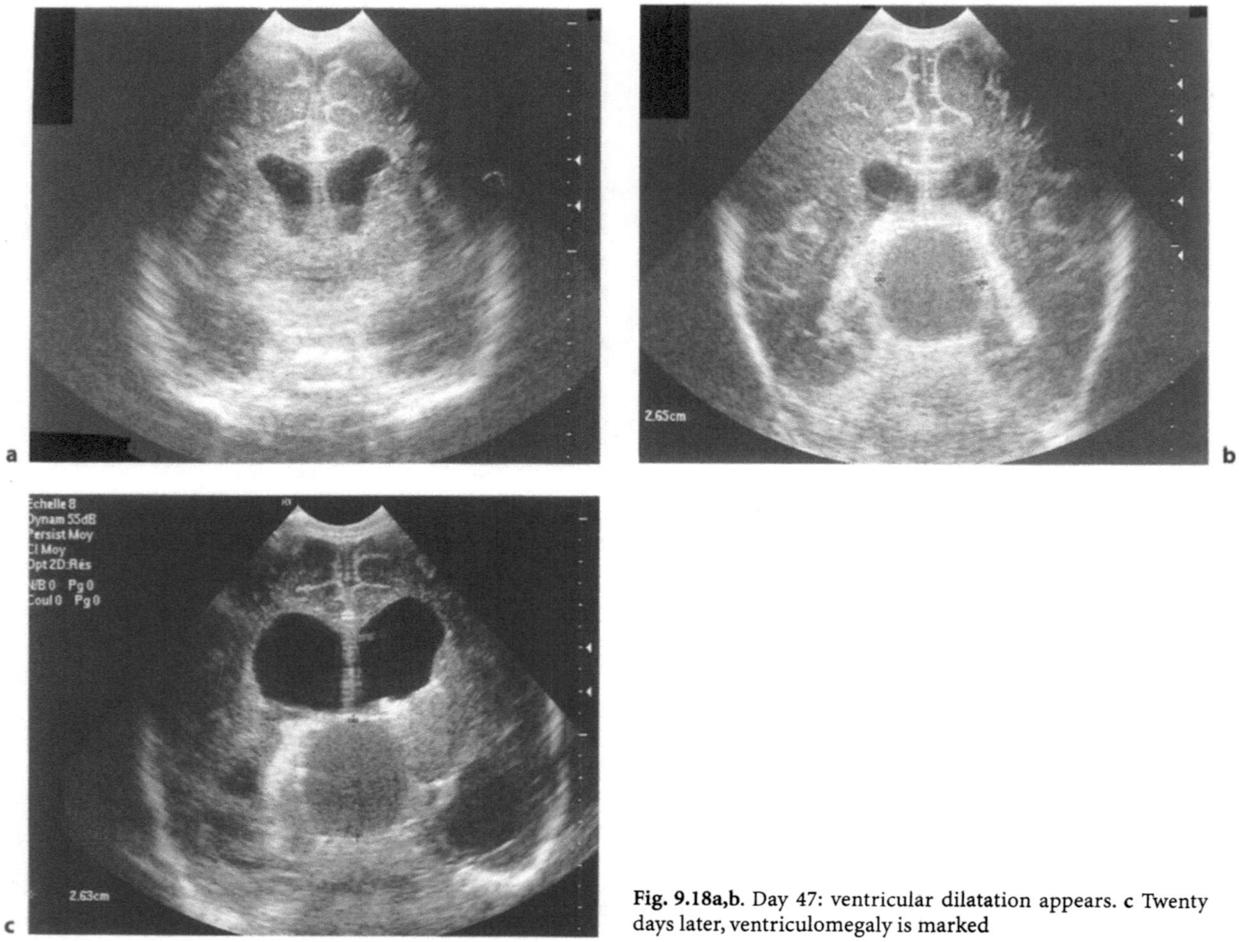

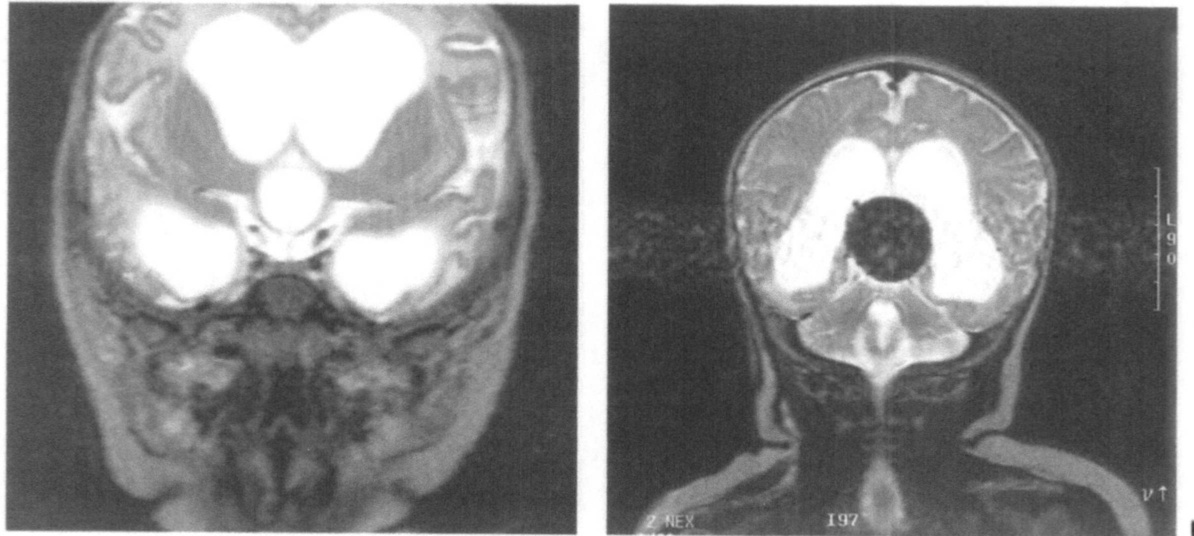

Fig. 9.18a,b. Day 47: ventricular dilatation appears. c Twenty days later, ventriculomegaly is marked

Fig. 9.19a,b. Day 80: pretreatment assessment.T2-weighted MRI confirms the severe triventricular dilatation (a) and the huge galenic aneurysm (b). Note that the brain parenchyma remains normal (Dr. Brunelle, Paris)

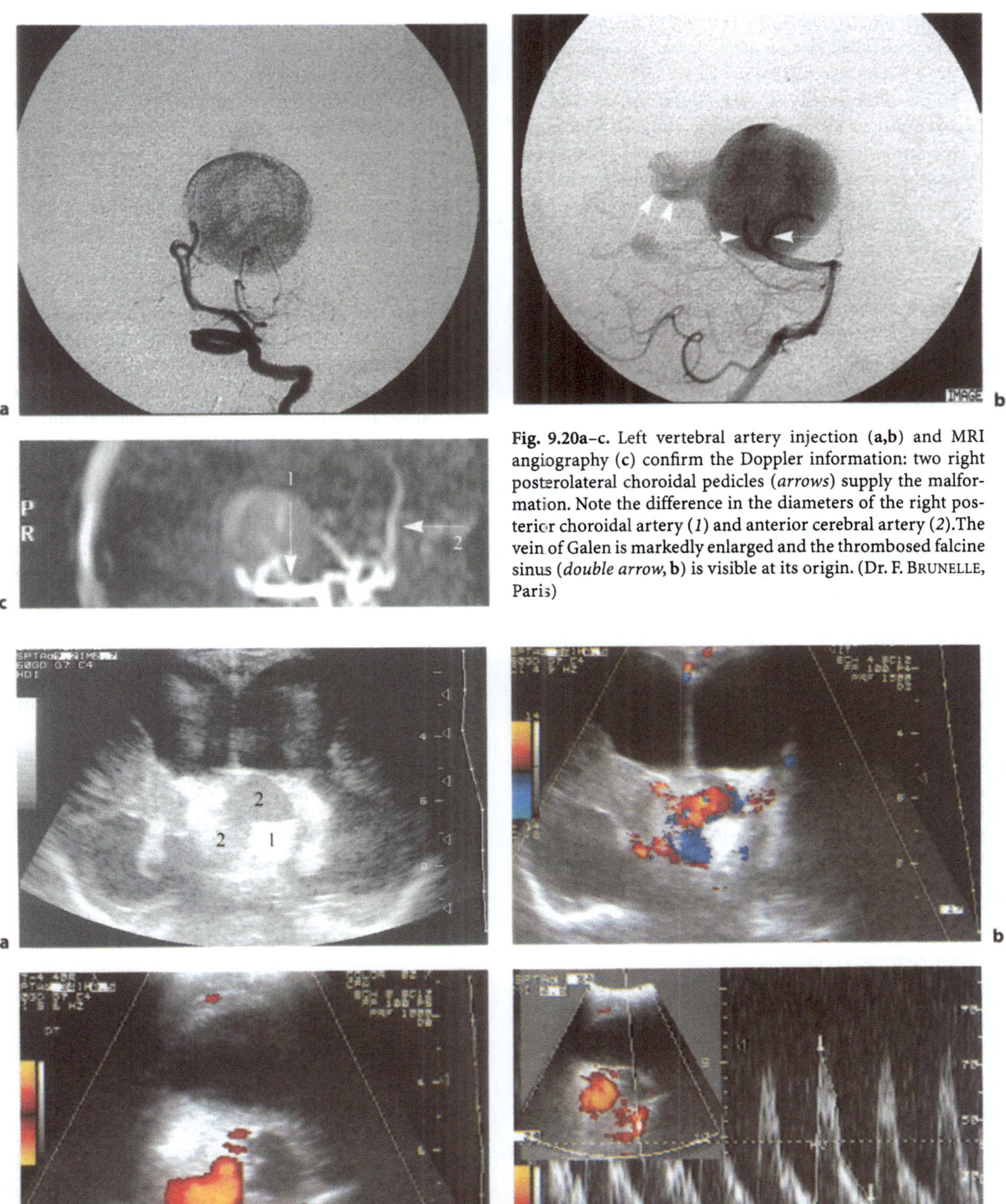

Fig. 9.20a–c. Left vertebral artery injection (**a,b**) and MRI angiography (**c**) confirm the Doppler information: two right posterolateral choroidal pedicles (*arrows*) supply the malformation. Note the difference in the diameters of the right posterior choroidal artery (*1*) and anterior cerebral artery (*2*).The vein of Galen is markedly enlarged and the thrombosed falcine sinus (*double arrow,* **b**) is visible at its origin. (Dr. F. BRUNELLE, Paris)

Fig. 9.21a–d. Sonographic follow-up 10 days after transarterial embolization. **a.** The aneurysmal sac (31 mm×34 mm) has a heterogeneous echostructure: its inferior part (*1*) is strongly echogenic and thrombosed, while its superior medial part (*2*) contains punctuate echoes and persistent flow (**b**) and is fed by the right posterior choroidal artery (arrow, **c**). However, basilar artery velocities have decreased (**d**): PSV=74 cm/s, EDV=28 cm/s, RI=0.72, compared with PSV=81 cm/s, EDV=37 cm/s, RI=0.54 before embolization

ventriculocisternostomy (Fig. 9.22), the patency of which was checked on MRI (pulsed sequence).

- *At 4.5 months, ultrasonography confirmed complete thrombosis of the aneurysmal sac. At 7 months, MRI demonstrated reduced volume of the embolized aneurysm, decreased ventricular enlargement, and patency of the sylvian aqueduct and ventriculocisternostomy. At 16 months of life, the infant exhibited normal psychomotor development.*

This case report summarizes the current principles of the diagnosis and management of ectasia of the vein of Galen.

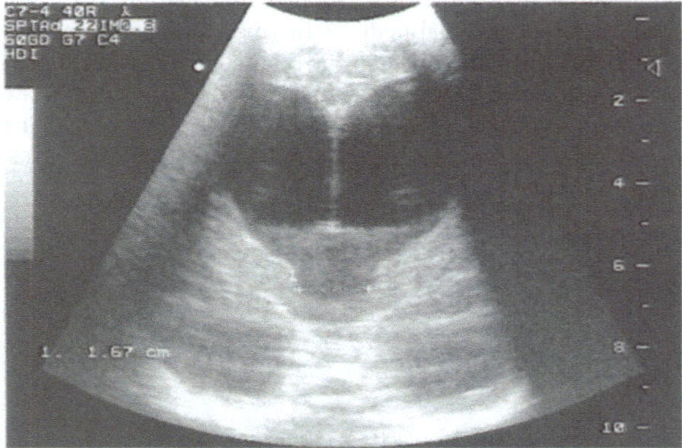

Fig. 9.22. At 3 months and 15 days of life: signs of increased intracranial pressure (vomiting, bulging fontanelle, severe triventricular dilatation). The aneurysm is completely thrombosed. Ventriculocisternostomy is decided upon

9.1.1.4.1
Diagnosis

The problem of diagnosis has been resolved, in both fetus and neonate, by the remarkable advances in imaging (color Doppler, spectral analysis, fetal brain MRI), so long as a strict protocol of analysis is followed.

- In the neonate, the value of color Doppler imaging is obvious to all authors (Brunelle 1997; Ciricillo 1990; Deeg 1990; Eltohami 1992; Horowitz 1994; Johnston 1987; Lasjaunias 1997; Saliba 1987; Stockberger 1993; Tessler 1989; Westra 1993; White 1992). Differential diagnosis is easy: supratentorial arachnoid cyst and cisternal dilatation are excluded. Color imaging enables accurate assessment of the aneurysmal sac and its feeding and draining vessels. The hemodynamic behavior of venous ectasia mainly depends on the number and communication of the supplying arteries. Tessler (1989) showed on color Doppler the presence of a swirling flow (Fig. 9.23) and high-velocity jets from feeding vessels within the aneurysm.

During the diagnostic evaluation, all brain vessels should be studied:

- Supplying arteries have increased diameter, contrasting with other vessels that have a normal or decreased diameter (Fig. 9.13).
- The mode of communication with the venous ectasia may also be assessed (Fig. 9.24).
- Draining veins are precisely depicted: straight sinus with a normal location, ectopic falcine sinus, or stenosis of venous drainage (Fig. 9.25).

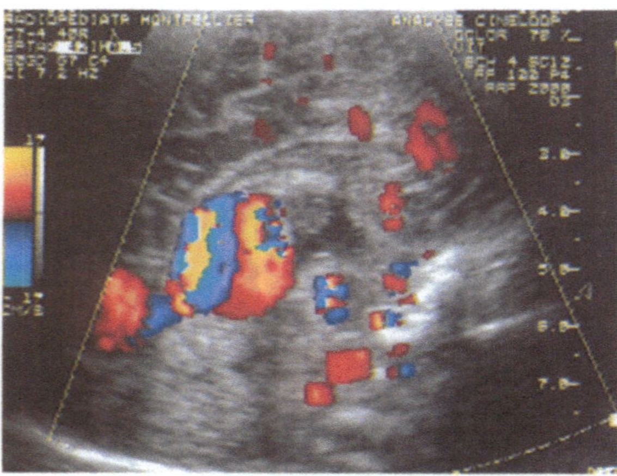

Fig. 9. 23. Aneurysm of the vein of Galen shown by neonatal color Doppler imaging. Counterclockwise swirling appearance, coded alternately *red* and *blue*

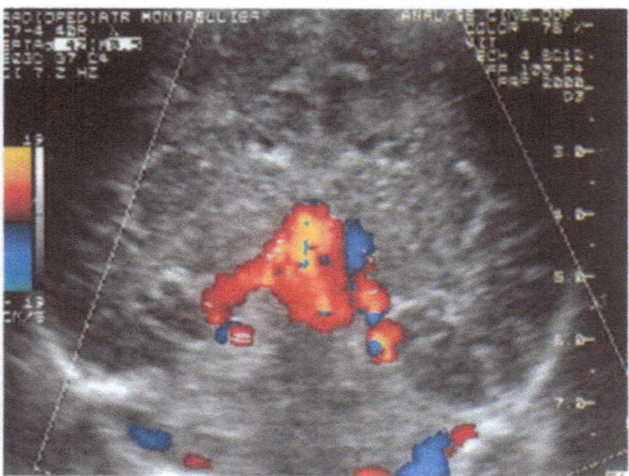

Fig. 9.24. Venous ectasia fed by posterior choroidal arteries

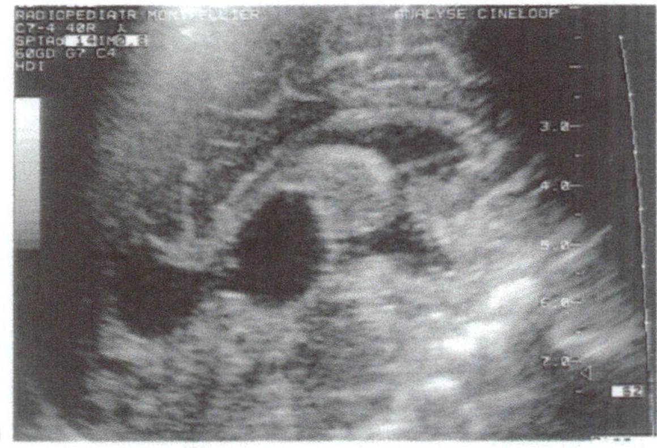
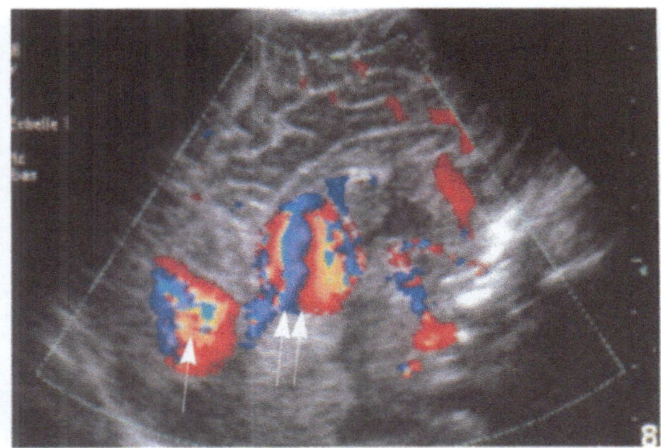

Fig. 9.25a,b. Stenosis of the straight sinus is possible (a) when a swirling flow (*arrow*) is seen before the proximal stenosis (*double arrow*) (b). It will be definitively demonstrated by pulsed Doppler

Color Doppler is only the first step in the diagnostic evaluation and is followed by pulsed Doppler, which demonstrates the hemodynamic abnormalities and measures their severity.

- Feeding arteries show two characteristic patterns: an increase (sometimes major) in peak-systolic, end-diastolic, and time-average velocities, and a decrease in resistive index. Doppler assessment should be as complete as possible, and relates mainly to the basilar artery, posterior cerebral arteries, and posterior choroidal arteries, but also to the transmesencephalic artery, middle cerebral arteries, and lenticulostriate and anterior choroidal arteries. The results are obvious: an abnormal spectral analysis (highly increased velocities, mainly diastolic) shows a supplying vessel; whereas if the spectral analysis remains normal, the vessel is not part of the malformation (Figs. 9.14, 9.15).

Within the galenic aneurysm, flow is frequently arterialized; velocities are most often accelerated, predominantly on the diastolic component, which explains the low resistive index (Fig. 9.16).

Finally, spectral analysis of venous drainage is essential. Venous pressure is constantly increased in correlation to the clinical pattern: when venous hyperpressure is severe, pre- or postnatal heart failure is the rule and subsequent hydrocephalus is frequent; when venous hyperpressure is minimal (where there is a protective stenosis of the straight sinus), heart failure is absent or minimal.

Pulsed Doppler findings in galenic venous ectasia are poorly documented (Eltohami 1992; Westra 1993). Westra (1993) pointed out the value of detecting a low resistive index to identify supplying vessels (average RI=0.38 in 51 vessels determined to be arterial feeders on angiography).

- Knowledge of these postnatal diagnostic data is essential, because the present resolution of US equipment should allow the same results in the fetus.

Almost invariably, the diagnosis is made during the third trimester, rarely in the second one (Ballester 1994; Ordorica 1990). All authors (Ballester 1994; Chisholm 1997, Dan 1992; Evans 1991; Hata 1988; Ishimatsu 1991; Mai 1996; Paumier 1998; Sepulveda 1995; Yuval 1997) agree on the decisive impact of color imaging for prenatal diagnosis, since the same sonographic appearance is seen as in the neonate (Fig. 9.26).

The great diagnostic value of pulsed Doppler (Fig. 9.27) has been documented too (Ballester 1994; Chisholm 1996; Evans 1991; Hata 1988; Reiter 1986; Rizzo 1987; Strauss 1991; Worswick 1992; Yamagushi 1991).

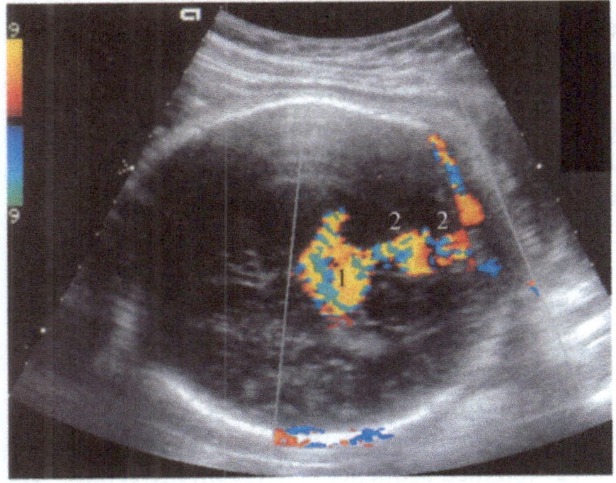

Fig. 9.26. Galenic aneurysm. The characteristic racket shape corresponds to the aneurysm (*1*) joining the draining sinus (*2*). (Dr. Deschamps, Montpellier)

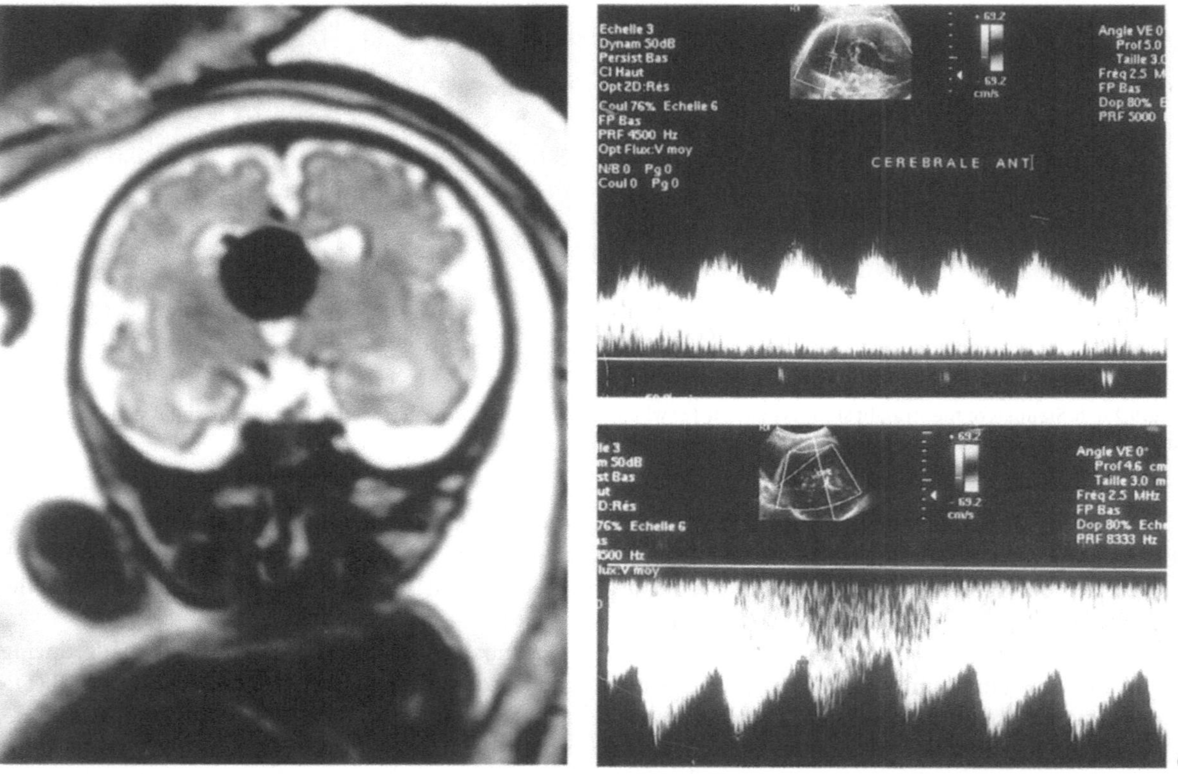

Fig. 9.27a–c. A 32-weeks' fetus with galenic aneurysm. MRI (**a**) shows a minimal ventricular dilatation and normal brain paren-chyma. The spectral analysis curve allows mapping of the vascular malformation: the velocities in the anterior cerebral artery (**b**) (PSV=51 cm/s, EDV=30 cm/s, RI=0.40) and in a posterior choroidal artery (**c**) (PSV=124 cm/s, EDV=70 cm/s, RI=0.44) prove that these two vessels contribute to the malformation. (Dr. SIMON, Paris)

All authors describe the resistive index distur-bances (SEPULVEDA 1995), but few report on the importance of studying velocities. MAI (1996) has shown increased velocities within the galenic ectasia (PSV=44 cm/s) and the communicating vessels (PSV=59 cm/s, EDV=46 cm/s) in a 38-weeks' gesta-tion fetus.

Spectral analysis may also show arterial-type (WORSWICK 1992) or turbulent flow (BALLESTER 1994; ISHIMATSU 1991; DAN 1992) in the aneurysmal cystic structure.

– Antenatal MRI is evaluated in the diagnosis and prognosis of galenic aneurysm. Although its essential role is to detect ischemic brain damage, MRI provides good-quality diagnostic informa-tion (BRUNELLE 1997; CAMPI 1996; MARTINEZ-LAGE 1993; PAUMIER 1998; YAMASHITA 1992). On T2-weighted sequences (HASTE), the ectatic vein appears hypointense and its drainage is well visu-alized (Fig. 9.28).

The arterial vessels are more difficult to identify because of their small size, but the feeding arteries appear as multiple hypointense spots: the anterior cerebral, posterior choroidal, and transmesencepha-lic arteries are excellently shown (Fig. 9.29), and this improves the prognostic evaluation.

9.1.1.4.2
Evolution

When the diagnosis has been made and the neonate is hemodynamically stable, neurosurgical and neuro-radiological teams usually propose endovascular embolization, ideally performed at 5 months of life. This requires a protocolized sonographic follow-up in order to detect changes or complications during this period.

– *Spontaneous thrombosis* (BELTRAMELLO 1991; DI ROCCO 1983; HEINZ 1968; KUROKI 1995; SIX 1980; WHITAKER 1987)

Spontaneous thrombosis remains infrequent and unpredictable. HEINZ (1968) reported that it may occur in utero; heart failure is absent in the case of a throm-

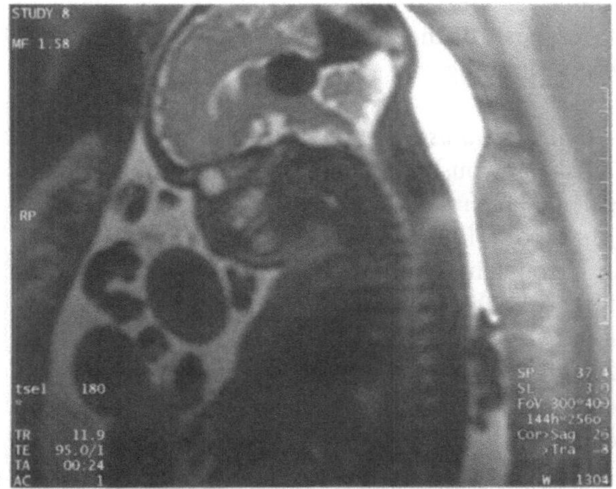

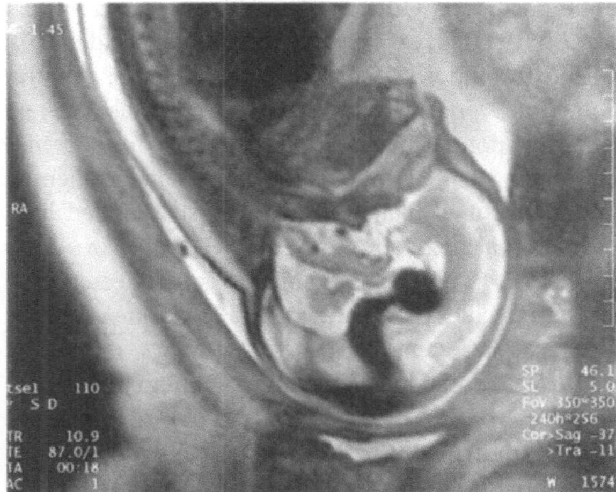

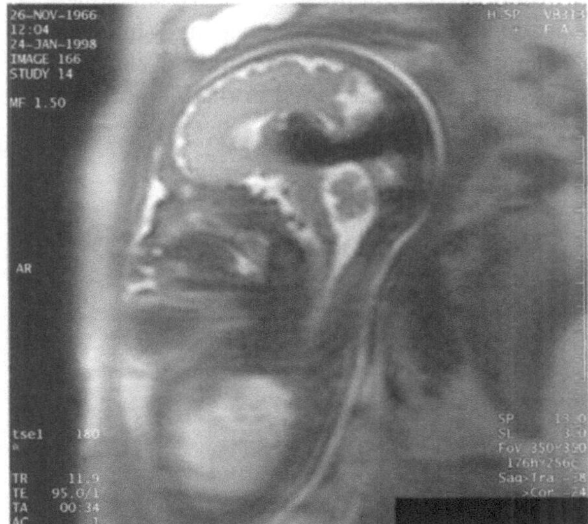

Fig. 9.28a–c. MRI (T2 HASTE sequence) provides precise imaging of venous drainage. a A 37-weeks' fetus. Proximal stenosis of straight sinus. b A 32-weeks' fetus. Ectopic falcine sinus (Dr. QUERE, Nantes). c. A 37-weeks' fetus. Large draining vein, severe congestive heart failure; the pregnancy was terminated

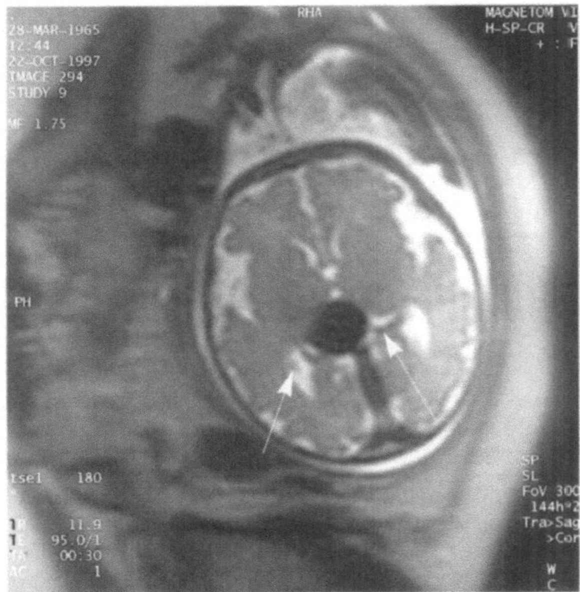

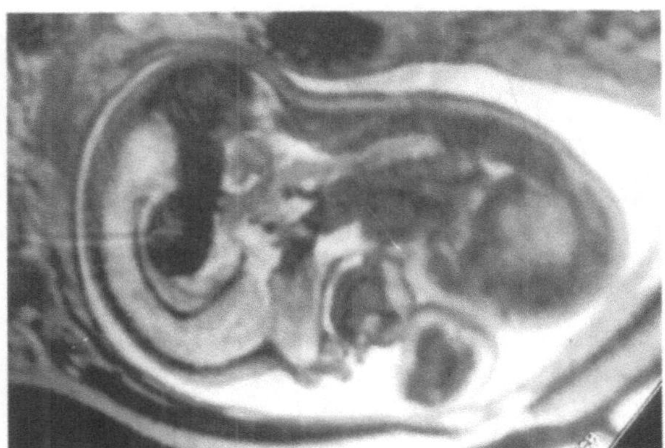

Fig. 9.29. a A 37-weeks' fetus with galenic aneurysm. The two feeding posterior choroidal arteries are excellently individualized (arrows). Confirmation by neonatal color Doppler. b A 37-weeks' fetus. On T2-weighted MRI the hypointense anterior cerebral artery is markedly enlarged and is involved in the malformation. Confirmation by fetal pulsed Doppler (Dr. SIMON, Paris)

botic aneurysm. Other authors (CHAPMAN 1989; DI ROCCO 1983) have provided convincing evidence of galenic thrombosis occurring between 5 and 7 months. Sometimes preceded by progressive irritability and lethargy, spontaneous thrombosis is easy to recognize on imaging. On CT, there is no longer enhancement of the aneurysmal dilatation, which is surrounded by a partially calcified rim (CHAPMAN 1989; MANCUSO 1989; WHITAKER 1987); the malformation decreases in size and calcifies (CHAPMAN 1989). This pattern may be also recognized on US (Fig. 9.30).

Surgical excision of a thrombotic aneurysm is conceivable (LAZAR 1974; WEIR 1968). LASJAUNIAS (1997) confirmed the infrequency of spontaneous thrombosis, which developed in only 5 out of 120 patients (i.e., 4%) in his series. He pointed out that spontaneous thrombosis should not be considered a favorable outcome, and that waiting for it to occur is a dangerous therapeutic strategy. Finally, hemody-namic factors probably further the spontaneous thrombosis of the malformation, especially stenosis of the draining vein.

– Hydrocephalus
This is obviously the most frequent complication of galenic aneurysm. In the 245 cases reported by JOHNSTON (1987), in the 43 cases of ZERAH (1992), and from a literature review (AL WATBAN 1987; CIRICILLO 1990; CRAWFORD 1990; MAHEUT 1987; MAYBERG 1988; O'DONNABHAIN 1989; WISOFF 1990; ZAMPELLA 1988), the incidence of hydrocephalus is 46.8%. Two hypotheses have been proposed to explain its development.
– The best known is obstruction: the aneurysmal sac progressively compresses the sylvian aqueduct, leading initially to reversible and intermittent stenosis, and later on to permanent occlusion. This theory has been accepted in the literature (AGEE

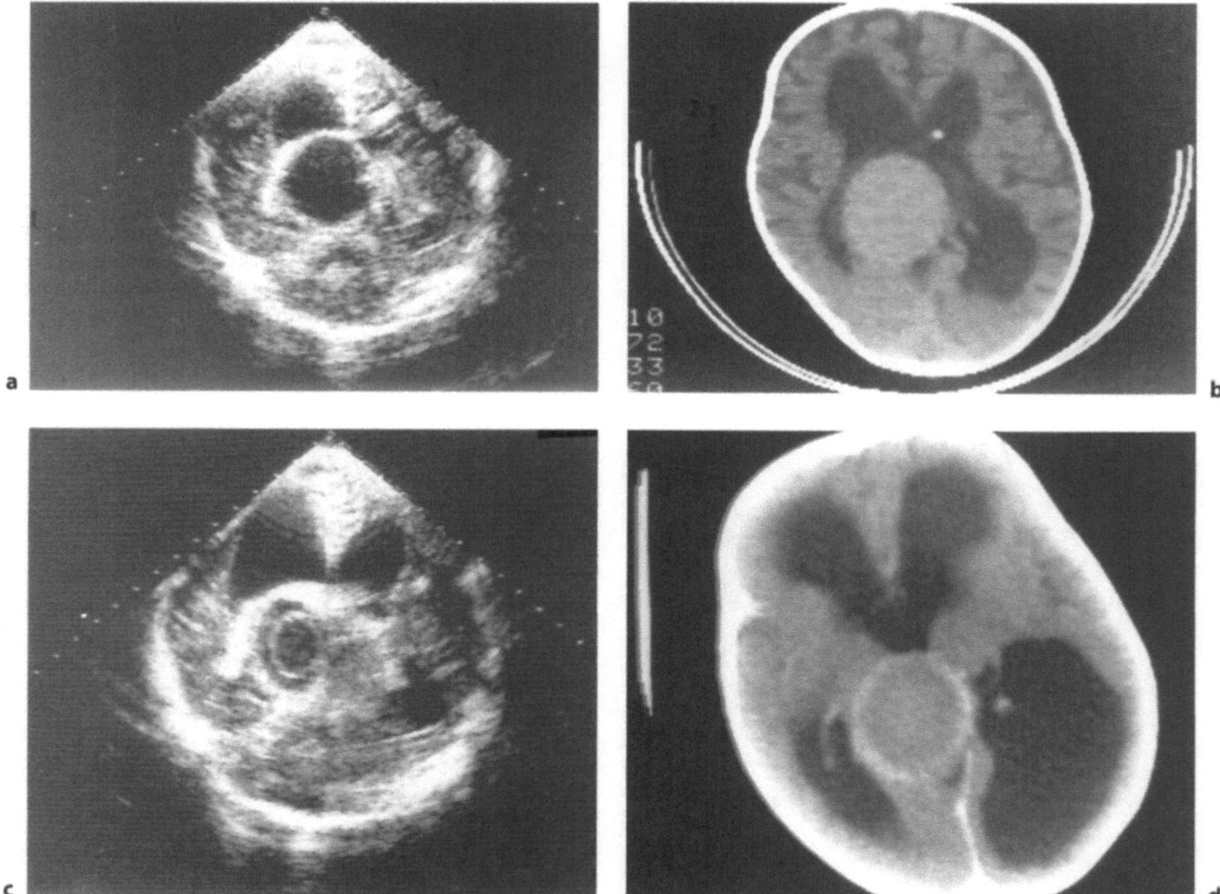

Fig. 9.30a–d. a A 4-month-old infant with macrocrania, without heart failure. A galenic aneurysm was detected and confirmed by CT (**b**). Ultrasound follow-up at 6 months of age. The aneurysmal dilatation was markedly reduced (**c**), contained intraluminal echoes, and showed a thickened wall with echogenic outer rim: calcified thrombosis. **d** CT confirmation. Note the severe hydrocephalus despite the aneurysmal thrombosis, suggesting aqueductal compression. (Dr. WILLI, Zurich)

1969; Bartal 1975; Hoffman 1982; Johnston 1973; Littvak 1969; Yasargil 1976), but has also been criticized. For example, Diebler (1981) noted that the aqueduct is usually patent on pneumoencephalography. Quisling (1989) reported hydrocephalus in five of six patients with a small, noncompressive aneurysm on CT, and in only six of nine patients with large aneurysm. Roosen (1986) described a case of fetal hydrocephalus and galenic malformation without aqueductal stenosis at pathological examination. Finally, Zerah (1992), reporting on a series of 17 shunted patients, underlined the frequency of postshunt complications: abnormal enlargement of the aneurysm in 7, subdural hematoma in 6, seizures in 3, and mechanical disorders in 3; moreover, more than 15% of the patients developed significant mental retardation.

Thus this theory needs to be supported by incontrovertible imaging evidence, such as phase contrast MRI to study CSF circulation.

– In the second hypothesis, high venous pressure plays a critical role. Although experimental studies in dogs and monkeys (Bedford 1934; Hammock 1971; Schlesinger 1940) do not seem to confirm this theory, this is probably because vein of Galen ligation does not reproduce the embryogenesis of the malformation: we know that the abnormal sac is not the vein of Galen, but its forerunner, the median prosencephalic vein.

Clinical facts are more significant. Secondary hydrocephalus from increased venous sinus pressure has been proposed in various situations (De Lange 1970; Haar 1975; Hooper 1961; Rosman 1978; Sainte Rose 1984; Young 1979), especially in high-flow arteriovenous fistulas. In these cases, hydrocephalus often starts with enlargement of the subarachnoid spaces, followed by mild ventricular dilatation.

In galenic aneurysm, venous pressure is consistently increased: Quisling (1989) reported pressures above 50 cm H_2O with a 1:5 ratio between intraventricular pressure and superior sagittal sinus pressure. This abnormal ratio explains why it is so difficult for CSF to enter from the subarachnoid space into the venous compartment. After transarterial embolization, venous pressure falls, and the ventricular dilatation and the amount of subarachnoid CSF decrease.

Ventriculoperitoneal shunting does not solve the problem that results from venous hyperpressure, and represents a simplistic answer to a complex problem. The shunting procedure induces a flow of water toward the brain, and increases the stagnation of water in white matter. It may produce a striking enlargement of the aneurysmal sac, which fills the free space created by the ventricular shrinkage. On the other hand, embolization treats the cause of the venous hyperpressure and allows maturation of the pacchionian granulations. These physiopathological explanations seem attractive; in the case of galenic aneurysm, the secondary hydrocephalus should initially be treated by embolization and not by shunt.

In fact, treatment (Lasjaunias 1997; Zerah 1992) should be discussed individually for each case.

In the case of Anthony, everything suggests obstruction of the sylvian aqueduct by the galenic malformation. Velocities were only moderately increased in the straight sinus (Fig. 9.16) and superior sagittal sinus, suggesting a slight venous overpressure; moreover, they quickly fell and normalized; the onset of progressive triventricular dilatation led to performance of early transarterial embolization; this did not improve the hydrocephalus and ventriculostomy was required at 3 months; and, finally, phase-contrast MRI provided strong evidence of an obstructive mechanism (Fig. 9.31): invisible aqueduct, compressed by a large aneurysmal sac, absence of flow and reduced velocities in the sylvian aqueduct immediately before the shunting procedure. At 7 months of life, ventricular enlargement had markedly decreased, the aneurysmal sac was small, and the sylvian aqueduct was visible. MRI confirmed patency of the aqueduct (8 cm/s) and ventriculocisternostomy (3 cm/s).

This example demonstrates that hydrocephalus may be due to obstruction and emphasizes the importance of imaging (Doppler measurement of draining venous velocities, MRI appearance of sylvian aqueduct, MRI analysis of CSF velocities in the aqueduct) in guiding the choice of treatment.

9.1.1.4.3
Prognostic Assessment

Determination of prognostic factors is important in the neonate as in the fetus. Lasjaunias (1996), in a recent multicenter study of 120 patients with galenic malformation, proposed a neonatal evaluation score (at 8 days of life), established on the basis of cardiac, cerebral, hepatic, respiratory, and renal functions (Table 9.1).

In the opinion of this author, embolization should be refused if the score is less than 8, or if ischemic brain damage is detected; emergency embolization should be performed if the score is more than 8 but less than 12; while a score of more than 12 indicates

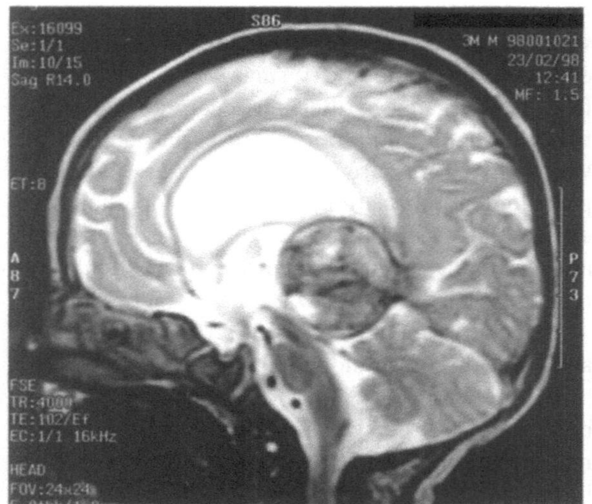

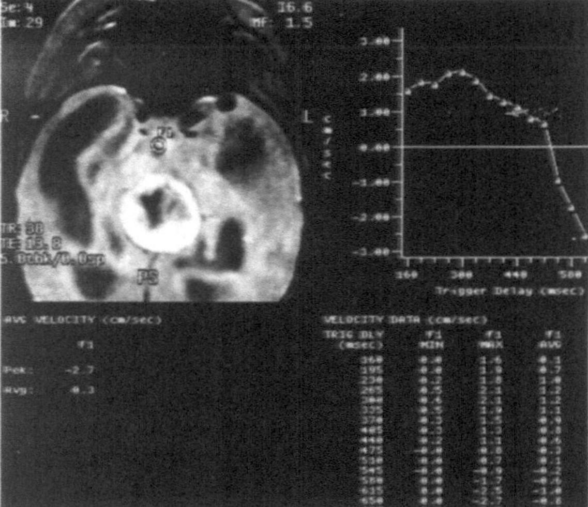

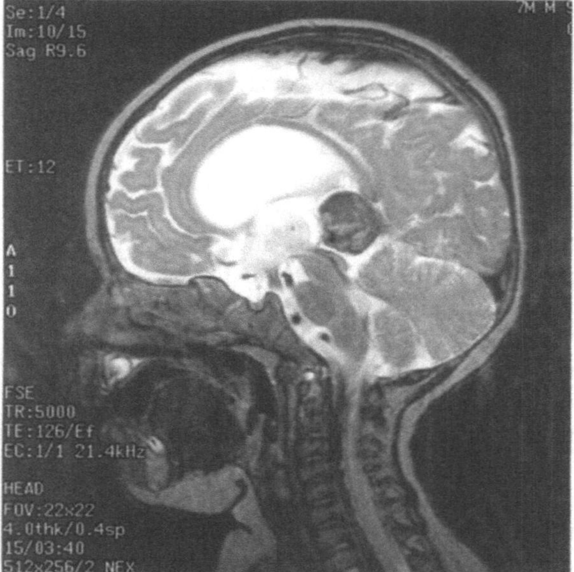

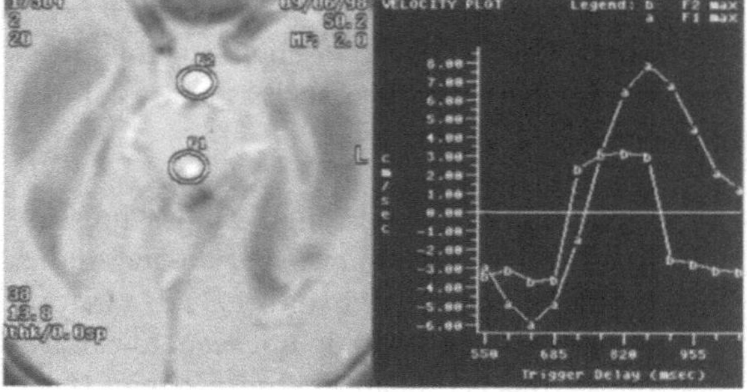

Fig. 9.31. a,b Preshunt evaluation. The large thrombosed aneurysm compresses the aqueduct of Sylvius. Phase-contrast MRI shows absence of flow within the aqueduct, with extremely reduced velocities (b). Ventriculocisternostomy is performed. Four months later: the ventricular enlargement has decreased, the thrombosed aneurysm is small, and the sylvian aqueduct is visible (c). Phase-contrast MRI shows normal patency of the sylvian aqueduct and the ventriculocisternostomy; maximal velocities are slightly higher in the aqueduct (8 cm/s) (d) than in the ventriculocisternostomy (3 cm/s). (Dr. BRUNELLE, Paris)

Table 9.1. Neonatal evaluation score (from LASJAUNIAS 1996)

Score	Cardiac function	Cerebral function	Hepatic function	Respiratory function	Renal function
5	Normal	Normal	–	Normal	–
4	Nontreated overload	Infraclinical isolated EEG anomalies	–	Polypnea Finishes bottle	–
3	Failure stable under treatment	Nonconvulsive Intermittent neurological signs	No hepatomegaly Normal function	Polypnea Does not finish bottle	Normal
2	Failure not stable under treatment	Isolated convulsive episode	Hepatomegaly Normal function	Assisted ventilation Normal saturation $Fi\,O_2 < 25\%$	Transitory anuria
1	Ventilation necessary	Seizures Constant neurological signs	Moderate or transient hepatic insufficiency	Assisted ventilation Normal saturation $Fi\,O_2 > 25\%$	Unstable diuresis under treatment
0	Resistant to treatment	–	Coagulation disorder Elevated enzymes	Assisted ventilation Desaturation	Anuria

delayed embolization, with maximum efficacy at 5 months of age.

Applying these selection criteria, 78 patients (65%) were embolized, with striking results: the mortality rate was 9% (7 cases), but neurological development was normal in 71 patients (i.e., 66%). These data completely change the pessimistic opinion held previously. Now, when a newborn shows good tolerance of extrauterine life, his or her prognosis after endovascular embolization is greatly improved. It is therefore obvious that an accurate prognosis should be established in order to optimize management.

However, the diagnosis is increasingly often made in the antenatal period, and the main challenge is to determine prognostic criteria in the fetus. Recognition of a galenic aneurysm during the third trimester of pregnancy shortens the diagnostic delay and allows the newborn to be referred to a specialist center. But which baby should be sent to the neurosurgeon or the neuroradiologist, and when? These questions explain the great importance of fetal imaging (morphological ultrasonography, pulsed and color Doppler imaging, fetal MRI).

- Obviously, the complexity and density of the arteriovenous anastomotic network is the main prognostic factor, responsible for the presence or absence of heart failure and of ischemic brain damage. Thus, color Doppler should analyze the vascular anatomy of the malformation precisely (Fig. 9.32).On morphological color imaging, a poor prognosis correlates to the presence of more than five feeding vessels (Fig. 9.33), large dilated draining veins (straight or falcine sinus), and small or absent noncontributing arterial vessels. However, these findings remain insufficient for a precise prognosis to be established. A hemodynamic component, provided by pulsed Doppler, is also required. Highly increased velocities within draining veins closely reflect the venous hyperpressure and predict a poor outcome. In the fetus, all brain arteries should be depicted, not only the dilated supplying vessels. These stealing arteries demonstrate a characteristic hemodynamic pattern: increased peak-systolic and, especially, end-diastolic velocities, associated with decreased resistive index. The future will tell whether the severity of these changes may be considered as a prognostic factor.

It is also important to depict the arteries that have been stolen from: either their spectrum and velocities are normal and brain ischemic damage is probably absent, or their velocities are decreased and their

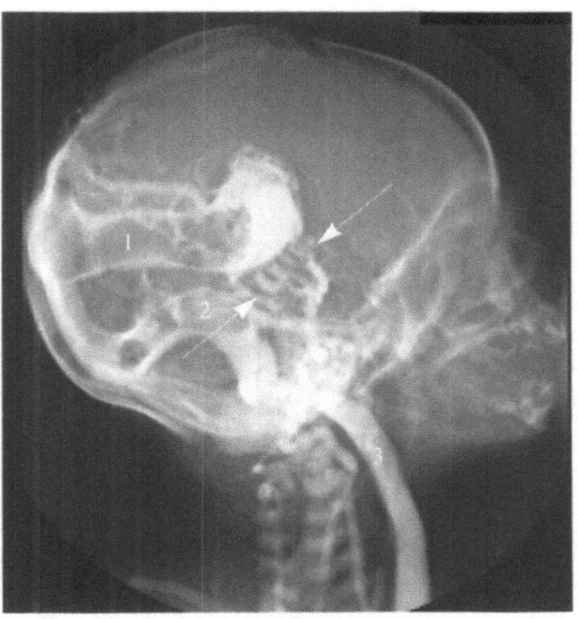

Fig. 9.32. A 34-weeks' fetus with galenic aneurysm. Color Doppler demonstrates multiple feeding arteries and severe congestive heart failure. The pregnancy was terminated (35 weeks' gestation). Post-mortem angiography showed several arteries (at least six) coming from the basilar system to join the aneurysm (*arrows*). Note the extreme dilatation of the draining vein (*1*), lateral sinus (*2*), and jugular vein (*3*). The anterior cerebral artery is not visualized: vascular steal? Thrombosis?

resistive index increased, and the risk of ischemic brain damage is obvious. Direct measurement of velocities seems to be a promising research trend, but it has yet to be validated, since it is not been reported in the literature (MAI 1996).

- Detection of congestive heart failure (GARCIA-MONACO 1991), which reflects the hemodynamic disturbances is essential. Its presence is easily understood, since up to 80% of left ventricular output may be shunted to the low-resistance arteriovenous malformation (PELLEGRINO 1987). In the prenatal period, the low resistance of the placenta protects the fetus by competing with the galenic ectasia, reducing the amount of blood shunted and preventing fetal heart failure. The onset of cardiomegaly or hydrops fetalis despite this protective mechanism characterizes a large shunt and a poor prognosis. This can only be assessed by echocardiography. Heart disease appears mainly in the form of dilated cardiomegaly (BALLESTER 1994; EVANS 1991; MENDELSOHN 1984; WORSWICK 1992), with right cardiac decompensation, dilated right cavities (JEANTY 1990), and enlarged jugular veins (Fig. 9.34). These signs

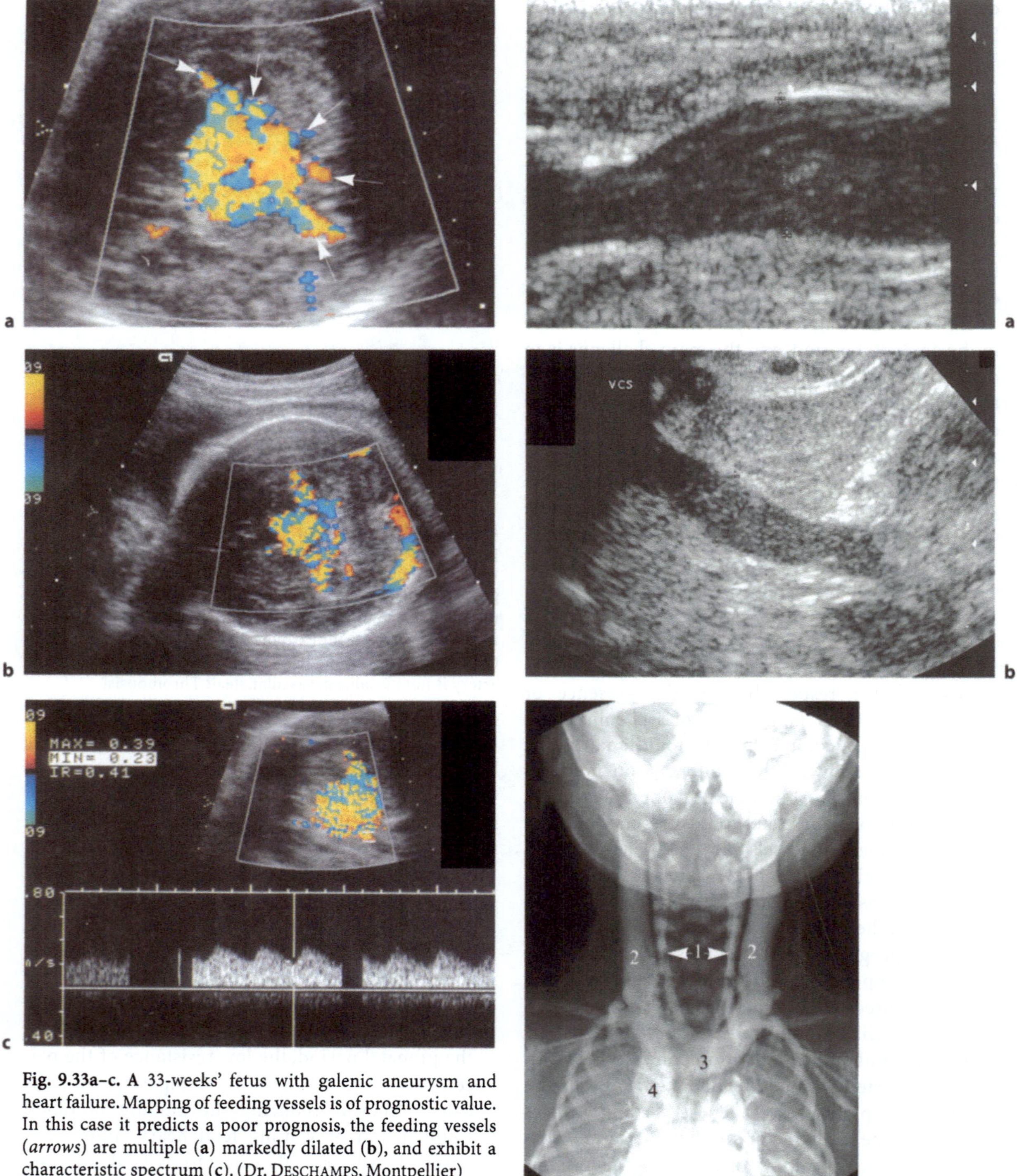

Fig. 9.33a–c. A 33-weeks' fetus with galenic aneurysm and heart failure. Mapping of feeding vessels is of prognostic value. In this case it predicts a poor prognosis, the feeding vessels (*arrows*) are multiple (**a**) markedly dilated (**b**), and exhibit a characteristic spectrum (**c**). (Dr. DESCHAMPS, Montpellier)

Fig. 9.34a,b. A 36-weeks' fetus with galenic aneurysm, severe heart decompensation, and enlarged jugular vein. The pregnancy was terminated. Post-mortem ultrasonography confirmed right heart failure and showed an extremely dilated jugular vein (**a**) (6.9 mm on left) and superior vena cava (6.8 mm). **b** Confirmation after carotid injection: carotid artery (*1*), jugular vein (*2*), left brachiocephalic vein (*3*), superior vena cava (*4*)

appear early, are pathognomonic, and reflect a decompensated right-to-left shunt through the foramen ovale. Liver enlargement and pleural effusions (BALLESTER 1994) appear later. A retrograde aortic diastolic flow is the first sign of left heart failure, and hydrops fetalis the ultimate stage (BALLESTER 1994; DOREN 1995; JEANTY 1990; JOHNSON 1998).

– Finally, detection of ischemic brain damage is a critical part of the fetal assessment. Although ultrasonography is very valuable, the search for brain ischemic lesions relies on fetal MRI. Ischemic injury of the fetal brain is well documented in the literature (BAEZINGER 1993; DEKONING 1997; DELEZOIDE 1997; NORMAN 1974; REICHMAN 1993; SWANSTROM 1994; TAKASHIMA 1980). NORMAN (1974) reported the presence of antenatal cortical infarction or periventricular

leukomalacia in seven neonates with vein of Galen malformation (at pathological examination).

In the neonate, lesions consist of microcephaly, laminar cortical necrosis, periventricular leukomalacia, and hemorrhagic infarction. Brain damage is mainly attributed to the vascular steal phenomenon (GROSSMAN 1984), but also to ischemic injury resulting from cardiac failure, to the atrophy due to compression of areas close to the aneurysmal sac (BAENZIGER 1993), and to the thrombosis within the vein of Galen. These lesions most often occur in utero, as is shown by fetal pathological examination, and therefore, they should be carefully searched for in the antenatal period (DELEZOIDE 1997; REITER 1996), ideally by MRI (BRUNELLE 1997; CAMPI 1996; YAMASHITA 1992) (Fig. 9.35); nevertheless, they may be discovered only after birth (DE KONING 1997).

In this malformation, the notion of vascular steal phenomenon was introduced by GROSSMAN (1984) on

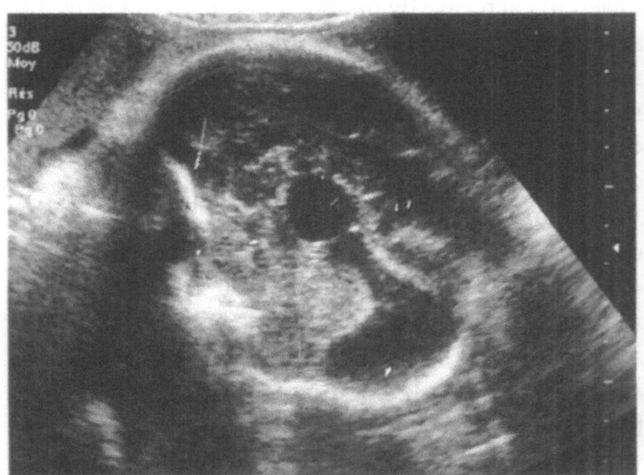

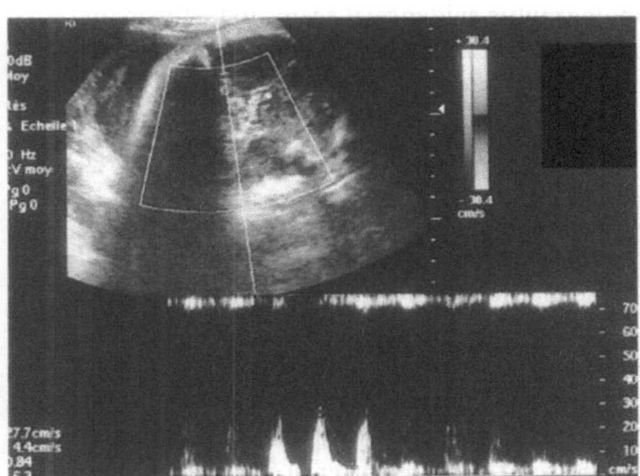

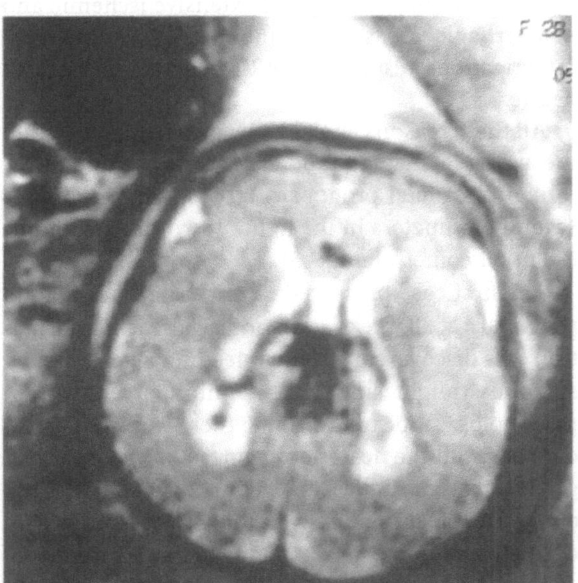

Fig. 9.35a–c. A 33-weeks' fetus with galenic aneurysm and severe congestive heart failure: cardiomegaly, dilated jugular vein, and liver enlargement. Ultrasonography reveals an enlarged draining vein and several feeding arteries (a). Pulsed Doppler on the middle cerebral artery shows a characteristic pattern of deprived artery: PSV=27 cm/s, EDV=4.4 cm/s (intense vascular diastolic steal), RI=0.84. b These velocities are markedly below the normal range: for example, anterior cerebral artery velocities in a 33-weeks' premature baby are PSV=47 cm/s, EDV=9 cm/s, RI=0.80. T2-weighted MRI demonstrates abnormal gyral development with small, thin, poorly differentiated sulci (c). In sum, cortical ischemic damage due to vascular steal. The pregnancy was terminated. (DRS. SIMON, BRUNELLE, PARIS).

Table 9.2. Hemodynamic evaluation of cerebral vascular steal

Stage I	
Stealing arteries	↑ Velocities. Mainly EDV ↓ Resistive index
Deprived arteries	Normal data
Stage II	
Stealing arteries	↑↑ Velocities. Mainly EDV ↓ Resistive index
Deprived arteries	↓ Velocities. Diastolic steal ↑ Resistive index
Stage III	
Stealing arteries	↑↑↑ Velocities. Mainly EDV ↓ Resistive index
Deprived arteries	Not visualized

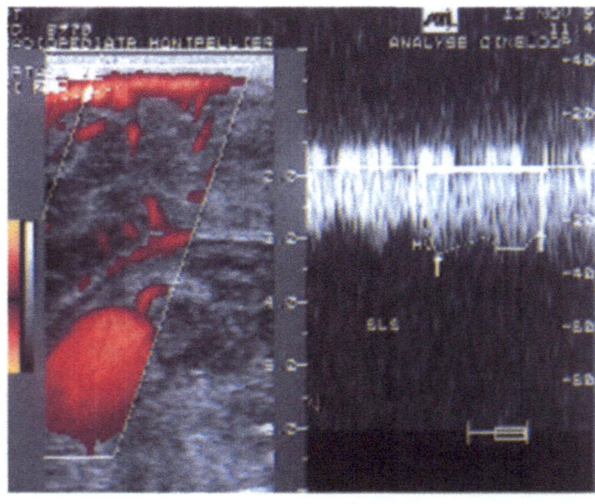

Fig. 9.36. Day 20. Pulsed Doppler on the superior sagittal sinus: velocity (28 cm/s) is at the upper limit of the normal range for a 42-weeks' neonate. Venous hyperpressure is not intense

angiographic evidence; it seems to be the main cause of ischemic brain damage when discovered early, and may be assessed using Doppler techniques (Table 9.2).

Three stages of stepwise increasing severity are described:

- *Stage I:* There is no hemodynamic effect on the artery stolen from: diameter, peak-systolic and end-diastolic velocities, and resistive index remain normal (Fig. 9.15).
- *Stage II:* There is vascular steal (Fig. 9.36); the deprived arteries velocities are reduced, with increased diastolic leakage, and the resistive index is raised. Decreased arterial diameter is only a subjective appreciation on color imaging.
- *Stage III:* The last phase of vascular steal; the deprived arteries are indetectable.

This hemodynamic staging might help to suggest a prognosis, since stage I appears to be related to a good outcome, unlike stages II and III. Of course, these new hemodynamic data require further evaluation, as some literature reports are contradictory. WESTRA (1993), comparing stealing and deprived arteries, noted that the usual response in deprived arteries is vasodilatation and reduced downstream resistance, in order to compensate for the vascular steal of feeding arteries.

To sum up, advances in imaging help prognostic assessment not only in the neonate but also in the fetus. In the literature, the importance of detecting indicators of poor prognosis has been emphasized. RODESCH (1994), in a detailed study of 18 fetuses with galenic ectasia, found 4 with severe heart failure, fol-

lowed in each case by neonatal death. In the fetus, the severity of the disease may be underestimated, and moderate fetal cardiomegaly may lead to severe neonatal decompensation: it is well known that cessation of blood flow to the placenta induces a sudden rise in cardiac output (SEPULVEDA 1995).

Similarly, antenatal detection of brain ischemic damage justifies abstaining from treatment. However, there is a delay before fetal ischemic injury induces lesions that are detectable on imaging (ultrasonography or MRI). PAUMIER (1998) reported the case of a fetus with galenic malformation and cerebral integrity on MRI; 2 weeks later, the pregnancy was terminated because of hydrops fetalis, and pathological examination revealed extensive ischemic and hemorrhagic areas. Thus the timing of antenatal investigations (especially MRI) remains difficult to define.

All these reasons explain why we attempt to use all the available imaging modalities and suggest indicators of poor fetal prognosis. YUVAL (1997) proposes several parameters in the light of two cases with different outcomes (Table 9.3).

The first case presented all the criteria of a good prognosis: at 38 weeks' gestation a galenic malformation was discovered, with two feeding arteries and a stenotic straight sinus with a minimal flow. Brain morphology appeared normal; there was mild cardiomegaly, and the descending aorta showed no retrograde steal diastolic flow. Four days after birth, congestive heart failure developed; it responded to digitalic and diuretic treatment; and at 19 months of age the infant was clinically healthy.

Table 9.3. Prognostic significance of fetal sonographic characteristics (from YUVAL 1997)

Characteristics	1	2	3
Brain damage*	+		
Hydrops*		+	
Many supplying vessels (5 or more)		+	
Dilated jugular veins and vena cava		+	
Retrograde aortic diastolic flow*		+	
Normal-sized or narrowed straight sinus			+
Normal brain			+
Few supplying vessels (2 or less)			+
Absence of heart failure*			+

* Highly significant prognostic factor
1 = Severe prognosis: therapeutic abstention
2 = Neonatal heart failure: immediate arterial embolization required
3 = Good prognosis: arterial embolization around 5–6 months of age.

The second case presented several criteria of a poor prognosis. At 33 weeks' gestation, a galenic aneurysm was discovered, with a large feeding pericallosal artery and blood draining into an enlarged straight sinus with high velocities. There was obvious cardiomegaly, cervical vessels were dilated, retrograde diastolic flow was observed in the descending aorta, and venous hyperpressure was confirmed in the transverse sinus. Soon after delivery, the baby developed a severe heart decompensation that failed to respond to medical treatment. Two days later he died.

This study by YUVAL (1997) determined effective prognostic parameters on the basis of which to adapt the future management of the baby. Our initial experience shows that integrating hemodynamic criteria will surely be extremely valuable (Table 9.4).

Precise definition during fetal life of the severity of a galenic malformation is critical to planning postnatal management in a center that includes obstetricians, pediatric cardiologists, resuscitators, and trained neuroradiologists (MAI 1996; SEPULVEDA 1995).

Neuroradiological imaging can and should answer all the following questions:

– What are the vascular anatomy and hemodynamic characteristics of the aneurysmal malformation? (Color and pulsed Doppler)
– What is the hemodynamic behavior of the fetus? (Echocardiography)
– Is the fetal brain normal? (Ultrasonography and MRI)

Table 9.4. Hemodynamic criteria of poor prognosis

1. Increased velocities in draining vessels, a sign of increased venous pressure.

2. Markedly increased velocities in supplying vessels, a sign of a wide shunt.

3. Decreased velocities and increased resistive index in deprived arteries or nonvisualized deprived arteries, signs of cerebral vascular steal.

9.1.1.4.4
Ultrasound in Pre- and Post-Treatment Assessment
Detailed analysis of the case of Anthony demonstrates how important it is to following the changes in the malformation:

– The hemodynamic data (velocities in arteries not involved in the malformation) show that this brain was well supplied from birth to endovascular embolization (day 80) (Table 9.5). This confirms the favorable fetal pattern and the good neonatal clinical status.
– Pulsed Doppler assessment of feeding arteries and draining veins showed a gradual decrease in velocities. This occurred quickly and strikingly within the aneurysmal sac (Table 9.6): from 104 cm/s on day 2, it reached 30 cm/s on day 19. In the draining straight sinus, velocities were only moderately increased at birth (40 cm/s) and rapidly normalized on day 19 (14 cm/s).

This makes it possible (Fig. 9.36) to understand and predict the subsequent thrombosis. On day 67, straight sinus flow was indetectable, and velocities in the aneurysm were low (20 cm/s). Probably, endovascular embolization would not have had to be per-

Table 9.5. Velocities in arteries not involved in the malformation

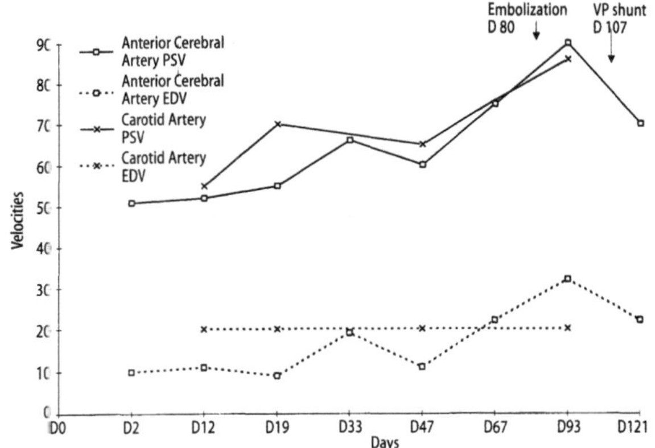

Table 9.6. Velocities in venous drainage

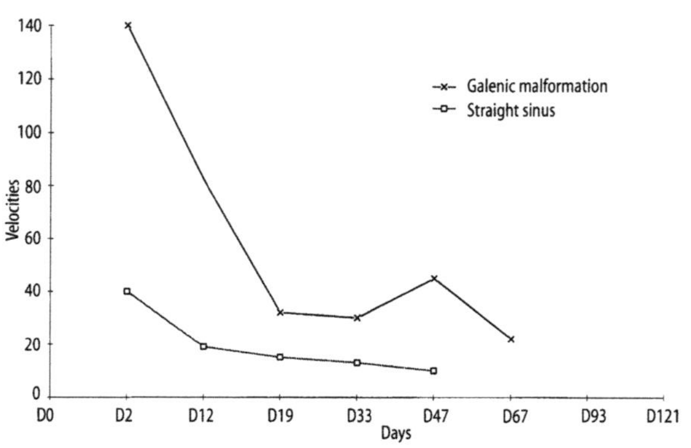

Table 9.7. Velocities in arteries feeding the malformation

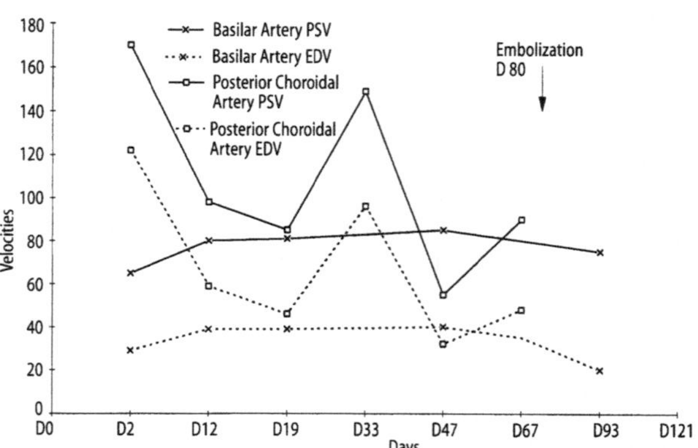

formed early (day 80) if progressive hydrocephalus had not appeared.

Thrombosis was complete in the straight sinus and left posterior choroidal artery and would probably extend to the whole malformation (HURST 1992). Decreased and more irregular afferent vessel velocities (Table 9.7) accompanied reduced venous velocities. While the appearance of the basilar artery remained characteristic of a feeding vessel (high diastolic amplitude, unchanged velocities), the velocities of the posterior choroidal arteries gradually decreased (Fig. 9.37): in the right one, the initial peak-systolic and end-diastolic velocities were 166 cm/s and 124 cm/s respectively, whereas immediately before embolization they were 90 cm/s and 48 cm/s respectively.

– Ventriculocisternostomy was decided on in good conditions: absence of hemodynamic signs of intracranial hypertension, usually characterized by decreased end-diastolic velocities in the anterior cerebral artery and internal carotid artery.

– Finally, color and pulsed Doppler may demonstrate the efficacy of treatment:

. Color Doppler confirms complete or partial thrombosis of the galenic ectasia.

. Pulsed Doppler depicts a residual feeding vessel in the case of partial thrombosis, and demonstrates the hemodynamic pattern of a good outcome in the case of complete thrombosis (Fig. 9.38): for example, in our patient, the basilar artery lost its stealing artery spectrum (EDV=40 cm/s) and took on a normal hemodynamic appearance (EDV=20 cm/s) (Table 9.7). Changes in the resistive index were also significant: it increased from 0.50 to 0.72 after embolization (Table 9.8).

The treatment of a galenic malformation has always been a difficult challenge. Until 1980, mortal-

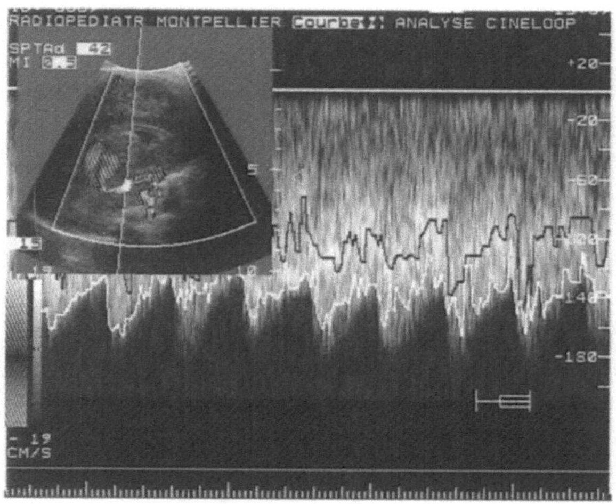

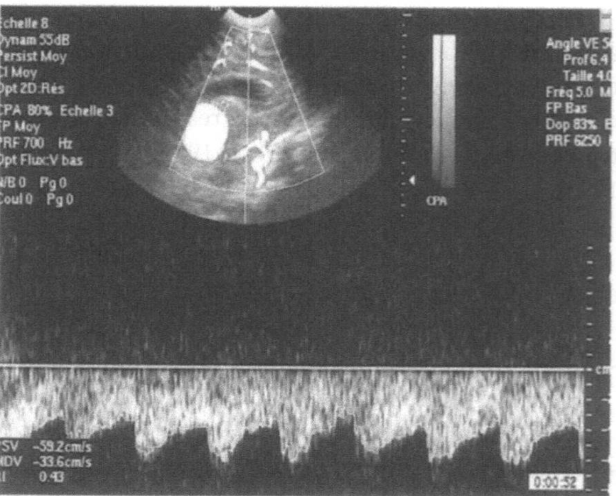

Fig. 9.37a,b. Velocities in a feeding right choroidal artery decrease markedly: on day 3, PSV=166 cm/s (**a**) on day 47, PSV = 59 cm/s (**b**)

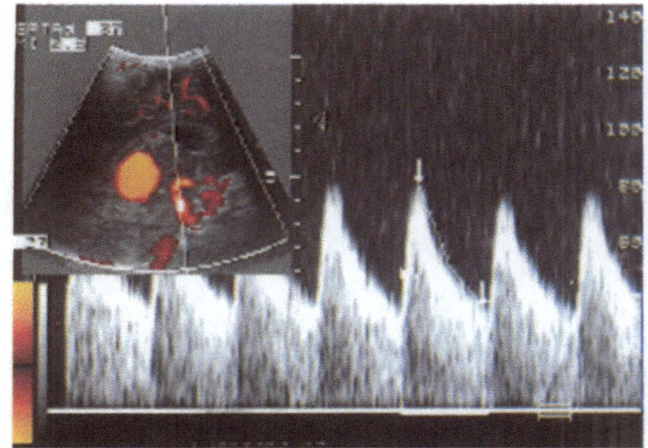 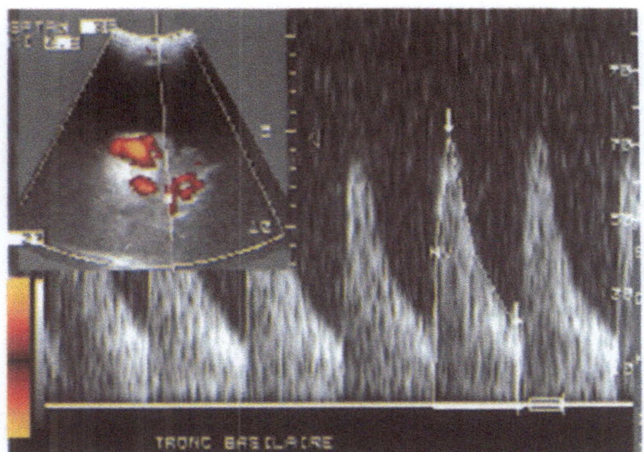

Fig. 9.38a,b. The spectral analysis curve is completely different before and after endovascular embolization. On day 13 (**a**), EDV=37 cm/s, RI= 0.53. After treatment, on day 93 (**b**), EDV=20 cm/s, RI=0.71

ity was up to 100% in severe cases of neonatal presentation (PEIBLER 1981). Control of this vascular maze was inconceivable: surgery was impossible and endovascular embolization ineffective. Recent years have shown advances in treatment: the principle is to control the shunt flow and venous hyperpressure by endovascular embolization, and it is now well accepted that interventional neuroradiology is the modality of choice. The final goal is to preserve normal circulation to the brain.

Two techniques have been described: a transvenous and a transarterial approach.

Transtorcular embolization of the aneurysmal sac was proposed by HANNER (1988) and HAWKINS (1986), with striking hemodynamic results and disappearance of congestive heart failure in 11 of 15 patients treated (HANNER 1988). Their technique includes transtorcular placement of coils (a variable amount) and, as an accessory, detachable microballoons, depending on the severity of the shunt, previously defined by cerebral angiography. However, HANNER (1988) reported 3 neonatal deaths out of 15

Table 9.8. Resistive index in the basilar artery

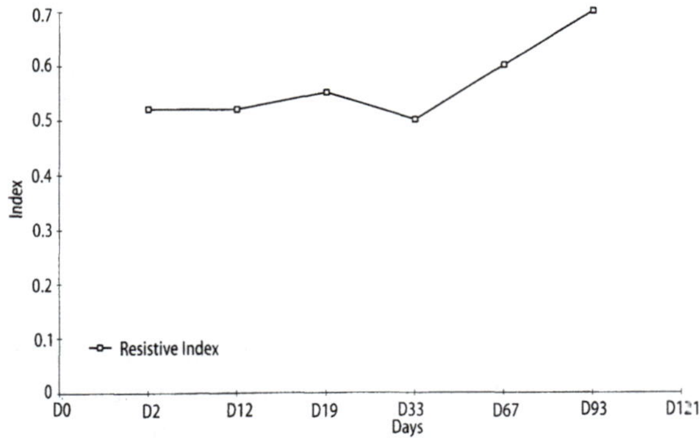

cases despite the treatment, and LYLYK (1993) confirmed alarming mortality rates (3 deaths among 8 venous embolizations). Moreover, although the cardiac situation appears to be definitely improved, the long-term neurological outcome remains unknown, since the quality of cerebral circulation after treatment is difficult to assess. Finally, in the opinion of LASJAUNIAS (1997), coils and detachable microballoons are inappropriate materials for the treatment of such lesions. Thus, the transvenous approach has not shown enough benefit as a primary form of treatment.

Most authors (CIRICILLO 1990; BRUNELLE 1997; KAWAGUCHI 1997; LASJAUNIAS 1996; RAO 1994; REICHMAN 1993; RODESCH 1994; SWANSTROM 1994; YAMASHITA 1992) prefer a transarterial approach that consists in selective catheterization of feeding vessels and embolization with butylcyanoacrylate. This method has been proven to offer convincing results, and the recent multicenter study of LASJAUNIAS (1996) is impressive: out of 120 patients with galenic malformation, 78 were embolized, 47 (i.e., 66%) with a normal neurological outcome, 10 (i.e., 14%) with transient neurological symptoms, 8 (i.e., 11.5%) with persistent mild neurological disorders, 6 (i.e., 8.5%) with severe neurodevelopmental deficit, while 7 patients (i.e., 9%) died. The antenatal group well reflected the true aggressivity of the malformation and showed the efficacy of transarterial embolization (LASJAUNIAS 1996): among 21 cases, 5 already exhibited irreversible brain damage and were not treated. Neurodevelopment was normal in 12 out of 14 embolized patients; the other 2 had some degree of neurological deficit.

In conclusion, the neonatal management seems clear:

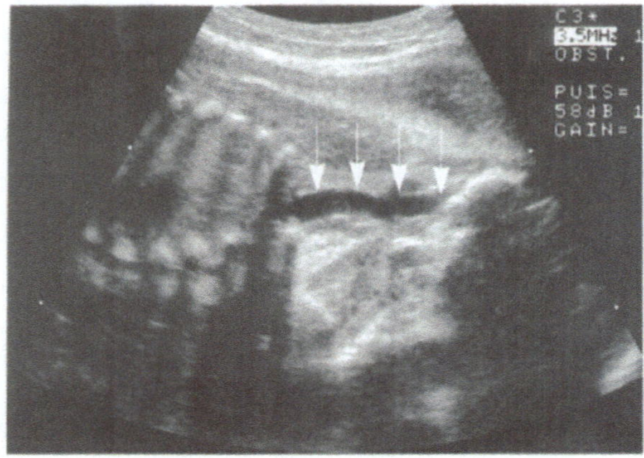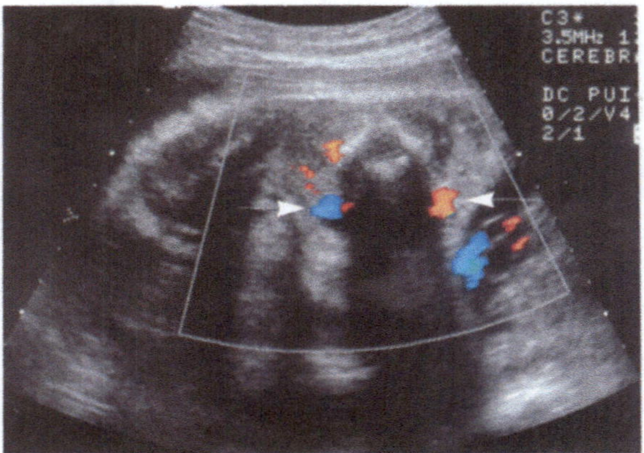

Fig. 9.39a,b. A 37-weeks' gestation fetus with galenic aneurysm and heart failure. Ultrasonography (**a**) shows a significant enlargement of the internal jugular vein (*arrows*), confirmed on color Doppler (**b**). Several feeding vessels are visualized. The pregnancy was terminated (Dr. DESCHAMPS, Montpellier)

- Embolization should not be carried out in a neonate with irreducible congestive heart failure or/ and irreversible ischemic brain damage. Ideally, modern imaging (color, pulsed Doppler, echocardiography, MRI) should detect these poor-prognosis cases in utero, leading to discussion of terminating the pregnancy.
- In the neonate, heart failure must be quickly controlled by common digitalic and diuretic medications. The immediate goal is to restore a satisfactory systemic physiology, to avoid development of macrocrania and significant retardation and to gain time before endovascular treatment has to be carried out. If cardiac decompensation fails to respond to medical treatment, early embolization should be considered.
- In all other circumstances, and especially when hemodynamic criteria of poor prognosis are absent, the best management is to wait until the child is at least 5 months old, and to proceed with transarterial embolization. The importance of imaging for the follow-up of newborns that are in fragile equilibrium during the first months of life is easy to conceive. The role of ultrasonography is to define the degree and duration of hemodynamic stability after birth, to carefully depict the arterial and venous vessels involved in the malformation, and to assess the efficacy of embolization (either immediate or delayed).

Finally, regarding imaging strategy, several comments may already be made:
- Diagnostic angiography has disappeared, angiography is only performed with the transarterial embolization.

- MRI is important during the antenatal period, since it allows an appreciation of the brain parenchyma and can demonstrate irreversible ischemic damage. It is even more useful for the morphological and prognostic assessment of the malformation itself: the volume of the aneurysm, and visualization of supplying arteries and draining veins. Some authors (BRUNELLE 1997) propose routine neonatal MRI, emphasizing its excellent ability to provide morphological information. In our experience, given the known high potentialities of ultrasound, it seems justified to keep MRI for unexplained manifestations, such as the mechanism of a progressive hydrocephalus.

Thanks to the quality of imaging today and to advances in therapeutic modalities, a fetus or a neonate with a galenic aneurysm can become a healthy baby with normal neurological development and cardiovascular status; this is now a reality.

9.1.2
Other Intracranial Vascular Malformations

Some observations explain the poor value of ultrasound techniques in the detection of nongalenic intracranial vascular malformations.

9.1.2.1
A Rare Abnormality

In the fetus, the neonate, and the young infant, these congenital vascular malformations are extremely rare (KAPLAN 1984; KUCHELMEISTER 1993; LEE 1978; MUCZYNSKI 1994). THRUSH (1988) described the case of a neonate with cerebral arterial aneurysm and found only seven other similar cases in the literature. More recently, ALLISON (1998) reported a collaborative study over 20 years, in which 21 children were diagnosed with intracranial aneurysm, but only 6 of them were younger than 1 year of age. VENTUREYRA (1980) estimated that intracranial arterial aneurysms in children account for approximately 1–2% of all cases, and even less in the newborn. Similar findings have been obtained in the other types of vascular malformation. BRUNELLE (1983), in a CT and angiographic study of 39 children with vascular malformations (34 arteriovenous malformations, 3 cavernous hemangiomas, 2 venous angiomas), found only 5 patients younger than 1 year of age. WESTRA (1993), and RODESCH (1995) observed that neonatal presentation of pial arteriovenous malformation remained extremely rare. Finally, LASJAUNIAS (1997) and others (GARCIA-MONACO 1991), from a case of antenatal detection, confirmed the extreme rarity of dural arteriovenous shunts.

9.1.2.2
Polymorphic Presentation

The clinical symptoms that reveal a vascular malformation in a neonate or infant are not well known. Congestive heart failure in a neonate suggests a pial or dural arteriovenous malformation (MENOVSKY 1997; RODESCH 1995), but the manifestations of an arterial aneurysm may be extremely variable, depending on its location, volume, and whether it ruptures (HULSMANN 1998; KASAHARA 1996; NEWCOMB 1999; PICKERING 1970; TAN 1998): irritability, vomiting, seizures, and stroke are the most usual findings. In the report by FERRANTE (1988), subarachnoid hemorrhage was the commonest presentation in the infant. THOMSON (1969) described a 9-month-old infant with an internal carotid artery aneurysm, revealed by masquerading features (ophthalmoplegia, quadriparesis). RODESCH (1995), studying 13 neonatal arteriovenous malformations, reported the occurrence of seizures as the presenting sign in 31% of cases and hemorrhage in 15%. Finally, nongalenic vascular malformations are commonly latent.

9.1.2.3
Diagnostic Strategy

The neuroradiological imaging of intracranial vascular malformations in the newborn and infant is based on angiography (ALLISON 1998; BRUNELLE 1983; KAPLAN 1984; LITTLE 1986), on CT (SCHIJMANE 1983, THRUSH 1988) on MRI (PUTTY 1990), especially MR angiography, which will develop further in the future (ALLISON 1998; ROSS 1990). Ultrasonography does not seem to have any place in this strategy.

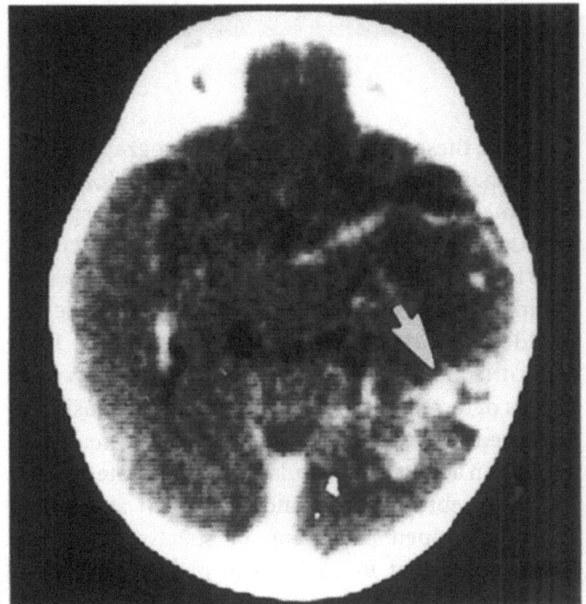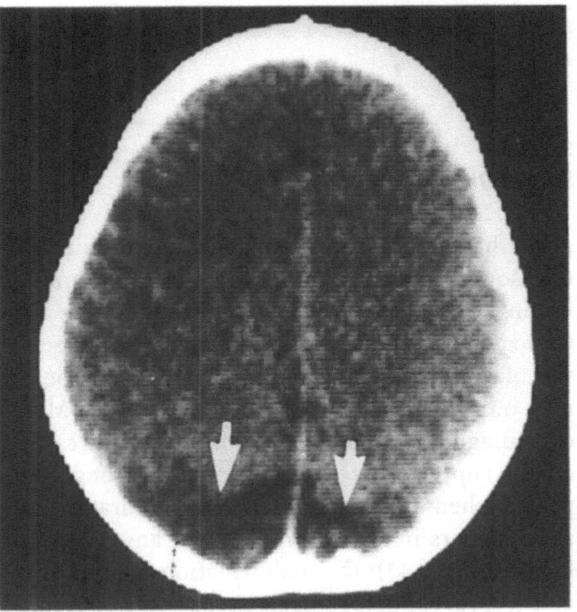

Fig. 9.40a,b. A 10-day-old infant with left retroauricular thrill and focal intense intracranial bruit. Brain ultrasonography is considered normal. CT easily demonstrates a superficial left arteriovenous fistula (*arrowhead*) (a). b Notice a posterior ischemic area (*arrowheads*), probably due to vascular steal. The infant quickly died

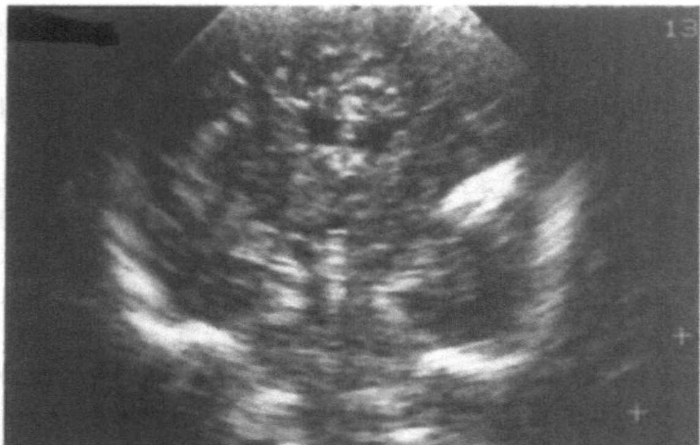

a

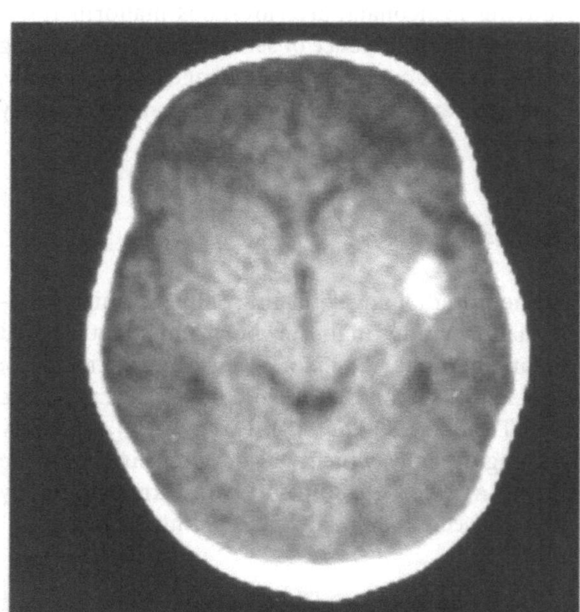

c

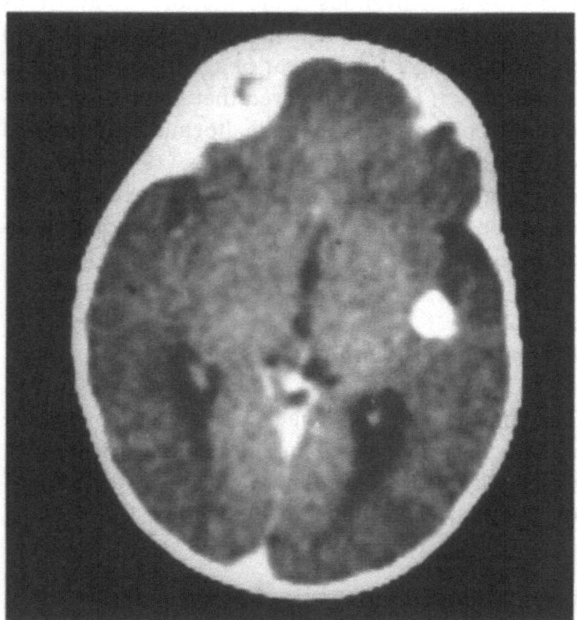

b

Fig. 9.41a–c. A 2-month-old infant with right hemicorporeal seizures. **a** Ultrasonography reveals a hyperechoic entity with acoustic shadow in the left parenchyma. Etiological diagnosis is impossible and the only credit due to ultrasound is to suggest a lesional cause of the clinical manifestation. CT demonstrates the vascular nature of the calcified lesion: hyperdensity within the left sylvian area (**b**), with post-contrast enhancement (**c**). Final diagnosis: calcified cavernous angioma

9.1.2.4
Role of Ultrasonography

As we have said, in this clinical context the role of ultrasound appears extremely modest. Sonographic findings are disappointing: ultrasonography may fail to detect the lesion (Fig. 9.40) or to recognize the vascular nature of a lesion (Fig. 9.41), and at best it may only suggest the diagnosis (Fig. 9.42). Moreover, diagnosis is not always possible in the case of a small ruptured vascular abnormality strongly suspected when an acute or recurrent cerebral hemorrhage occurs in a newborn without any particular history (Fig. 9.43): the malformation is often difficult to prove, unrecognized because it is obscured by the hematoma. Delayed angiography should be preferred.

In fact, these limitations of ultrasonography relate to the imaging of the past, in contrast to color-coded assessment of brain vessels. Since the case reported by VAKSMANN (1990), in which color Doppler was used to describe a peripheral cerebral arteriovenous aneurysm in a 6-week-old infant, the literature has included reports (HAYASHI 1996; HEGGESA 1991; PALADINI 1996) of three patients with arteriovenous fistulas detected by color Doppler. The diagnosis was suggested in two neonates with congestive heart failure, and in a fetus with fistula involving posterior and middle cerebral arteries and confirmed at autopsy. These data open promising perspectives. RODESH (1995) noted that in 26 cases of pial arteriovenous malformation, no diagnosis was made antenatally by means of gray-scale ultrasonography. However, color Doppler imaging should be attempted in cases of con-

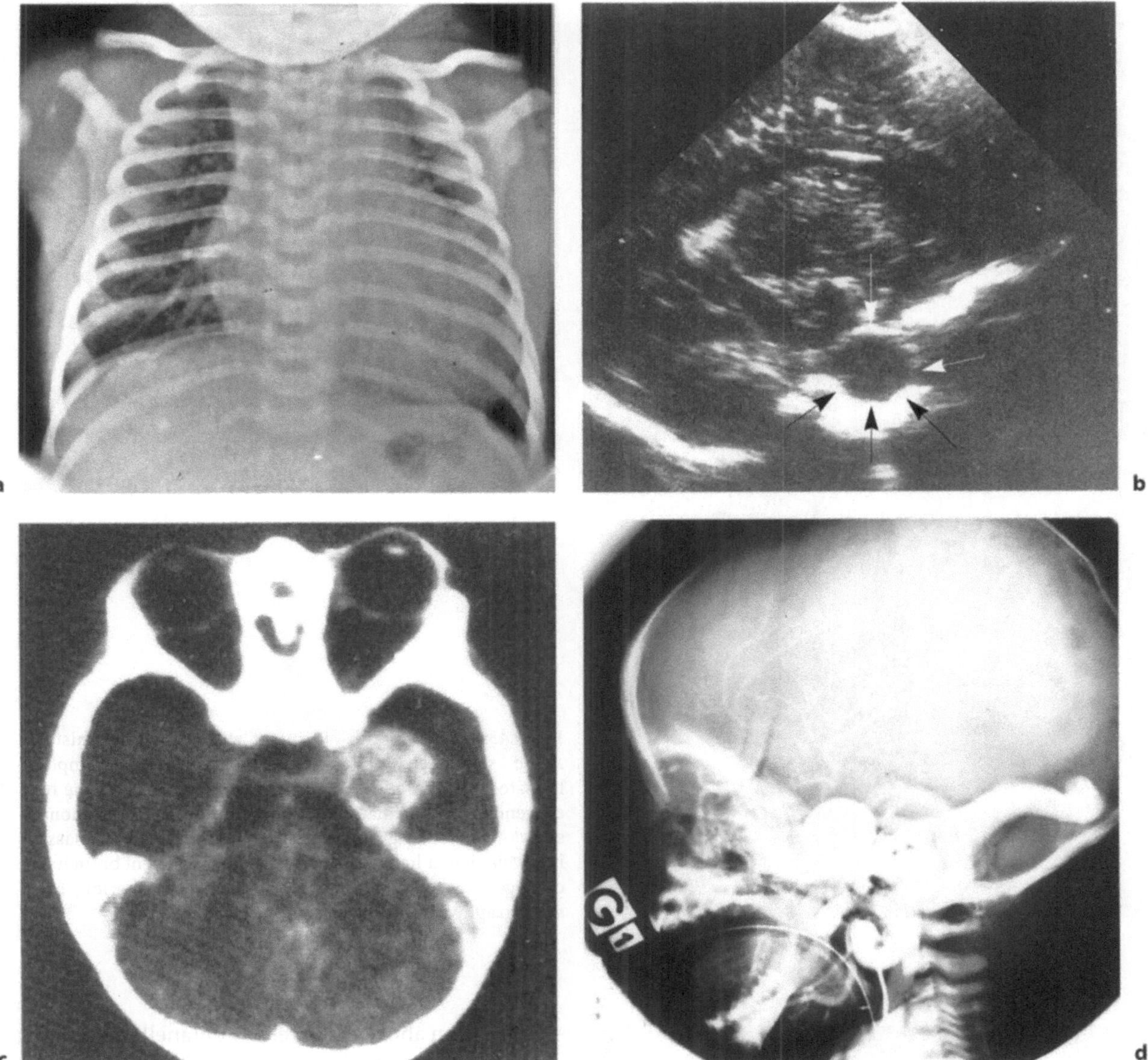

Fig. 9.42a–d. A 2-day-old newborn with tachycardia and cardiomegaly (**a**). At 3 months, left exophthalmia and intracranial bruit are noted. Ultrasound detects a parasellar, rounded, nonpulsatile fluid structure (*arrows*, **b**). A vascular malformation is suspected and proved by CT (**c**, rounded enhanced lesion). Selective angiography shows a megadolichocarotid artery and an aneurysmal sac within the cavernous sinus with a major arteriovenous shunt draining into the left lateral sinus (**d**). Summary: carotidocavernous fistula. (Dr. DIDIER, Nancy)

gestive heart failure or neonatal seizures, before more invasive investigations are performed (angiography, CT, MR angiography).

Along the same lines, it seems valuable to suggest a routine color Doppler analysis of the whole fetal brain vasculature: early detection of arterial, venous, or arteriovenous malformation may benefit the diagnostic and prognostic assessment.

9.1.3
Extracranial Vascular Malformations

There exists a wide spectrum of extracranial lesions and malformations: sinus pericranii, cavernous hemangioma, meningocele, meningoencephalocele, leptomeningeal cyst, dermoid cyst, eosinophilic granuloma, and others. Several clinical characteristics are suggestive:

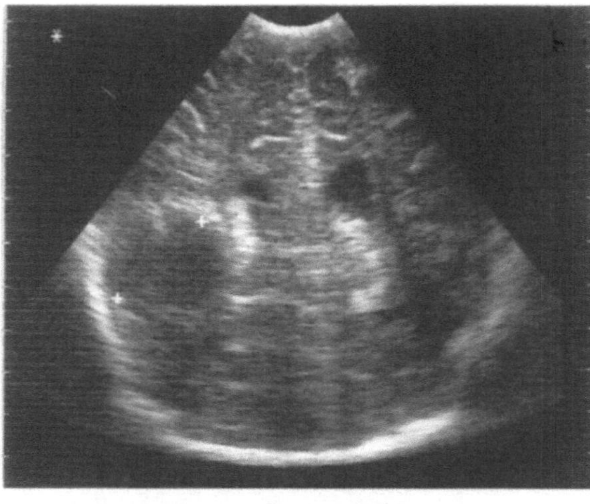

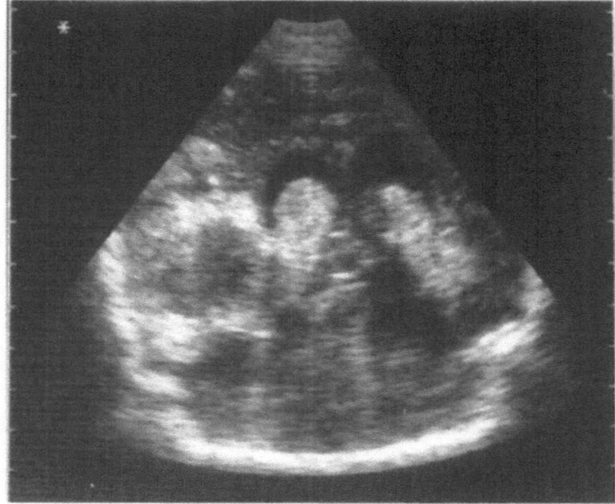

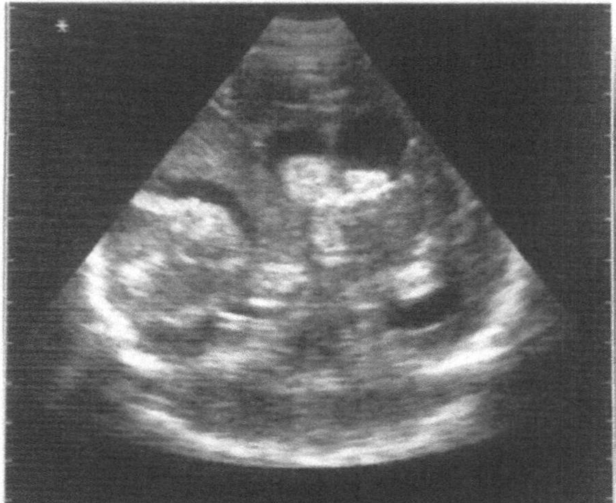

Fig. 9.43a–c. A 2-month-old infant without relevant history. Acute status epilepticus. CT reveals a right temporal hematoma. Initial ultrasonography (a) demonstrates the heterogenous right hematoma. Routine follow-up at 2.5 months shows recurrent right temporal hematoma (b) with massive intraventricular hemorrhage (c). In sum: recurrent brain hemorrhage suggesting a cerebral vascular malformation; early angiography was normal. Death rapidly ensued

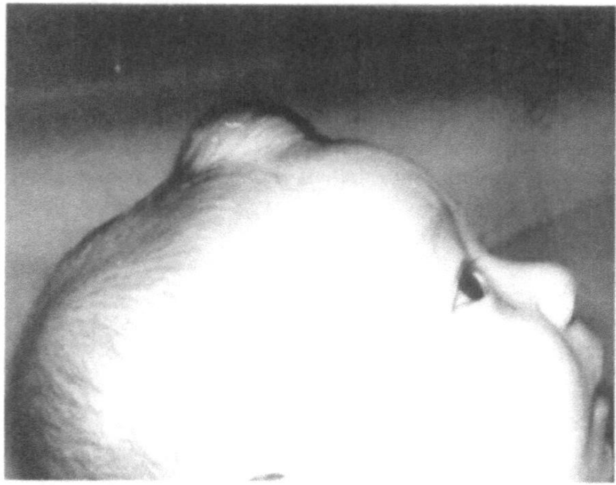

Fig. 9.44. A 3-month-old infant with a small smooth mass on top of the anterior fontanelle. Skull X-rays (bony defect on the sagittal suture) and brain ultrasonography (extracranial cystic mass) suggest a diagnosis of meningocele or dermoid cyst. Histological diagnosis after surgical excision was dermoid cyst

- A location above the anterior fontanelle suggests a meningocele or a dermoid cyst (Fig. 9.44), less frequently a cavernous hemangioma (YANAKA 1992).
- A history of traumatic injury suggests a leptomeningeal cyst, but this mechanism is also discussed for the sinus pericranii (ANTOUN 1997).
- A round, fluctuating mass, enlarging with increased intracranial pressure, is typical of sinus pericranii, but differential diagnosis against cavernous hemangioma can be difficult.

Thus imaging is important, not only to define the extracranial location, but also to guide the etiological diagnosis.

9.1.3.1
Sinus Pericranii

Sinus pericranii is a rare extracranial vascular malformation, characterized by multiple sinusoid vessels that communicate directly with the intracranial dural venous sinus via diploic and emissary veins across the calvarium (BUXTON 1999; DAVID 1998; VINAS 1994). The superior sagittal and transverse sinuses are the most frequent sites of communication (BONIOLI 1994; SPEKTOR 1998). A bony defect may be found beneath the mass, as may small erosions in the outer table (BONIOLI 1994).

Its cause is unknown. Two hypotheses are under discussion:
- A congenital etiology, because other associated vascular malformations are often encountered: venous angioma (CERQUEIRA 1995; SAKAI 1997),

aneurysm of the internal cerebral vein (NAKASU 1993).
- A traumatic etiology, with direct injury to a dural sinus or tearing of emissary veins (KIHARA 1991).

Examination under the microscope may help to define the mechanism: endothelial tissue lines the lesion in a congenital sinus, while it is absent in an acquired anomaly (BOLLAR 1992; VINAS 1994).

LUKER (1995) observed that the frontal bone near the central and posterior thirds of the superior sagittal sinus is the most commonly affected (40–70% of cases), followed by the parietal, occipital, and temporal bones. The malformation is usually isolated, but

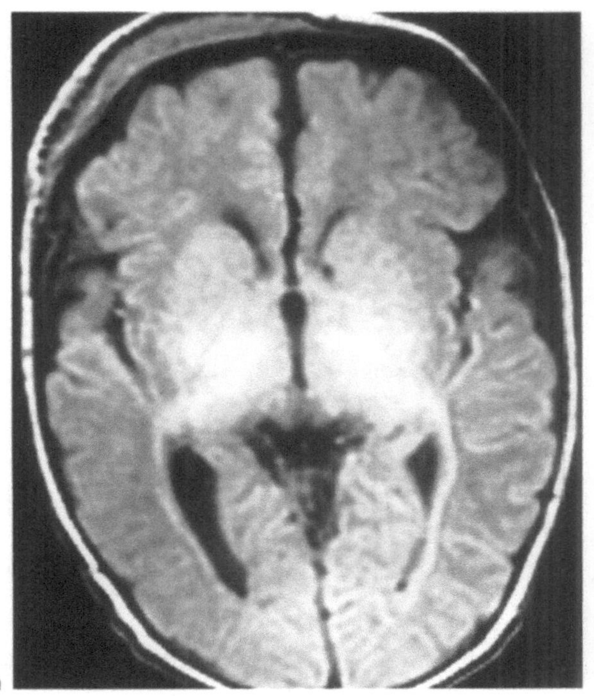

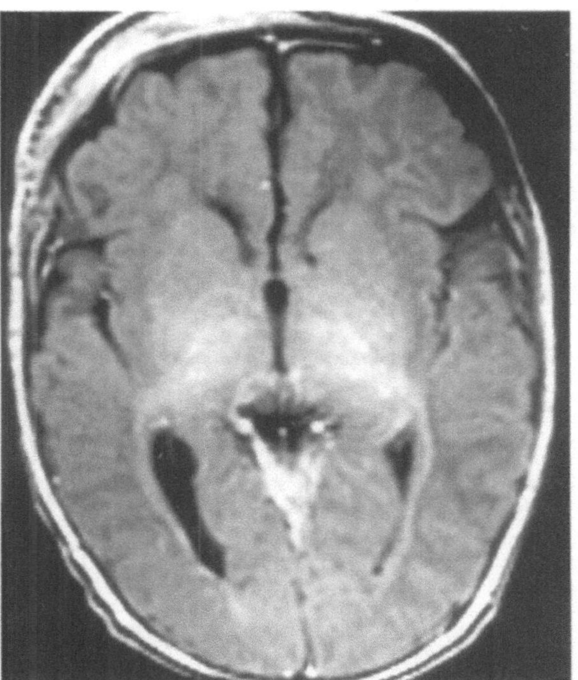

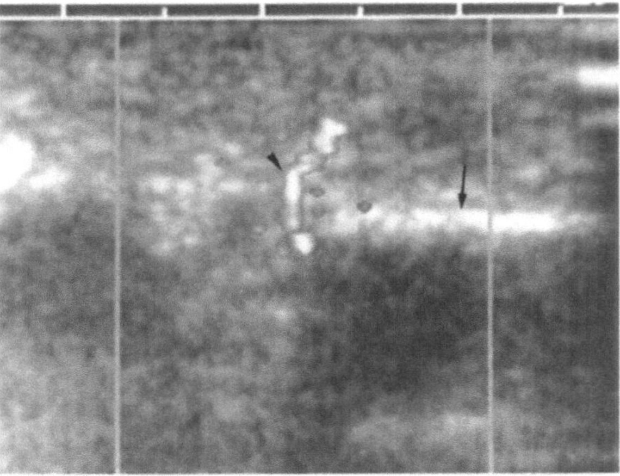

Fig. 9.45a–c. A 7-month-old infant with a right frontopalpebral mass present since birth; the mass is smooth, painless, nonpulsatile, fluctuates in volume, and increases with crying. Intermediate signal on T1 weighted MRI (a), heterogeneous postgadolinium enhancement (b). On postcontrast CT, several vascular structures are detected. Color Doppler ultrasonography (c) shows the vascular character of the mass, depicts low velocity flow, and displays a vessel (*arrowhead*) crossing a hyperechoic cranial vault (*arrow*). (Dr. ADAMSBAUM, Paris)

lateral or multiple lesions have been reported (NAKASU 1993). Most patients are asymptomatic and present with a nonpulsatile fluctuating mass that enlarges when intracranial pressure is increased (Valsalva maneuver, crying, jugular compression) and decreases when the head is elevated.

Imaging is required to assess the extracranial situation and vascular nature of the lesion. CT and MR show postcontrast enhancement (Fig. 9.45) and may identify the bone defect. MRI shows a heterogeneous hyperintense signal due to turbulent slow flow (SALDER 1990). Angiography (or direct transcutaneous puncture) is performed during the preoperative phase (VINAS 1994; WITRAK 1986) and demonstrates the connection of the vascular mass to an intracranial dural venous sinus.

Color Doppler is obviously underused in this abnormality (ANTOUN 1997; LUKER 1995); this is a shame since it may show the same findings and provide decisive diagnostic evidence by showing the transosseous pathway of a venous vessel (Fig. 9.46).

9.1.3.2
Other Malformations

In the neonate, the diagnosis and entire assessment of a superficial hemangioma relies on color and pulsed Doppler imaging. An immature hemangioma during its proliferative phase shows obvious arterial and venous hypervascularization. Typically, arteries exhibit a low resistance and high diastolic amplitude, with resistive index ranging from 0.40 to 0.70 (Fig. 9.47). Color imaging allows antenatal diagnosis (BOULOT 1996), which is confirmed by fetal MRI and postnatal ultrasonography (Fig. 9.48).

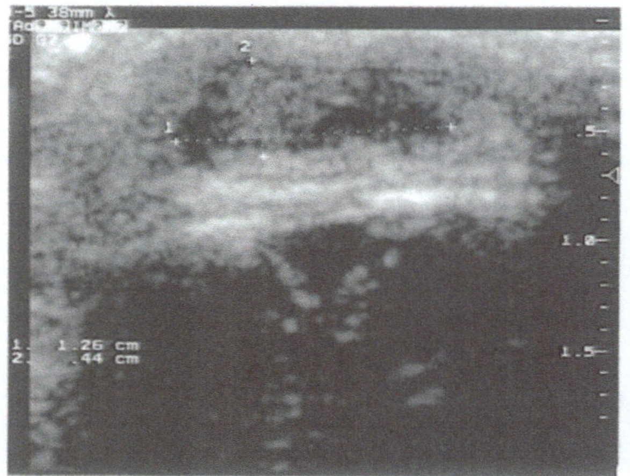

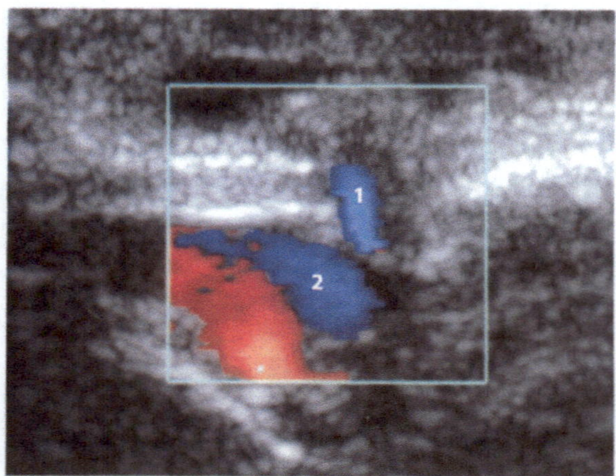

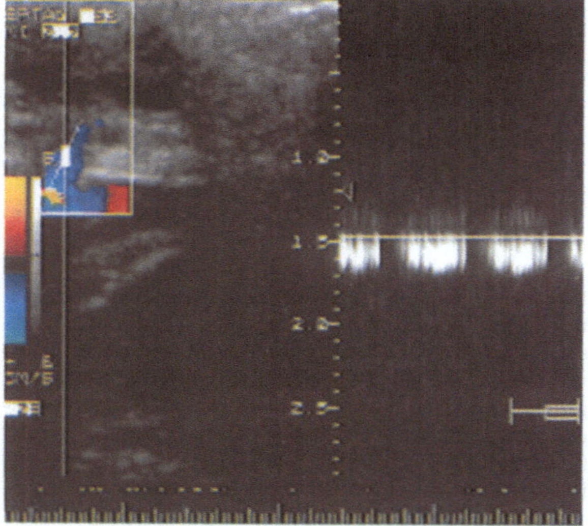

Fig. 9.46a–c. A 7-day-old neonate with a nonpulsatile, silent, midline posterior mass. The extracranial structure (**a**) is slightly heterogeneous and located above the superior sagittal sinus; it contains colored dots that define its vascular nature. The diagnosis of sinus pericranii is provided by color Doppler (**b**), which demonstrates the transcranial vessel (*1*) joining the superior sagittal sinus (*2*); venous flow is proved by spectral analysis (**c**)

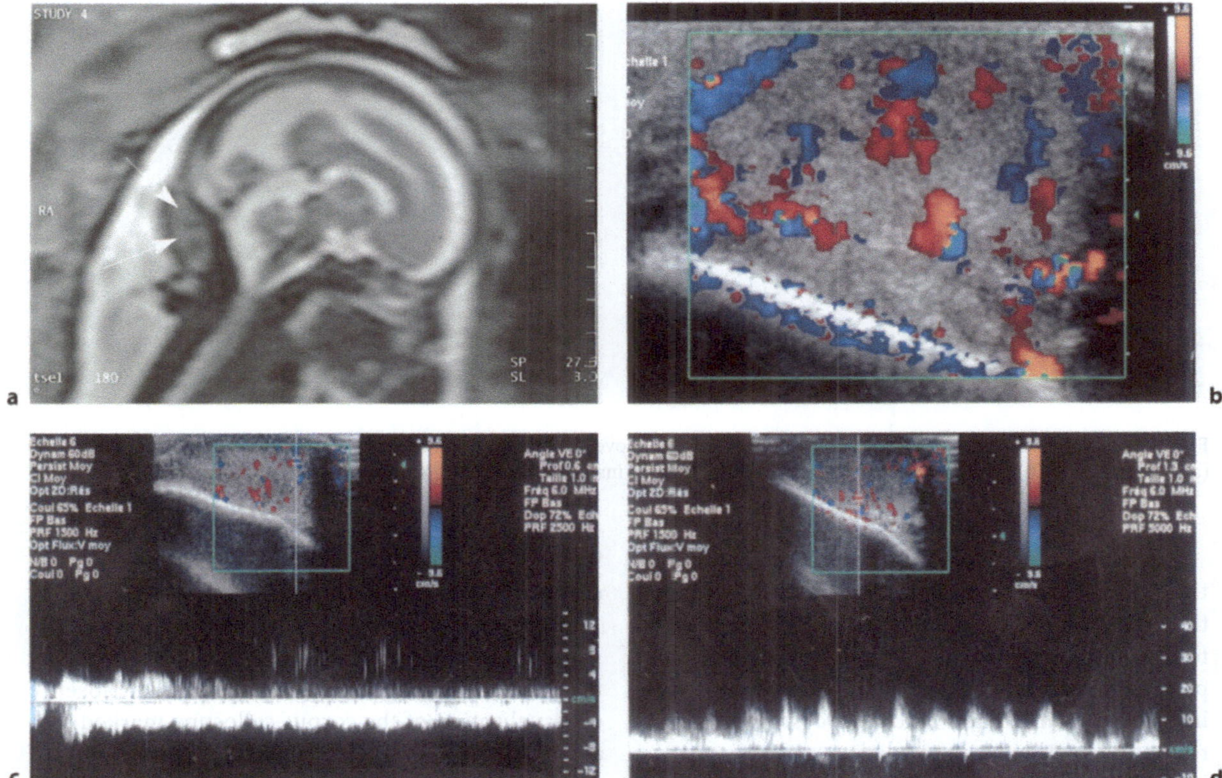

Fig. 9.47a–d. At 25 weeks' gestation, fetal ultrasonography reveals a subcutaneous cervical hypervascular mass suspected to be a hemangioma. The location of the lesion is confirmed by MRI at 26 weeks (*arrows*, **a**). At birth, all the characteristics of a hemangioma are present: a retro-occipital hypervascular mass (**b**) containing venous (**c**) and arterial (**d**) flows, with a low RI (0.40)

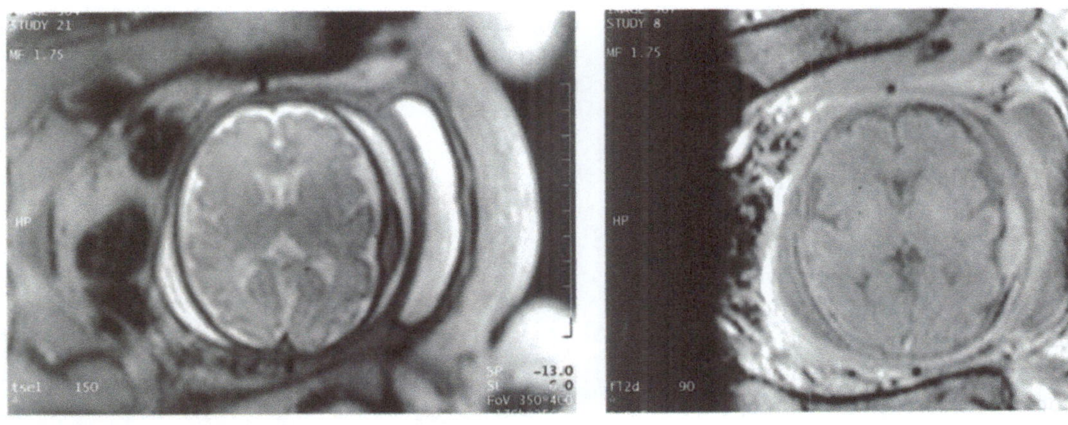

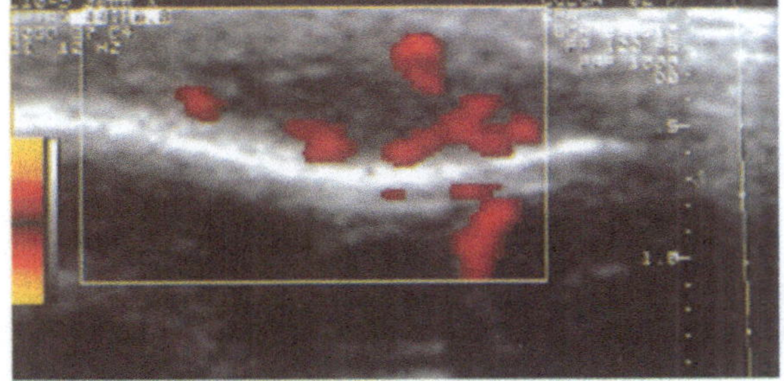

Fig. 9.48a–c. A 35-weeks' fetus with a right subcutaneous hypervascular mass discovered on ultrasonography. Angioma is suspected but there are atypical anatomic characteristics (deformity of the parietal bone, presence of intracranial hyperemia). Fetal MRI (**a,b**) assesses the extracranial location of the lesion, which appears hyperintense on T1-weighted and hypointense on T2-weighted images, and induces a depression on the skull. At birth, the neonate presented with an angiomatous disease that involved the right temporal tissue but also the groin and the bowel (BALACI 1999). Note the hypervascularization on power Doppler and the concave parietal bone (**c**)

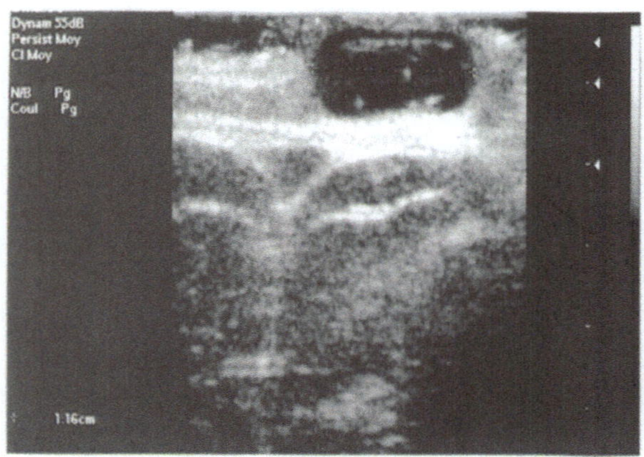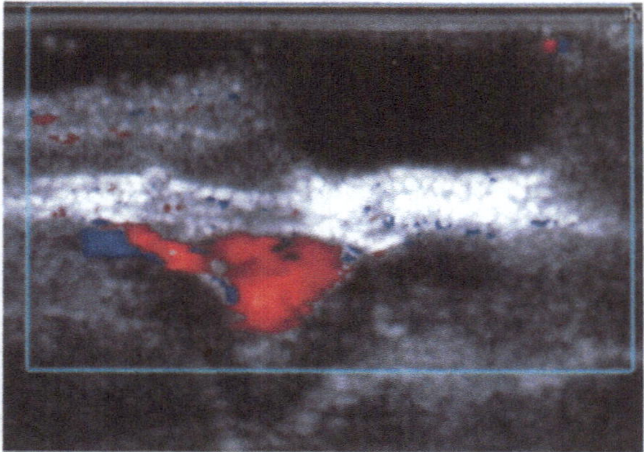

Fig. 9.49a,b. A 2-month-old infant with an extracranial mass above the anterior fontanelle; hemangioma is suspected. The cystic (**a**) and avascular (**b**) appearance excludes this hypothesis, and instead a meningocele or dermoid cyst is suggested

Literature review reveals other interesting indications provided by color Doppler. VOET (1992) reports the case of a neonate with post-traumatic mass; a leptomeningeal cyst was suspected because color Doppler visualized an arterial connection between the intracranial circulation and the cyst; posthemorrhage liquefaction was excluded.

Finally, the absence of any colored signal in an extracranial mass guides the diagnostic hypothesis (Fig. 9.49).

9.2
Cerebral Nonvascular Malformations

In the neonate, ultrasonography coupled to MRI allows accurate diagnosis and complete assessment of all cerebral malformations. Why, then should color imaging be used and developed to diagnose brain malformations?

It is in fact the case that, in the newborn, Doppler techniques do not add to the information provided by the morphological diagnosis; most often, they are useless. In the fetus, however, the diagnosis of brain malformation is often not precise enough on ultrasound. In these circumstances, color Doppler may be useful in orientating and complementing a suspected diagnosis: this is especially the case in callosal abnormalities, holoprosencephaly, neuronal migration disorders, and schizencephaly.

9.2.1
Abnormalities of the Corpus Callosum

Agenesis of corpus callosum is easily diagnosed by neonatal ultrasonography (COUTURE 1994): absence of visualization of the corpus callosum, marked separation of the lateral ventricles, colpocephaly, upward extension of the roof of the third ventricle, and a radial arrangement of the medial cerebral sulci. Ultrasound diagnosis of posterior partial callosal agenesis is also easy (COUTURE 1994). This neonatal sonographic pattern has improved the in utero diagnosis of these malformations. However, antenatal diagnosis may be difficult, mistakes and uncertainties remain possible, especially due to the use of axial transverse planes. Finally, when callosal malforma-

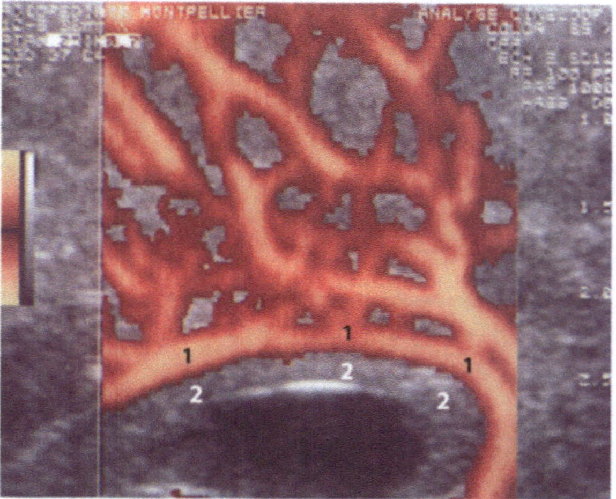

Fig. 9.50. Normal newborn, power Doppler imaging. The pericallosal artery (*1*) remains close to the surface of the corpus callosum (*2*)

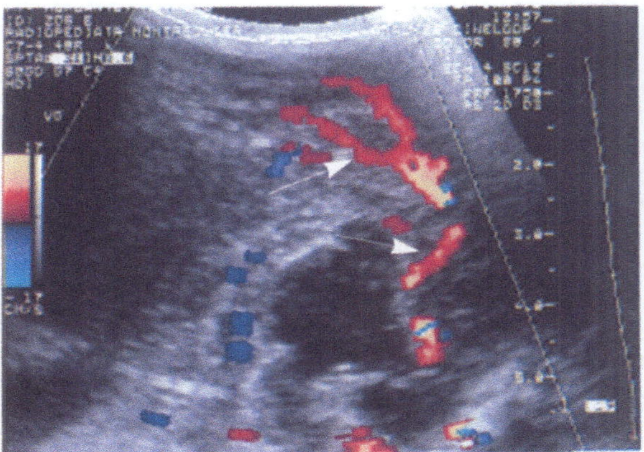

Fig. 9.51. Antenatal MRI diagnosis of cerebral malformation with lissencephaly, hydrocephalus, cerebellar hypoplasia, and complete agenesis of the corpus callosum, suggesting Walker-Warburg syndrome. At birth, color imaging confirms the presence of callosal agenesis: the pericallosal artery (*arrows*) remains far from the third ventricle and takes an upward oblique direction

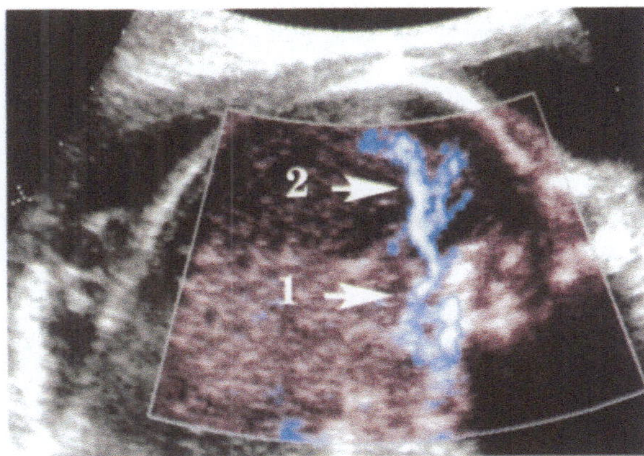

Fig. 9.52. A 24-weeks' gestation fetus with absent corpus callosum. The pericallosal artery (*2*) has a typical upward direction in continuity with anterior cerebral artery (*1*). (Dr. Deschamps, Montpellier)

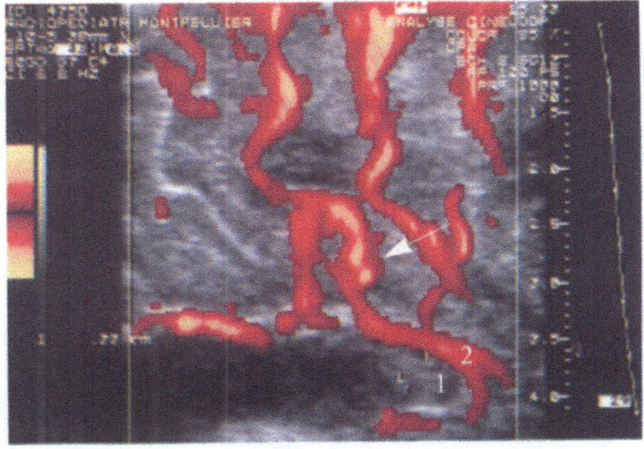

Fig. 9.53. Neonate with partial agenesis of corpus callosum. The genu (*1*) has a normal shape and thickness (3.3 mm) but the body and splenium are absent. The pericallosal artery (*2*) is close to the genu but loses its normal course where the corpus callosum disappears; at this level it takes an upward posterior oblique direction (*arrow*)

tion is suspected on ultrasound, further evaluation by fetal MRI is required (Brisse 1998).

These obvious difficulties of prenatal diagnosis (Bennett 1996; Droulle 1995) indicate the value of color Doppler as a complementary investigation.

In the normal neonate, the anterior cerebral artery and pericallosal artery closely follow the surface of the corpus callosum, from rostrum to splenium (Fig. 9.50).

In complete agenesis, the pericallosal artery takes an abnormal upward direction (Fig. 9.51).

This appearance was already described, before the advent of color Doppler imaging, by Baarsma (1987), who noticed the missing pulsatile echoes from the pericallosal artery; it relates to the well-known angiographic findings of callosal agenesis (Decker 1975). The artery is not absent, as described in the literature (Maheut-Lourmière 1998), but abnormally directed. The diagnostic value of this sign in the fetus is evident (Fig. 9.52).

Its value is yet greater in the case of partial callosal agenesis: the pericallosal artery closely follows the normal corpus callosum, and takes an abnormal upward orientation immediately after it disappears (Fig. 9.53).

Thus, in utero, color imaging helps the positive diagnosis of callosal abnormality, and the differential diagnosis between complete and partial agenesis. In a personal study, post-mortem angiography has shown the abnormal direction of the pericallosal artery in each of ten fetuses with callosal agenesis (Fig. 9.54).

Color Doppler mapping of brain vessels, which is routinely performed in the case of callosal abnormality, also allows differentiation between primitive agenesis and secondary destruction of callosal tissue. When the corpus callosum has been damaged after the 20th week of gestation, most often from ischemic injury, the course of the pericallosal artery remains normal (Fig. 9.55).

Callosal hypoplasia develops after the 20th week, from an insult (vascular, obstructive, or ischemic) to a normally formed corpus callosum. After birth, the diagnosis is based on ultrasonography (morphological analysis and thickness measurement). The prognosis is usually poor: in our experience, out of 37

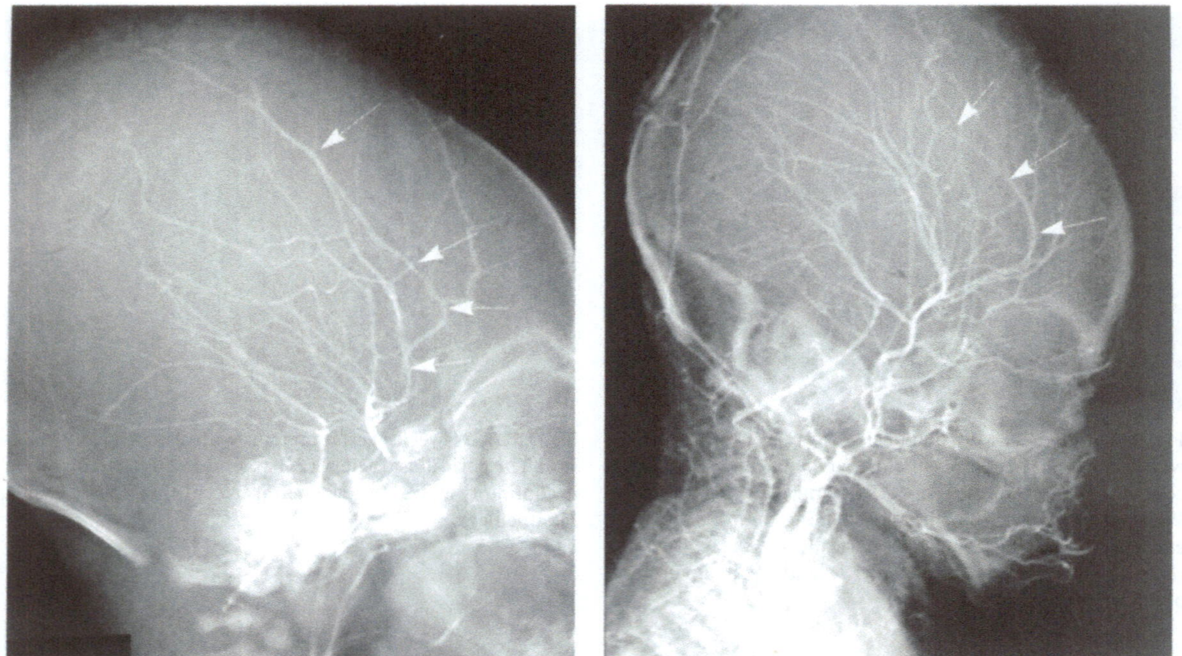

Fig. 9.54a,b. Antenatal ultrasound and MRI diagnosis of callosal agenesis. The pregnancy was terminated at 30 weeks. The diagnosis was confirmed by post-mortem ultrasonography. Cerebral angiography after umbilical catheterization (**a**) showed a characteristic upward and backward oblique course of the pericallosal artery (*arrows*). **b** Normal brain in a 25-week fetus: normal curved course of the pericallosal artery (*arrows*)

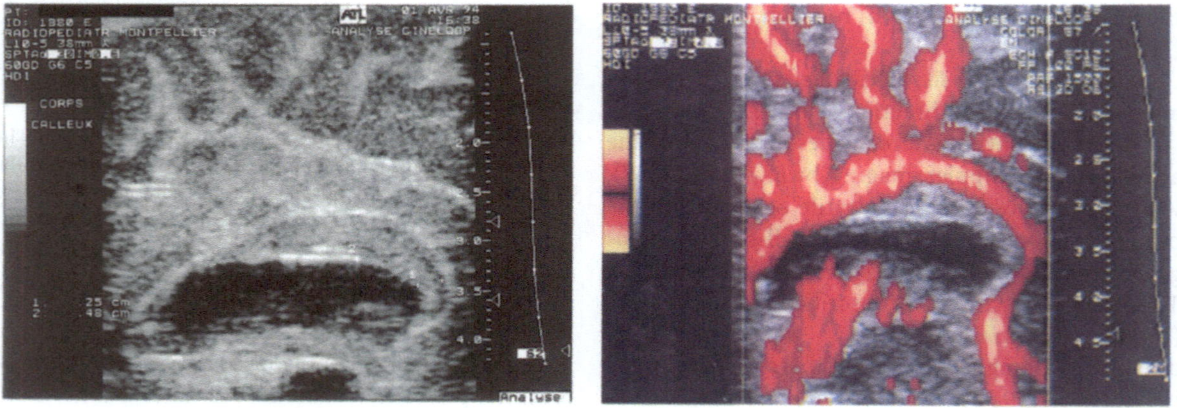

Fig. 9.55 a Cerebral malformation with infratentorial arachnoid cyst, dysmorphic lateral ventricles, and dysgenesis of the corpus callosum. The genu is small (2.5 mm), the body abnormally enlarged (4.8 mm), and the splenium absent, but the medial cerebral sulci do not follow a radial arrangement. **b** Color Doppler: the pericallosal artery has a normal course even at the level of the absent splenium. This pattern rules out partial callosal agenesis and suggests that a secondary process occurred after previously normal development of the complete corpus callosum

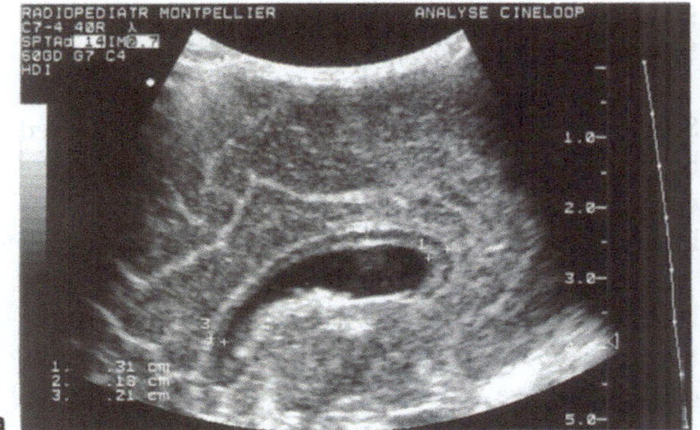

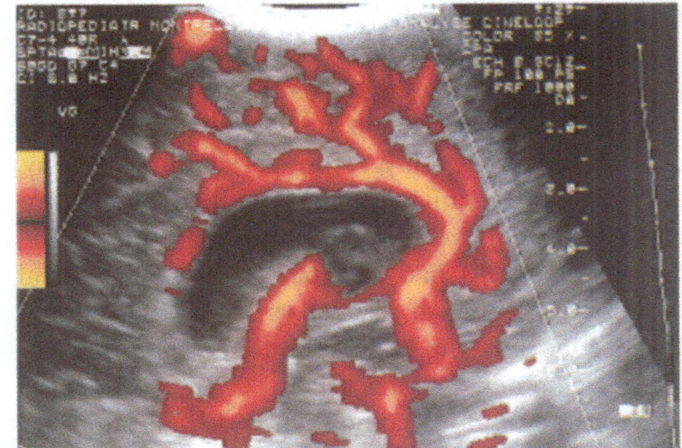

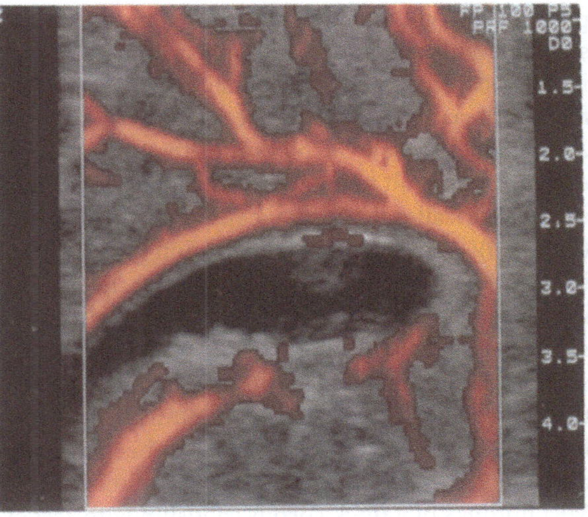

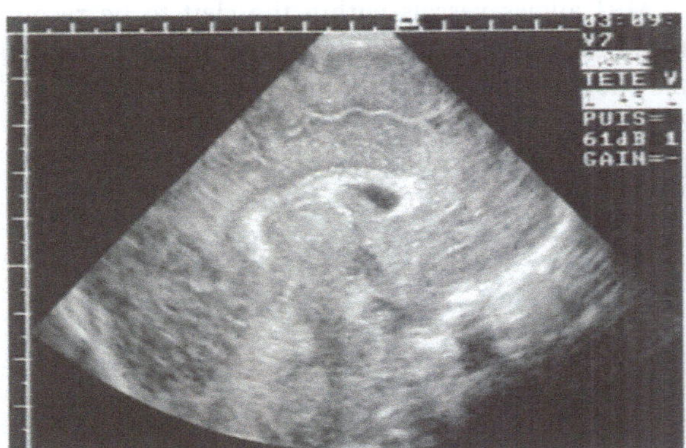

Fig. 9.56a–c. A 3-month-old infant with psychomotor retardation. The corpus callosum is hypoplastic (a) (genu 3 mm, body 1.8 mm, splenium 2 mm), but the pericallosal artery maintains a normal course (b). c Major hypoplasia of the corpus callosum associated with a normal course of the pericallosal artery

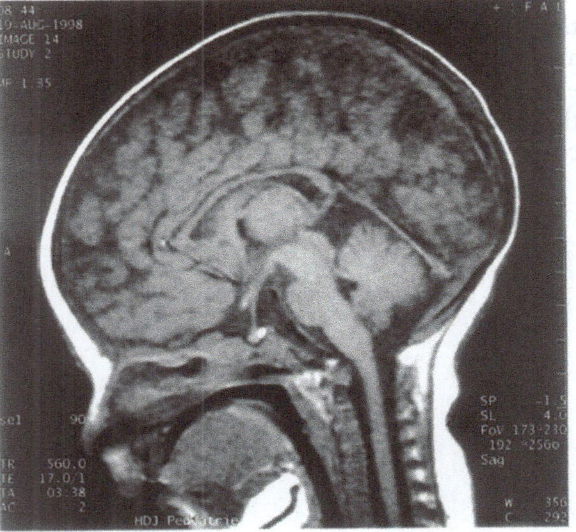

Fig. 9.57a,b. Ischemic injury in a full-term newborn. Hyperechoic white matter; the whole corpus callosum is strongly hyperechoic but of normal thickness (a). At 2 months of age, MRI (b) shows diffuse post-ischemic hypoplasia of the corpus callosum

patients with callosal hypoplasia diagnosed by ultrasound, a multiple malformation syndrome was seen in 15, a chromosomal abnormality in 7, and white matter disease in 2 (Krabbe disease, and Van Bogaert-Alexander disease). Corpus callosum hypoplasia is extremely difficult to diagnose antenatally, especially as the pericallosal artery keeps a normal course (Fig. 9.56); however, demonstration of callosal ischemic injury (COLEY 1997; HAYAKAWA 1996) leading to secondary hypoplasia is now an undisputed sonographic reality (Fig. 9.57).

Finally, color imaging seems to help diagnosis of a thick corpus callosum. This rare entity (GOHLICH-RATHMANN 1998; RYPENS 1996) has been recently documented by RYPENS (1996), who reported fetal MRI findings of a thick corpus callosum with associated neuronal migration disorder, confirmed at postmortem macroscopic examination (the corpus callosum was 10 mm thick, and multiple neuronal heterotopias were observed). In our experience of three cases with callosal thickening (Goldenhar syndrome in 1, Down syndrome in 1, and karyotype 48 XXXX in 1), the pericallosal artery exhibited a particular course: it did not follow the corpus callosum closely, but a wavy course above it (Fig. 9.58).

To sum up, routine use of color Doppler seems to improve the diagnosis and evaluation of callosal dysgenesis. The course and direction of the pericallosal artery allow a distinction between complete and partial agenesis. They also give information as to the timing of callosal injury: when the splenium is absent, the course of the pericallosal artery indicates either late destruction, after the 20th week of gestation (normal course), or early damage (abnormal course).

9.2.2
Schizencephaly

Schizencephaly is a rare malformation characterized by a hemispheric cleft extending from the pia to the ependymal lining of the lateral ventricles. The cleft is lined by abnormal thick gray matter.

Schizencephaly is frequently bilateral, and usually located in or near the sylvian region. Two anatomic types have been described by BIRD (1987): the walls of the cleft are either in apposition (closed lip or type I) or separated by a wide CSF cavity (open lip or type II).

The clinical pattern depends on the severity of the parenchymal defect. In bilateral open-lipped cleft, clinical disturbances begin in the neonate and mainly consist of microcephaly, severe developmental delay, and seizures. In unilateral closed-lipped clefts, BIRD (1987) reported that first symptoms may appear late; his eight patients had hemiparesis or contralateral monoparesis. In such cases, CASTILLO (1996) noted that seizures are the main symptoms when intellectual development is normal.

The sonographic diagnosis of wide open-lip schizencephaly is easy in the neonate (SUCHET 1994) and fetus (KLINGENSMITH 1986; LITUANIA 1989). Obviously, it is much more difficult in the case of type I cleft, but color Doppler may provide decisive evidence.

MRI allows vessels within the cleft to be recognized (BIRD 1987). In the same way, color Doppler may demonstrate a colored vessel within the hyperechoic linear image of the cleft: this constitutes a pathognomonic finding of schizencephaly (Fig. 9.59).

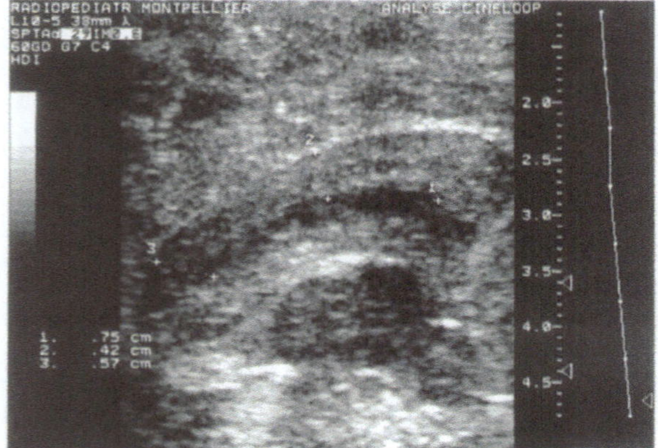
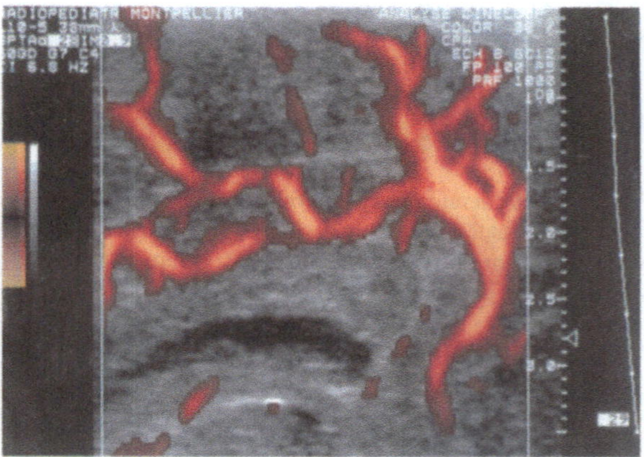

Fig. 9.58a,b. Neonate with intrauterine growth retardation and karyotype 48 XXXX. Thick corpus callosum (genu 7.5 mm, body 4.2 mm, splenium 5.7 mm) and agenetic rostrum (**a**). At birth, the normal thickness of corpus callosum is: genu 4.2 mm, body 3.3 mm, splenium 2.2 mm. On color Doppler (**b**) the pericallosal artery is shown running away from the genu and appears wavy

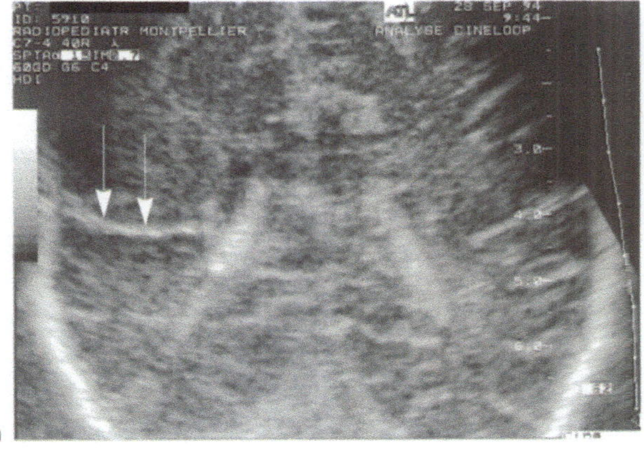

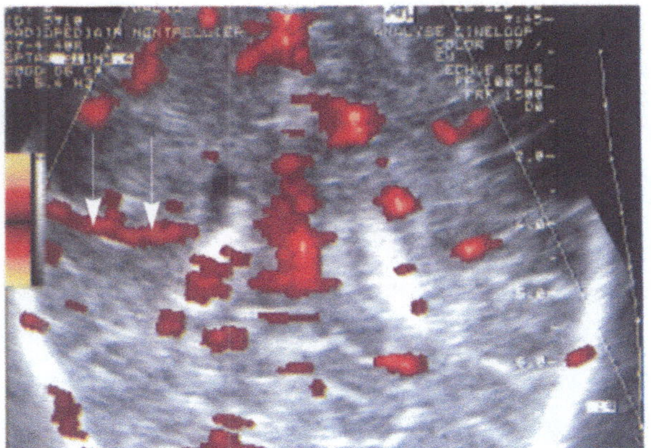

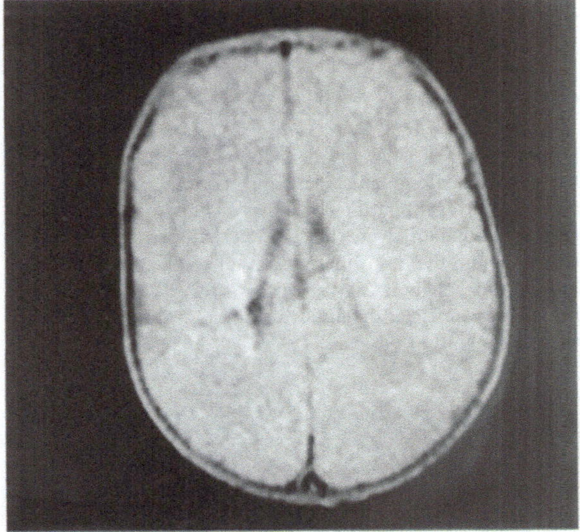

Fig. 9.59a–c. A 15-day-old neonate with unexplained seizures. Ultrasonography contributes information since it detects a thin, linear, hyperechoic image (*arrows*) transversely directed to the right ventricle (**a**). On color Doppler (**b**) this line contains a vessel (*arrows*) that reaches the ventricular wall (**c**). Closed-lip schizencephaly is suspected. Diagnosis confirmed by MRI (**c**)

9.2.3
Holoprosencephaly

Alobar or semilobar holoprosencephaly is known to be easily diagnosed antenatally: a single horseshoe-shaped ventricle, fused thalami and hemispheres, and common facial abnormalities (Fig. 9.60) are observed.

Lobar holoprosencephaly is the least severe form, often difficult to diagnose. Hypotelorism is suggestive but may be absent. Lateral ventricles assume an almost normal shape with well-differentiated occipital and temporal horns, but the frontal horns are fused and the septum pellucidum absent. Thus, differentiating lobar holoprosencephaly from septal agenesis and hydrocephalus with necrosed septum pellucidum is never easy. The morphological diagnosis rests on subtle features: squared frontal horns or incomplete interhemispheric fissure and falx cerebri suggest lobar holoprosencephaly.

In this difficult diagnosis, it is important to know the angiographic anomalies of holoprosencephaly. All authors (ARNOLD 1996; KHODADAD 1969; MAKI 1974; MANELFE 1982; OSAKA 1977; OVERBEEKE 1994; WISEN 1965; ZINGESSER 1966) have emphasized the characteristic nature of the vasculature in alobar holoprosencephaly: either there is a main, dysgenetic arterial trunk that supplies the whole brain, or there is an azygous system with a single median anterior cerebral artery and two lateral middle cerebral arteries (often hypoplastic) arranged in a fan shape on the anterolateral sides of the holosphere. There are associated venous anomalies, since the midline venous structures may be absent [superior sagittal sinus, inferior sagittal sinus, internal cerebral vein, and straight sinus (ZINGESSER 1966)]; the basal ganglia and thalami drain directly into the lateral sinuses (OSAKA 1977).

This abnormal vascular distribution is observed not only in alobar holoprosencephaly, but also in the

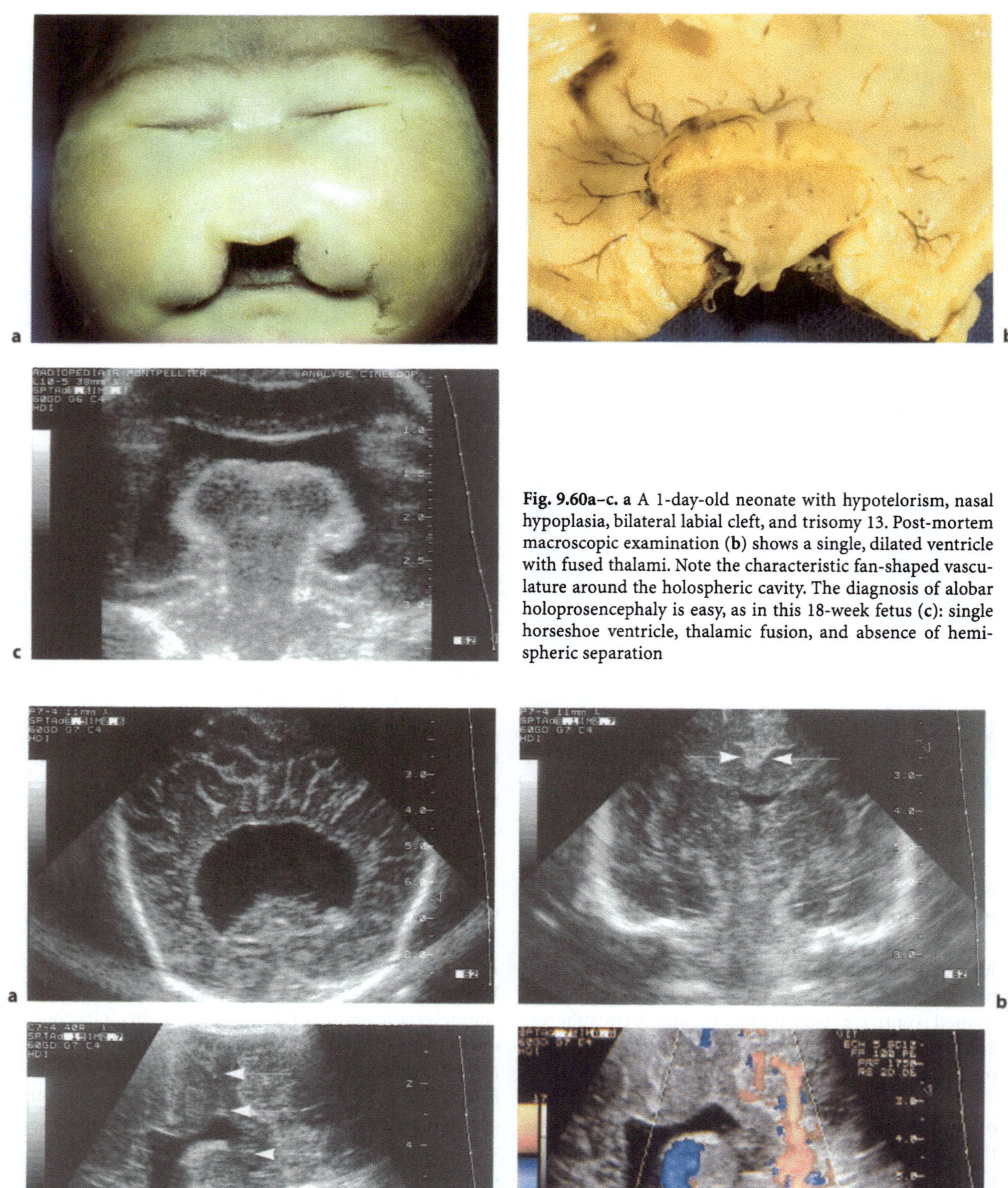

Fig. 9.60a–c. a A 1-day-old neonate with hypotelorism, nasal hypoplasia, bilateral labial cleft, and trisomy 13. Post-mortem macroscopic examination (**b**) shows a single, dilated ventricle with fused thalami. Note the characteristic fan-shaped vasculature around the holospheric cavity. The diagnosis of alobar holoprosencephaly is easy, as in this 18-week fetus (**c**): single horseshoe ventricle, thalamic fusion, and absence of hemispheric separation

Fig. 9.61a–d. Maternal diabetes; semilobar holoprosencephaly. Single ventricle and fused hemispheres are typical (**a**). The incipient hemispheric division (**b**, *arrows*) appears as changing echogenicity of midline structures (**c**, *arrows*). Color Doppler imaging demonstrates suggestive abnormalities of the arterial distribution: a single anterior cerebral artery, and an abnormal course of the pericallosal artery, which runs far from the midline because of the incomplete hemispheric division (**d**). On a coronal plane, fan-shaped vasculature is seen

semilobar and lobar forms, and recognizing it can help the diagnosis of these malformations (MANELFE 1982; OSAKA 1977). The course of the abnormal artery reflects the severity of the brain malformation: it remains close to the internal table of the calvarium in the case of alobar holoprosencephaly because of the absence of the interhemispheric fissure, but runs away from the vault in the semilobar and lobar forms.

The description of these angiographic findings underlines the potentialities of color Doppler imaging, which can show the abnormal vascular anatomy and is of great value in differentiating lobar holoprosencephaly (Fig. 9.61) from septal agenesis.

9.2.4
Other Indications for the Use of Doppler Techniques

Other examples show well how little the capacities of Doppler imaging are known in relation to the diagnosis of brain malformations.

IQBAL (1994) suggested using transcranial Doppler in the assessment of outcome following surgery for *craniosynostosis*. In all operated patients, velocities increased significantly in the cerebral arteries, especially the anterior cerebral arteries.

DOI (1990) reported color Doppler demonstration of the absent supraclinoid portion of the internal carotid artery in patients with *hydranencephaly*.

Finally, PELLICER (1995) showed that the diagnosis of neuronal migration disorders may be helped by color imaging: sulcal arteries on the brain surface are scanty and the middle cerebral artery loses its branching pattern. In our experience of 22 neonates with migrational disorders (lissencephaly in 17,

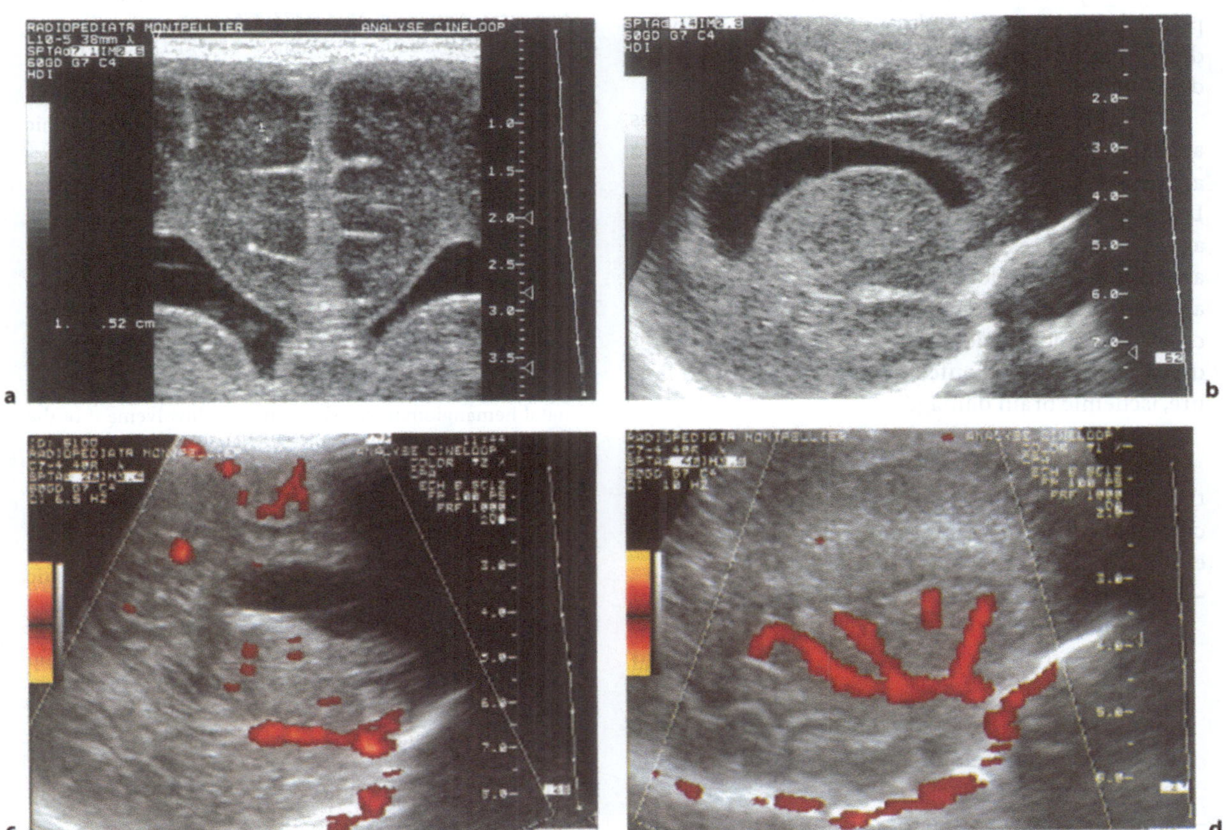

Fig. 9.62a–d. A 6-day-old newborn with seizures: abnormal neuronal migration, characterized by cortical thickening (**a**), disappearance of the insular pattern, which is replaced by a single hyperechogenic sulcus (**b**), and a single vessel (**c**). In a normal newborn (**d**), hyperechogenic cortical sulci exhibit a branching pattern in the insular gyrus, each of them containing a colored vessel. This color imaging is not very useful after birth, but can obviously provide considerable information in the antenatal assessment and diagnosis of a migrational disorder

pachygyria in 5), the main diagnostic evidence was the presence of a rudimentary sylvian fissure with absent or incomplete operculation. This appearance is associated with a reduction of insular vasculature (Fig. 9.62) and constitutes for the future, a good screening method for lissencephaly and fetal pachygyria.

9.3
Conclusion

Doppler techniques provide obvious innovative solutions to diagnostic and prognostic problems in the assessment of cerebral malformations.

● Color and pulsed Doppler are necessary to diagnose and estimate the prognosis of a galenic aneurysm: this much is certain. Ideally, they should be used antenatally; all the criteria of postnatal ultrasonography may be applied to the fetus: color Doppler diagnosis, and color and pulsed Doppler determination of the prognosis (feeding arteries, draining veins, degree of heart failure).

The concept of stealing and deprived arteries appears extremely valuable. It is already essential to analyze the entire intracerebral vasculature by pulsed Doppler and to define the risk of ischemic brain damage. This requires a protocolized study – prolonged and difficult, therefore – of the fetal brain (arterial and venous network) in order to distinguish between cases with a good and a poor prognosis, and to predict a poor postnatal outcome (wide shunt, heart failure, ischemic brain damage).

● Knowledge and color Doppler demonstration of the abnormal vascular anatomy of cerebral nonvascular malformations represents a promising advance, especially in the fetus. It is important to know:
- How to confirm callosal agenesis on the basis of the abnormal course of the pericallosal artery, how to differentiate complete from partial callosal agenesis, how to appraise the time at which a callosal injury occurred (before or after 20 weeks' gestation), and to understand physiopathogenesis of the lesion.
- How to recognize in a fetus or neonate the vascular characteristics of lobar holoprosencephaly or of closed-lip schizencephaly, the morphological diagnosis of which is difficult.

● Color Doppler allows the extracranial location of a lesion to be determined and guides its etiological diagnosis: hemangioma, sinus pericranii, and others.

● Finally, specialists in antenatal diagnosis should perform routine screening of fetal brain vessels using color Doppler coupled to pulsed Doppler. This would obviously improve the early detection of rare but potentially progressive vascular malformations such as arteriovenous aneurysm, cavernous hemangioma, and others.

References

Agee OF, Musella R, Tweed CG (1969) Aneurysm of the great vein of Galen: report of two cases. J Neurosurg 31:346-350

Allison JW, Davis PC, Yutaka S, James CA, Haque SS, Angtuaco EJC, Glasier CM (1998) Intracranial aneurysms in infants and children. Pediatr Radiol 28:223-229

Al-Watban J, Banna M (1987) Infantile cardiomegaly as a complication of vascular malformations of the brain: report of two cases. Ann Saudi Med 8:373-376

Antoun H, Adamsbaum C, Kalifa G (1997) Quid? J Radiol 78:593-595

Arnold WH, Sperberg H, Machin GA (1996) Anatomy of the circle of Willis in three cases of human fetal synophthalmic holoprosencephaly. Anat Anz 178:553-558

Aube M, Tenner M, Brown J, Sher J (1975) Arteriovenous malformation of the vein of Galen. Acta Radiol 347:23-30

Baarsma R, Martjin A, Okken A (1987) The missing pericallosal artery on sonography: a sign of agenesis of the corpus callosum in the neonatal brain? Neuroradiology 29:47-49

Baenziger O, Martin E, Willi U, Fanconi S, Real F, Boltshauser E (1993) Prenatal brain atrophy due to a giant vein of Galen malformation. Neuroradiology 35:105-106

Balaci E, Sumner TE, Auringer ST, Cox TD (1999) Diffuse neonatal hemangiomatosis with extensive involvement of the brain and cervical spinal cord. Pediatr Radiol 29:441-443

Ballester MJ, Raga F, Serra-Serra V, Bonilla-Musoles F (1994) Early prenatal diagnosis of an ominous aneurysm of the vein of Galen by color Doppler ultrasound. Acta Obstet Gynecol Scand 73:592-595

Barkovich AJ, Fram EK, Norman D (1989) MR of septooptic dysplasia. Radiology 171:189-194

Barkovich AJ (1990) Apparent atypical callosal dysgenesis: analysis of MR findings in six cases and their relationship to holoprosencephaly. AJNR Am J Neuroradiol 11:333-337

Barkovich AJ, Kjos B (1992) Gray matter heterotopias: MR characteristics and correlation with developmental and neurological manifestations. Radiology 182:483-487

Bartal AD (1975) Classification of aneurysm of the great vein of Galen. J Neurosurg 42:617-618

Bedford TH (1934) The venous system of the velum interpositum of the rhesus monkey and the effect of experimental occlusion of the great vein of Galen. Brain 57:255-265

Beltramello A, Perini S, Mazza C (1991) Spontaneously healed vein of Galen aneurysm. Child's Nerv Syst 7:129-134

Bennett GL, Bromley B, Benacerraf BR (1996) Agenesis of the

corpus callosum: prenatal detection usually is not possible before 22 weeks of gestation. Radiology 199:447-452

Bird CR, Gilles FH (1987) Type I schizencephaly: CT and neuropathologic findings. AJNR Am J Neuroradiol 8:451-454

Bonioli E, Bellini C, Palmieri A, Fondelli MP, Donati PT (1994) Sinus pericranii. Arch Pediatr Adolesc 148:607-608

Bollar A, Allut 1AG, Prieto A, Gelabert M, Becerra E (1992) Sinus pericranii: radiological and etiopathological considerations. Case Report. J Neurosurg 77:469-472

Boulot P, Deschamps F, Montoya F, Montoya P, Couture A, Ferran JL, Lefort G (1996) Prenatal aspects of giant fetal cranial haemangioendothelioma. Prenat diagn 16:357-359

Bouvaist H, Rossignol AM, Rocca C, Andrini P, Durand C, Bost M (1998) Anevrysme de l'ampoule de Galien et insuffisance cardiaque. Attitude thérapeutique actuelle. Arch Mal Coeur Vaiss 91:637-643

Brisse H, Sebag G, Fallet C, Elmaleh M, Garel C, Rossler L, Vuillard E, Oury JF, Hassan M (1998) IRM anténatale des agénésies calleuses. Etude de 20 cas avec corrélations neuropathologiques. J Radiol 79:659-666

Bronstein M, Bar-Hava I, Blumenfeld Z (1992) Early second trimester sonographic appearance of occipital haemangioma simulating encephalocele. Prenat Diagn 12:695-698

Brunelle F (1997) Arteriovenous malformation of the vein of Galen in children. Pediatr Radiol 27:501-513

Brunelle F, Harwood-Nash D, Fitz C, Chuang S (1983) Intracranial vascular malformations in children: computed tomographic and angiographic evaluation. Radiology 149:455-461

Buxton N, Vloeberghs M (1999) Sinus pericranii. Report of a case and review of the litterature. Pediatr Neurosurg 30:96-99

Campi A, Scotti G, Filipp M, Gerevini S, Stigimi F, Lasjaunias P (1996) Antenatal diagnosis of vein of Galen aneurysmal malformation: MR study of fetal brain and postnatal follow-up. Neuroradiology 38:87-90

Campi A, Rodesch G, Scotti G, Lasjaunias P (1998) Aneurysmal malformation of the vein of Galen in three patients: clinical and radiological follow up. Neuroradiology 40:816-821

Castillo M, Mukherji SK (1996) Imaging of pediatric head, neck and spine. Lippincott-Raven, Philadelphia 155-157

Cerqueira L, Reis FC (1995) Sinus pericranii and developmental venous anomalies: a frequent association. Acta Med Port 8:239-242

Chapman S, Hockley AD (1989) Calcification of an aneurysm of the vein of Galen. Pediatr Radiol 19:541-542

Chisholm CA, Kuller JA, Katz VL, McCoy MC (1996) Aneurysm of the vein of Galen: prenatal diagnosis and perinatal management. Am J Perinatol 13:503-506

Ciricillo SF, Schmidt KG, Silverman NH, Hieshima GB, Higashida RT, Halbach VV, Edwards MSB (1990) Serial ultrasonographic evaluation of neonatal vein of Galen malformations to assess the efficacy of interventional neuroradiological procedures. Neurosurgery 27:544-547

Coley BD, Hogan MJ (1997) Cystic periventricular leucomalacia of the corpus callosum. Pediatr Radiol 27:583-585

Couture A, Ferran JL, Senac JP, Castan-Tabouriech E, Bonnet H (1981) Image ultrasonore d'un anévrysme de la veine de Galien. Arch Fr Pediatr 38:55-57

Couture A, Veyrac C, Baud C (1994) Les malformations cérébrales. In: Echographie cérébrale. Du foetus au nouveau-né. Imagerie et hémodynamique. Couture A, Veyrac C, Baud C. Sauramps Medical, Montpellier. 267-370

Crawford JM, Rossitch EK, Oakes WJ, Alexander E (1990) Arteriovenous malformation of the great vein of Galen associated with patent ductus arteriosus. Report of 3 cases and review of the literature. Child's Nerv Syst 6:18-22

Cubberley DA, Jaffe RB, Nixon GW (1982) Sonographic demonstration of galenic arteriovenous malformations in the neonate. AJNR Am J Neuroradiol 3:435-439

Dan U, Shalev E, Greif M, Weiner E (1992) Prenatal diagnosis of fetal brain arteriovenous malformation: the use of color Doppler imaging. J Clin Ultrasound 20:149-151

David LR, Argenta LC, Venes J, Wilson J, Glazier S (1998) Sinus pericranii. J Craniofac Surg 9:3-10

Decker K, Backmund H (1975) Paediatric Neuroradiology. Georg Thieme, Stuttgart, pp 132-135

Deeg KH, Scharf J (1990) Color Doppler imaging of arteriovenous malformation of the vein of Galen in a newborn. Neuroradiology 32:60-63

De Koning T, Gooskens R, Veenhoven R, Meijboom E, Jansen G, Lasjaunias P, De Vries L (1997) Arteriovenous malformation of the vein of Galen in three neonates: emphasis on associated early ischaemic brain damage. Eur J Pediatr 156:228-229

De Lange SA, Vlieger M (1970) Hydrocephalus associated with raised venous pressure. Dev Med Child Neurol 12 :28-32

Delezoide AL, Fallet-Blanco C, Narcy F, Frappat S, Esculpavit C (1997) L'anévrysme de la veine de Galien: point de vue du foetopathologiste. Méd Foet Echogr Gynécol 30:28-32

Diebler C, Dulac O, Renier D (1981) Aneurysms of the vein of Galen in infants aged 2 to 15 months. Diagnosis and natural evolution. Neuroradiology 21:185-197

Di Rocco C (1991) Vein of Galen aneurysm and hydrocephalus. Child's Nerv Syst 7:359

Di Rocco C, Iannelli A, Puca A, Colosimo C (1983) Spontaneous thrombosis of an aneurysm of the great vein of Galen. Eur Neurol 22:293-299

Doi H, Tatsuno M, Mizushima H, Matsumoto K (1990) The use of two-dimensional Doppler sonography (color Doppler) in the diagnosis of hydranencephaly. Child's Nerv Syst 6:456-458

Dören M, Tercanli S, Holzgreve W (1995) Prenatal sonographic diagnosis of a vein of Galen aneurysm: relevance of associated malformations for timing and mode of delivery. Ultrasound Obstet Gynecol 6:187-289

Dowd CF, Halbach VV, Barnwell SL, Higashida RT, Edwards MSB, Heishima GB (1990) Serial transfemoral venous embolization of vein of Galen malformation. AJNR Am J Neuroradiol 11:643-648

Droulle P, Didier F (1995) L'agénésie calleuse. Problèmes diagnostiques. Point de vue de l'échographiste. Med Foet Echogr Gynecol 24:8-10

Eide J, Folling M (1978) Malformation of the great vein of Galen with neonatal heart failure. Acta Paediatr Scand 67:529-531

Eiras J, Carcavilla LI, Gomez J, Goni A, Salazar J, Marco A (1985) Surgical treatment of an aneurysm of the vein of Galen in a newborn with heart failure. Child's Nerv Syst 1:126-129

Eltohami EA, Robida A (1992) Arteriovenous malformation of the vein of Galen in a newborn diagnosed with color Doppler examination. A case report. Angiology 43:443-447

Evans AJ, Twining P (1991) Case report: in utero diagnosis of a vein of Galen aneurysm using colour flow Doppler. Clin Radiol 44:281-282

Ferrante L, Fortuna A, Celli P, Santioro A, Fraiou O (1988) Intracranial hemorrhage in children and adolescents. Surg Neurol 29:39-56

Garcia-Monaco R, De Victor D, Mann C, Hannedouche A, Terbrugge K, Lasjaunias P (1991) Congestive cardiac manifestations from cerebrocranial arteriovenous shunts. Endovascular management in 30 children. Child's Nerv Syst 7:48-52

Garcia-Monaco R, De Victor D, Alvarez H, Lasjaunias P (1991) Congestive cardiac manifestations from cerebral arteriovenous shunts. Neuroradiology 33:659-660

Garcia-Monaco R, Rodesch G, Terbrugge K, Burrows P, Lasjaunias P (1991) Multifocal dural arteriovenous shunts in children. Child's Nerv Syst 7:425-431

Georgy BA, Hesselink JR, Jernican TL (1993) MR Imaging of the corpus callosum. AJR Am J Roentgenol 160:949-955

Glatt BS, Rowe RD (1960) Cerebral arteriovenous fistula associated with congestive heart failure in the newborn. Pediatrics 26:596

Goelz R, Mielke G, Gonser M, Schoning M (1996) Prenatal assessment of shunting blood flow in vein of Galen malformations. Ultrasound Obstet Gynecol 8:210-212

Gohlich-Ratmann G, Baethmann M, Gartner J, Goebel HH, Engelbrecht V, Christen HJ, Lenard HG, Voit T (1998) Megalencephaly, mega corpus callosum and complete lack of motor development: a previously undescribed syndrome. Am J Med Genet 79:161-167

Gomez MR, Whitten CF, Nolke A, Berstein J, Meyer JS (1963) Aneurysm malformation of the great vein of Galen causing neonatal heart failure. Pediatrics 31 :400

Grossman RI, Bruce DA, Zimmerman RA (1984) Vascular steal associated with vein of Galen aneurysm. Neuroradiology 26:381-386

Haar FI, Miller CA (1975) Hydrocephalus resulting from superior vena cava thrombosis in an infant. Case report. J Neurosurg 42:597-601

Hammock MK, Milhorat TH, Earle K (1971) Vein of Galen ligation in the primate. Angiographic, gross and light microscopic evaluation. J Neurosurg 34:77-83

Hanner JS, Quisling RG, Mickle JP, Hawkins JS (1988) Giant urco coil embolization of vein of Galen aneuryms: technical aspects. Radiographics 8:935-946

Hata T, Hata K, Senoh D, Aoki S, Takamiya O, Yamamoto K, Kitao M (1988) Antenatal Doppler color flow mapping of arteriovenous malformation of the vein of Galen. J Cardiovasc Ultrasonogr 7:301-303

Hayakawa K, Kanda T, Hashimoto K, Okuno Y, Yamori Y, Yuge M, Ando R, Ozaki N, Tamamoto A (1996) MR imaging of spastic diplegia. The importance of corpus callosum. Acta Radiol 37:830-836

Hayashi T, Ishiyama T, Nishikawa M, Furukawa S, Kashiwagi S, Kondoh O, Mito H, Tsuha M (1996) A case of large neonatal arteriovenous malformation with heart failure. Color Doppler sonography MRI and MR angiography as early noninvasive diagnostic procedures. Brain Dev 18:236-238

Haynes R, Sobel DF, Holeman G (1987) Cranial arteriovenous hemangioma in a neonate. AJNR Am J Neuroradiol 8:916-918

Hawkins J, Quisling RG, Mickle JP, Hawkins IF (1986) Retrievable Gianturco-coils introducer. Radiology 158:262-264

Hegesh J, Kuint J, Frand M, Setton A, Tadmor R, Nass D,Kaplinsky E, Motro M (1991) Cerebral arteriovenous malformation diagnosis by two dimensional color coded Doppler ultrasonography of the head. Pediatr Cardiol 12:107-109

Heinz ER, Schwartz CF, Sear RA (1968) Thrombosis in the vein of Galen malformation. Br J Radiol 41:424-428

Hill MC, Lande LM, Larsen JW (1988) Prenatal diagnosis of fetal anomalies using ultrasound and MRI. Radiol Clin North Am 26:287-307

Hirsch JH, Cyr D, Eberhardt H, Zunkel D (1983) Ultrasonographic diagnosis of an aneurysm of the vein of Galen in utero by duplex scanning. J Ultrasound Med 2:231-233

Hoffman HJ, Chuang S, Hendrick EB, Humphreys RP (1982) Aneurysms of the vein of Galen. Experience at the hospital of Sick Children Toronto. J Neurosurg 57:316-322

Hooper R (1961) Hydrocephalus and obstruction of the superior vena cava in infancy: clinical study of the relationship between cerebrospinal fluid pressure and venous pressure. Pediatrics 28:792-799

Horowitz MB, Jungreis CA, Quisling RG, Pollack I (1994) Vein of Galen aneurysms: a review and current perspective. AJNR Am J Neuroradiol 15:1486-1496

Houdart E, Gobin YP, Merland JJ (1993) A proposed angiographic classification of intracranial arteriovenous fistulae and malformations. Neuroradiology 35:381-385

Hulsmann S, Moskopp D, Wassmann H (1998) Management of a ruptured cerebral aneurysm in infancy. Report of a case of ten month old boy. Neurosurg Rev 21:161-166

Hungerford GD, Marzluff JM, Kempel G, Powers JM (1981) Cerebral arterial aneurysm in a neonate. Neuroradiol 21:107-110

Hurst RW, Kagetsu NJ, Berenstein A (1992) Angiographic findings in two cases of aneurysmal malformation of vein of Galen prior to spontaneous thrombosis: therapeutic implications. AJNR Am J Neuroradiol 13:1446-1450

Iqbal JB, Hockley AD, Wake MJ, Goldin JH (1994) Transcranial Doppler sonography in craniosynostosis. Child's Nerv Syst 10:259-263

Ishimatsu J, Yoshimura O, Tetshou M, Hamada T (1991) Evaluation of an aneurysm of the vein of Galen in utero by pulsed and color Doppler ultrasonography. Am J Obstet Gynecol 164:743-744

Jeanty P, Kepple D, Rousis P, Shah D (1990) In utero detection of cardiac failure from an aneurysm of the vein of Galen. Am J Obstet Gynecol 163:50-51

Johnson W, Berry JM, Einzig S, Bass JL (1988) Doppler findings in nonimmune hydrops fetalis and cerebral arteriovenous malformation. Am Heart J 115:1138-1140

Johnston IH, Whittle IR, Besser M, Morgan MK (1987) Vein of Galen malformation: diagnosis and management. Neurosurgery 20:747-758

Johnston H (1973) Reduced CSF absorption syndrome. Reappraisal of benign intracranial hypertension and related conditions. Lancet 2:418-420

Jones RK, Shearburn EW (1961) Intracranial aneurysm in a four week old infant. Diagnosis by angiography and successful operation. J Neurosurg 18:122-124

Kachaner J, Nouaille JM, Batisse A (1977) Les cardiomégalies massives du nouveau-né. Arch Fr Pediatr 34:297-307

Kalifa GL, Chiron C, Sellier N (1987) Hemimegalencephaly: MR imaging in five children. Radiology 165:29-34

Kaplan PA, Hahn FJ (1984) Aneurysms of the posterior cerebral artery in children. AJNR Am J Neuroradiol 5:771-774

Kasahara E, Murayama T, Yamane C (1996) Giant cerebral arterial aneurysm in an infant: report of a case and review of 42 previous cases in infants with cerebral arterial aneurysm. Acta Paediatr Jpn 38:684-688

Kawaguchi T, Kawano T, Kazekawa K, Honma T, Kaneko Y, Koizumi T, Dousaka A (1997) Transarterial embolization of a vein of Galen aneurysm: a case report. No Shinku Geka 25:739-743

Khodadad G, Putschar WG (1969) The cerebral arteries in cyclopia and arhinencephaly. An angiographic and anatomical study. Acta Anat 72:12-24

Kihara S, Koga H, Tabuchi K (1991) Traumatic sinus pericranii. Case report. Neurol Med Chir 31:982-985

Klingensmith WC, Cioffi-Ragan DT (1986) Schizencephaly: diagnosis and progression in utero. Radiology 159:617-618

Komarnishi CA, Cyr DR, Mack LA, Weinberger E (1990) Prenatal diagnosis of schizencephaly. J Ultrasound Med 9:305-307

Kuchelmeister K, Schulz R, Bergmann M, Schwuchow R, Vollmer E (1993) A probably familial saccular aneurysm of the anterior communicating artery in a neonate. Child's Nerv Syst 9:302-305

Kuroki K, Uozami T, Arita K, Takeschi A, Matsuura R, Fujidaka M (1995) Spontaneous disappearance of an aneurysmal malformation of the vein of Galen. Neuroradiology 37:244-246

Langer R, Kaufmann HJ (1987) Arteriovenous malformation of the great cerebral vein of Galen in a newborn. Eur J Pediatr 147:87-89

Lasjaunias P, Alvares H, Rodesh G, Garcia-Monaco R, Brugge K, Burrows P, Taylor W (1996) Aneurysmal malformation of the vein of Galen. Follow-up of 120 children treated between 1964 and 1994. Intervent Neuroradiol 2:15-26

Lasjaunias P (1997) Vein of Galen aneurysmal malformation. In: Vascular Diseases in Neonates, infants and children. Springer, Berlin 75:202

Lasjaunias P (1997) Dural arteriovenous shunts in vascular diseases in neonates, infants and children. Springer, Berlin 321-371

Lazar ML (1974) Vein of Galen aneurysm: successful excision of a completely thrombosed aneurysm in an infant. Surg Neurol 2:22-24

Lee JY, Kandall SR, Ghali VS (1978) Intracerebral arterial aneurysm in a newborn. Arch Neurol 35:171-172

Levine D, Barnes PD, Madsen JR, Li W, Edelman RR (1997) Fetal central nervous system anomalies: MR imaging augments sonographic diagnosis. Radiology 204:635-638

Little JR, Larkins MV, Luders H, Hahn JF, Erenberg G (1986) Fusiform basilar artery aneurysm in a 33 month old child. Neurosurgery 19:631-634

Littvak J, Yahr MD, Ransohoff J (1960) Aneurysm of the great vein of Galen and midline cerebral arteriovenous anomalies. J Neurosurg 17:945-954

Lituania M, Passamonti U, Cordone MS, Magnano GM, Toma P (1989) Schizencephaly: prenatal diagnosis on sonography and magnetic resonance imaging. Prenat Diag 99:649-655

Luker GD, Siegel MJ (1995) Sinus pericranii: sonographic findings. AJR Am J Roentgenol 165:175-176

Lylyk P, Vinuela CF, Dion JE, Duckwiler G, Guglielmi G, Peacock W, Martin N (1993) Therapeutic alternatives for vein of Galen vascular malformations. J Neurosurg 78:438-445

Maheut J, Satini JJ, Barthez MA (1987) Anévrysme de l'ampoule de Galien. Résultats thérapeutiques de l'étude multicentrique nationale. Neurochirurgie. 33:337-340

Maheut-Lourmiere J, Paillet C (1998) Prenatal diagnosis of anomalies of the corpus callosum with ultrasound: the echographist's point of view. Neurochirurgie 44:85-92

Mai R, Rempen A, Kristen K (1996) Prenatal diagnosis and prognosis of a vein of Galen aneurysm assessed by pulsed and color Doppler sonography. Ultrasound Obstet Gynecol 7:228-230

Maki Y, Kumagai K (1974) Angiographic features of alobar holoprosencephaly. Neuroradiology 6:270-276

Mancuso P, Chiaramonte I, Pero G, Tropea R, Guarnera F (1989) A case of thrombosed aneurysm of the vein of Galen associated with superior sagittal sinus thrombosis. J Neurosurg Sci 33:305-309

Manelfe C, Sevely A (1982) Etude neuroradiologique des holoprosencéphalies. J Neuroradiology 9:15-45

Martinez-Lage JF, Garcia-Santos JM, Poza M, Sanchez FG (1993) Prenatal magnetic resonance imaging detection of a vein of Galen aneurysm. Child's Nerv Syst 9:377-378

Mattison DR, Angtuaco T (1988) Magnetic resonance imaging in prenatal diagnosis. Clin Obstet Gynecol 31:353-389

Mayberg M, Zimmerman CH (1988) Vein of Galen aneurysm associated with dural AVM and straight sinus thrombosis. J Neurosurg 68:288-291

Mendelsohn D, Hertzanu Y, Butterworth A (1984) In utero diagnosis of a vein of Galen aneurysm by ultrasound. Neuroradiology 26:417-418

Menovsky T, Van Overbeeke JJ (1997) Cerebral arteriovenous malformations in childhood: state of the art with special reference to treatment. Eur J Pediatr 156:741-746

Mickle JP, Quisling RG (1986) The transtorcular embolization of vein of Galen aneurysms. J Neurosurg 64:731-735

Mullaart RA, Daniels O, Hopan J, Krijgman JB, Kollee LA, Roteveel JJ, Sotelinga GB, Slool JL, Thijssen HO (1982) Ultrasound detection of congenital arteriovenous aneurysm of the great cerebral vein of Galen. Eur J Pediatr 139:195-198

Muszynski CA, Carpenter RJ, Armstrong DL (1994) Prenatal sonographic detection of basilar aneurysm. Pediatr Neurol 10:70-72

Nakasu Y, Nakasu S, Minouchi K (1993) Multiple sinus pericranii with systemic angiomas: case report. Surg Neurol 39:41-45

Newcomb AL, Munns G (1999) Rupture of aneurysm of the circle of Willis in the newborn. Pediatrics 3:769-772

Newlin NS, Seeger JF, Stuck KJ (1981) Vein of Galen aneurysm: diagnosis by real time ultrasound. J Can Assoc Radiol 32:224-226

Norman MG, Becker LE (1974) Cerebral damage in neonates resulting from arteriovenous malformation of the vein of Galen. J Neurol Neurosurg Psychiatry 37:252-258

O'Donnabhain D, Duff DF (1989) Aneurysm of the vein of Galen. Arch Dis Child 64:1612-1617

Okamura K, Murotsuki J, Sakai T (1993) Prenatal diagnosis of lissencephaly by magnetic resonance image. Fetal Diagn Ther 8:56-59

Ordorica SA, Marks F, Frieden FJ, Hoskins IA, Young BK (1990) Aneurysm of the vein of Galen: a new cause for Ballantyne syndrome. Am J Obstet Gynecol 162:1166-1167

Osaka K, Sato N, Yamasaki S, Fujita K, Matsumoto S, Kodama S (1977) Dysgenesis of the deep venous system as a diagnosis criterion for holoprosencephaly. Neuroradiology 13:231-238

Paladini D, Palmieri S, D'Angelo A, Martinelli P (1996) Prenatal ultrasound diagnosis of cerebral arteriovenous fistula. Obstet Gynecol 88:678-681

Paumier A, Winer N, Joubert M, Yvinec M, Aubron F, Sagot S, Quere MP, Boog G (1998) Anévrysme de la veine de Galien. Revue de la litterature à propos de 2 cas. J Gynecol Obstet Biol Reprod 27:814-820

Pellegrino PA, Milanesi O, Saia OS, Carollo C (1987) Congestive heart failure secondary to cerebral arteriovenous fistula. Child's Nerv Syst 3:141-144

Pellicer A, Cabanas F, Perez-Higueras A, Garcia-Alix A, Quero J (1995) Neural migration disorders studied by cerebral ultrasound and colour Doppler flow imaging. Arch Dis Child 73:F51-F61

Pickering LK, Hogan GR, Gilbert EF (1970) Aneurysm of the posterior inferior cerebellar artery. Rupture in a newborn. Am J Dis Child 119:155-158

Pile-Spellman JMD, Baker KF, Liszczak TM, Sandrew BB, Oot RF, Debrun G, Zervas NT, Taveras JM (1986) High-flow angiopathy: cerebral blood vessel changes in experimental chronic arteriovenous fistula. AJNR Am J Neuroradiol 7:811-815

Putty TK, Luerssen TG, Campbell RL, Boaz JC, Edwards MK (1990) Magnetic resonance imaging diagnosis of a cerebral aneurysm in an infant. Pediatr Neurosurg 91:48-51

Quisling RG, Mickle PJ (1989) Venous pressure measurements in vein of Galen aneurysms. AJNR Am J Neuroradiol 10:411-417

Rao VR, Ravimandalam K, Gupta AK, Joseph S, Unni M, Rao AS (1994) Angiographic analysis and results of endovascular therapy of aneurysm of vein of Galen. J Neuroradiol 21:213-222

Raybaud C, Hald JK, Strother C, Choux M, Jiddane M (1987) Les anévrysmes de la veine de Galien. Etude angiographique et considération morphogénétique. Neurochirurgie 33:302-314

Raybaud CA, Strother CM, Hald JK (1989) Aneurysms of the vein of Galen. Embryonic considerations and anatomical features relating to the pathogenesis of malformation. Neuroradiology 31:109-128

Reichman A, Vinuela F, Duckwiller GR, Peacock WJ, Vinters HV (1993) Pathologic findings in a patient with a vein of Galen aneurysm treated by staged endovascular embolization. Child's Nerv Syst 9:33-38

Reiter A, Hutha J, Carpenter R, Segall G, Hawkins C (1986) Prenatal diagnosis of arteriovenous malformation of the vein of Galen. J Clin Ultrasound 14:623-628

Rizzo G, Arduini D, Colosimo C, Boccolini MR, Mancuso S (1987) Abnormal fetal cerebral blood flow velocity waveforms as a sign of an aneurysm of the vein of Galen. Fetal Ther 2:75-79

Rodesch G, Malherbe V, Alvares H, Zerah M, Devictor D, Lasjaunias P (1995) NonGalenic cerebral arteriovenous malformations in neonates and infants. Review of 26 consecutives cases. Child's Nerv Syst 11:237-241

Rodesch G, Hui F, Alvarez H, Tanaka A, Lasjaunias P (1994) Prognosis of antenatally diagnosed vein of Galen aneurysmal malformation. Child's Nerv Syst 10:79-83

Roosen N, Schirmer M, Lins E, Bock WJ, Stork W, Gahlan D (1986) MRI of an aneurysm of the vein of Galen. AJNR Am J Neuroradiol 7:733-735

Rosman NP, Shands KN (1978) Hydrocephalus caused by increased intracranial venous pressure: a clinicopathological study. Ann Neurol 3:445-450

Ross DA, Walker J, Edwards MS (1986) Unusual posterior fossa dural arteriovenous malformation in a neonate: case report. Neurosurgery 19:1021-1024

Ross JS, Masaryk TJ, Modic MT (1990) Intracranial aneurysms: evaluation by MR angiography. AJNR Am J Neuroradiol 11:449-456

Ruchoux mm, Renjaro L, Monegier du Sorbier C, Raybaud C, Santini JJ, Lhuintre Y (1987) Histopathologie de la veine de Galien. Neurochirurgie 33:272-284

Rypens F, Sonigo P, Aubry MC, Delezoide AL, Cessot F, Brunelle F (1996) Prenatal MR diagnosis of a thick corpus callosum. AJNR Am J Neuroradiol 17:1918-1920

Sainte-Rose C, Lacombe J, Pierre-Kahn A (1984) Intracranial venous sinus hypertension: cause or consequence of hydrocephalus in infants? J Neurosurg 60:727-736

Sakai K, Namba K, Meguro T, Mandai S, Gohda Y, Sakurai M, Matsumoto Y (1997) Sinus pericranii associated with a cerebellar venous angioma. Case report. Neurol Med Chir (Tokyo) 37:464-467

Salder LR, Tarr RW, Jungreis CA, Sekhar L (1990) Sinus pericranii: CT and MR findings. J Comput Assist Tomogr 14:124-127

Saliba E, Santini JJ, Chantepie A, Pottiff JM, Cheliakine C, Gold F, Bloc D, Laugier J (1987) Retentissement cardiaque et cérébral de l'anévrysme de l'ampoule de Galien. Apport de l'échographie et du Doppler cérébral en période néonatale. Neurochirurgie 33:296-301

Schijman E, Monges JA (1983) Giant arteriovenous aneurysm of the posterior fossa in a three month old infant. Child's Brain 10:121-129

Schlesinger B (1940) The tolerance of the blocked Galenic system against artificially increased intravenous pressure. Brain 63:178-183

Sepulveda W, Platt CC, Fisk NM (1995) Prenatal diagnosis of cerebral arteriovenous malformation using color Doppler ultrasonography: case report and review of the literature. Ultrasound Obstet Gynecol 6:282-286

Sivakoff M, Nouri S (1982) Diagnosis of vein of Galen arteriovenous malformation by two-dimensional ultrasound and pulsed Doppler method. Pediatrics 69:84-86

Six EG, Cowley AR, Kelly DL (1980) Thrombosed aneurysm of the vein of Galen. Neurosurgery 7:274-278

Snider A, Soifer S, Silverman N (1981) Detection of intracranial arteriovenous fistula by two dimensional ultrasonography. Circulation 63:1179-1185

Sonigo P, Elmaleh A, Fermont L, Delezoide AL, Mirlesse V, Brunelle F (1996) Prenatal MRI diagnosis of fetal cerebral tuberous sclerosis. Pediatr Radiol 26:1-4

Sonigo P, Rypens FF, Carteret M, Delezoide AL, Brunelle F (1998) MR imaging of fetal cerebral anomalies. Pediatr Radiol 28:212-222

Spektor S, Weinberger G, Constantini S, Gomori JM, Beniadani L (1998) Giant lateral sinus pericranii. Case report. J Neurosurg 88:145-147

Stockberger S, Smith R, Don S (1993) Color Doppler sonography as a primary diagnostic tool in the diagnosis of vein of Galen aneurysm in a critically ill neonate. Neuroradiology 35:616-618

Strauss S, Weinraub Z, Goldberg M (1991) Prenatal diagnosis of vein of Galen arteriovenous malformation by duplex sonography. J Perinat Med 19:227-230

Suchet IB (1994) Schizencephaly: antenatal and postnatal assessment with color flow Doppler imaging. Can Assoc Radiol J 45:193-200

Swanstrom S, Flodmark O, Lasjaunias P (1994) Conditions for treatment of cerebral arteriovenous malformation associated with ectasia of the vein of Galen in the newborn. Acta Paediatr 83:255-257

Swischuk LE, Crowe JE, Mewborne EB (1977) Large vein of Galen aneurysms in the neonate. A constellation of diagnostic chest and neck radiologic findings. Pediatr Radiol 6:4-9

Takashima S, Becker LE (1980) Neuropathology of cerebral arteriovenous malformations in children. J Neurol Neurosurg Psych 43:380-385

Tan MP, McConachie NS, Vloeberghs M (1998) Ruptured fusiform cerebral aneurysm in a neonate. Child's Nerv Syst 14:467-469

Tessler FN, Dion J, Vinuela F, Perrella RR, Duckwiller G, Hall T, Boechat MI, Grant EG (1989) Cranial arteriovenous malformations in neonates: color Doppler imaging with angiographic correlations. AJR Am J Roentgenol 153:1027-1030

Thompson RA, Pribam HF (1969) Infantile cerebral aneurysm associated with ophtalmoplegia and quadriparesis. Neurology 19; 903-906

Thrush AL, Marano GD (1988) Infantile intracranial aneurysm: report of a case and review of the literature. AJNR Am J Neuroradiol 9:903-906

Vaksmann G, Jardin M, Mauran P, Brevière GM, Rey C, Dhellemmes P, Duduis C (1990) Peripheral cerebral arteriovenous malformation in an infant: assessment by transcranial color flow mapping. J Clin Ultrasound 18:215-217

Van Overbeeke JJ, Hillen B, Vermeij-Keers C (1994) The arterial pattern at the base of arhinencephalic and holoprosencephalic brains. J Anat 185:51-63

Van Zalen-Sprock RM, Van vugt JM, Van Geijn HP (1995) First and early second trimester diagnosis of anomalies of the central nervous system. J Ultrasound Med 14-8:603-607

Ventureyra CG, Choo SH, Benoit BG (1980) Super giant globoid intracranial aneurysms in an infant. J Neurosurg 53:411-416

Vinas FC, Valenzuela S, Zuleta A (1994) Literature review: sinus pericranii. Neurol Res 16:471-474

Vintzileos AM, Eisenfeld LI, Campbell WA, Herson VC, Dileo PE, Chameides L (1986) Prenatal ultrasonic diagnosis of arteriovenous malformation of the vein of Galen. J Clin Ultrasound 14:623-628

Voet D, Govaert P, Caemaert J, De Lille L, D'Herbe K, Afschrift M (1992) Leptomeningeal cyst: early diagnosis by color Doppler imaging. Pediatr Radiol 22:417-418

Weir BKZ, Allen PBR, Miller JDR (1968) Excision of thrombosed vein of Galen aneurysm in an infant: case report. J Neurosurg 29:619-622

Westra SJ, Curran JG, Duckwiler GR, Zaninovic AC, Hall TR, Martin NA, Boechat MI, Vinuela F (1993) Pediatric intracranial vascular malformations: evaluation of treatment results with color Doppler US. Radiology 186:775-783

Whitaker JB, Latack JT, Venes JL (1987) Spontaneous thrombosis of a vein of Galen aneurysm. AJNR Am J Neuroradiol 8:1134-1136

White BD, Bis KG, Cacciarelli A, Madrazo BL (1992) Ultrasound case of the day. Radiographics 12:396-400

Wierdis T, Biannini V, Jala E (1965) Fetal and neonatal cerebrovascular disease. Panminerva Med 7:325-339

Wisen M, Demyer W, Campbell R (1965) Unique angiographic and ventriculographic pattern of alobar holoprosencephaly. Radiology 84:945-949

Wisoff JH, Berenstein A, Choi IS (1990) Management of vein of Galen malformations. In: Martin AE (ed) Concepts in pediatric neurosurgery, vol 10, Karger, Basel, 137-155

Witrak BJ, Davis PC, Hoffman JC (1986) Sinus pericranii. A case report. Pediatr Radiol 16:55-56

Worswick L, Lamont R, Thomas R, Gordon H (1992) Prenatal ultrasonographic diagnosis of an aneurysm of the vein of Galen. Br J Radiol 65:609-610

Yamagushi M, Kaneko M, Miyakawa I, Mori N, Ohba K, Hayakawa K (1991) Prenatal diagnosis of the aneurysm of the vein of Galen by pulsed Doppler unit. Am J Perinatol 8:244-246

Yamashita Y, Abe T, Ohara N, Maruoka T, Toyada O, Inoue O, Kojima K, Kato H (1992) Successful treatment of neonatal aneurysmal dilatation of the vein of Galen: the role of prenatal diagnosis and transarterial embolization. Neuroradiology 34:457-459

Yanaka K, Enomoto T, Fujimori H, Nose T (1992) Cavernous hemangioma over the anterior fontanelle. Surg Neurol 37:380-383

Yasargil MG, Antic J, Laciga R (1976) Arteriovenous malformations of the vein of Galen. Microsurgical treatment. Surg Neurol 6:195-200

Yokota A, Oota T, Matsukado T, Okudera T (1978) Structures and development of the venous system in congenital malformation of the brain. Neuroradiol 16:23-30

Young B (1979) Hydrocephalus and elevated intracranial venous pressure. Case report. Child's Brain 5:73-80

Yuval Y, Lerner A, Lipitz S, Rotstein Z, Hegesh J, Achiron R (1997) Prenatal diagnosis of vein of Galen aneurysmal malformation: report of two cases with proposal for prognosis indices. Prenat diagn 17:972-977

Zampella EJ, Aronin PA, Odrezin GT (1988) Conservative management of thrombosed vein of Galen malformations. Report of two cases and review of the literature. Pediatr Neurosci 14:264-271

Zerah M, Garcia-Monaco R, Rodesch G, Terbrugge K, Tardieu M, De Victor D, Lasjaunias P (1992) Hydrodynamics in vein of Galen malformations. Child's Nerv Syst 8:111-117

Zingesser LH, Schechter M, Medina M (1966) Angiographic and pneumoencephalographic features of holoprosencephaly. AJR Am J Roentgenol 97:561-574

10 Quiz

Case 1

A. Couture, C. Veyrac

Chanel, a 12-day-old full-term newborn, was admitted to our hospital in poor neurological condition (marked hypotonia, weak crying). Brain ultrasonography was performed immediately, including morphological (Figs. 10.1, 10.2) and color Doppler (Fig. 10.3) imaging.

What is your diagnosis?

Ultrasonography demonstrates several findings:

- The lateral ventricles are moderately enlarged (Fig. 10.2); they contain thin intraluminal echoes (Fig. 10.2a) and a mobile strand on the right side (Fig. 10.1a). The abnormal intraventricular presence of cells is confirmed by color Doppler imaging, which detects a CSF flow alternately colored red and blue (Fig. 10.3a) within the aqueduct of Sylvius.
- High-frequency imaging demonstrates parenchymal lesions: cortico-subcortical differentiation has disappeared and some echodense areas involve the cortex and subcortical white matter. This is especially obvious in the median part of the left frontal lobe (Fig. 10.2). On color Doppler, these lesions do not show any detectable flow (Fig. 10.3b).
- Finally, there are hyperechoic areas in the basal ganglia (Fig. 10.1b) and right thalamus.

Everything suggests a severe intracerebral infection: the intraventricular echoes and color Doppler findings demonstrate meningitis with ventriculitis.

A. Couture, MD; C. Veyrac, MD
Service de Radiologie Pédiatrique, Hôpital Arnaud de Villeneuve, 371 av. Doyen Gaston Giraud, 34295 Montpellier Cedex, France

Intraventricular hemorrhage may reasonably be excluded since the clinical pattern is not suggestive in this full-term newborn. The multifocal parenchymal involvement (cortex, subcortical white matter, basal ganglia, and thalamus) may be considered to be ischemic damage, known as a frequent complication of neonatal bacterial meningitis.

Finally, the nature of the infective agent may be discussed: Escherichia coli tends to be responsible for ventriculitis, *Proteus mirabilis* for brain abscess, while *Streptococcus pneumoniae*, *Hemophilus influenzae*, and *Neisseria meningitidis* affect older infants. *Streptococcus* group B may be suspected, with its associated high risk of ischemic injury.

The diagnosis is provided by lumbar puncture: *Streptococcus* group B meningitis. The newborn soon dies.

This example demonstrates the value of ultrasound imaging in cases of neonatal brain infection:

● This easy, noninvasive investigation guides the diagnosis and the prognostic assessment by answering the question: Is any ischemic brain damage present? In the case of this newborn, the diagnosis and poor prognosis were clearly established before the lumbar puncture was performed. In this situation there is no need for any other imaging procedure (CT or MRI).

● Color Doppler provides valuable information. Winkler (1992) and Tatsuno (1993) were the to first show the great sensitivity of color Doppler imaging for detecting scattered particles as a colored flow within the ventricular lumen (red blood cells, leukocytes, gas, etc.). In our experience, color Doppler seems more sensitive than intraventricular echogenicity and enables the detection of minimal intraventricular hemorrhage or infection. If this colored CSF flow can be found in the third and fourth ventricles as well as in the foramina of Monro and Magendie (Winkler 1992), its investigation should preferably be at the level of the sylvian aqueduct, which is the narrowest point of the ventricular system. Spectral

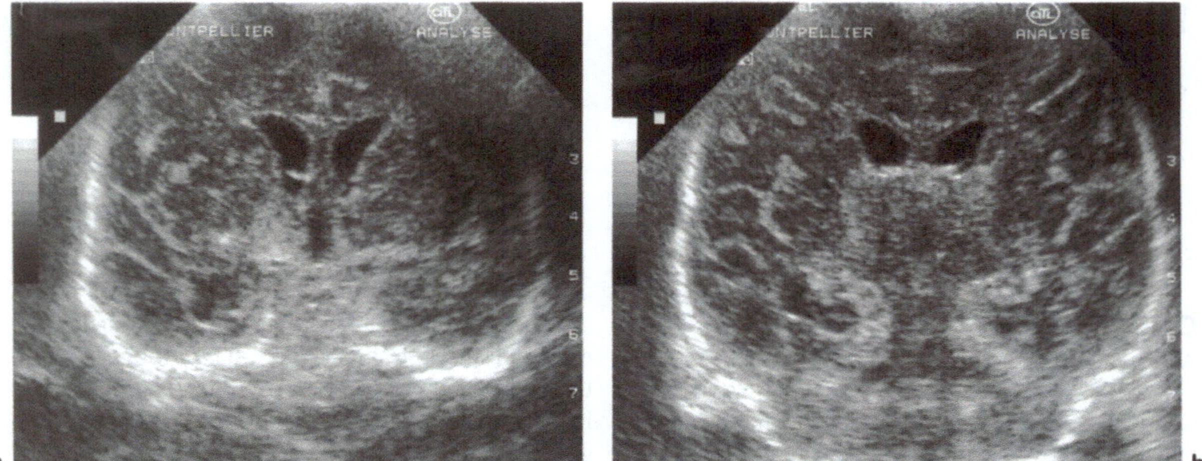

Fig. 10.1. a Coronal scan at the level of the third ventricle. **b** Coronal scan at the level of the basal ganglia.

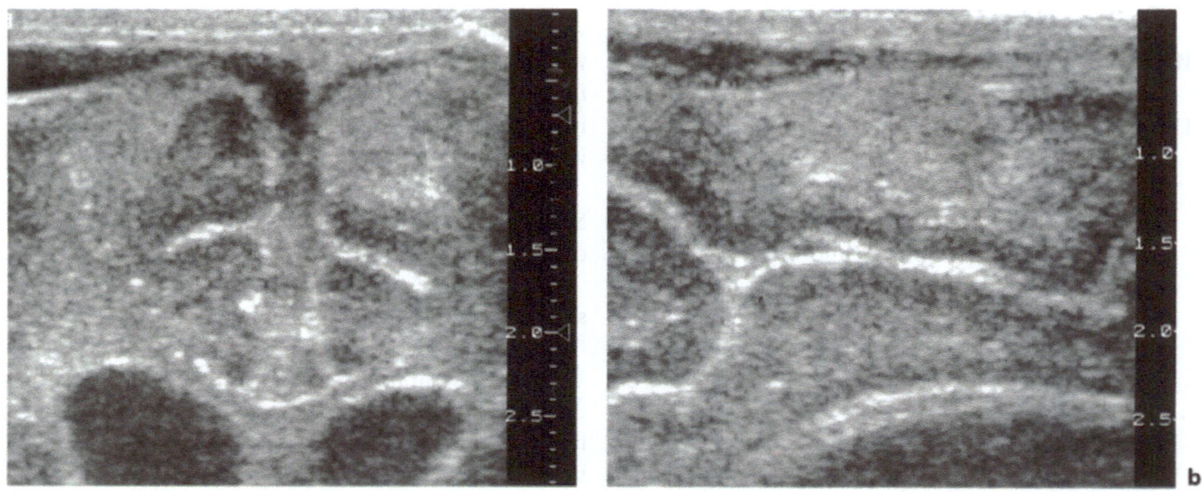

Fig. 10.2a, b. High-frequency probe. **a** Coronal scan, **b** left parasagittal scan

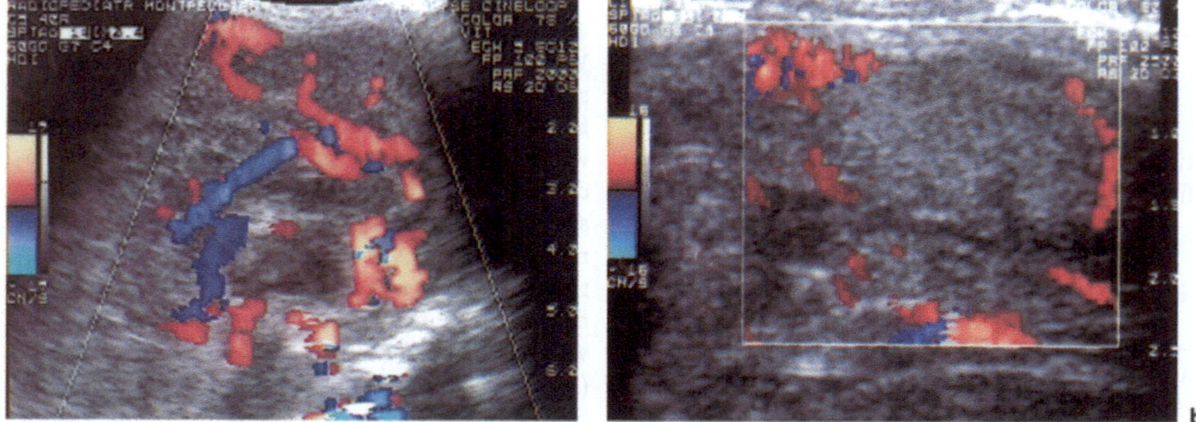

Fig. 10.3a, b. Color Doppler imaging. **a** Midline sagittal scan, **b** left parasagittal scan.

analysis of this ventricular flow confirms the color Doppler findings and shows alternately positive and negative velocities, usually synchronous with respiration. It may be sensitized by several stimuli: fontanellar compression (retrograde flow), abdominal pressure (antegrade flow), crying, sucking, and lower limb motion.

Finally, we have not enough experience to assess color Doppler in the evaluation of parenchymal ischemic lesions. Color imaging may show hyperemia in the early phase (STEVENSON 1997), but most often ischemic lesions appear as avascular areas (OREY 1999) (Fig. 10.3b). The sonographic diagnosis of ischemic brain damage continues to be based on morphological imaging.

References

D'Orey MC, Melo MJ, Ramos I, Guimaraes H, Alves AR, Silva JS, Vasconcelos G, Costa A, Silva G, Santos NT (1999) Cerebral ischemic infarction in newborn infants. Diagnosis using pulsed and color Doppler imaging. Arch Pediatr 6:457–459

Stevenson D, John P (1997) Power Doppler ultrasound appearances of neonatal ischaemic brain injury. Pediatr Radiol 27:147–149

Tatsuno M, Hasegawa M, Okuyama K (1993) Ventriculitis in infants: diagnosis by color Doppler flow imaging. Pediatr Neurol 9:127–130

Winkler P (1992) Colour-coded echographic flow imaging and spectral analysis of CSF in meningitis and hemorrhage. Part I. Clinical evidence. Pediatr Radiol 22:24–30

Case 2

A. COUTURE, C. VEYRAC, F. DESCHAMPS

In a 30-year-old gravida I, para I woman, fetal ultrasonography detected, at 22 weeks of gestation, a 3×3 cm highly vascularized occipital mass (Fig. 10.4) with a low resistive index on arterial pulsed Doppler.

At 26 weeks, repeat ultrasonography demonstrated marked growth of the tumor (now 7 cm in diameter), involving the whole right parieto-occipital area (Fig. 10.5).

At the end of pregnancy, the lesion was unchanged, it was a huge hypervascular tumor (Fig. 10.6), and cesarean delivery was decided on at 37 weeks of gestation.

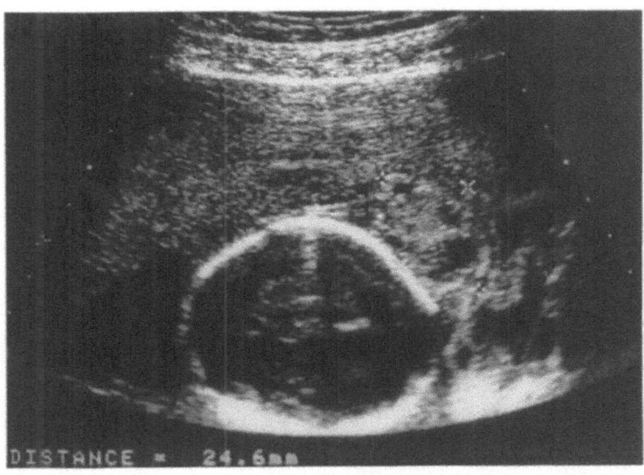

Fig. 10.4. Twenty-two weeks of gestation: axial transverse scan of fetal head

What should be done?

What is your diagnosis?

In this case, the diagnosis was as difficult as assessment of the prognosis. There was obviously a solid, highly vascularized tumor with a homogeneous echostructure (Figs. 10.5, 10.6) and located extracranially (Fig. 10.4). The mass was covered by normal

A. COUTURE, MD; C. VEYRAC, MD
Service de Radiologie Pédiatrique, Hôpital Arnaud de Villeneuve, 371 av. Doyen Gaston Giraud, 34295 Montpellier Cedex, France
F. DESCHAMPS, MD
Service d'Echographie, Maternité, Hôpital Arnaud de Villeneuve, 371 av. Doyen Gaston Giraud, 34295 Montpellier Cedex, France

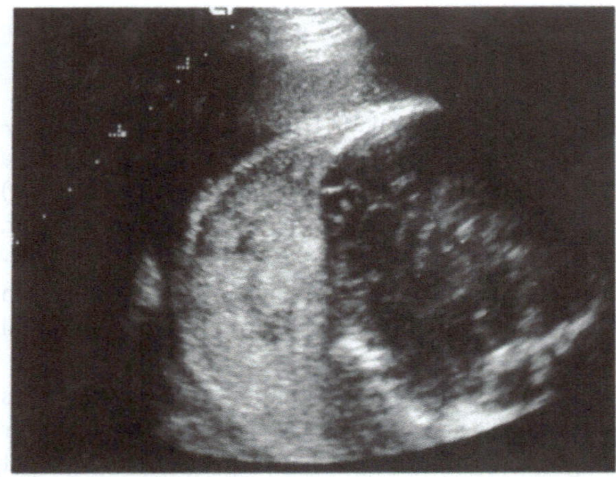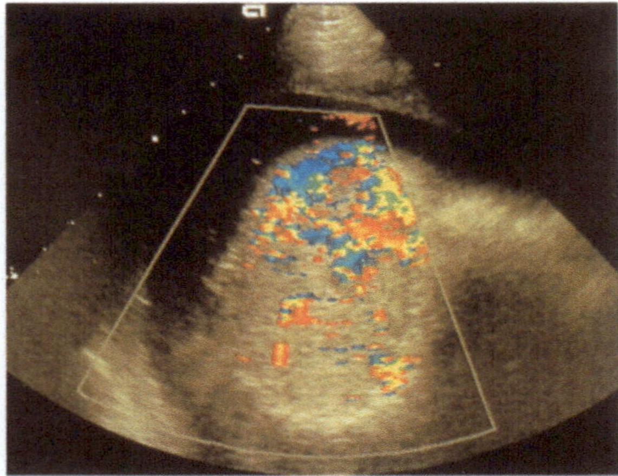

Fig. 10.5a, b. Twenty-six weeks of gestation: **a** focalized scan of the tumor, **b** with color Doppler

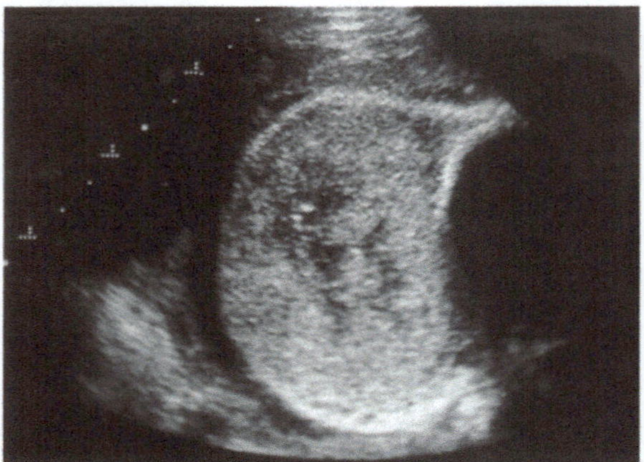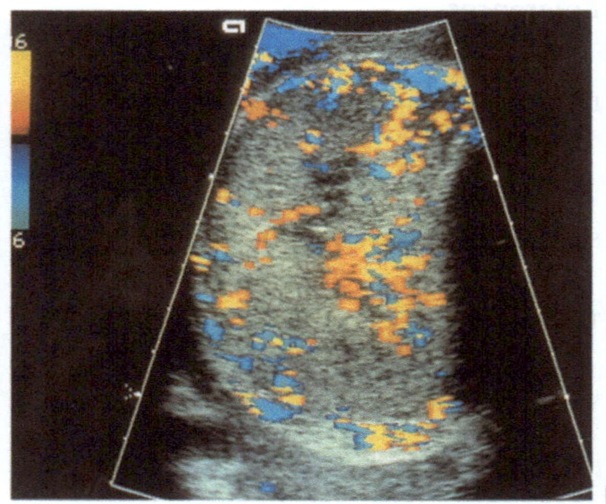

Fig. 10.6a, b. Thirty-six weeks of gestation: **a** gray scale and **b** color Doppler appearance

skin and was not associated with any bony skull defect. Intracranial structures were normal (Fig. 10.4). These anatomical characteristics did not change throughout the pregnancy.

The echostructure, anarchic vascularization of the mass, and absence of bony defect ruled out an encephalocele, while the homogeneous appearance did not suggest a teratoma. An angiomatous tumor might be reasonably suspected, especially since intratumoral arteries exhibited high diastolic flow velocity.

The explosive growth of the tumor from 22 to 26 weeks of gestation was worrying and points up the difficulty of determining a prognosis, since there was no information as to whether the tumor was benign or malignant.

What should be done?

In agreement with the parents and after multidisciplinary discussion, it was decided to allow the pregnancy to continue since the fetal brain and bony skull remained normal in appearance.

At 37 weeks, a cesarean delivery was performed in order to avoid dystocia and intrapartum cephalic pole laceration which might result from fetal anemia and thrombopenia.

At birth, the infant presented with a 8–6 cm violaceous tumor with markedly dilated superficial veins (Fig. 10.7).

A transient moderate heart failure was observed. Skull X-rays was normal. On Doppler US, the mass was mainly supplied by branches of the external

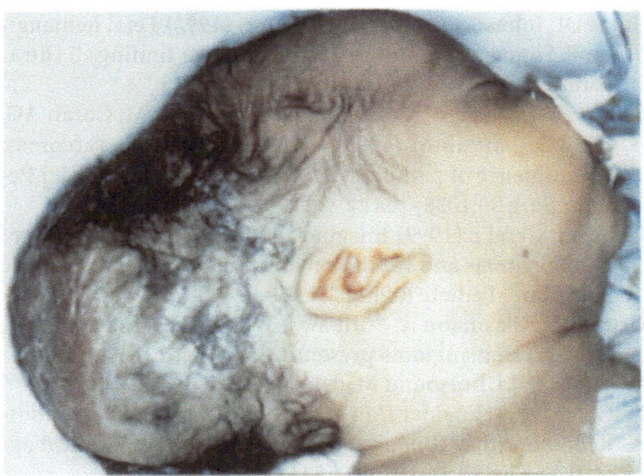

Fig. 10.7

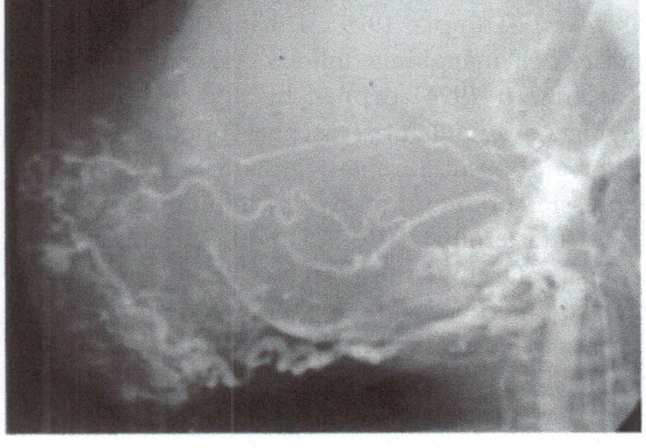

Fig. 10.8

carotid artery, what was confirmed by angiographic investigation (Fig. 10.8).

Surgical biopsy and ligation of supplying pedicles were performed at 4 days of life. The tumor was a *benign giant hemangioma.*

At day 7, a Kasabach-Merritt syndrome occurred, requiring surgical excision of the tumor with a cutaneous graft. The outcome was favorable and the infant is normal at a 4-year follow-up.

This observation prompts several comments:

● In the literature, antenatal diagnosis of congenital hemangioma is rare. TREADWELL (1993) reported six patients with congenital hemangioma in a craniocervical location, while BOON (1996) proposed this diagnosis in 3 out of 13 fetuses with angioma. Diagnostic errors are frequent in utero: congenital hemangioma may be confused with venous malformation (GRUNDY 1985), malignant tumor (BONN 1995), teratoma (AZIZKHAN 1995), or encephalocele (BRONSHE-TEIN 1992; MITCHELL 1999; SHERER 1993). Although the tumoral echostructure and bony skull integrity allow hemolymphangioma and encephalocele to be ruled out, the differential diagnosis against a teratoma may be less easy. Rapid tumoral growth is common in the evolution of a fetal teratoma, but its heterogeneous echostructure, with fluid areas, solid tissue, and calcifications, is usually suggestive.

Similarly, the morphology and evolution of the mass cannot rule out a malignant tumor. Hypothesizing this, rhabdomyosarcoma and hemangiopericytoma should be discussed since some rare prenatal cases have been reported (AHMED 1999; DILLAN 1995; ONDEROGLU 1999; PAUTARD 1999). They are usually heterogeneous, but the different patterns of these unusual fetal neoplasms are little known and decisive grounds for the differential diagnosis are lacking.

Color imaging and pulsed Doppler assessment (BOON 1996; BOULOT 1996; BULAS 1992) of a craniocervical mass provide obviously valuable information: any highly vascularized tumor may be reasonably suspected as angiomatous. The vascular distribution is homogeneous and diffuse in congenital hemangioma, while in other tumors it is more heterogeneous and incomplete, but these vascular characteristics are not specific. All this shows how difficult it is to give an accurate etiological diagnosis in the fetus.

These real insufficiencies set into relief the recent discovery of a new immunohistochemical marker for hemangioma (NORTH 2000). In a retrospective study, this author found intense endothelial GLUT 1 immunoreactivity (erythrocyte-type glucose transporter protein) in 97% of 143 juvenile hemangiomas and considered this high reactivity to be a specific feature of juvenile hemangiomas. This offers interesting diagnostic perspectives.

● Since antenatal ultrasonography has come into routine use, congenital hemangioma has been recognized as a special entity resulting from early antenatal proliferation: detection of such a tumor at 12 weeks of gestation has been documented (BOON 1996). The specific evolution of congenital hemangioma is known: the rapid development of fetal angiogenesis explains the large volume of the tumor, followed by early involution, usually after birth. This makes it very different from postnatal hemangioma, which appears in the first week of life and is then characterized by rapid proliferation (3–9 months) followed by variable stability and slow involution (18 months to 10 years) (DUBOIS 1999). During its proliferative phase, a hemangioma follows a complex process (TAKAHASHI 1994) defined by high expression of angiogenic stimulators (vascular endothelial growth factor and basic fibroblast growth factor) and low expression of interferon-β (which inhibits angiogenesis). Interferon-α is found in the amniotic fluid, fetoplacental unit, and placental blood; the trophoblast produces a six-fold higher level of interferon in the first trimester than in the third. BOON (1996) proposed that intrauterine hemangioma results from a low concentration of trophoblastic interferon in a localized area of the developing fetus.

● Antenatal diagnosis of hemangioma is important for several reasons:

- Sonographic monitoring is recommended to detect the occurrence (though rare) of hydrops fetalis (MCGAHAN 1986) and track tumoral growth. The delivery, which in some cases may be by cesarean section, can be planned.

- At birth, the diagnosis should be confirmed and complications looked for: congestive heart failure, platelet trapping coagulopathy, tumoral necrosis, or compression of a vital organ. Although the evolution of hemangioma is usually spontaneously regressive, a complication may require urgent treatment, either pharmacological (corticoid or/ and interferon), or by embolization, or by surgical excision, as in our case.

References

Ahmed OA, Hussain A, King DJ, Holmes JD (1999) Congenital rhabdomyosarcoma. Br J Plast Surg 52:304–307

Azizkhan RG, Haase GM, Applebaum H, Dillon PW, Coran AG, King PA, King DR, Hodge DS (1995) Diagnosis, management and outcome of cervicofacial teratomas in neonates: a Children's Cancer Group Study. J Pediatr Surg 30:312-316

Boon LM, Fishman S, Lund DP, Mulliken JB (1995) Congenital fibrosarcoma masquerading as congenital hemangioma: report of two cases. J Pediatr Surg 30:1378–1381

Boon LM, Enjolras O, Mulliken JB (1996) Congenital hemangioma: evidence of accelerated involution. J Pediatr 128:329–335

Boulot P, Deschamps F, Montoya F, Montoya P, Couture A, Ferran JL, Lefort G (1996) Prenatal aspects of giant fetal cranial haemangio-endothelioma. Prenat Diagn 16:357–359

Bronshtein M, Bar-Hava I, Blumenfeld Z (1992) Early second trimester sonographic appearance of occipital haemangioma simulating encephalocele. Prenat Diagn 12:695–698

Bulas DI, Johnson D, Allen JF, Kapur S (1992) Fetal hemangioma. Sonographic and color flow Doppler findings. J Ultrasound Med 11:499–501

Dillon PW, Whalen TV, Azizkhan RG, Haase GM, Coran AG, King DR, Smith M (1995) Neonatal soft tissue sarcomas: the influence of pathology on treatment and survival. J Pediatr Surg 30:1038–1041

Dubois J, Garel L (1999) Imaging and therapeutic approach of hemangiomas and vascular malformations in the pediatric age group. Pediatr Radiol 29:879–893

Grundy H, Glasmann A, Burlbaw J, Waltan S, Dannar C, Doan L (1985) Hemangioma presenting as a cystic mass in the fetal neck. J Ultrasound Med 4:147–150

McGahan JP, Schneider JM (1986) Fetal neck hemangioendothelioma with secondary hydrops fetalis: sonographic diagnosis. J Clin Ultrasound 14:384–388

Mitchell CS (1999) Vertex hemangioma mimicking an encephalocele. J Am Osteopath Assoc 99:626–627

North PE, Waner M, Mizeracki A, Mihm MC (2000) Glut 1: a newly discovered immunohistochemical marker for juvenile hemangiomas. Hum Pathol 31:11–22

Onderoglu LS, Yucel A, Yuce K (1999) Prenatal sonography features of embryonal rhabdomyosarcoma. Ultrasound Obstet Gynecol 13:210–212

Pautard B, Canarelli JP, Gontier MF, Risbourg B, Piussan C, Flamant F (1990) Rhabdomyosarcome embryonnaire de découverte anténatale. Arch Fr Pediatr 47:433–435

Sherer DM, Perillo AM, Abramowicz JS (1993) Fetal hemangioma overlying the temporal occipital suture, initially diagnosed by ultrasonography as an encephalocele. J Ultrasound Med 12:691–693

Takahashi K, Mulliken JB, Kozakewich HPW, Rogers RA, Folkman J, Ezekowitz RA (1994) Cellular markers that distinguish the phases of hemangioma during infancy and childhood. J Clin Invest 93:2357–2364

Treadwell MC, Sepulveda W, Le Blanc LL, Romero R (1993) Prenatal diagnosis of fetal cutaneous hemangioma: case report and review of the literature. J Ultrasound Med 12:683–687

Case 3

A. Couture, MP Quere, C. Talmant

Routine ultrasonography was performed at 22 weeks' gestation and showed normal fetal brain. The examination was repeated at 25 weeks (Figs. 10.9, 10.10).

What is your diagnosis?

There was a hyperechoic, rounded, extracerebral mass surrounded by pericerebral fluid, posterior to the occipital lobes and superior to the tentorium cerebelli, without any colored signal on color Doppler.

Galenic aneurysm was easily ruled out: the lesion was too posteriorly located, and no afferent or draining vessel could be detected. A meningeal or bony tumor was unlikely, because of acute angles with the bony skull.

A sinusal thrombosis should be suspected, but the color Doppler analysis was incomplete – it failed to answer the questions: Does the venous thrombosis involve the distal part of the superior sagittal sinus or the torcular? Is there an associated deep vein thrombosis? The ultrasound study was complemented by brain MRI which confirmed the sonographic hypothesis and demonstrated an ovoid thrombus that appeared hyperintense on T1- and hypointense on T2-weighted sequences (Fig. 10.11).

The thrombus was located low on the midline, which excluded transverse sinus involvement and suggested a torcular thrombosis. The deep venous sinuses and proximal part of the superior sagittal sinus remained patent. Finally, the fetal brain had a normal appearance (Fig. 10.12).

The pregnancy was interrupted at 26 weeks in accordance with the parents' wishes. Pathological examination revealed hemorrhagic subarachnoid fluid surrounding an ovoid mass that corresponded to the thrombosed torcular (Fig. 10.13). The brain was normal.

This case of *fetal thrombosis of the torcular* is exceptional and as yet undescribed in the literature.

A. Couture, MD
Service de Radiologie Pédiatrique, Hôpital Arnaud de Villeneuve, 371 av. Doyen Gaston Giraud, 34295 Montpellier Cedex, France
MP Quere, MD
Service de Radiopédiatrie, Centre Hospitalier Universitaire, Nantes, France
C. Talmant, MD
Centre d'échographie de l'ile Gloriette, Nantes, France

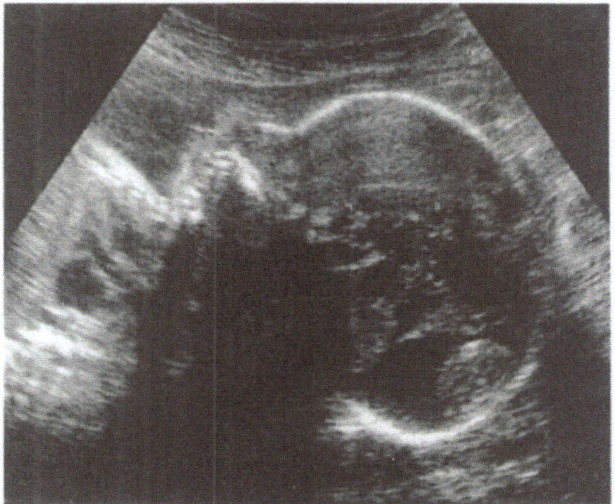

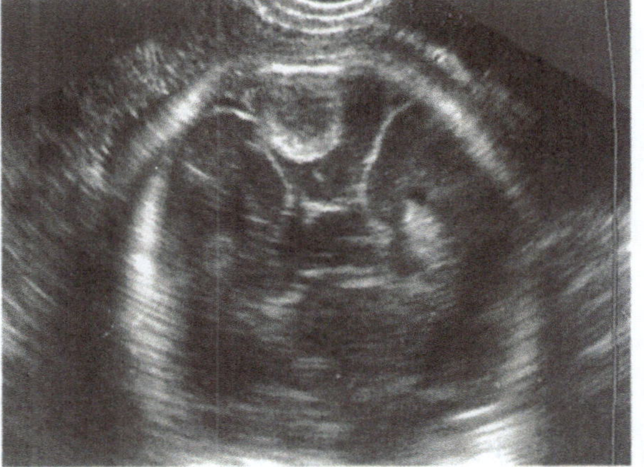

Fig. 10.9. Sagittal **a** and axial transverse **b** scans of the fetal head

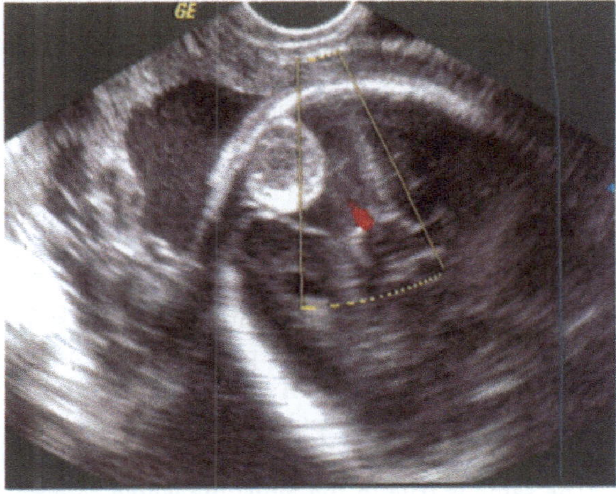

Fig. 10.10. Color Doppler, axial transverse plane

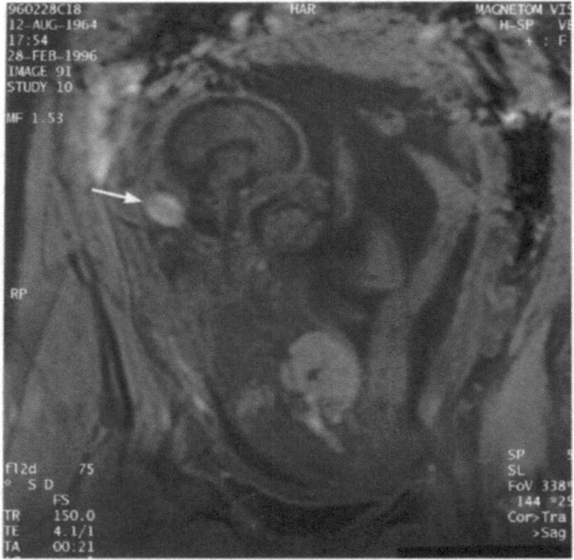

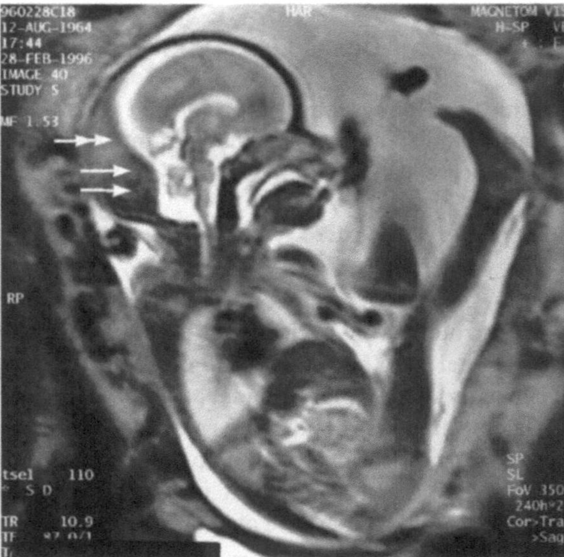

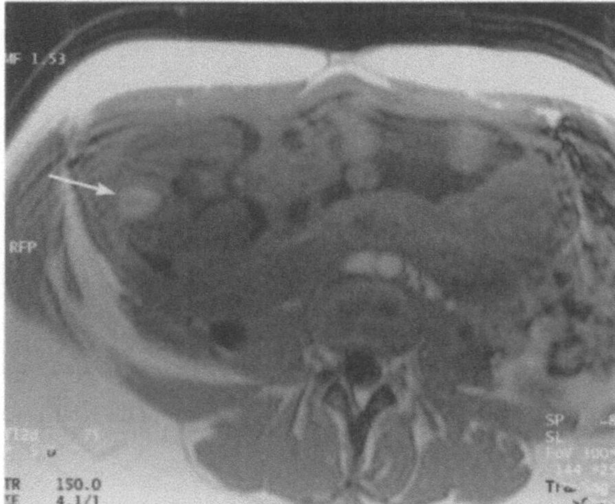

Fig. 10.11a–c. Subacute clot with hypersignal on T1- (*arrow*) (**a, b**) and hyposignal on T2-weighted MR images (*double arrow*) (**c**) on the midline. The intermediate signal of surrounding fluid is well recognized on the T2-weighted sequence (*double arrow*)

In children, cerebral vein thromboses are infrequent, but their diagnosis has widely benefited from modern imaging (CT and, especially, MRI). More recently, ultrasonography (DEAN 1995; LAM 1995; PEDESPAN 1996) has increased the diagnostic imaging potentialities: in the neonate, initial diagnosis and follow-up are easily assessed by gray-scale and color Doppler imaging. Several pieces of information may be gained:

● In the healthy newborn, the superior sagittal sinus and deep sinuses are always depicted by color imaging. Failure to see them on color Doppler and to obtain a spectrum on pulsed Doppler is always abnormal and the sign of a venous thrombosis.

The same is true in the fetus: the whole cerebral venous system may be demonstrated by color imaging (LAURICHESSE-DELMAS 1999). If the integrity of the venous circulation is doubtful, it should be evaluated in its entirely by color Doppler, in order to accurately locate the clotted focus, detect an extensive thrombosis, and assess the sinusal blood flow. Because of the exceptional nature of our case, the vasculature was studied not by Doppler but by MRI. However, this example demonstrates the value of combining arterial and venous mapping with the morphological assessment of the fetal brain.

● What is the etiology? In the neonate, many conditions may affect the cerebral venous blood flow. Instability of arterial blood pressure in a preterm infant, postinfectious or hemorrhagic distress, and congenital heart disease cause disturbances of cerebral venous blood flow. Patent ductus arteriosus, congen-

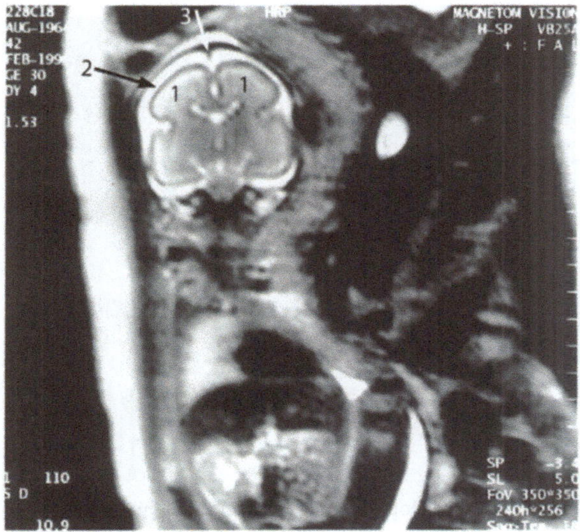

Fig. 10.12. HASTE sequence, frontal plane. Normal brain with hyperintense white matter (*1*) and hypointense peripheral cortical ribbon (*2*). Notice the normal pattern of the superior sagittal sinus (*3*)

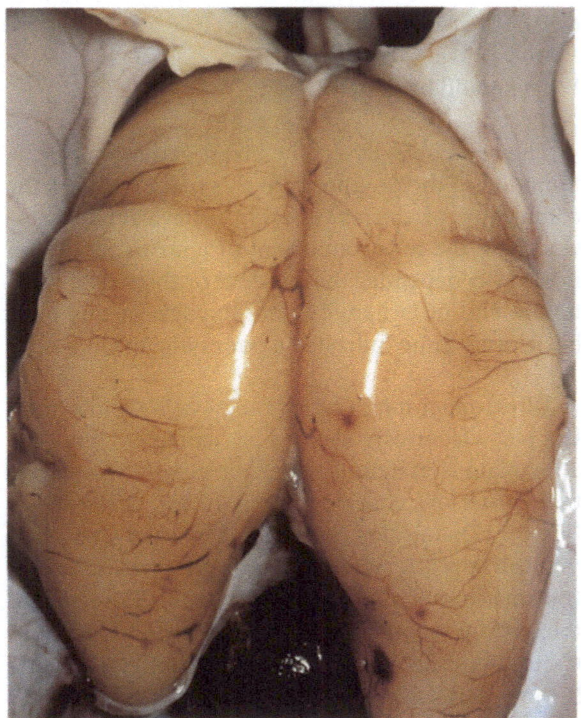

Fig. 10.13. Gross examination of the brain: thrombosis of the torcular is visible as a blackish ovoid node

ital (IBRAHIM 2000) or acquired hypercoagulate states, hemoconcentration, and polyglobuly are also factors for developing cerebral vein thrombosis. Beside these high-risk situations, vein thrombosis

may also occur as an isolated event. In our 25-week fetus, etiological investigations remained negative.

● What is the prognosis? This is obviously the main question. The consequences of neonatal cerebral venous thrombosis combine meningeal (subarachnoid, subdural hemorrhage) and parenchymal damage (capillary congestion, edema, hemorrhage, ischemia, necrosis). These data explain the sonographic (Fig. 10.9) and MR (Fig. 10.11) images: the fluid surrounding the thrombosis relates to meningeal hemorrhage.

Although the prognosis is difficult to establish, cerebral venous thrombosis seems infrequently to be associated with ischemic brain damage (VOLPE 1995). There is an apparent relationship between the site of the thrombus and the location and severity of ischemic-hemorrhagic lesions: parasagittal hemorrhagic infarct with superior sagittal sinus thrombosis (exceptionally), and gangliothalamic ischemic hemorrhage with deep vein thrombosis. In our case, the venous thrombosis remained superficial as it involved only the torcular, and brain MRI excluded parenchymal injury. Thus, there were no ground for predicting a poor neurological outcome. It would have been more appropriate to monitor the brain integrity by serial MRI.

This case illustrates how difficult it is to make an accurate prognosis in the presence of exceptional fetal disease.

References

Dean LM, Taylor GA (1995) The intracranial venous system in infants: normal and abnormal findings on duplex and color Doppler sonography. AJR Am J Roentgenol 164:151-156

Ibrahim A, Damon G, Teyssier G, Billiemaz K, Rayet I, Tardy B (2000) Deficit heterozygote en protéine C: à propos de deux cas avec thromboses veineuses cérébrales en période néonatale. Arch Pediatr 7:158-162

Lam AH (1995) Doppler imaging of superior sagittal sinus thrombosis. J Ultrasound Med 14:41-47

Laurichesse-Delmas H, Grimaud O, Moscovo G, Ville Y (1999) Color Doppler study of the venous circulation in the fetal brain and hemodynamic study of the cerebral transverse sinus. Ultrasound Obstet Gynecol 13:34-42

Pedespan JM, Chateil JF, Pedespan-Joly L, Fontan D, Demarquez JL, Guillard JM (1996) Thromboses du sinus longitudinal supérieur chez l'enfant au cours de la première année de vie: aspects cliniques, imagerie et évolution. Arch Fr Pediatr 3:561-565

Volpe JJ (1995) Hypoxic ischemic encephalopathy: neuropathology and pathogenesis. In: Volpe JJ Neurology of the newborn. Saunders, Philadelphia, pp 279-313

Case 4

A. Couture and C. Veyrac

This newborn was admitted with heart failure. Chest X-ray showed cardiomegaly and a widened upper mediastinum. Complete assessment demonstrated multivisceral distress: an enlarged liver with coagulation disturbances and cytolysis, renal insufficiency, and subclinical EEG disorders.

Brain ultrasonography, with gray-scale (Fig. 10.14) and color imaging (Fig.10.15), was performed on day 6.

What is your diagnosis?

What should be done?

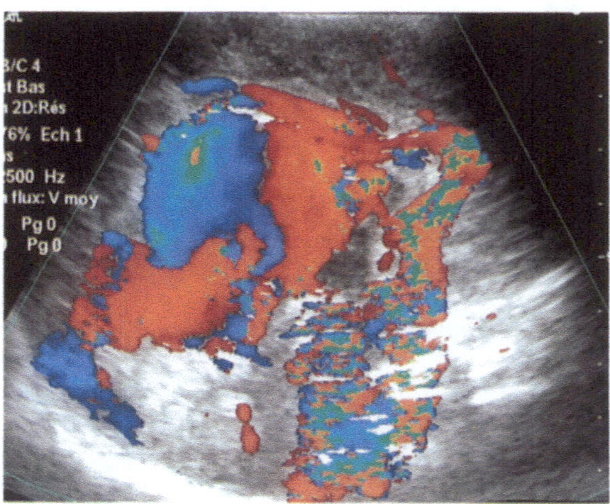

Fig. 10.15. Color Doppler imaging: sagittal plane

The diagnosis was obvious: the posterior cystic structure that anteriorly displaced the third ventricle (Fig. 10.14) and was highly vascular on color Doppler (Fig. 10.15) was clearly an *aneurysm of the vein of Galen.*

What should be done?

The main objective of the investigation was determination of the prognosis. In this malformation, the complexity of the anastomotic arteriovenous network was the most important prognostic factor: on its severity depended the presence or absence of heart failure and of ischemic brain damage. In this newborn, everything indicated a poor outcome:

- Ultrasonography (morphology, color and pulsed Doppler features) showed a complex multiple angiomatous matrix. The galenic ectasia was fed by the posterior choroidal (Fig. 10.16), pericallosal (Fig. 10.17), anterior choroidal (Fig. 10.18), and lenticulostriate arteries together with a multitude of transmesencephalic vessels (Fig. 10.19). Moreover, all the feeding vessels were greatly enlarged; their contribution to the malformation was confirmed by the hemodynamic investigation (Fig. 10.20).

- The presence of a markedly dilated draining vein with high blood flow (Fig. 10.21) is a second element arguing for a poor outcome.

- Finally, neonatal MRI confirms the severity of the vascular steal by showing periventricular ischemic damage (Fig.10.22) and abnormal signal in basal ganglia.

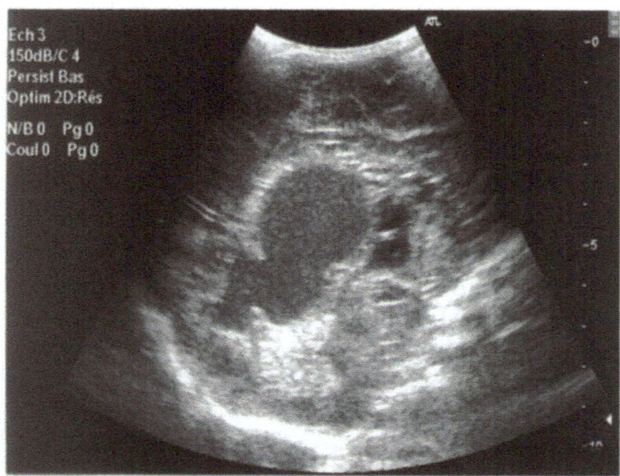

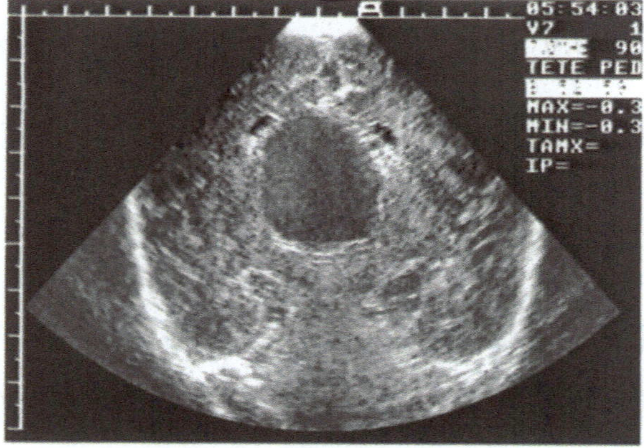

Fig. 10.14. Sagittal (**a**) and posterior frontal planes (**b**)

A. Couture, MD; C. Veyrac, MD
Service de Radiologie Pédiatrique, Hôpital Arnaud de Villeneuve, 371 av. Doyen Gaston Giraud, 34295 Montpellier Cedex, France

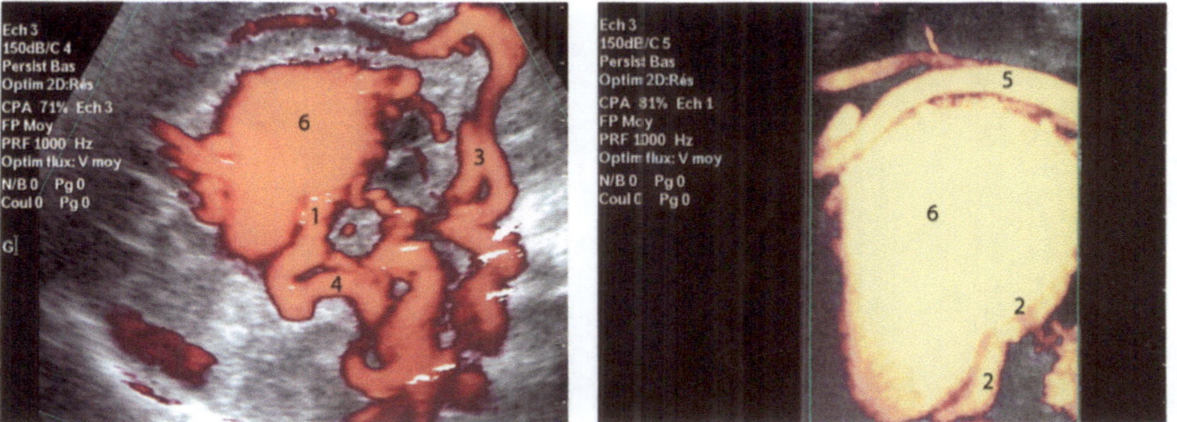

Fig. 10.16. The branches of the posterior cerebral arteries are extremely dilated, e.g., the posterior choroidal artery (*1*) on the left parasagittal plane (**a**), and the posterior and medial choroidal artery (*2*) on the sagittal plane (**b**). *3* Anterior cerebral artery, *4* posterior cerebral artery, *5* pericallosal artery, *6* aneurysm of the vein of Galen

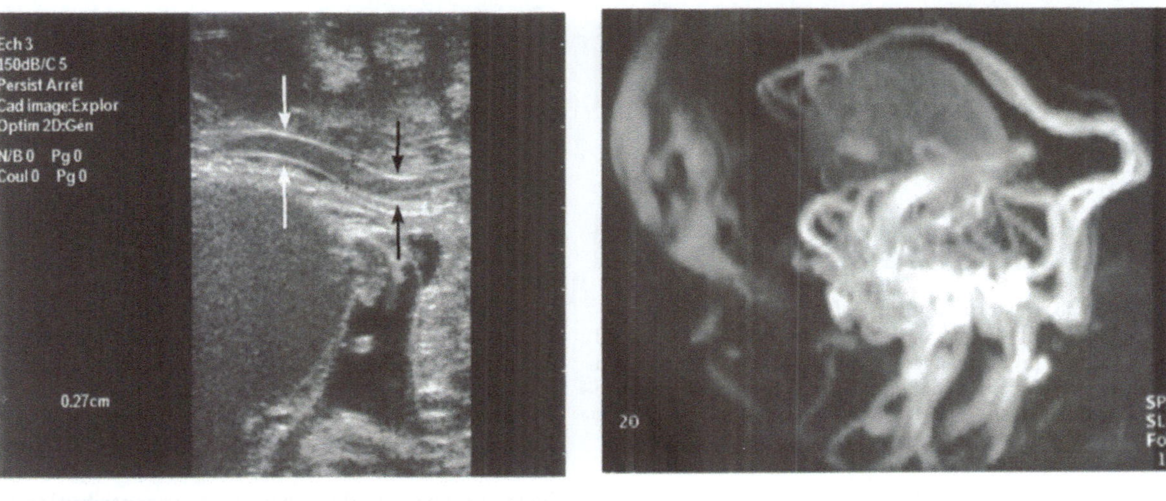

Fig. 10.17a–c. In a healthy newborn, the pericallosal artery lumen is never visualized since it is always less than 1 mm in diameter. In this newborn (**a**) it measures 2.7 mm (*arrow*) and drains fully into the galenic ectasia (*6*) via trigonal distal branches (*1*) (**b**). Notice the major dilatation of the great feeding vessels: anterior cerebral artery (*2*), pericallosal artery (*3*), basilar artery (*4*), posterior medial choroidal artery (*5*). MR angiography (**c**) confirms the sonographic findings

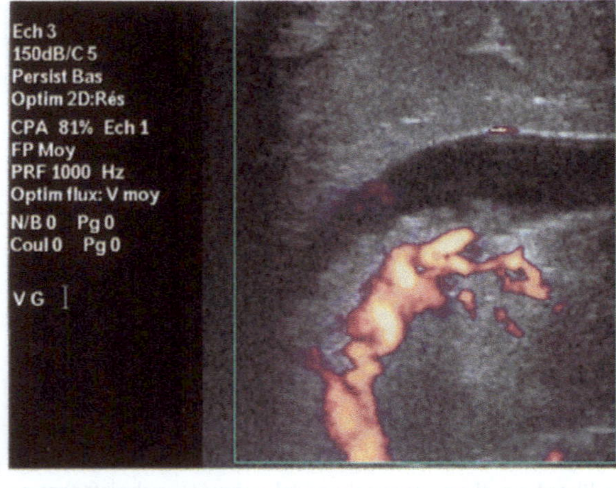

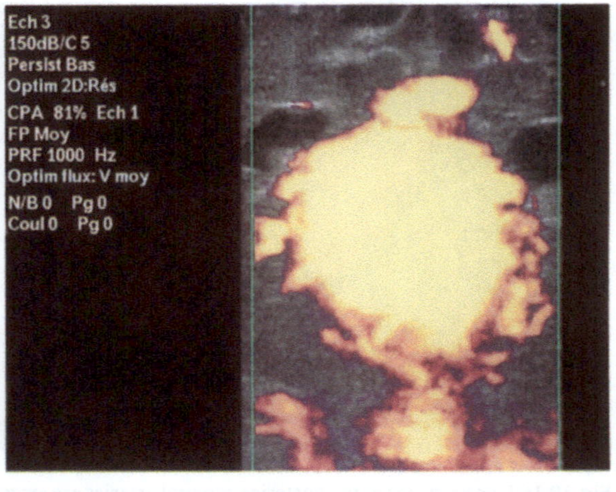

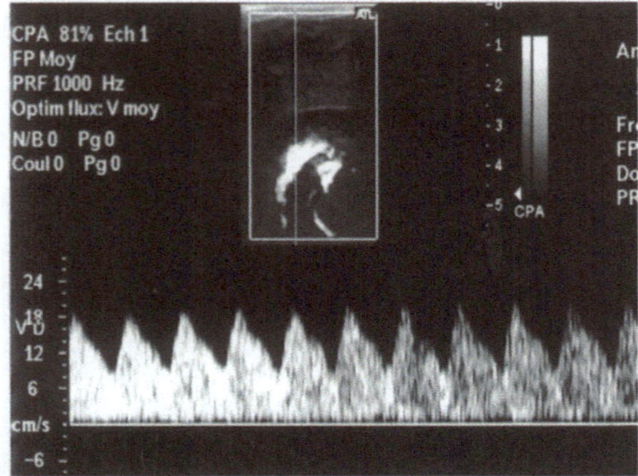

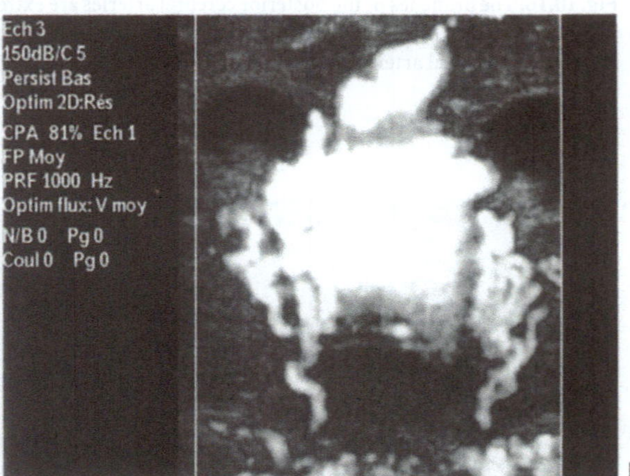

Fig. 10.18a,b. The tortuous course of the dilated anterior choroidal artery (**a**), a branch of the internal carotid artery, is well seen. Its part in the aneurysmal malformation is assessed on the basis of its hemodynamic spectrum (**b**), with a resistive index less than 0.50

Fig. 10.19a,b. On either side of the aneurysm, the transmesencephalic arteries constitute a striking vascular matrix, made up of a cluster of multiple enlarged tortuous vessels

Taken all together, all the criteria of poor prognosis were present in this newborn: multivisceral distress, multiple feeding vessels, large draining vein, ischemic brain damage. Transarterial embolization was rejected and the infant died at 24 days of life.

Some valuable conclusions may be drawn from this case report:

● The diagnosis is easy in the neonate. The same may be applied to the fetus, where diagnosis only requires the use of an ultrasound machine with pulsed and color Doppler functions.

● Today, neonatal evaluation of the malformation is well defined, combining color imaging, hemodynamic assessment, and brain MRI. Appreciation of the vascular malformation relies mainly on ultrasonography, which can provide a complete, accurate map of the feeding vessels, demonstrate their contribution by pulsed Doppler, and quantify the draining flow.

Several authors (BRUNELLE 1997; CAMPI 1996; SENER 1996) have emphasized the value of neonatal brain MRI. However, this technique has some disadvantages: it does not permit any hemodynamic analysis and the participation of an artery in the aneurysm cannot be proven. Complete, accurate determination of the arterial supply is made difficult by the multiple vascular superpositions. For example, in our case, MRI demonstrated well the contribution of the pericallosal arteries (Fig. 10.17), the draining vein (Fig. 10.21), and the dilatation of the transverse sinus and jugular veins, but the course of other feeding vessels such as the choroidal and transmesencephalic arteries (Fig. 10.22) was much less easy to determine precisely.

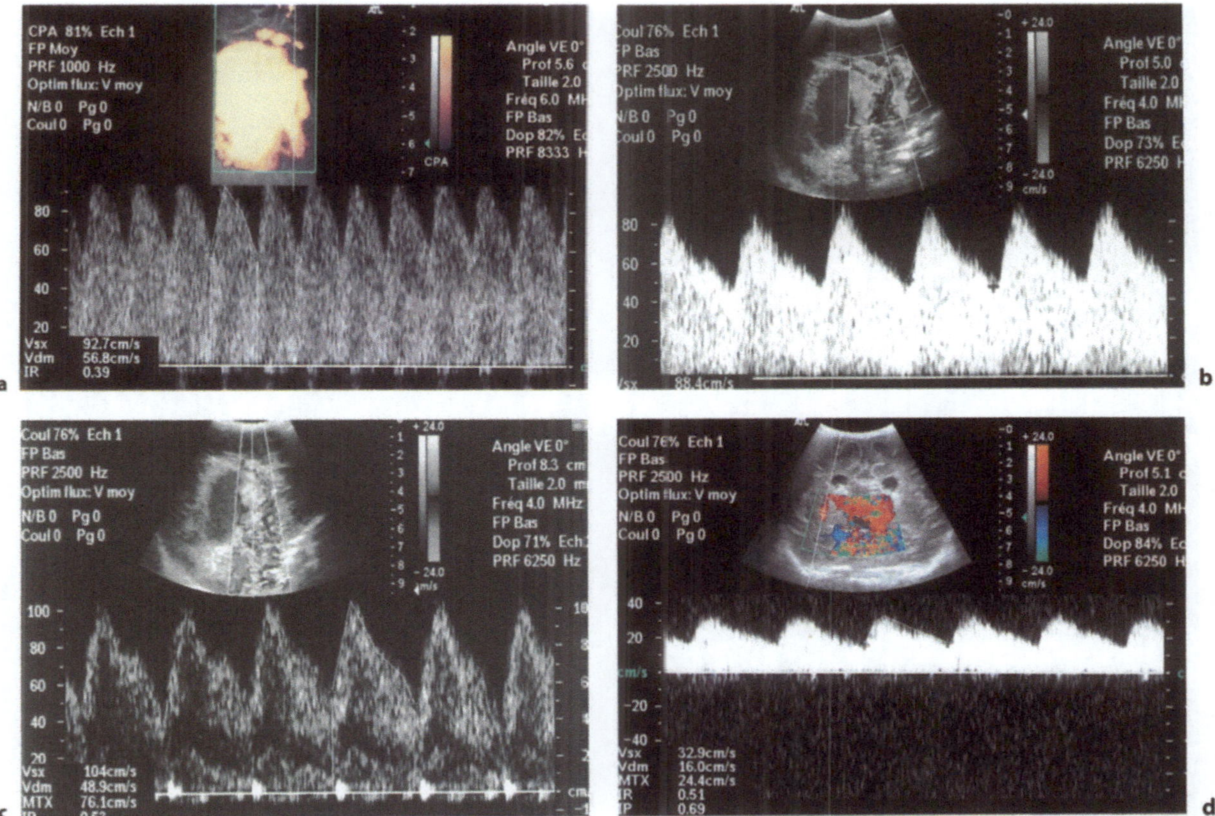

Fig. 10.20a–d. The feeding arteries exhibit a specific hemodynamic pattern with increased peak-systolic velocities, extremely high end-diastolic velocities, and low resistive index. This is obvious in: **a** the posterior choroidal artery: PSV: 92.7 cm/s, EDV: 56.8 cm/s, RI: 0.39; **b** the anterior cerebral artery: PSV: 88.4 cm/s, EDV: 47 cm/s, TAV: 63.9 cm/s, RI: 0.47; **c** the basilar artery: PSV: 104 cm/s, EDV: 48.9 cm/s, TAV: 76 cm/s, RI: 0.53; **d** the lenticulostriate arteries, branches of the middle cerebral artery: PSV: 32.9 cm/s, EDV: 16 cm/s, TAV: 24.4 cm/s, RI: 0.51. Values (*not shown*) for the anterior choroidal artery were: PSV: 55 cm/s, EDV: 31 cm/s, TAV: 42.3 cm/s, RI: 0.44; and those for the carotid artery were: PSV: 120 cm/s, EDV: 75.5 cm/s, TAV: 92 cm/s, RI: 0.41

Ischemic brain injury is mainly attributable to the vascular steal phenomenon, more infrequently to congestive heart failure or to atrophy of adjacent structures due to compression. Neonatal brain lesions are well documented (DE KONING 1997; TAKASHIMA 1980): microcephaly, laminar cortical necrosis, periventricular leukomalacia, and hemorrhagic infarction. It is important to know that these lesions may be moderate, progressive, and difficult to diagnose: brain MRI is obviously the most efficient imaging tool (Fig. 10.23).

● The prognosis may be reliably established in the neonate on the basis of a complete protocolized study: color and pulsed Doppler are used to assess the morphological and hemodynamic pattern of the malformation and MRI demonstrates any ischemic brain damage. These data provide objective grounds for proposing or rejecting interventional treatment.

The same methods may be applied in the fetus, and prenatal recognition of a galenic aneurysm has become essential: the delay to diagnosis is shortened and the prognostic assessment permits selection of patients who can be treated by transarterial embolization: the criteria are absence of severe heart failure, a vascular matrix supplied by only one or two arteries, and absence of ischemic brain damage. This assessment is important, because psychomotor development seems to be improved in infants who have undergone embolization (LASJAUNIAS 1996).

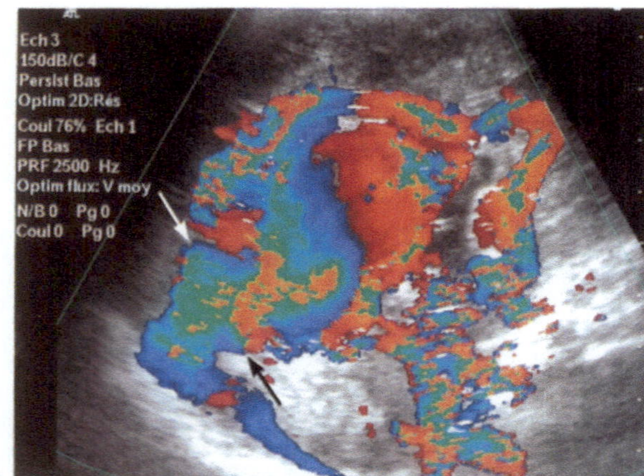

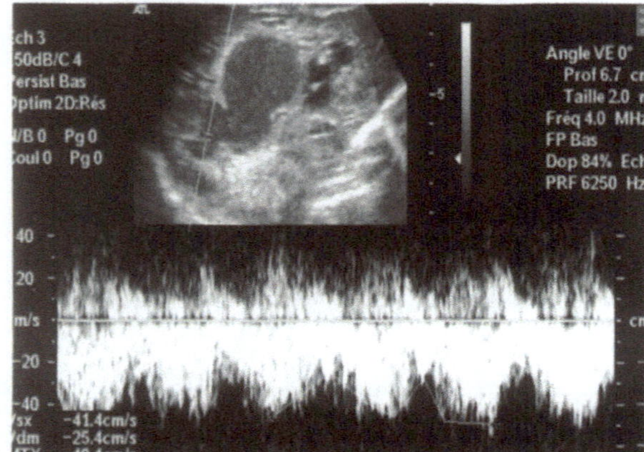

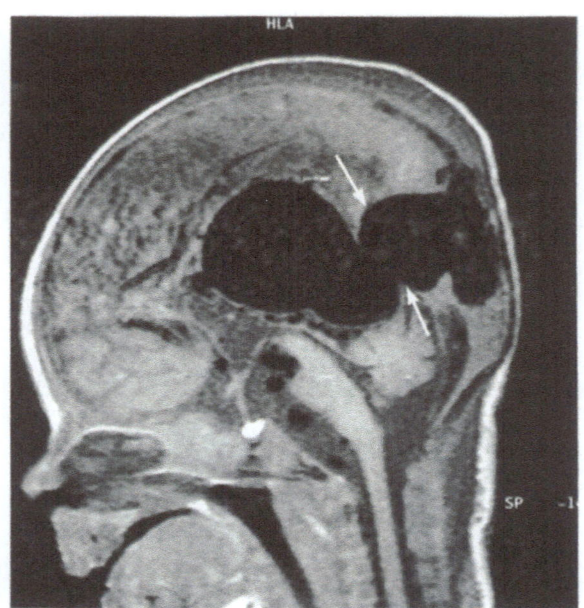

Fig. 10.21. Color imaging (**a**) and T1-weighted MRI (**b**) show the major dilatation of the draining vein (*arrows*). Its blood flow velocity (**c**) is very high (40 cm/s), as are those in the straight sinus and jugular veins

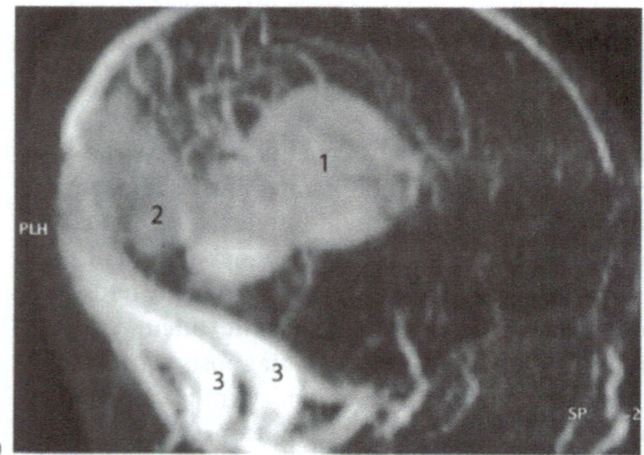

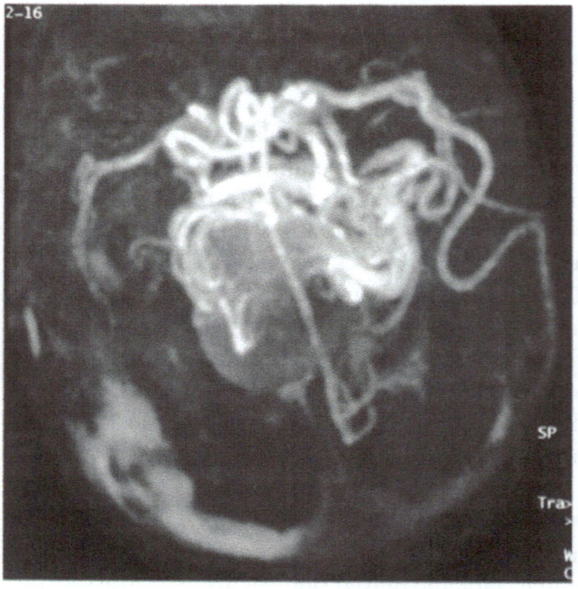

Fig. 10.22a,b. On the venous MRI (**a**), the aneurysm (*1*), draining vein (*2*), and transverse sinus (*3*) are easily recognized. On the arterial MRI (**b**), on the other hand, it is difficult to determine the course of the feeding vessels because of the superpositions

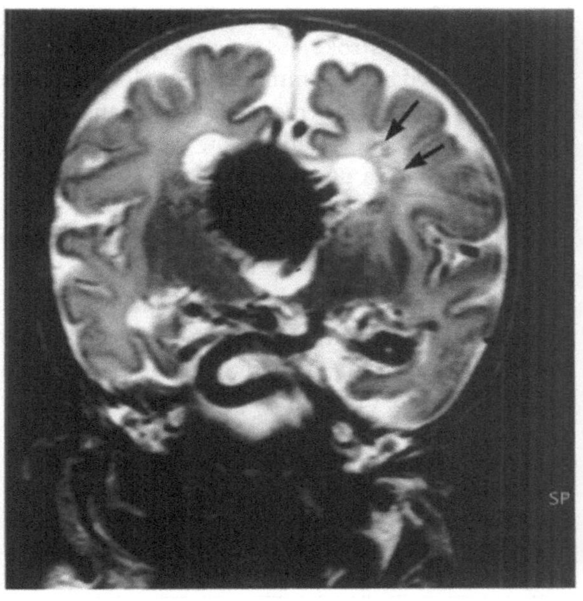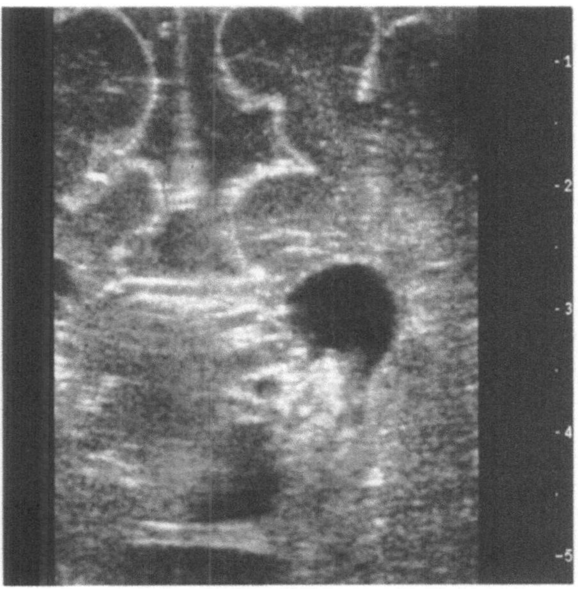

Fig. 10.23. On T2-weighted MRI (**a**), periventricular leukomalacia is evident (*arrow*); the sonographic appearance (**b**) is equivocal

References

Brunelle F (1997) Arteriovenous malformation of the vein of Galen in children. Pediatr Radiol 27:501-503

Campi A, Scotti G, Filipp M, Gereveni S, Stigimi F, Lasjaunias P (1996) Antenatal diagnosis of vein of Galen aneurysmal malformation: MR study of fetal brain and postnatal follow-up. Neuroradiology 38:87-90

De Koning T, Godskens R, Veenhoven R, Meijboom E, Jansen G, Lasjaunias P, De Vries L (1997) Arteriovenous malformation of the vein of Galen in three neonates: emphasis on associated early ischaemic brain damage. Eur J Pediatr 156:228-229

Lasjaunias P, Alvarez H, Rodesh G, Garcia-Monaco R, Brugge K, Burrows P, Taylor W (1996) Aneurysmal malformation of the vein of Galen. Follow-up of 120 children treated between 1964 and 1994. Interv Neuroradiol 2:15-26

Sener RN (1996) MR angiography of the vein of Galen malformation. Clin Imaging 20:243-246

Takashima S, Becker LE (1980) Neuropathology of cerebral arteriovenous malformations in children. J Neurol Neurosurg Psychiatry 43:380-385

Case 5

C. VEYRAC

Gregory was a full-term baby born by cesarean section after premature rupture of membranes, but without any sign of fetal distress.

At 10 min of life, he suffered respiratory distress syndrome requiring intubation and mechanical ventilation. He was admitted in the intensive care unit with a noncompressive right pneumothorax, but also clonic seizures. Brain ultrasonography was immediately performed: the morphological examination was normal and a Doppler spectrum of the anterior cerebral artery was obtained (Fig. 10.24).

What is your interpretation?

What diagnosis should be suspected?

What investigations should be performed?

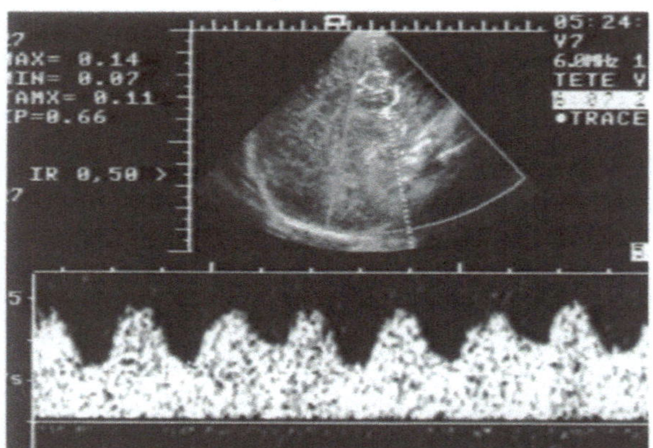

Fig. 10.24

1. What is your interpretation?

The Doppler spectrum showed several anomalies:

- It had a fluctuating pattern.
- Peak-systolic velocities (14 cm/s) were reduced (compared to normal values in a full-term newborn), suggesting low blood flow, and the resistive index was moderately decreased (0.50).

C. VEYRAC, MD
Service de Radiologie Pédiatrique, Hôpital Arnaud de Villeneuve, 371 av. Doyen Gaston Giraud, 34295 Montpellier Cedex, France

- The waveform contour was striking, characterized by a delayed upstroke and slow upslope. This could be quantified by determining the acceleration time that is prolonged (mean=175 ms, range=145–195 ms), and the relative flow rate index (area under the curve up to the peak-systolic velocity divided by the area under the curve down to the end-diastolic velocity), which was markedly increased (0.50).

The abnormal results were particularly obvious when compared with the spectra for healthy infants and for distressed infants with low blood flow and a similar heart rate (Table 10.1, Figs. 10.25, 10.26).

Table 10.1. Acceleration time of the anterior cerebral artery in three full-term newborns

	Heart rate beats/min	PSV cm/s	Acceleration time ms
Healthy newborn	150	35	66
Low blood flow	136	17	67
Our patient	159	14	175

2. What diagnosis should be suspected? What investigations should be performed?

The slow acceleration slope, the delayed upstroke, and the decreased peak systolic velocity should first suggest severe deficiency of left ventricular ejection: left heart hypoplasia, critical aortic valve stenosis, aortic arch interruption, and coarctation of the ascending aorta. Echocardiography should be performed as an emergency procedure. In our patient, it

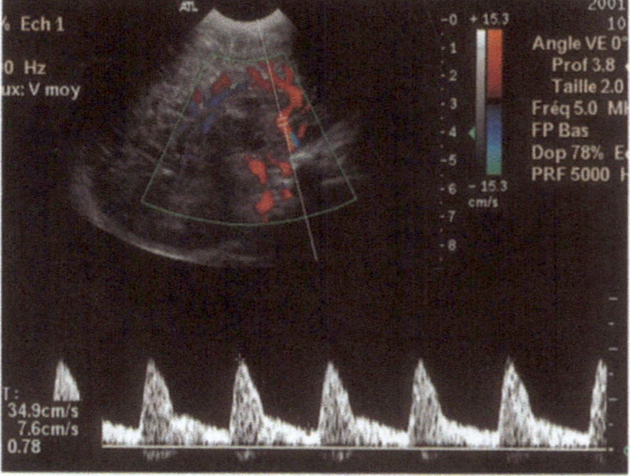

Fig. 10.25. Healthy full-term newborn: Doppler spectrum of the anterior cerebral artery (PSV = 34.9 cm/s, EDV = 7.6 cm/s, RI = 0.78, acceleration time = 65 ms)

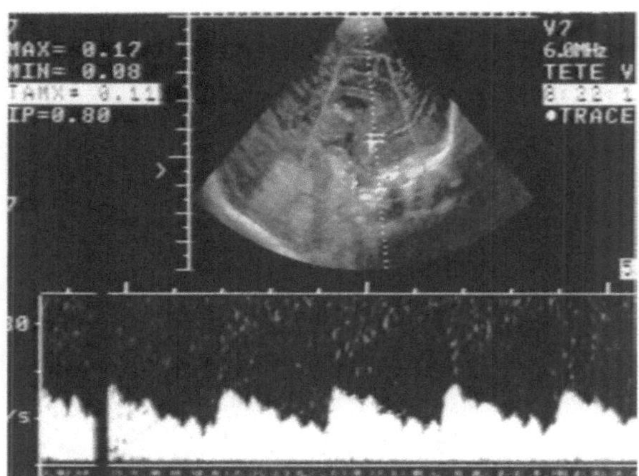

Fig. 10.26. Full-term newborn with acute distress: low blood flow (PSV = 17 cm/s, EDV = 8 cm/s, TAV = 11 cm/s, RI = 0.53, acceleration time = 66 ms)

was done immediately after brain ultrasonography and confirmed the diagnosis of hypoplastic left heart: an extremely small, akinetic left ventricle, atretic mitral valve, hypoplastic aorta, absence of antegrade flow, and large patent ductus arteriosus with bidirectional shunt.

Prostaglandin treatment was begun to maintain the patency of the ductus arteriosus, and improved the hemodynamic situation. Follow-up brain ultrasonography did not detect any subsequent hemorrhagic or ischemic brain lesion. The infant was operated on with good short-term outcome.

Little has been published about the consequences of congenital heart disease for cerebral hemodynamics in the neonate, except those of patent ductus arteriosus. SNIDER (1985) compared the Doppler spectrum of cerebral arteries in 20 healthy neonates and 54 newborns with various forms of congenital heart disease, describing different abnormal flow signals. In her series, she reported four newborns with critical aortic valve stenosis and two newborns with hypoplastic left heart syndrome. These six infants exhibited a Doppler curve similar to that of our patient, i.e., with decreased peak-systolic frequency, very slow upslope, and prolonged acceleration time.

Acceleration time was measured in 145 nondistressed preterm and term infants by VAN DE BOR (1990), who found values of 33±9 ms in the pericallosal artery of term newborns, and a positive correlation with the peak-systolic velocity and heart rate.

In adults with isolated aortic stenosis, carotid artery duplex waveform abnormalities have been documented, combining increased acceleration time, decreased peak velocity, delayed upstroke, rounded waveform, which correlated with the severity of the aortic stenosis (O'BOYLE 1996). Obviously, the hemodynamic situation in the adult cannot be compared with that in the neonate who maintains a patent ductus arteriosus at birth.

In the neonate with congenital heart disease where blood flow in the descending aorta is ensured by the persistent patency of ductus arteriosus, decreased or even reverse diastolic flow is observed in the cerebral arteries. This was not the case in our infant, since the absence of antegrade flow in the proximal ascending aorta and akinesis of the left ventricle induced a bidirectional shunt through the large ductus arteriosus.

This case report shows how, exceptionally, a cerebral hemodynamic disorder may be the initial presentation of severe congenital heart disease. In our experience, only major abnormalities of left heart ejection produce a suggestive profile on brain Doppler ultrasonography.

References

O'Boyle MK, Vibhakar NI, Chung J, Keen WD, Gosink BB (1996) Duplex sonography of the carotid arteries in patients with isolated aortic stenosis: imaging findings and relation to severity of stenosis. AJR Am J Roentgenol 166:197-202

Snider AR (1985) The use of Doppler ultrasonography for the evaluation of cerebral artery flow patterns in infants with congenital heart disease. Ultrasound Med Biol 11:503-514

Van De Bor M, Walther FJ, Sims ME (1990) Acceleration time in cerebral arteries of preterm and term infants. J Clin Ultrasound 18:167-171

Subject Index

The most important pages are indicated by bold type.

MEDICAL RADIOLOGY
Diagnostic Imaging and Radiation Oncology

Titles in the series already published

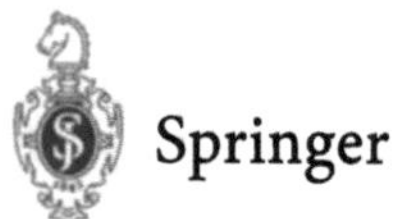
Springer

FSC
www.fsc.org
MIX
Papier aus verantwortungsvollen Quellen
Paper from responsible sources
FSC® C105338